Library Queen's Hospital
Burton on Trent

00004826

KW-380-134

Library (MEC), Queens Hospital Burton
Library.bur@burtonft.nhs.uk
01283 511511 x2104

This book is due for return on or before the last date shown below.

Withdrawn

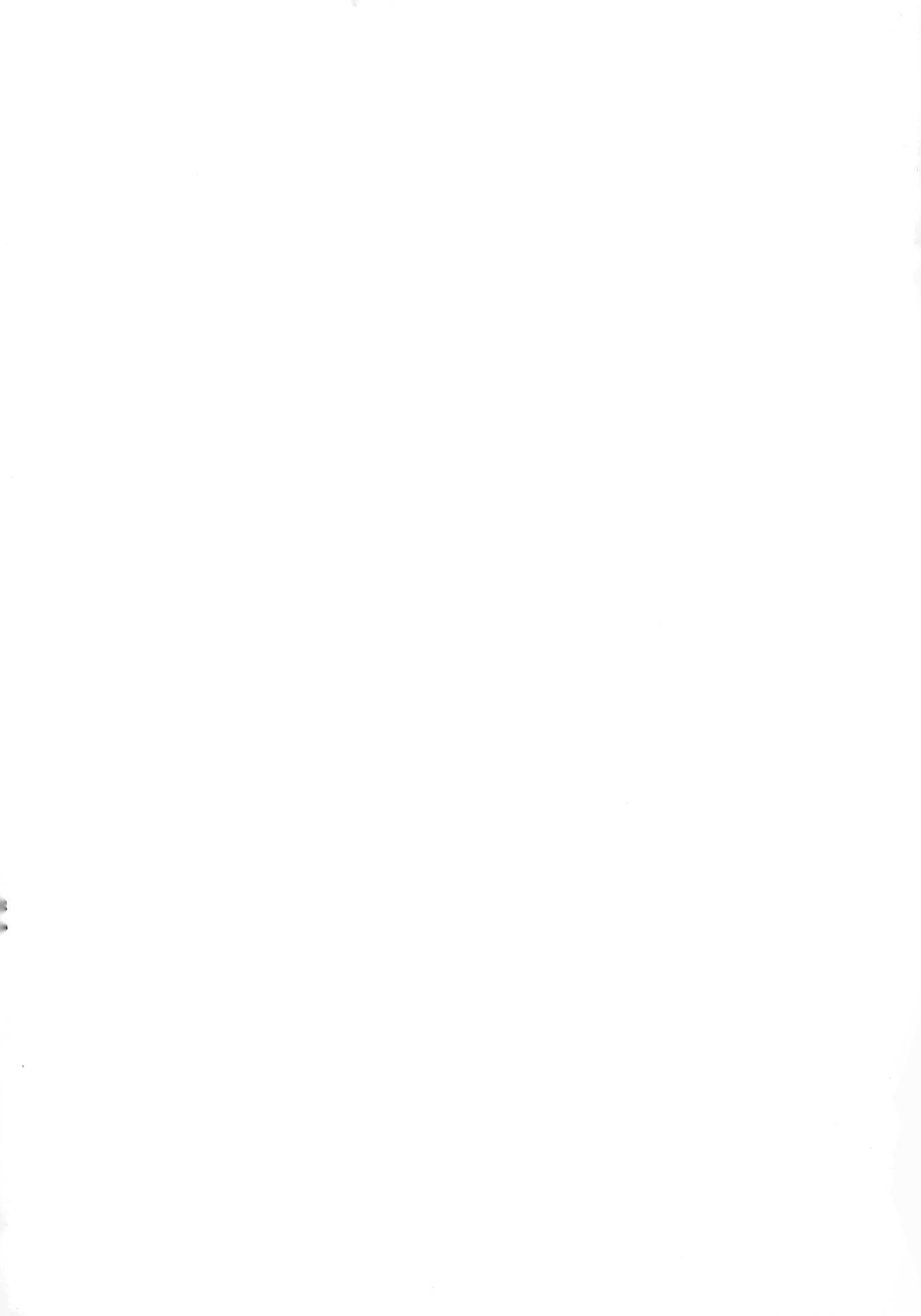

CUTANEOUS
MANIFESTATIONS
of
HIV DISEASE

Clay J. Cockerell, MD
Clinical Professor, Dermatology & Pathology
Director, Division of Dermatopathology
University of Texas Southwestern Medical Centre
Director, Cockerell & Associates Dermpath Diagnostics, Dallas, Texas, USA

Antoanella Calame, MD
Director, Compass Dermatopathology
La Jolla, California, USA

⧓ **MANSON**
PUBLISHING

Copyright © 2013 Manson Publishing Ltd

ISBN: 978-1-84076-142-9

All rights reserved. No part of this publication may be reproduced, stored in a retrieval system or transmitted in any form or by any means without the written permission of the copyright holder or in accordance with the provisions of the Copyright Act 1956 (as amended), or under the terms of any licence permitting limited copying issued by the Copyright Licensing Agency, 33–34 Alfred Place, London WC1E 7DP, UK.

Any person who does any unauthorized act in relation to this publication may be liable to criminal prosecution and civil claims for damages.

A CIP catalogue record for this book is available from the British Library.

For full details of all Manson Publishing Ltd titles please write to:
Manson Publishing Ltd, 73 Corringham Road, London NW11 7DL, UK.
Tel: +44(0)20 8905 5150
Fax: +44(0)20 8201 9233
Website: www.mansonpublishing.com

Commissioning editor: Jill Northcott
Project manager: Paul Bennett
Copy-editor: Ruth Maxwell
Design and layout: DiacriTech, Chennai, India
Colour reproduction: Tenon & Polert Colour Scanning Ltd, Hong Kong
Printed by: Grafos SA, Barcelona, Spain

CONTENTS

PREFACE

Skin diseases are common problems in patients with human immunodeficiency virus (HIV) infection and acquired immunodeficiency syndrome (AIDS). In many cases, the Dermatologist may be the first medical professional to encounter an individual with HIV infection. It is, therefore, vital that Dermatologists recognize the cutaneous manifestations of HIV infection and AIDS so that the diagnosis can be established as early as possible and appropriate therapy can be instituted soon thereafter. In times past, this was important to lessen the likelihood of a patient developing a life-threatening opportunistic infection. Today, following diagnosis of HIV infection, highly active antiretroviral therapy (HAART) is instituted, which can essentially eradicate HIV viral loads, rendering them undetectable and significantly lessening the patient's chance of developing a complication, infectious or otherwise. Many different skin disorders may be seen in these patients ranging from infections such as lues and mycobacterial infections, to other inflammatory conditions such as drug eruptions, psoriasis, and sarcoidosis. Depending on the patient's immune status, skin disorders may appear similar to those seen in immunocompetent patients or they may be unusual and bizarre especially when CD4 cell counts are low. In any event, the skin is a very common site where diseases are manifest in HIV infected patients and any medical professional who takes care of these individuals must be cognizant of these manifestations and know how to manage them.

Fortunately, HAART has transformed HIV infection and AIDS so that patients are living longer with less sequelae today than when the AIDS pandemic was rampant. Unfortunately, in some populations, individuals have developed a 'cavalier' attitude about HIV infection thinking, erroneously, that if they become infected, they can be 'cured' by simply taking HAART. While indeed, 'highly active', these medications do have side-effects and are not a cure for HIV infection. Thus, while the number of patients who present with severe infectious complications or profoundly depressed CD4 cell counts is lower than in the past, there are still a significant number of individuals who are newly-infected with HIV each year and who may present with severe immunosuppression and even life-threatening opportunistic infections. Clinicians cannot 'lower their guard' and must maintain a high index of suspicion as HIV is still significantly endemic.

In this book, we cover the entire spectrum of HIV-associated cutaneous diseases and emphasize how they present in immunocompromised patients. Each entity is discussed in detail including its clinical presentation, histopathologic findings, and treatment. As Dermatology is a specialty that emphasizes morphology, numerous clinical and histopathological images are included in each chapter.

The book is written for any provider caring for HIV patients. It will also serve as an excellent reference for the experienced Dermatologist who may encounter these individuals either on occasion or frequently, and it will also serve as a reminder of some of the serious sequelae that may be encountered in severely immunocompromised patients.

Clay J. Cockerell, MD
Antoanella Calame, MD

CONTRIBUTORS

Cindy Berthelot, MD
Department of Internal Medicine, University of Texas
Houston Health Science Center, Houston, USA

Gabriela M. Blanco, MD
Department of Dermatology, University of Texas
Southwestern Medical Center, Dallas, USA

Molly V. Burns, BS
University of Texas Health Science Center San
Antonio, San Antonio, USA

Antoanella Calame, MD
Director, Compass Dermatology, La Jolla,
California, USA

Clay J. Cockerell, MD
Department of Dermatology, University of Texas
Southwestern Medical Center, Dallas, USA

Robert H. Cook-Norris, MD
Department of Dermatology, Mayo Rochester
Medical School, University of Texas, Houston, USA

Mary Feldman, MD
Department of Dermatology, University of Texas
Southwestern Medical Center, Dallas, USA

Bryan Gammon, MD
Department of Dermatology, University of Texas
Northwestern University, Chicago, USA

Deborah B. Henderson, MD
Department of Dermatology, University of Texas
Northwestern University, Chicago, USA

Loebat Kamalpour, MD
Department of Dermatology, Loyola University,
Maywood, USA

Shadi Kourosh, MD
Department of Dermatology, University of Texas
Southwestern Medical Center, Dallas, USA

I would like to express my appreciation to Dr. Clay
Cockerell, Dr. Mary Feldman, and Dr. Antoanella
Calame for the opportunity to contribute to this
book, and for their encouragement and exceptional
mentorship throughout the process of writing. It has
been a very enriching experience to serve on this
team. I would also like to thank Dr. Emitis and
Sadato Hosoda, Dr. Atoosa Kourosh, and Dr.
Charlotte Glenn for their support and invaluable
assistance with ideas and editing.

Kumar Krishnan, MD
Department of Dermatology, University of Texas
Southwestern Medical Center, Dallas, USA

Saira B. Momin, DO
Department of Dermatology, University of Texas
Southwestern Medical Center, Dallas, USA

Peter Morrell, DO
University of North Texas Health Science Center,
Texas College of Osteopathic Medicine, USA

Frankie G. Rholdon, MD
Department of Dermatology, University of Texas
Southwestern Medical Center, Dallas, USA

Benjamin K. Stoff, MD
Department of Dermatology, Emory University,
Atlanta, USA

Wei Su, MD
Department of Dermatology, University of Texas
Southwestern Medical Center, Dallas, USA

ABBREVIATIONS

AA	alopecia areata
ABPA	allergic bronchopulmonary aspergillosis
ADR	adverse drug reaction
AGEP	acute generalized eruptive pustulosis
AIDS	aquired immunodeficiency syndrome
ALT	alanine transferase
ANA	antineutrophilic antibody
APC	antigen-presenting cell
AR	actinic reticuloid
ARC	AIDS-related complex
ARS	acute retroviral syndrome
ATRA	all-trans-retinoic acid
AZT	azidothymidine (zidovudine)
BA	bacillary angiomatosis
BCC	basal cell carcinoma
BCG	bacillus Calmette–Guérin
b-FGF	basic fibroblastic growth factor
BP	bowenoid papulosis
CAD	chronic actinic dermatitis
CDC	Centers for Disease Control
CF	complement fixation
CMV	cytomegalovirus
CNS	central nervous system
CRABP	cytoplasmic retinoic acid binding protein
CSF	cerebrospinal fluid
CT	computed tomography
CTCL	cutaneous T cell lymphoma
CTL	cytotoxic T-lymphocyte
DEAFF	detection of early antigen fluorescent foci
DNA	deoxyribonucleic acid
DNCB	dinitrochlorobenzene
DRESS	drug rash with eosinophilia and systemic symptoms
DSO	distal subungual onychomycosis
DTH	delayed type hypersensitivity
EBV	Epstein–Barr virus
EDV	epidermodysplasia verruciformis
EED	erythema elevatum diutinum
EF	eosinophilic folliculitis
EIA	enzyme immunoassay
ELISA	enzyme linked immunosorbent assay
EM	erythema multiforme
EPF	eosinophilic pustular folliculitis
FDA	Food and Drug Administration
FI	fusion inhibitor
FLICE	Fas-associated death domain-like interleukin-1β-converting enzyme
FTA-abs	fluorescent treponemal antibodies
GA	granuloma annulare
GMS	Gomori methenamine silver
GSH	glutathione
GUD	genital ulcerative disease
H&E	hematoxylin and eosin
HAART	highly active antiretroviral therapy
HBV	hepatitis B virus
hCG	human chorionic gonadotropin
HCV	hepatitis C virus
HDV	hepatitis D virus
HHV	human herpesvirus
HLA	human leucocyte antigen
HIV	human immunodeficiency virus
HP	hyperalgesic pseudothrombophlebitis
HPV	human papillomavirus
HR-HPV	high oncogenic risk HPV
HSP	Henoch–Schönlein purpura
HSV	herpes simplex virus
HTLV	human T cell lymphotrophic virus
HZ	herpes zoster
HZO	herpes zoster ophthalmicus
ICAM	intercellular adhesion molecule
ID	immunodiffusion
IFN	interferon
Ig	immunoglobulin
IGDR	interstitial granulomatous drug reaction
IK	infectious keratitis
IL	interleukin
IRIS	immune reconstitution inflammatory syndrome
ITP	idiopathic thrombocytopenic purpura
IVDU	intravenous drug use
IVIG	intravenous immunoglobulin
KOH	potassium hydroxide
KS	Kaposi's sarcoma
KSHV	KS-associated herpesvirus

LANA	latency-associated nuclear antigen		PK	pitted keratolysis
LCV	leukocytoclastic vasculitis		PKDL	postkala-azar dermal leishmaniasis
LDH	lactate dehydrogenase		PI	protease inhibitor
LE	lupus erythematosus		PLC	pityriasis lichenoides chronica
LGDA	lichenoid and granulomatous dermatitis of AIDS		PLEVA	pityriasis lichenoides et varioliformis acuta
LGV	lymphogranuloma venereum		PLR	persistent light reaction
LN	lichen nitidus		PPD	purified protein derivative
LP	lichen planus		PPE	pruritic papular eruption
LPP	large plaque parapsoriasis		PPV	positive predictive value
LRP	lipoprotein-related protein		PR	pityriasis rosea
LS	lichen striatus		PRP	pityriasis rubra pilaris
LGSIL	low-grade squamous intraepithelial lesion		PSO	proximal subungual onychomycosis
			PTD	photodynamic therapy
LyP	lymphomatoid papulosis		PUVA	psoralen with ultraviolet A light
MAI	*Mycobacterium avium-intracellulare*		RA	rheumatoid arthritis
MC	molluscum contagiosum		RNA	ribonucleic acid
MCV	molluscum contagiosum virus		ROS	reactive oxygen species
MED	minimal erythema dose		RPR	rapid plasma reagin
MF	mycosis fungoides		RT-PCR	real-time polymerase chain reaction
MMP	matrix metalloproteinase inhibitor		RXR	retinoic X receptor
MRI	magnetic resonance imaging		SCC	squamous cell carcinoma
MRSA	methicillin-resistant *Staphylococcus aureus*		SCCIS	squamous cell carcinoma *in situ*
			SD	seborrheic dermatitis
MSM	men who have sex with men		SJS	Stevens–Johnson syndrome
NCAP	N-acetyl-4-cystaminylphenol		SMX	sulfamethoxazole
NHL	non-Hodgkin's lymphoma		SPP	small plaque parapsoriasis
NNRTI	non-nucleoside reverse transcriptase inhibitor		SSSS	staphylococcal scalded skin syndrome
NRTI	nucleoside reverse transcriptase inhibitor		STD	sexually transmitted disease
			TB	tuberculosis
NSAID	nonsteroidal anti-inflammatory drug		TEN	toxic epidermal necrolysis
NUPD	necrotizing ulcerative periodontal disease		TMP	trimethoprim
			TMP–SMX	trimethoprim–sulfamethoxazole
OHL	oral hairy leukoplakia		TNF	tumor necrosis factor
PA	pityriasis alba		TPPA	*T. pallidum* particle agglutination
(c)-PAN	(cutaneous) polyarteritis nodosa		US	United States
PAS	periodic acid-Schiff		UV	ultraviolet
PBMC	peripheral blood mononuclear cell		VDRL	Venereal Disease Research Laboratory
PCM	paracoccidioidomycosis		VEGF	vascular endothelial growth factor
PCP	*Pneumocystis carinii* pneumonia		vIRF	viral interferon regulatory factor
PCR	polymerase chain reaction		VZIG	varicella-zoster immune globulin
PCT	porphyria cutanea tarda		VZV	varicella-zoster virus
PD	photosensitive 'eczema'		WBC	white blood cell
PDGF	platelet-derived growth factor		WHO	World Health Organization
			WSO	white superficial onychomycosis

CHAPTER 1

INTRODUCTION

Antoanella Calame and Clay J. Cockerell

The world became aware of a new epidemic almost three decades ago, largely a consequence of cutaneous manifestations which were among the first to be recognized. Reports of Kaposi's sarcoma occurring in association with *Pneumocystis carinii* pneumonia in select subpopulations, especially homosexual men, ushered in a new era in infectious diseases, eventually leading to the definition of the condition now known as the acquired immunodeficiency syndrome (AIDS) and subsequently to the discovery of the human immunodeficiency virus (HIV). The first reports of this new syndrome were made in the United States (US) in 1981 in the Morbidity and Mortality Weekly Report from the Centers for Disease Control, and in a preliminary report by Gottlieb *et al.* describing widely disseminated Kaposi's sarcoma in young homosexual men.[1,2] In the following months, a number of other reports published in prominent journals described other signs and symptoms associated with severe immunodeficiency, including many of the now well-recognized cutaneous manifestations of HIV infection.[3–12]

As the severity of the disease began to be understood and it became apparent that a worldwide pandemic was underway, our resourcefulness in the face of a new infectious agent was soon to be tested. In the early years following its description, AIDS was universally fatal and there seemed to be no cure in sight. Even after discovery of HIV, the causative agent of AIDS, treatment was primarily supportive and mortality rates continued to be high. While initially hopes for development of more effective therapy and an effective vaccine were high, progress remained slow. Furthermore, biased and negative public perceptions about AIDS and HIV

infection as well as lack of political interest delayed much needed research funding. The first anti-retroviral medication, azidothymidine (AZT), was approved in 1987, 6 years after the first reports of AIDS. Over the next 10 years, better understanding of the disease, both scientifically and publicly, led to greater funding and accelerated research. Multiple new medications were approved by the Food and Drug Administration (FDA) in the US, and by 1997, regimens known as highly active antiretroviral therapy (HAART) gave new hope of transforming HIV infection from a death sentence to a chronic, manageable disease. With more effective long-term treatment and the ability to prevent or reduce transmission of HIV via early treatment after exposure and prenatal prophylaxis for affected mothers, a more optimistic view has arisen in the fight against HIV. Although development of an effective HIV vaccine remains elusive, worldwide focus on prevention, early diagnosis, and treatment have made significant impacts on the HIV pandemic, especially in developed countries. However, significant challenges remain, especially in developing countries that are often fraught with problems of political unrest, general lack of education regarding HIV/AIDS, and social and cultural stigmata that hinder safe sex practices. Furthermore, side-effects of HAART, many of which are addressed in other chapters in this book, may cause individuals with HIV infection to discontinue taking medications, which can result in a recrudescence of immunodeficiency. Finally, and potentially most disheartening, recent data show that many men who have sex with men have begun practicing unsafe sex with the erroneous idea that they can use HAART as a foolproof way to prevent infection if they are exposed. Thus, it behoves physicians and caretakers to maintain a high degree of vigilance about the possibility of HIV/AIDS in their patients as the virus continues to maintain a high degree of prevalence in many countries, including the US.

Skin diseases are extremely common in HIV-infected individuals and, as noted above, are often the first sign of infection. The correct diagnosis of a cutaneous disease is, therefore, often instrumental in early detection and treatment of HIV infection. Skin diseases continue to be among the most recognizable signs of HIV infection, although the types of dermatologic problems observed in these individuals have changed over the years. HAART-compliant patients have significantly reduced incidence of many skin diseases although they may develop medication-related side-effects which may affect the skin (Chapters 6 and 11). Skin diseases almost exclusively seen in HIV-infected patients such as Kaposi's sarcoma and eosinophilic folliculitis were seen much more frequently before the advent of HAART

(Chapters 9 and 12). While other sexually transmissible diseases (STDs) have been associated with HIV/AIDS since its description, recently, a resurgence of STDs in the HIV-infected population has been observed. As HIV/AIDS changed from a virtually universally fatal illness to a chronic disease following the development of HAART, fear of acquiring HIV infection through unsafe sexual practices has decreased in certain groups as noted above, leading to new epidemics of diseases such as syphilis and gonorrhea (Chapter 13).

The ensuing chapters in this book review the spectrum of dermatologic manifestations associated with HIV/AIDS ranging from infectious and neoplastic conditions considered pathognomonic for HIV/AIDS, to skin diseases seen in the general population but which often present atypically in this group. It is our hope that caregivers will learn to diagnose skin diseases correctly in these individuals and by so doing, especially in early stages, help decrease rates of transmission, improve treatment, and increase the quality of life for these patients.

CHAPTER 2

VIRAL INFECTIONS IN HIV DISEASE

Wei Su, Cindy Berthelot, and Clay J. Cockerell

ACUTE HIV SYNDROME

DEFINITION/OVERVIEW

Acute HIV infection, also known as acute retroviral syndrome (ARS) and seroconversion illness, is the period from the initial infection with HIV to complete seroconversion. It is often subclinical and asymptomatic, and therefore may escape diagnosis. Symptomatic ARS is a transient illness that is associated with robust HIV replication followed by an expansive immunologic response to the virus.[1] The estimated incidence of symptomatic primary HIV infection ranges from 25% to 75%.[2,3] ARS has been described in all populations at risk for HIV infection: homosexual men, heterosexual men and women, recipients of contaminated blood, recipients of organs from infected donors, and those acquiring HIV from accidental occupational exposure and contaminated body fluids.[4] Acute HIV infection is a period of extreme infectiousness, and the occurrence and severity of symptoms during ARS may correlate with the severity of clinical decline. It has been shown that early identification and treatment of patients with ARS may preserve immune function. Therefore, timely recognition of the ARS is imperative for patients and for public health as it allows for early initiation of antiviral therapy and prevention of subsequent transmission.

PATHOGENESIS/PATHOPHYSIOLOGY

HIV primarily infects CD4+ T-lymphocytes and, soon after primary infection, the virus rapidly concentrates in lymphoid tissue. During primary HIV infection, billions of virions are produced and destroyed each day. CD4+ lymphopenia ensues and T-lymphocyte function is diminished. There is also an expansion of CD8+ T-lymphocytes resulting in a reversal of the CD4:CD8 ratio. Decreased viremia and p24 antigenemia seen during primary infection is thought to be the consequence of the development of cellular and humoral immune responses combined with virus sequestration in lymphoid tissue. The rapid decline in HIV viremia is temporarily correlated with the development of HIV-specific CD8+ cytotoxic T-lymphocyte (CTL) responses. HIV infection is unique among human viral infections in that, despite robust cellular and immune responses that are mounted after primary infection, the virus is not completely cleared from the body. One of the most important reasons for this is thought to be antigenic exhaustion of the HIV-specific CTL responses. Chronic infection develops that persists with varying degrees of virus replication for a median of 10 years before an individual becomes clinically ill. Most adults and adolescents infected with HIV remain symptom free for long periods although viral replication continues to occur at a high pace.

CLINICAL FEATURES

When primary HIV infection is symptomatic, the clinical manifestation resembles an acute nonspecific viral infection with fever, lethargy, malaise, arthralgias, myalgias, headache, sore throat, night sweats, anorexia, and lymphadenopathy.[5,6] These symptoms, thought to be related to the immune response to HIV, peak at the same time as the viremia and develop days to weeks after the virus has been acquired. Some patients may experience weight loss, retro-orbital pain and/or depression.[7,8]

Less common complaints include gastrointestinal problems such as nausea, vomiting, and/or diarrhea, or neurologic symptoms such as headache. The duration of symptoms typically is less than 2 weeks; however, in rare instances it may persist for as long as 10 weeks.[9]

Cutaneous manifestations are seen in up to 75% of symptomatic patients and usually appear several days after the onset of symptoms. The most common is a morbilliform eruption with pink macules and papules up to 1 cm in diameter (**1**). The trunk is most commonly involved, followed by the face, lower limbs, and upper limbs.[6] Vesicles, pustules, urticaria, alopecia, desquamation of the palms and soles, and Stevens–Johnson syndrome (SJS) have also been reported.[10] It has been suggested that the exanthem could be secondary to infection of Langerhans cells in the epidermis. In approximately 25% of ARS, the exanthem is accompanied by painful erosions and ulcerations of the mucous membranes. Ulcers range in size from 5 mm to 10 mm in diameter, are round to oval, shallow with white bases surrounded by a red halo, and can involve the tonsils, palate, buccal, and/or esophageal mucosa. Although the oral cavity is most commonly involved, genital lesions have been reported rarely.[11]

The presentation of ARS is nonspecific and the differential diagnosis includes many infectious diseases including exanthems caused by primary cytomegalovirus (CMV) infection, primary Epstein–Barr virus (EBV) infection, influenza, streptococcal infection, secondary syphilis, toxoplasmosis, rubella, brucellosis, and malaria.[12] Drug reactions, early toxic shock syndrome, Rocky Mountain spotted fever, Lyme disease, herpesvirus infection, and viral hepatitis should also be considered.

DIAGNOSIS

It is unknown how many patients seek medical attention for ARS. It is likely that the initial visit is with a primary care clinician because the symptoms mimic those of more common illnesses.[4] Because ARS may simulate many other conditions, awareness is requisite for diagnosis. It is also important that the condition be recognized for a number of reasons. First, several studies have demonstrated that patients with ARS have a more aggressive disease course and earlier onset of AIDS than those who do not develop the syndrome.[13,14] It has also been observed that the severity of the seroconversion illness may predict the subsequent course of HIV infection. Among patients with illnesses lasting longer than 2 weeks, 78% had an AIDS-related diagnosis within 3 years versus 10% of those whose primary illness lasted less than 2 weeks.[15] Furthermore, symptomatic primary HIV infection may be a period in which initiation of treatment allows immune reconstitution which may improve the subsequent clinical course and CD4+ count[16,17] as treatment with antiretroviral agents results in rapid remission of ARS in the majority of patients. Lastly, patients are highly infectious during primary HIV infection due to pronounced viremia.

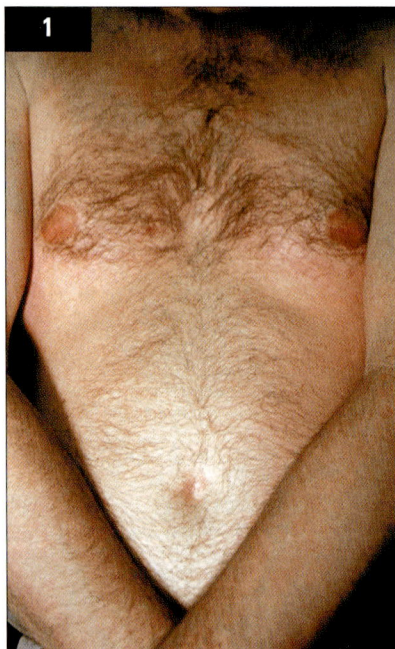

1 Acute exanthem of HIV infection. There is a diffuse pink morbilliform eruption associated with fever and malaise that developed approximately 3 weeks following exposure to HIV. The eruption coincided with seroconversion.

The risk of acquiring HIV when exposed to an individual with symptomatic primary HIV infection may be 500-fold greater than when exposure occurs in the period of clinical latency.[18] Thus, it is of prime importance to identify newly infected patients to prevent further spread of the disease.

The diagnosis of primary HIV infection is usually made by documentation of HIV seroconversion, the development of anti-HIV antibodies, with the enzyme linked immunosorbent assay (ELISA) technique confirmed by Western blot assays. In early disease, however, tests for viral antigen itself must be used as antibodies will not appear for a number of weeks. Established HIV infection can be confirmed by these serologic tests but can also be documented by isolation of HIV from blood or cerebrospinal fluid (CSF), or demonstration of p24 antigen.

In those with a morbilliform eruption, physicians can inquire about risk factors for acquisition of HIV including having unprotected intercourse with someone at risk, possible occupational exposure, and intravenous drug use. The absence of any HIV risk factors lessens the likelihood of ARS; however, it is important to appreciate that sexual and substance abuse histories may not be readily volunteered. Screening for other sexually transmitted diseases (STDs) including syphilis and hepatitis B infection should be performed.

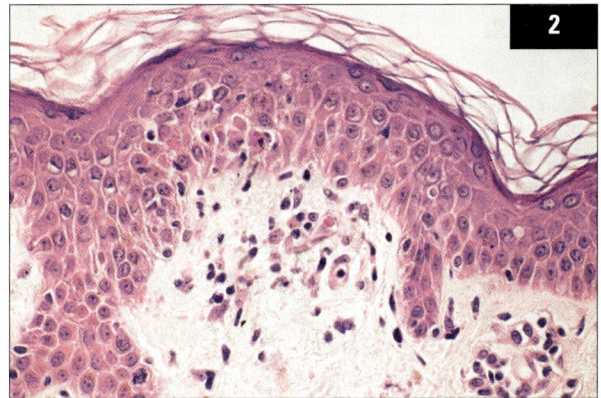

2 Sparse infiltrate of lymphocytes and scattered plasma cells with slight spongiosis and scattered dyskeratotic keratinocytes, characteristic of the acute exanthem of HIV seroconversion. H&E, ×100.

HISTOPATHOLOGY

The histologic findings are nonspecific and resemble those of other acute viral exanthems.[19] Perivascular lymphohistiologic infiltrates in the superficial dermis with minimal epidermal alterations are most common (2). In some cases, there may be scattered individually necrotic keratinocytes in the epidermis as well as scattered plasma cells in the infiltrate in the dermis.

MANAGEMENT

Treatment protocols for ARS are similar to those used in patients with advanced AIDS although because relatively few cases have been treated, there is little data about which protocols may be optimal for this form of HIV infection. As noted previously, early treatment often leads to immune preservation and reconstitution. Treatment during primary infection also appears to restore the balance between naïve and memory CD4+ T cells and improves lymphoproliferative responses to candidiasis and tetanus.[20] Furthermore, neutralizing antibodies appear more rapidly in treated patients than in untreated patients. In some patients, however, by the time acute symptoms arise, treatment may already be too late to prevent the accumulation of a large pool of infectious virus in CD4+ T-lymphocytes.[21] In addition, it has been suggested that removal of HIV antigen before the evolution of a complete immune response may impair future immune control. Because of the complexities of treating ARS, it is recommended that expert consultation be obtained as soon as the diagnosis of primary HIV infection is made. The availability of comprehensive services including social workers, pharmaceutical assistance, psychosocial counseling, and patient education is crucial to a successful management strategy.

MOLLUSCUM CONTAGIOSUM

DEFINITION/OVERVIEW

Molluscum contagiosum (MC) is a viral infection almost universally encountered in sexually active individuals with HIV. Although most lesions are self-limiting, patients with weakened immune systems have increased difficulty clearing lesions, which may persist for prolonged periods. The association between MC and HIV was first noticed in 1983 through an autopsy study of 10 patients with AIDS.[22] MC has surfaced as one of the three most common reasons nondermatologists referred HIV patients to a university-based immunosuppression skin clinic.[23] Molluscum contagiosum virus (MCV) is present worldwide and is passed by direct skin-to-skin contact to produce cutaneous, and rarely, mucosal lesions. It occurs predominately in preadolescent children, sexually active adults, participants in sports with skin-to-skin contact, and in individuals with impaired cellular immunity.

PATHOGENESIS/PATHOPHYSIOLOGY

The virus (genus *Molluscipoxvirus*) causing MC is a member of the family Poxviridae of which smallpox is also a member. MCV is a large double-stranded deoxyribonucleic acid (DNA) virus with a brick-shaped morphology. Four subtypes have been identified, all of which have a similar clinical presentation and are not localized to a particular region of the body.[24] MCV type 1 (MCV-1) is the most common subtype, detected in 98% of infected patients, whereas MCV-3 and 4 are rarely observed.[25] MCV-2 and 3 are slightly more prevalent in Europe, and significantly more prevalent in Australia and in patients with HIV. In HIV-infected patients, MC occurs most commonly when immune function has been dramatically reduced, especially when the CD4+ count falls below 200 × 10^6/l. Several studies have documented that MC is a sign of HIV progression and very low CD4+ counts[26,27] and is correlated with poor prognosis and a median survival time of 12 months.[28] However, the presence of MC is not an independent prognostic indicator after accounting for immunosuppression.[28] The development of MC in AIDS patients is believed to

reflect reactivation of latent infection, although others propose that it is due to recently acquired infection complicating progressive immuno-suppresion.[29] MCV commonly infects the general population with 23% of individuals having antibodies to the virus.[30]

In adolescents and adults, MC is most commonly transmitted by sexual contact and is considered a STD. However, MCV may be transmitted by casual contact, fomites (e.g. underwear), or self-inoculation.[24] The incubation time for MCV has not been well established; however, the average incubation period for MCV in humans ranges from 14 to 50 days.[24]

CLINICAL FEATURES

In AIDS patients, the prevalence of MC skin lesions ranges from 5% to 18%.[31–33] In sero-positive individuals, MC can occur at any time of HIV disease.[34] They typically appear as white, pink, or skin-colored, umbilicated, raised papules (1–5 mm in diameter) or nodules (6–10 mm in diameter). MC may occur as single or multiple lesions. Although most patients are asymptomatic, they may present with a dermatitis surrounding lesions and may experience pruritus or tenderness due to host immune responses, so-called 'molluscum dermatitis'. Gentle pressure on a MC lesion will often cause the central plug to be extruded. In children, the cutaneous lesions of MC are commonly located on the extremities, often as grouped lesions in the axillae, antecubital fossa, and less commonly the popliteal fossa, due to auto-inoculation.[35] In adults, where they are often sexually transmitted, they are located in the genital region, lower abdomen, and thighs. In dark-skinned individuals, significant postinflammatory hyperpig-mentation may occur after treatment.

Immunocompromised patients may present with atypical features of MC including unusual mor-phology and growth patterns (3–7). HIV-positive patients may develop giant (>1 cm) lesions or may have clusters of several hundred lesions. In young men and immunocompromised patients, facial involvement commonly occurs and is spread by shaving (auto-inoculation) which may result in a diffuse infection that simulates a beard. Rarely,

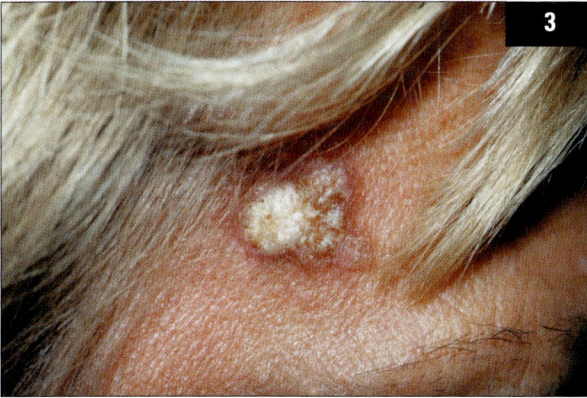

3 Molluscum contagiosum may assume many different patterns in patients with HIV infection. Here, a lesion resembling a keratoacanthoma is seen.

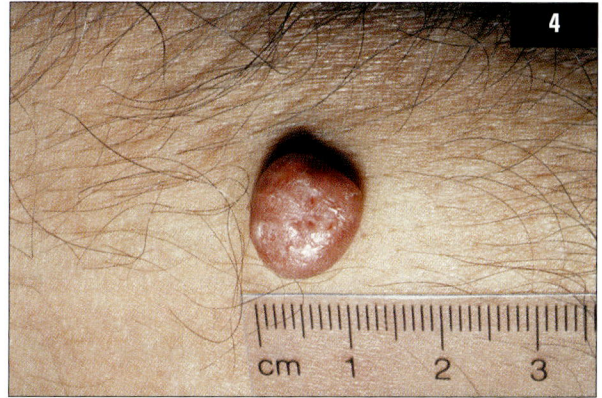

4 Giant molluscum lesion on the forearm.

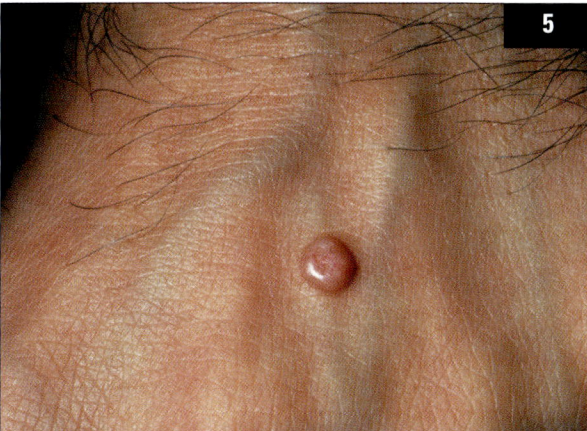

5 Molluscum contagiosum lesion resembling a basal cell carcinoma.

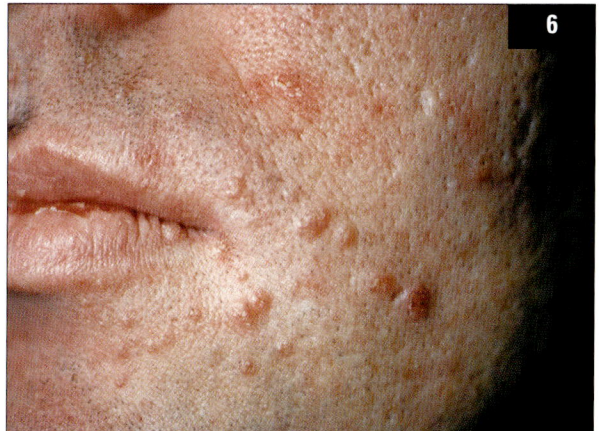

6 Inflammatory molluscum lesions on the face.

7 Multiple clustered, umbilicated papules of molluscum with areas of scarring from previously treated lesions on the flank.

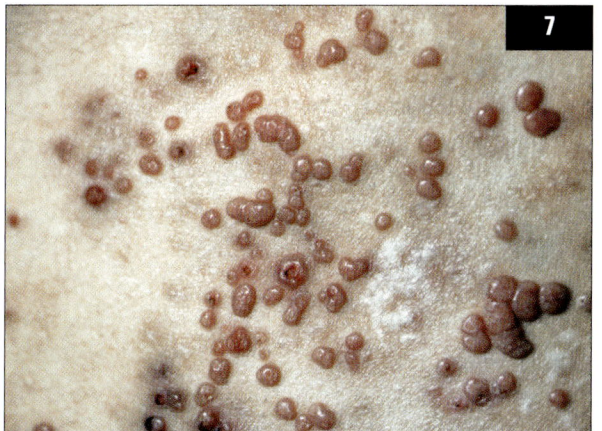

sexual transmission may also result in intraoral or perioral involvement, especially in immunocompromised patients. MC can also develop on the conjunctiva causing conjunctivitis.

The clinical differential diagnosis of MC includes flat warts, condylomata acuminata, vulvar syringomata, and sebaceous hyperplasia for multiple small MC lesions. Disseminated infections including *Cryptococcus*, histoplasmosis, penicilliosis, and pneumocystosis may also appear similar to MC. Larger lesions may appear similar to squamous or basal cell carcinoma, keratoacanthoma, and epidermoid cysts.

Histopathology

Studies evaluating the microscopic and ultrastructural features of MC identify no major differences between samples taken from healthy individuals and from AIDS patients. Direct microscopic examination of Giemsa-stained smears of the keratotic plug reveals 'molluscum bodies' (Henderson–Patterson bodies).[36] Histologically, epidermal cells contain large inclusion bodies that appear as single, ovoid eosinophilic structures in the lower cells of the stratum malpighii (8). Each body contains large numbers of maturing virions. The epidermis invaginates into the dermis and infection involves the epithelium of the hair follicles which eventually coalesce producing a small cyst-like structure. Early transcription of MCV occurs within the basal cell layer, and MCV viral colonies first become visible by light microscopy approximately four layers higher. Because MCV characteristically proliferates within the follicular epithelium, routine fixation produces an area of retraction artifact separating the one to three layers of CD34+ stromal cells that immediately surround the follicle. This feature may be obscured when the lesions are inflamed, usually after rupture, into the surrounding dermis. One study noted ultrastructural presence of viral particles in adjacent normal appearing skin adjacent to mollusca in HIV-positive patients.[37] It has been suggested that this may partially explain the high rate of reoccurrence after destructive treatment.

Diagnosis

Diagnosis of genital MC is generally made by clinical examination of the patient. However, because of the atypical nature of MC in the HIV-positive patient, diagnosis may be dependent on biopsy. Studies evaluating the microscopic and ultrastructural features of MC did not identify any major differences between samples taken from healthy patients as compared to patients with AIDS.[38,39] One exception to this is that AIDS patients may lack the inflammation and lymphocytic infiltration seen in ruptured lesions. If genital MC lesions are identified, patients should be tested for other STDs as a precautionary measure.

Management

Preventative management includes avoidance of skin-to-skin contact with individuals infected with MV. HIV patients with MC in the beard area should also be advised to minimize shaving facial hair to grow a beard.[40] MC in HIV patients is notoriously difficult to treat, and there is little evidence that lesions spontaneously resolve.[40] Perhaps the most widely used methods are curettage and cryosurgery.[41] Small mollusca may be removed with a small curette with minimal discomfort. Freezing lesions for 10–15 seconds is effective using either a cotton-tipped applicator or liquid nitrogen spray. For MC refractory to cryosurgery, especially in HIV-infected individuals, electrodesiccation or laser surgery is the treatment of choice. Large lesions typically require anesthesia either applied topically or intralesionally. Giant MC may require several cycles of electrodessication and curettage.

While destructive treatment is the mainstay, several topical agents have demonstrated efficacy in treating MC. Daily topical tretinoin application may serve as an adjunctive therapy to local destructive treatment[42] and studies have also reported success with cantharidin with or without curettage for resistant lesions.[43] Although tretinoin appears to diminish the appearance of new lesions and helps eliminate older lesions, its use is limited by local irritation. Trichloroacetic acid peels yielded an

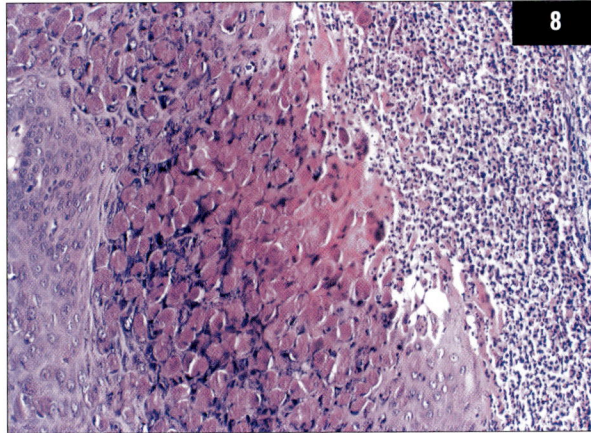

8 Histology of molluscum contagiosum with characteristic intranuclear inclusions (Henderson–Patterson bodies).

average reduction in MC lesion counts of 40.5% in seven HIV-infected individuals.[44] Immune therapy with systemic and intralesional interferon (IFN) has been used with moderate success in treating AIDS patients with MC.[45] Topical application of imiquimod enhances functional maturation of Langerhans cells and their migration to regional lymph nodes, thereby enhancing cutaneous adaptive responses, as well as innate and adaptive immunologic response.[46] It has been studied for treatment of MC in AIDS patients and has shown moderate success although its use is limited by local inflammation.[47] Podophyllin is also effective but may be a poor choice in patients with HIV given their predisposition for development of cancer and its being mutagenic.[48] If applied, it should be left on for only a minimal period (1–4 hours) and then thoroughly washed off. Because podophyllin is caustic and causes irritation, only a small area should be treated at one time. A nucleotide analog of deoxycytidine monophosphate, cidofovir, is an antiviral with activity against a broad variety of DNA viruses, including MCV. It is most commonly used for the treatment of CMV retinitis in AIDS patients, and is useful as topical or intravenous treatment for recalcitrant MC although it is quite expensive. Patients with concurrent MC and CMV treated with intravenous cidofovir have experienced clearance of MC lesions.[49] Finally, several case reports have described the reduction in MC after beginning antiretroviral treatment.[50]

HUMAN PAPILLOMAVIRUS INFECTIONS

DEFINITION/OVERVIEW

Human papillomavirus (HPV) infections are extremely common in humans and cause a wide variety of clinical lesions of the skin and mucous membranes (9–12). HPV is a double-stranded DNA virus of the papovavirus class that induces hyperproliferative lesions of cutaneous and mucosal epithelia.[51] Many viral strains play roles in oncogenesis of epithelial neoplasms including squamous cell carcinoma *in situ* (SCCIS) and invasive squamous cell carcinoma (SCC). More than 150 types of HPV have been identified and many are associated with distinct clinical syndromes. Transmission is by skin-to-skin contact and minor breaks in the stratum corneum facilitate epidermal infection.

PATHOGENESIS/PATHOPHYSIOLOGY

Three cutaneous HPV infections are encountered most frequently: common warts (verrucae vulgaris), plantar warts, and flat warts. While they may be of minimal consequence, they often cause significant cosmetic and functional abnormalities. Genital warts (condyloma acuminatum), although less common in the general population, are seen with higher frequency in HIV-infected individuals.

Plantar warts located over pressure points of the feet, may be extremely painful and may limit normal daily activities. Common warts are firm papules 1–10 mm in diameter with a verrucous, hyperkeratotic surface. Characteristic red or brown dots, representing thrombosed capillary loops, are best seen with a hand lens. Early plantar warts (verruca plantaris) are small, shiny, sharply defined papules. The papules evolve into plaques with a rough hyperkeratotic surface studded with red-brown dots. As with common warts, normal dermatoglyphics are disrupted in plantar warts. 'Kissing' lesions may occur on opposing surfaces of two toes. Flat warts (verruca plana) are sharply defined, skin-colored to brown, flat papules 1–5 mm in diameter. They may be round, oval, polygonal, or linear due to self-inoculation by scratching. Epidermodysplasia verruciformis (EDV) is a HPV-associated genodermatosis with autosomal recessive inheritance. Regarded as a model of cutaneous HPV oncogenesis, it is caused by several HPV types including 2, 3, 5, 8, 9, 10, 12, and 14. EDV lesions are extensive flat warts of the face, trunk, and extremities primarily, that often coalesce and may simulate tinea versicolor[52] (12). They often involve sun-exposed surfaces and may be erythematous. The condition represents a genetic inability of the host to destroy HPV and is associated with development of SCC.

Oncogenic HPV may cause SCCIS and SCC in immunocompromised hosts, especially those with HIV. Immunocompromise also causes an increased incidence, and more widespread nature, of cutaneous warts.[53] Histology reveals acanthosis, papillomatosis, and hyperkeratosis. The characteristic and pathognomonic feature is the koilocyte which is a vacuolated cell with pale-staining cytoplasm and clumped basophilic keratohyaline granules often seen near the surface of the epidermis. There are also vertical tiers of parakeratotic cells overlying epidermal digitations and often hemorrhage within the parakeratotic foci. The diagnosis is typically made on clinical findings alone, but in HIV-infected patients lesions with unusual features or failure to respond to treatment should be biopsied to rule out SCC.

MANAGEMENT

Traditional treatment modalities include podophyllin resin, podophyllotoxin, salicylic acid, trichloroacetic acid, bichloroacetic acid, cryotherapy, laser, and surgical techniques.[54,55] Recently, topical application of immunomodulatory compounds such as imiquimod have demonstrated good efficacy with clearance rates up to 77% and low recurrence rates. A vaccine to prevent acquisition of oncogenic HPV has also recently been released although it is unclear how useful this will be in those with established HPV infection.[55] Unfortunately, in immunocompromised hosts, cutaneous HPV infections may be very resistant to all modalities of therapy.

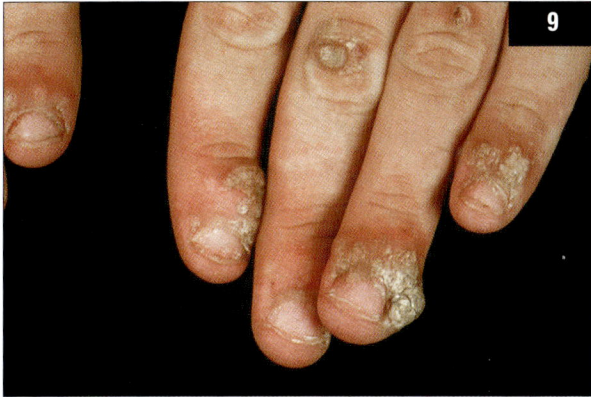

9 Human papilloma virus infection, showing periungual coalescing verrucae.

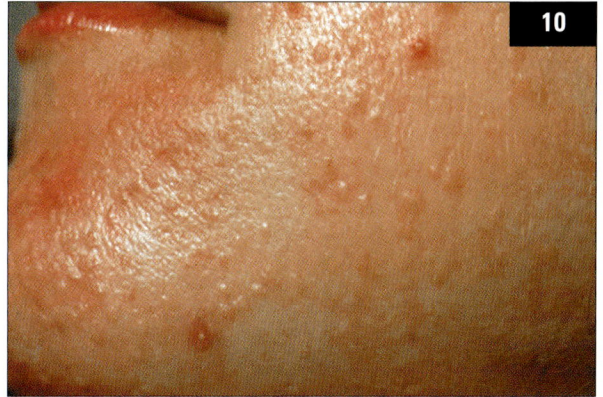

10 Verrucae plana on the face.

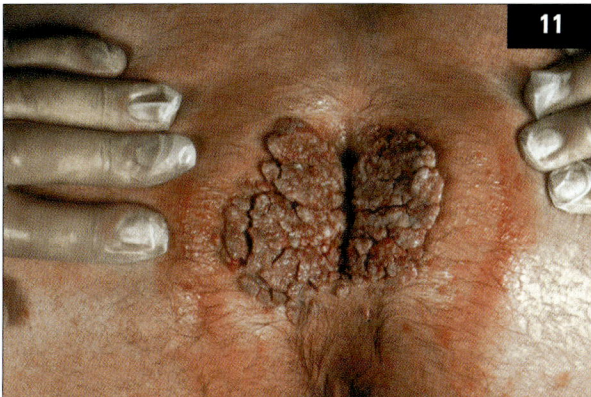

11 Perianal condyloma acuminata.

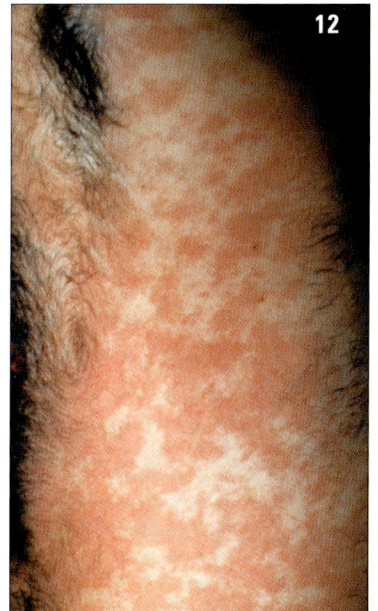

12 Epidermo-dysplasia verruciformis. Hyperpigmented, slightly erythematous, flat, coalescing plaques on the trunk of an HIV-infected patient.

HERPESVIRIDAE

DEFINITION/OVERVIEW

The herpesviridae are double-stranded DNA viruses that are somewhat arbitrarily classified into three subfamilies: the alpha, the beta, and the gamma subgroups.[56] There are eight human herpesviruses. Members of alphaherpesviruses replicate rapidly *in vitro* and *in vivo* and lead to lytic destruction of infected cells. Herpes simplex virus (HSV)-1, HSV-2 and varicella-zoster virus (VZV) belong to this group.

Betaherpesvirus, on the other hand, has a relatively long reproductive cycle and grows slowly in culture. CMV is the only human pathogen in this group. CMV typically causes a chronic nonlytic cellular infection resulting in cytomegalic changes (cellular enlargement). The gamma herpesviruses of humans include four lymphotropic agents: EBV and herpesviruses 6, 7, and 8.

Members of the herpesvirus family share a common structure. They all have an icosahedral nucleocapsid composed of 162 subunits called 'capsomeres'.

The nucleocapsid is surrounded by a membranous envelope that is largely derived from host cell membrane with modification of virus-coded glycoprotein. A layer called 'tegment', which is comprised of amorphous protein largely encoded by the virus itself, is present between the nucleocapsid and the envelope. The whole virion measures approximately 120–300 nm in diameter with the alphaviridae being the smallest and CMV being the largest.

The genome of the herpesvirus is a linear double-stranded DNA molecule 80–220 kilobasepairs in length.[56] Although many functionally important genes are conserved among the members of herpesviruses family (such as DNA polymerase and thymidine kinase), there is still considerable variation in their DNA sequences. Herpesvirus genes and their protein products can be divided into those coding for 'early' virus events in the replication cycle such as DNA replication and transcription and those involved in 'late' events such as translation for viral structural proteins and proteins responsible for viral assembly.

All herpesviruses share the property of being able to establish life-long latent infection in humans, but the cell types in which individual viruses achieve latency vary.[57,58] Alphaherpesviridae remain dormant in dorsal root ganglion, CMV in lymphoreticular cells, kidney cells and secretory glands, and gamma herpesviruses in lymphoid tissue. When the host immune status declines, the latent virus may reactivate to cause overt clinical diseases.[57,58] In immunocompromised individuals, reactivation of dormant virus can lead to severe clinical presentations with widespread and persistent infections. Five human herpesviridae commonly cause mucocutaneous infections in AIDS patients: HSV-1, HSV-2, VZV, CMV, and EBV.

ANTIVIRAL AGENTS DIRECTED AGAINST HERPESVIRIDAE

The majority of current antiherpetic drugs are designed to antagonize the function of protein products of viral 'early genes' such as viral DNA polymerase. Acyclovir is the prototypic antiherpetic agent and is effective against HSV- 1 and -2, VZV, and somewhat against EBV.[59] Acyclovir is a guanosine analog that is selectively phosphorylated by the herpes virus-encoded enzyme thymidine kinase

in infected cells.[59,60] Cellular enzymes then convert acyclovir monophosphate to acyclovir triphosphate, which preferentially inhibits viral DNA polymerase. Acyclovir resistance results mostly from mutations in viral thymidine kinase and rarely from altered viral DNA polymerase.[61,62] The side-effects of acyclovir are generally mild and include headache, diarrhea, nausea, vomiting and, rarely, transient renal toxicity.

Since acyclovir has low oral bioavailability (20%), several compounds have been developed to overcome this shortcoming. Valacyclovir is a prodrug of acyclovir that is converted to acyclovir after absorption.[63] Similarly, famciclovir is a prodrug of penciclovir.[64] The latter is an acyclic guanosine nucleoside derivative that has a similar mode of action as acyclovir. All three drugs, capable of achieving higher blood concentration than acyclovir after absorption, permit less frequent dosing. They are approved for treatment of HSV and zoster infections.

Foscarnet is an analog of pyrophosphate that inhibits viral DNA and ribonucleic acid (RNA) polymerases at the pyrophosphate binding site at a concentration that does not affect cellular DNA polymerases.[65] Although foscarnet has a broad antiviral activity *in vitro*, it is approved only for CMV retinitis and HSV/VZV infections. Foscarnet does not require phosphorylation by thymidine kinase to be activated and is therefore active against acyclovir-resistant VZV mutants that have deficient thymidine kinase activity.[66] Foscarnet exhibits poor oral bioavailability and has to be administrated intravenously. Significant side-effects are nephrotoxicity and anemia.[65,67]

Ganciclovir, similar in structure to famciclovir, is an acyclic nucleoside analog approved only for treatment and prophylaxis of CMV infection.[68–70] Ganciclovir has 8- to 20- times greater activity against CMV than acyclovir. Like acyclovir, ganciclovir needs to be converted to the triphosphate nucleoside for activation *in vivo*. The enzyme that carries out phosphorylation in CMV is the protein product of the viral gene UL 97 as CMV is deficient in thymidine kinase. The activated ganciclovir not only inhibits viral DNA polymerase but also causes premature termination of chain elongation. The major adverse effect is severe, dose-dependent neutropenia.[69,70]

Cidofovir is a nucleotide analog of cytosine that inhibits viral DNA polymerase.[71] It is given intravenously or intravitreally for treatment of CMV retinitis. Cidofovir exhibits significant renal toxicity.[72,73] In cases in which patients cannot tolerate cidofovir, intravitreal injection of fomivirsen, an antisense oligonucleotide directed against CMV mRNA, is given instead. The side-effects of fomivirsen include iritis, vitritis, and decreased visual acuity.[74]

HERPES SIMPLEX

PATHOGENESIS/PATHOPHYSIOLOGY

Cutaneous HSV infection is caused by two viruses: HSV-1 and HSV-2.[75] They share more than 50% DNA sequence homology and similar mechanistic action. Generally speaking, HSV-1 causes herpes labialis and HSV-2 causes anogenital disease. However, significant cross-over infection is present as 10% of herpes labialis cases are associated with HSV-2 and 22–29% of herpes genitalis are caused by HSV-1.[76,77] This overlap is presumably due to oral–genital exposure through practice of oral sex. Transmission occurs through exchange of body fluids including semen, cervical secretion, and saliva as well as direct contact with vesicular fluids of active herpetic lesions.[57,58]

The prevalence of HSV infection is increased among HIV-infected patients, with rates as high as 45% in some studies.[78] HSV may occur at any CD4 count but shows sharp rise in incidence when the CD4 count drops below $10 \times 10^7/l$.[79] Persistent, progressive lesions of HSV lasting more than 1 month with or without therapy are considered as AIDS-defining conditions. Although recurrent herpes infection has shown dramatic decrease since the advent of HAART, it remains one of the most common cutaneous opportunistic infections of AIDS.

CLINICAL FEATURES

In the early stages of HIV infection, clinical presentations of HSV are classical and similar to those in immunocompetent patients, namely grouped vesicles on erythematous bases on the labial or perigenital regions that not uncommonly ulcerate and crust and usually resolve within 2 weeks without treatment.[80] With deterioration of the immune status associated with either the onset or at advanced stages of AIDS, lesions of HSV often become clinically atypical[81,82] (13, 14). These atypical features can be roughly divided into three forms: chronic ulcerative HSV, generalized acute mucocutaneous HSV, and systemic HSV.

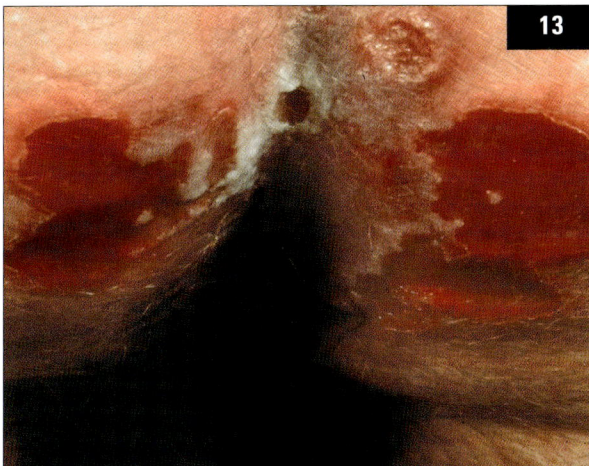

13 Herpes simplex virus infection with extensive perianal ulcerations in a patient with AIDS.

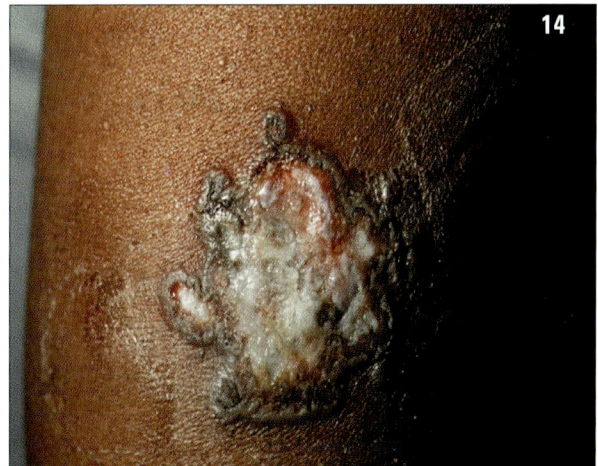

14 Chronic vegetative HSV lesion.

Chronic ulcerative HSV exhibits recalcitrant ulcerations most often occurring at perioral and perigenital regions that enlarge, deepen, and become confluent.[83] Without treatment, they can reach enormous sizes and clinically resemble pyoderma gangrenosum. Lesions with diameters of 20–100 cm have been reported.[84,85] These persistent, erosive lesions of HSV often last more than 1 month and are a clinical indicator of AIDS. Other than large sizes as a result of peripheral spreading, herpetic infections in immunocompromised patients may assume uncharacteristic verrucous or tumorous appearances caused by extensive infection of keratinocytes, including involvement of cutaneous adnexae, and marked crusting. Such lesions may simulate other infections or even neoplasms. Rarely, chronic perianal HSV may resemble an anal fissure.

In addition to oral and genital herpes, herpetic whitlow and herpetic folliculitis may develop in AIDS patients, albeit at lower frequency. Herpetic whitlow is manifested as a deep-seated, painful ulcer usually involving the volar aspect of distal phalanges. This form of herpetic infection most frequently occurs in young children who suck their fingers and in health workers who perform oral examinations or other medical procedures. Herpetic folliculitis refers to HSV inflammation of hair follicles that most commonly occurs on the face.

Generalized acute mucocutaneous lesions of HSV occur following a localized skin lesion. The disseminated, vesicular lesions clinically resemble varicella or, in some cases, smallpox infection. Patients exhibit high fever and other systemic symptoms. Death can ensue in some without obvious visceral involvement.

Systemic infection with HSV is a relatively rare event in AIDS patients. When it does supervene, it usually follows an outbreak of oral or genital herpes. The most commonly involved internal organs include the lungs, liver, adrenal glands, pericardium, and brain.[86–88]

In HIV-infected pediatric patients, larger facial lesions with gingivostomatitis are seen somewhat more frequently than in adult counterparts. Oral involvement is also the most common manifestation in recurrent and persistent herpetic infections in children. Ulcers are often deep and associated with severe pain which leads to diminished oral intake. In such cases, hospitalization is often necessary for treatment of dehydration and maintenance of adequate nutrition. Corneal involvement with herpes infection is a relatively common event in both pediatric and adult AIDS patients and often requires corneal transplantation.

HISTOPATHOLOGY

The major histopathologic manifestation of HSV and zoster infection is ballooning degeneration of keratinocytes and syncytia of nuclei resulting in the pathognomonic multinucleated epithelial giant cell.[89] Dyscohesion and acantholysis lead to the formation of an intraepidermal vesicle. Individually infected cells contain viral inclusions of which there are two types: a homogeneous slate gray inclusion that distends the entire nucleus and has a ground-glass appearance and a nuclear inclusion that is defined as a central, densely eosinophilic viral body separated from a thickened nuclear membrane by a clear halo (Cowdry type A). The nuclear membrane has a thickened appearance caused by condensation of chromatin beneath the nuclear membrane, a phenomenon known as 'margination' of nuclear chromatin. Keratinocytes infected by herpesvirus frequently merge and form multinucleated giant cells in which multiple nuclei exhibit nuclear molding where the contour of the nuclear membrane conforms to that of another cell. The molding, multinucleation, and margination constitute the so-called '3Ms' that summarize the diagnostic nuclear changes seen in HSV infection (15–17). Late lesions may be characterized by a lichenoid infiltrate or by a predominance of histiocytes with granulomatous inflammation. Verrucous HSV infections are characterized by extensive viral infection of large zones of the epithelium with extensive adnexal involvement, including necrosis of sebaceous glands, hair follicles, and sweat glands. There may be minimal inflammation associated with the extent of the infection which can serve as a clue that the patient may be immunocompromised. Usually patients with verrucous herpesvirus infections are profoundly immunocompromised with CD4 counts well below $2 \times 10^5/l$.[90]

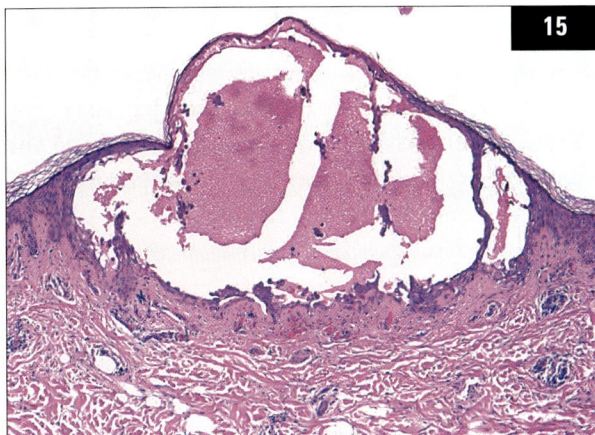

15 Low power histologic appearance of HSV infection showing an intraepidermal blister. H&E, ×40.

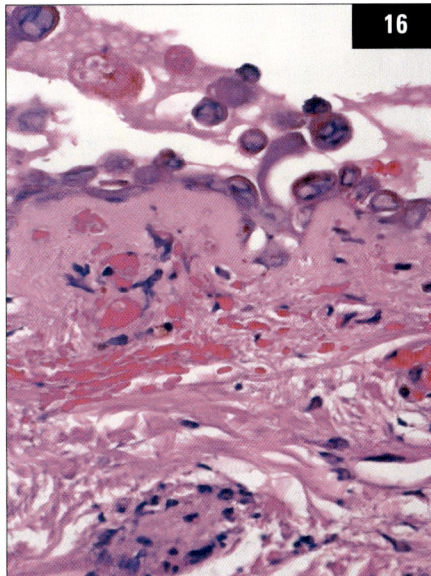

16 Higher power reveals multinucleated giant cells with nuclear molding and margination of chromatin, characteristic of herpesvirus infection. H&E, ×200.

DIAGNOSIS

Although typical clinical presentation of HSV usually points to the correct diagnosis, it is often necessary to confirm the clinical impression by either cytologic or histologic examination. A skin biopsy should be obtained from an early herpetic lesion such as an intact vesicle. Tzanck preparation is a more rapid and simple cytologic method to search diagnostic multinucleated giant cells[91] (**17**). Scrapings of an intact vesicle, preferably from the blister contents, the roof and the base, are smeared on a slide and stained with Giemsa, Wright's, Papanicolaou, or Sedi stains. If no intact blister is present, the base and edges of an ulcerated lesion can be scraped although the test may be artifactually negative. Neither finding multinucleated cells with the Tzanck smear nor the features seen on histologic evaluation can differentiate between HSV and herpes zoster infections. Viral-specific immunofluorescent or immunohistochemical antibody stains on tissue sections or tissue smears can be used to differentiate them, however.

For many years, viral culture has been the method considered to be the 'gold standard' for establishing a definitive diagnosis of HSV.[91] Both HSV-1 and HSV-2 replicate rapidly in cell culture with approxi-

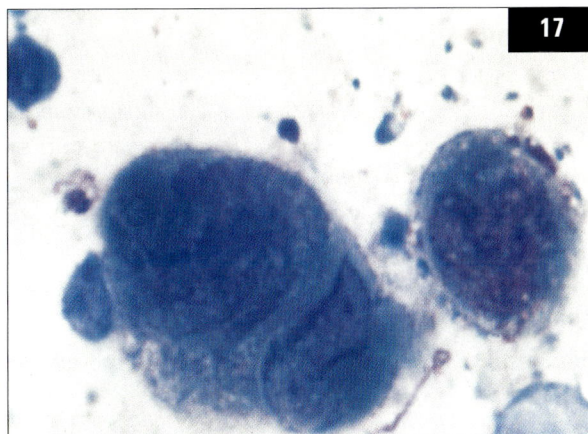

17 Tzanck smear showing multinucleated giant cells.

mately 50% of positive cultures being reported within 24 hours of inoculation, 85% within 48 hours, and more than 99% within 4 days. Distinction between HSV-1 versus HSV-2 can be readily achieved by virus-specific monoclonal fluorescent antibody staining performed on a positive culture. Methods using immunofluorescence techniques coupled with culture are now available for more immediate test results. Antibodies directed against protein products of viral immediate early genes are added into the tissue culture and the cells can be examined within 24 hours of inoculation for nuclear immunofluorescence staining. These methods are as sensitive and specific as conventional culture. However, the sensitivity of a cell culture depends greatly on techniques by which clinical samples are collected and the condition and speed at which the specimens are transported to laboratory. In the case of culture for HSV, fluids in intact vesicles should be sampled whenever possible, and in ulcerative lesions, the ulcer bed and edges should be vigorously swabbed. Calcium alginate swabs should not be used as it is inhibitory to HSV. The collected specimen should be placed in proper transport media and sent promptly to the laboratory.

In many settings, the polymerase chain reaction (PCR) has replaced traditional viral culture. The advantage of the PCR method over viral culture is threefold. First, it is more sensitive, detecting at least 25% more infections than culture. Second, simultaneous subtyping can be performed with easy distinction between HSV-1 and -2. Finally, it is faster with results being available in a matter of hours.[92]

MANAGEMENT

Acyclovir remains the drug of choice for HSV infection.[59] Acyclovir resistance, which has a prevalence of 6.4%, is encountered most commonly among AIDS patients in whom prolonged, low-dose administration for suppressive therapy is thought to play a role in the emergence of drug resistance.[93] Foscarnet (vidarabine) is effective for acyclovir-resistant strains although continuous high-dose acyclovir infusion (1.5–2 mg/kg/hour) and/or topical trifluridine may be used.[65] The selection of therapeutic regimens for treatment of HSV depends on the site of the lesions, the age of the patient, whether lesions are localized or disseminated, whether a primary or recurrent infection is being treated, or if suppressive therapy is considered. Intravenous rather than oral administration is required for severe local disease, disseminated cutaneous, or life-threatening systemic infection. Higher dose and longer duration suppressive therapy are the strategies for treatment of chronic HSV in HIV-infected patients.

Table 1 lists detailed treatment regimens for a wide range of clinical scenarios of HSV infection.

Lesions of documented HSV that fail to respond to acyclovir treatment should be biopsied and cultured to assess sensitivity to acyclovir. Since secondary infections or other cutaneous lesions commonly occur in HIV-positive patients infected with HSV, attention should be paid to rule out concurrent bacterial, fungal, and viral infections. Potassium permanganate solution soaked gauze may be topically applied to the ulcer beds of HSV to prevent secondary infection.

Table 1 Recommended regimens for the treatment of herpes simplex infections

DISEASE		ADULTS	PEDIATRIC[b]	DURATION	COMMENTS
		ACCEPTABLE REGIMEN ALTERNATIVES[a]			
Orofacial herpes	Primary infection	Acyclovir 200 mg PO five times/day Acyclovir 400 mg PO three times/day Valacyclovir 1000 mg PO twice/day Famciclovir 250 mg PO three times/day	Acyclovir 15 mg/kg PO five times/day	7–10 days or until resolution of symptoms	IV acyclovir for severely ill patients. No studies have been done in adults; regimens are extrapolated from their effectiveness in primary genital herpes
	Recurrent infection: episodic treatment	Topical penciclovir 1% cream q2h while awake Topical docosanol 10% cream five times/day Acyclovir 400 mg PO five times/day Famciclovir 500 mg PO two to three times/day Famciclovir 1500 mg single dose or 750 mg twice/day for 1 day Valcyclovir 2000 mg PO twice/day for 1 day		4–5 days or until lesions are healed. Valacyclovir and famciclovir were used for only 1 day	Generally not warranted
	Recurrent infection: prophylaxis	Acyclovir 400 mg PO twice/day			Start just before and during precipitating event such as intensive UV exposure
	Recurrent infection: suppression of confirmed frequent recurrences	Acyclovir 400 mg PO twice/day	There are no pediatric studies but children with confirmed frequent recurrences may benefit from suppressive oral acyclovir therapy		
Genital herpes	Primary infection	Acyclovir 200 mg PO five times/day Acyclovir 400 mg PO three times/day Valacyclovir 1000 mg PO twice/day Famciclovir 250 mg PO three times/day	Acyclovir 40–80 mg/kg/day PO divided in three to four doses (maximum 1 g/day)	7–10 days or until clinical resolution occurs	

[a] Doses are for patients with normal renal function.
[b] Oral dosage of acyclovir in children should not exceed 80 mg/kg/day. Children 40 kg and above should receive the adult dose.

(Continued overleaf)

Table 1 Recommended regimens for the treatment of herpes simplex infections (*continued*)

ACCEPTABLE REGIMEN ALTERNATIVES[a]

DISEASE		ADULTS	PEDIATRIC[b]	DURATION	COMMENTS
Genital herpes (*continued*)	Recurrent infection	Acyclovir 200 mg PO five times/day Acyclovir 400 mg PO three times/day Acyclovir 800 mg PO twice/day Valacyclovir 500 mg PO twice/day Valacyclovir 1000 mg PO once/day Valacyclovir 1000 mg PO twice/day[c] Famciclovir 125, 250, 500[c], mg PO twice/day Famciclovir 1000 mg PO twice/day for 1 day	Acyclovir 1000 mg/day PO in three to five divided doses	5–10 days or until clinical resolution occurs	
	Suppression of recurrences	Acyclovir 400 mg PO twice/day Acyclovir 800 mg PO once/day Valacyclovir 500, 1000 mg PO once/day[d] Valacyclovir 250 mg PO twice/day[d] Valacyclovir 500 mg PO twice/day or 1000 mg PO once/day[c] Famciclovir 250 mg PO twice/day Famciclovir 125, 250 mg PO three times/day	Acyclovir 400–1000 mg/day PO in two to three divided doses		Duration of therapy is controversial; some authors will offer treatment for 1 year, then reassess
	Suppression of recurrences in pregnant women	Acyclovir 400 mg PO three times/day from 36 weeks to delivery			Use is controversial
	Reduction of transmission	Valacyclovir 500 mg PO once/day			Safe sex practices should continue to be used
Ocular herpes	Therapy	Trifluridine drops 1%: 1 drop q2h during day, q4h during night, maximum 9 drops/day IDU drop 0.1%, 0.5% ointment; drop hourly during day, q2h during night, ointment q2h during day, q4h during night			Undertake in consultation with an ophthalmologist. Corneal and conjunctival toxicity of trifluridine is similar to that with IDU. IDU can cause corneal epithelial toxicity, follicular conjunctivitis and

Table 1 Recommended regimens for the treatment of herpes simplex infections (*continued*)

ACCEPTABLE REGIMEN ALTERNATIVES[a]

DISEASE		ADULTS	PEDIATRIC[b]	DURATION	COMMENTS
Ocular herpes (*continued*)		Vidarabine ointment 3% q3h during day Acyclovir 400 mg PO five times/day Valacyclovir 1000 mg PO twice/day			scarring, and closure of tear outflow channels. Vidarabine causes less corneal and conjunctival toxicity than IDU
	Suppression of recurrences	Acyclovir 400 mg PO twice/day	Acyclovir 80 mg/kg/ day PO in three divided doses (maximum 1 g/day) may be of benefit		Undertake in consultation with an ophthalmologist
Other cutaneous herpes (herpes gladiatorum, herpetic whitlow, etc)	Treatment	Acyclovir 200 mg PO five times/day Acyclovir 400 mg PO three times/day Valacyclovir 1000 mg PO twice/day Famciclovir 250 mg PO three times/day	Acyclovir 40–80 mg/kg/day PO in three to four doses (maximum 1 g/day)	7–10 days or until resolution of symptoms	No studies have been done. Regimens are extrapolated from the treatment of genital herpes. Consider suppressive antiviral therapy for patients with frequent recurrences
Neonatal herpes			Acyclovir 20 mg/kg IV q8h	14–21 days	The value of long-term suppression after initial treatment is being evaluated
Disseminated infection		Acyclovir 10–15 mg/kg IV three times/day	Acyclovir 10 mg/kg IV three times/day	14–21 days	
Encephalitis		Acyclovir 10–15 mg/kg IV three times/day	Acyclovir 10 mg/kg IV three times/day	14–21 days	
Eczema herpeticum		Acyclovir 200 mg PO five times/day Acyclovir 400 mg PO three times/day Valacyclovir 1000 mg PO twice/day Acyclovir 10–15 mg/kg IV three times/day	Acyclovir 40–80 mg/kg/day PO divided in three to four doses (maximum 1.2 g/day) Acyclovir 10 mg/kg IV three times/day	14–21 days	No studies have been done. Use IV acyclovir in severely ill patients. Consider suppressive antiviral therapy for patients with recurrences. Ocular involvement should be treated in consultation with an ophthalmologist

IDU: idoxuridine

[a] Doses are for patients with normal renal function.

[b] Oral dosage of acyclovir in children should not exceed 80 mg/kg/day. Children 40 kg and above should receive the adult dose.

[c] Human immunodeficiency virus patients.

[d] The high once/day and twice/day doses of valacyclovir are more effective in patients who present with more than 10 recurrences/year.

Note: valacyclovir and famciclovir are not approved by the US Food and Drug Administration for use in children.

(After Freedberg *et al*. 2003.)[141]

VARICELLA-ZOSTER VIRUS

PATHOGENESIS/PATHOPHYSIOLOGY

Prior to development of a specific vaccine, VZV infection was nearly universal with 95% of the general population being infected.[94,95] Transmission occurs via aerosol droplets or close contact. Primary infection with VZV (varicella or chickenpox) is manifest as successive crops of pruritic erythematous macules that quicky progress to clear, fluid-filled vesicles on red bases.[94] The lesions begin on the head and neck and spread caudally over the torso and extremities. While older lesions develop crusts, new crops emerge so that the simultaneous presence of lesions in various stages of evolution is seen. After the patient heals, VZV remains latent in dorsal root ganglia.[96] With depression of cellular immunity, the virus is reactivated and erupts as herpes zoster or shingles in a dermatomal-distribution pattern.[97,98]

While zoster is not considered an AIDS-defining condition itself, there are many associatons between VZV, HIV, and AIDS. The incidence of herpes zoster is much higher in AIDS patients than in general population, affecting 8–11%.[99–101] The age-adjusted relative risk of VZV infection is 15 times greater in HIV-positive individuals than in healthy persons (29.4 cases/1000/person-years versus 2.0 cases/1000 person-years). Reactivation of VZV can occur at either or both early and advanced stages of HIV infection. When herpes zoster occurs in the early stages of HIV infection, it is often the first manifestation of declining immune function, typically preceding oral thrush and oral hairy leukoplakia by an average of 1.5 years. The development of zoster infection in patients at risk for AIDS is a clinical indicator of progression of HIV infection as the incidence of AIDS following herpes zoster is about 1% per month, although it is not an independent predictor or progression when adjusted for CD4 count. It is associated with the development of HIV infection, especially in tropical, central, and east African areas where the positive predictive value of infection can reach 90%. Zoster in HIV-seropositive individuals commonly occurs with CD4 counts well above $200 \times 10^6/l$ and is a finding of the immune reconstitution syndrome seen in patients who receive HAART whose CD4 cells rise to this level. Finally, VZV infection in HIV-infected patients that is complicated by fever may signify faster progression of HIV disease.

CLINICAL FEATURES

VZV infection is often much more severe in immunocompromised hosts than in healthy individuals (18–21). The clinical manifestations of VZV infection in patients with depressed immunity can be classified as dermatomal zoster, recurrent zoster, chronic zoster, disseminated zoster with or without precedent dermatomal lesions, severe and persistent varicella.

When herpes zoster occurs early in the course of HIV infection, it presents as dermatomal zoster similar to that seen in HIV-seronegative individuals, with grouped and/or confluent papules, vesicles, and crusted erosions involving two or more contiguous dermatomes unilaterally.[99–101] The thoracic, cervical, and lumbar dorsal root ganglions are most commonly involved so that most eruptions involve the trunk or neck. The eruption usually spontaneously resolves in 2–3 weeks. Sensations of pain, numbness, or tingling often precede and accompany the eruption. Pain may be quite intense and severe during the attack and may persist after skin lesions have healed, so-called postherpetic neuralgia.[102] Postherpetic neuralgia and scarring of lesions are more common sequelae in HIV-infected individuals than in immunocompetent counterparts. Ocular herpes zoster occurs when the ophthalmic division of the trigeminal nerve is involved which happens in approximately 10–17.5% of cases.[103,104] It is clinically characterized by an eruption that extends from the level of the eye to the vertex of the skull but abruptly stops at the midline of the forehead. The presence of erythema and vesicles on the tip and sides of the nose indicate likelihood of eye infection as a result of involvement of the nasociliary nerve. Ocular complications range from 50–89% of cases of ophthalmic zoster and include conjunctivitis, keratitis, uveitis, and retinal necrosis that may eventuate in partial or total loss of eyesight. Early ophthalmologic intervention is mandatory to avoid long-term sequelae.[105]

Recurrent episodes of zoster are rare in

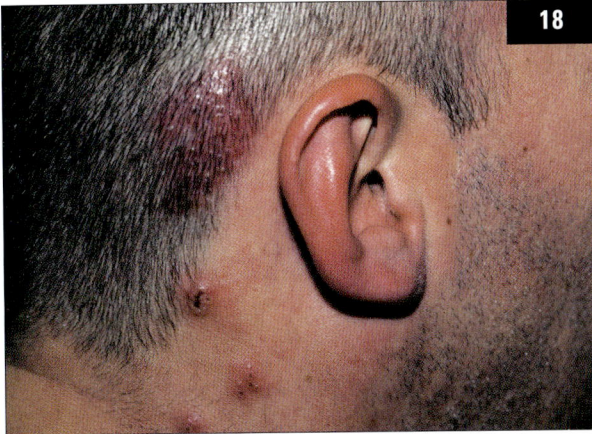

18 Herpes zoster infection with grouped vesicles on an erythematous base in dermatomal distribution.

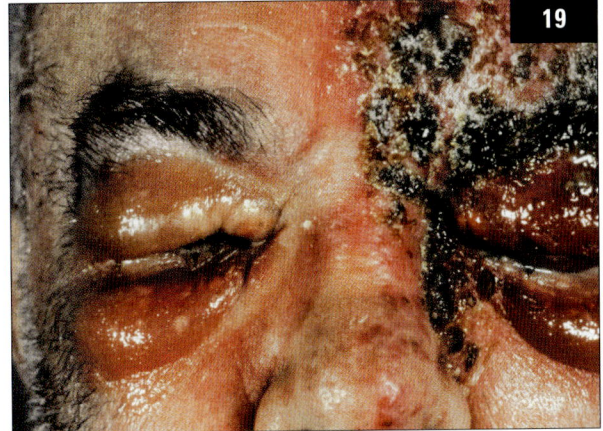

19 Severe VZV infection involving the V1 dermatome in a patient with AIDS.

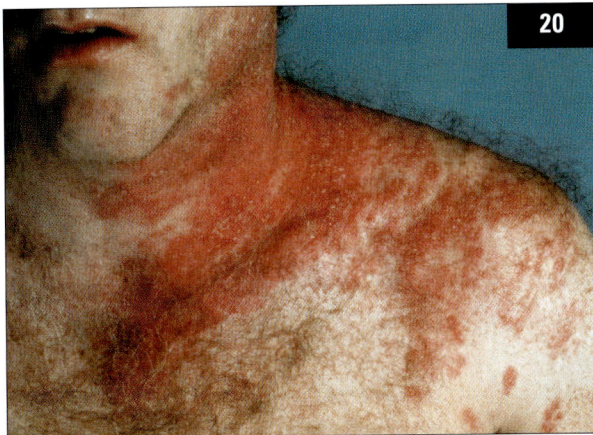

20 Widespread inflammatory VZV infection.

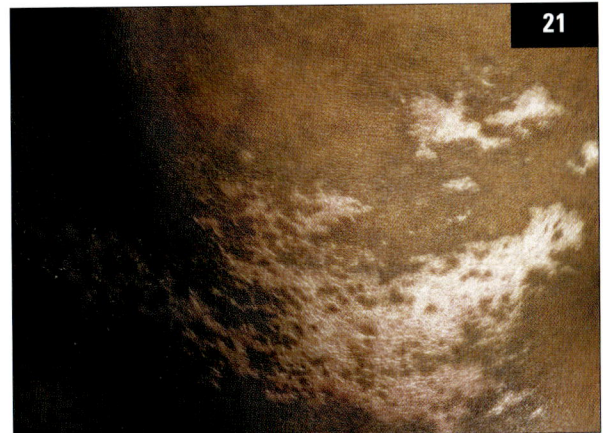

21 Hypopigmentation and scarring following zoster on the flank.

immunocompetent individuals but are dramatically increased in HIV patients: only 1–4% of the former group had more than one episode of zoster while 10–23% of the latter had one or more recurrence. Recurrent zoster signifies progression of HIV-related immunosuppression.[99]

In advanced HIV disease, multidermatomal lesions are more common. In addition, widespread dissemination of lesions as well as chronic lesions are frequently encountered. Disseminated zoster is defined as more than 20 lesions scattered outside the initial dermatome, cutaneous involvement by greater than three contiguous dermatomes, or systemic infections such as pneumonitis, hepatitis, and encephalitis. Dissemination occurs either with or without preceding dermatomal zoster. The latter is clinically indistinguishable from varicella in the absence of previous history of infection or serological evidence for VZV antibody. Chronic VZV infection has been described in both pediatric and adult AIDS patients. It manifests as hyperkeratotic papules and nodules ranging from 0.4–1 cm in diameter, some of which evolve to verrucous lesions or punched-out ulcerations. The chronicity is seen following either dermatomal zoster or disseminated varicella. Although the buttocks and lower extremities are most commonly reported sites, any body region can be involved with chronic VZV lesions. These persistent eruptions usually last from several weeks to months and often heal with atrophic, varicella-like scars.

Although varicella in HIV patients manifests as a benign primary VZV infection in most cases, higher rate of complications, and rarely death, have been reported compared to immunocompetent individuals. Perrone *et al.* reported that 12 out of 421 HIV-positive persons (2.9%) had varicella (in our view, three of the patients with so called 'atypical varicella' described in the paper were more consistent with disseminated zoster without antecedent dermatomal zoster).[107] Out of these 12 patients, six developed a profuse eruption, one a hemorrhagic eruption, one hepatitis, one pulmonary involvement with diffuse nodular infiltration, and one died due to fulminant varicella complicated by diffuse intravascular coagulopathy.

HISTOPATHOLOGY

The histopathologic features of varicella or herpes zoster cannot be distinguished from those of HSV infection: intraepithelial vesicles with ballooning degeneration and multinucleated keratinocytes containing nuclear inclusions are characteristics in both conditions.[90] However, it is generally felt that dermal changes are more pronounced in cutaneous VZV lesions than HSV lesions. In the former entity, dermal inflammation and vascular damage are more severe with frequent swelling of endothelial cells, microthrombi, hermorrhage, and fibrinopurulent exudates observed. Diagnostic eosinophilic nuclear inclusions can be seen in endothelial cells, fibroblasts, and neurilemmal cells of peripheral nerves in addition to epithelial cells.

Microscopically, the chronic verrucous VZV lesions seen in AIDS patients show marked orthokeratotic hyperkeratosis, verruciform acanthosis with prominent papillomatosis, and only mild dermal inflammatory infiltrate.[90] Although varying degrees of viral cytopathic changes can be seen including characteristic nuclear inclusions, multinucleated cells, and ballooning degeneration, acantholysis, a key histologic feature in HSV and

VZV infections, is conspicuously lacking in this wart-like form of chronic VZV lesions.

It is not uncommon to see involvement of hair follicles by viral cytopathic effects. However, cases with evidence of VZV infection limited to hair follicles are rare: only one case of VZV folliculitis has been reported to date in which the clinical manifestations are described as painful erythematous plaques without appearance of vesicles.[108]

A variety of reactive histopathologic patterns is seen in association with herpes zoster scars. They include lymphoid hyperplasia, sometimes resembling pseudolymphoma and cutaneous Rosai–Dorfman disease; granulomatous inflammation simulating granuloma annulare, and granulomatous vasculitis and folliculitis; lichenoid inflammation mimicking lichen planus and lichen sclerosus; fibrotic lesions having the appearance of reactive perforating collagenosis.[109–121]

DIAGNOSIS

Varicella or herpes zoster with typical clinical presentations poses no diagnostic challenge. The Tzanck smear, looking for nuclear inclusions and characteristic multinucleated cells, is usually all that is required to confirm the clinical impression.[122] Rarely, zoster is confused with HSV eruptions when the latter presents as a belt-like pattern simulating a dermatomal distribution. Since neither cytologic examination nor histologic examination is able to distinguish VZV from HSV infection and since immunocompromised patients not uncommonly present with atypical clinical characteristics, serologic testing, immunohistochemical studies, viral culture, or nuclear acid detection are often utilized to achieve the purpose of viral identification.

Specimen collection for culture of VZV follows the same rule as that in HSV culture. However, VZV is labile and may not grow properly even in the hands of experienced technical personnel. In addition, VZV grows much slower in cell culture than HSV and it generally takes 5–7 days before cytopathic effects are detectable in cultured cells. Rapid culture methods (such as shell vial assay) can improve the sensitivity and shorten the test time.

Immunofluorescent studies performed on tissue

scrapings or immunoperoxidase studies on biopsy specimens are now utilized by many as the test of choice to diagnose VZV. They are fast and have higher sensitivity than viral culture. DNA hybridization or PCR techniques are currently used to detect VZV DNA in CSF or ocular fluids in cases suspicious of central nervous system (CNS) or ocular infections. Viral nuclear acid testing has not been broadly used in detection of cutaneous VZV infection.

MANAGEMENT

Like HSV, the drug of choice for VZV infection is acyclovir, albeit at higher dosages.[59] Mild varicella/herpes zoster in the early stage of HIV infection, when the immune function is only mildly compromised, can be treated with oral acyclovir (or famciclovir or valacyclovir).[59,63,64] The oral acyclovir dosage is 800 mg five times a day for 7–10 days. Intravenous acyclovir is recommended as standard therapy for patients with varicella/zoster who are significantly immunocompromised, patients with severe clinical presentations of varicella or zoster, and patients with ocular or visceral complications. The intravenous dosage of acyclovir is 10 mg/kg three times a day for 7 days or longer.

Acyclovir-resistant VZV infections are rare, with fewer than 50 cases reported to date.[106] They are defined clinically by persistence of lesions for more than 10 days after initiation of acyclovir therapy. Acyclovir resistance may result from low-dosage suppressive therapy for prolonged periods of time. The clinical manifestations of acyclovir-resistant cases are usually verrucous or crusted lesions that are few in number and localized.[106] Saint-Leger et al. made the observation that acyclovir resistance correlates with poor prognosis. Based on their in vitro drug sensitivity study, the same authors recommended that duration of acyclovir therapy be extended to 3 weeks before ordering sensitivity tests.[106] Acyclovir-resistant VZV infection is treated with intravenous foscarnet (40 mg/kg three times a day until the lesions heal).[65]

VZV vaccine should not be administered to persons who have primary or acquired immunodeficiency except for HIV-seropositive children with no or mild clinical disease.[55] Children with HIV should be followed up closely after VZV vaccination because they have an increased risk of breakthrough infection.

Exposure to VZV should be avoided in HIV-positive patients, especially when those individuals do not have established immunity to VZV infection. The success in achieving this goal, however, cannot be guaranteed because the ongoing infection may not be recognized early enough to segregate the susceptible from infected persons (the disease is most contagious during the period 2 days before and 4–5 days after the appearance of the skin rash). In instances where immunocompromised persons have been exposed to varicella or zoster, varicella-zoster immune globulin (VZIG) can be given to either prevent clinical disease or alleviate its severity. VZIG should be administered as soon as possible after the presumed exposure in order to achieve maximum benefit.[123,124] However, VZIG given within 96 hours after exposure can still render some protection. Passive immunity established by VZIG administration may last for approximately 3 weeks.

CYTOMEGALOVIRUS
PATHOGENESIS/PATHOPHYSIOLOGY

Cytomegalovirus (CMV) is ubiquitously present in human populations with up to 90% of people demonstrating servoconversion by adulthood.[125] The natural history of a CMV infection can be sequentially described as primary infection, the latent infection, and reactivation. After the first bout of CMV infection (primary infection), the virus establishes a latent status in various tissues, such as peripheral blood leukocytes, salivary glands, and kidney. Reactivation may be caused by either changes in physiologic status such as pregnancy or pathologic alteration in immune status caused by immunodeficiency syndrome, immuno-suppressive drugs, chronic debilitating diseases, or operational procedures. Depending on the time of onset, primary infection may manifest as congenital infection transmitted through placenta, perinatal infection transmitted via contact with infected saliva, cervical secretions, or ingestion of breast milk, and postnatal infection contracted via exposure to a wide range of virus-containing bodily fluids including semen, feces, and urine.

CLINICAL FEATURES

Both primary infection and reactivation of CMV in most immunocompetent hosts result in subclinical diseases that pass unnoticed. When clinical symptoms do appear, they are mild and resemble a flu-like episode or a mononucleosis-like disease.[125] In HIV-infected patients, however, CMV infection represents one of the most common opportunistic infections that often results in disseminated, potentially fatal, systemic disease. The lungs, gastrointestinal tract, adrenal glands, and CNS are commonly involved and CMV retinitis is the most common complication.[126]

Cutaneous CMV infection is rare in both immuno-competent and immunocompromised hosts, with the vast majority of cases reported in the latter group. Cutaneous manifestations of CMV infection (**22–24**) are classified as specific and nonspecific types. The nonspecific type occurs as a result of immunologic derangement related to viral infection or of hyper-sensitivity reactions related to medical therapy. Clinically the nonspecific lesions may manifest as urti-carial, scarlatiniform, or generalized maculopapular eruptions. Other nonspecific eruptions include the diffuse, pruritic, morbilliform rash following ampicil-lin therapy, and the violaceous or dark red-blue papules and nodules seen in congenital or perinatal CMV infection ('blueberry muffin' rashes).

The specific dermatologic manifestation of CMV infection represents the skin lesions in which the presence of CMV can be demonstrated via various diagnostic modalities including morphological stud-ies, antigen detection, viral culture, and nuclear acid identification. Although information regarding clinical presentations of specific CMV eruptions are obtained from only a limited number of case reports with the vast majority of the involved patients being immunocompromised, the clinical characteristics are nevertheless protean. They include localized ulcerations, most commonly distributed on the genital area (30% of the cases) and also reported on the chest and oral mucosa; verrucous plaques of the heel; crusted papules on the face; hyperpigmented and indurated lesions on the thigh; granulation tissue overlying a burn; erythematous and purpuric morbilliform rash; perifollicular papulopustules; and generalized urticaria vesiculobullous eruptions.[127–130] Coexistence of CMV and HSV was described in two AIDS patients involving an ulcerated lesion on the lip and necrotic papules on the legs, respectively.[131]

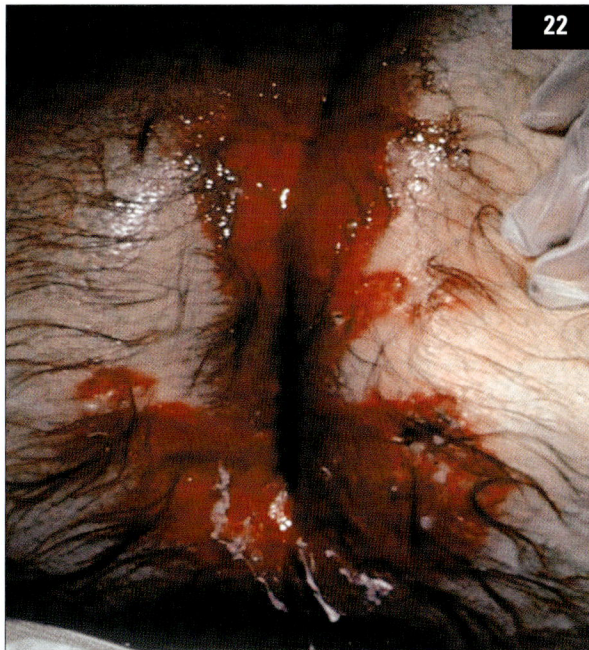

22 CMV infection with erosive perianal lesions in a patient with AIDS.

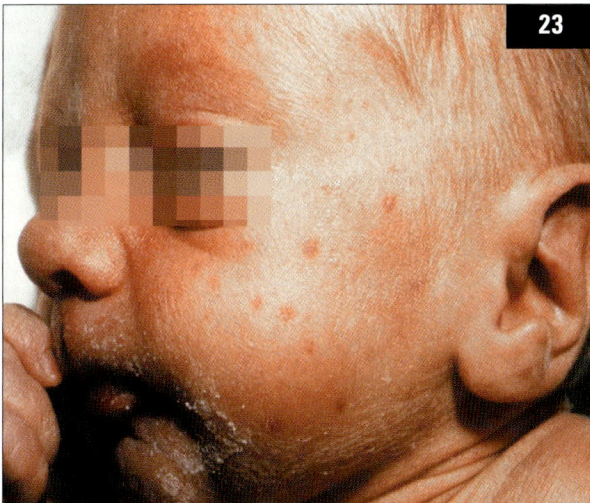

23 Congenital CMV infection causing 'blueberry muffin' lesions in an infant with HIV.

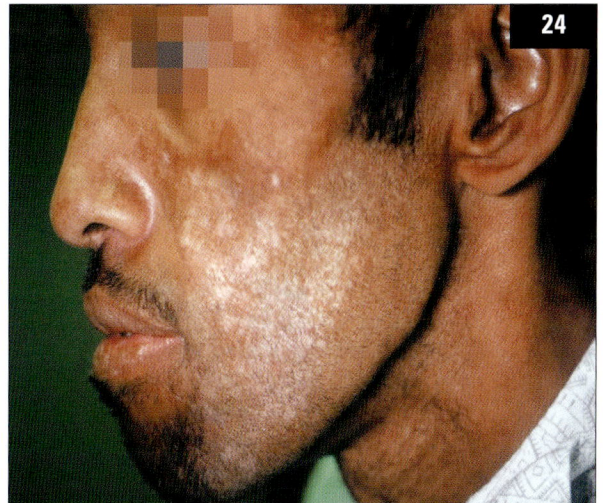

24 Hyperpigmentation secondary to CMV infection of the adrenal glands in a patient with AIDS.

HISTOPATHOLOGY

The histopathologic hallmark of CMV infection is the presence of cellular enlargement with both intranuclear and cytoplasmic inclusions in the infected human tissues (25, 26). The nuclear inclusions, morphologically resembling 'owl's eyes', are characterized by enlarged, often purple-staining intranuclear inclusions surrounded by a clear halo.[132] Smaller, basophilic, intracytoplasmic viral inclusions can be seen as well. In skin, the cytopathic effects of CMV are most commonly seen in endothelial cells lining the dermal vessels, although they are also described in dermal fibroblasts, macrophages, and eccrine ductal epithelial cells. In most cases there is a nonspecific perivascular lymphocytic infiltrate. Prominent neutrophils may be present with features of leukocytoclastic vasculitis reported in rare cases. The epidermal changes are nonspecific with frequent spongiosis, but no cytopathic changes of CMV. In vesiculobullous lesions, epidermal multinucleate giant cells containing viral inclusions are described in association with spongiotic vesicles and reticular degeneration in the epidermis. The 'blueberry muffin lesions' of CMV seen in neonates correlate with dermal erythropoiesis histologically.

DIAGNOSIS

Cutaneous CMV infection is difficult to diagnose clinically because of the variability of dermatologic manifestation. Although biopsy to assess for the presence of characteristic CMV inclusions is the most readily available method, this diagnostic modality is associated with low sensitivity (25).[133] The sensitivity of the traditional histologic examination can be increased, however, by application of immunoperoxidase staining using virus-specific monoclonal antibody (26). Alternatively, immunofluorescent antibodies can be utilized on various tissue specimens.

Conventional viral culture remains the gold standard method to detect CMV infection. Various body fluids as well as tissue biopsy samples are inoculated on human embryo lung fibroblasts. The CMV grows slowly in culture and it takes 1–3 weeks for the cytopathic effects to appear. Rapid culture methods such as shell vial assay and detection of early antigen fluorescent foci (DEAFF) are available for quick detection of CMV antigens. After inoculation of the patient's samples, immunofluorescent antibodies directed against protein products of viral immediate early genes are added into the culture, and the cultured cells can be examined within 24 hours of inoculation for nuclear immunofluorescent staining. These rapid viral culture methods appear as sensitive and specific as conventional culture.

HCMV pp65 antigenemia assay utilizes monoclonal immunofluorescent or immunoperoxidase antibody to detect pp65, a viral structural protein expressed on the surface of polymorphonuclear lymphocytes infected with CMV.[134] The test produces fast results (within the same day) and offers a rough estimation of viral burden that correlates with the severity of infection. As a result, this test is now widely used especially in monitoring invasive infection in HIV patients and transplant recipients. Direct quantification of pp65 protein by flow cytometry study is now used in practice.

PCR is a rapid and sensitive method to detect CMV DNA.[133] However, the results of this highly sensitive method do not distinguish between latent CMV genome versus active viral replication. Only quantitative PCR gives data on viral burden and can be used to monitor risk of active infection and efficacy of antiviral therapy. In situ hybridization offers an advantage to be able to locate viral genome in a specific cell type in a given tissue, but is a cumbersome test to perform. It is rarely used in routine practice.

Serologic tests are often complicated by false-positive and false-negative results in HIV-infected patients.[133] CMV immunoglobulin (Ig) M antibodies are detected in primary infection and persist for 3–4 months. In immunocompromised individuals, however, CMV IgM is frequently falsely negative during primary infection because the hosts are unable to mount an appropriate immune response. On the other hand, false-positivity takes place in the presence of infectious mononucleosis or a positive

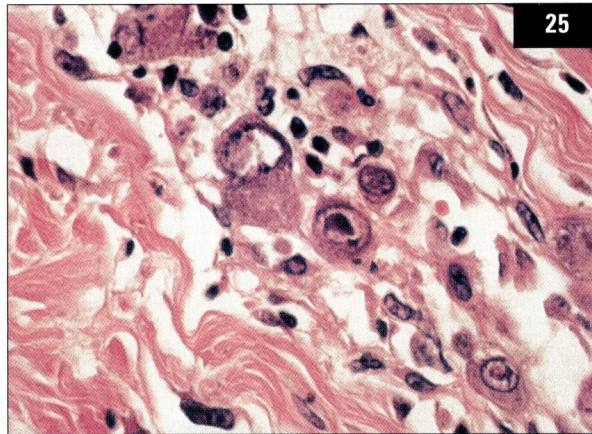

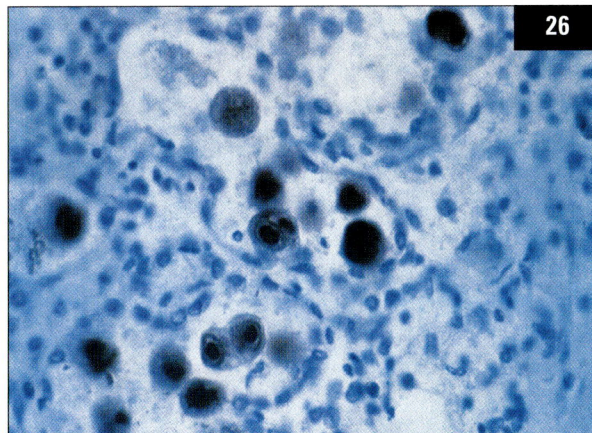

25, 26 Nuclear and intracytoplasmic inclusion bodies of cytomegalovirus infection, highlighted by immuno-peroxidase staining **(26)**, which emphasizes the 'owl-eye' appearance of infected cells.

rheumatoid factor. Detection of CMV IgG indicates past infection, whereas rising titers of IgG mark acute infection. The elevated CMV IgG is useful for the diagnosis of acute infection in immuno-compromised individuals in which CMV IgM antibodies often fail to develop. In cases in which the results of serologic tests are equivocal, viral culture often needs to be performed to confirm the presence of infection.

MANAGEMENT

Since cutaneous manifestations of CMV signify systemic infection, antiviral therapies are directed against various visceral and disseminated CMV infections. Ganciclovir is the drug of choice for visceral and systemic infection, whereas foscarnet is the second-line drug used.[65,68] Cidofovir and intravitreal injection of fomivirsen are approved for treatment of CMV retinitis.[71]

EPSTEIN–BARR VIRUS

PATHOGENESIS/PATHOPHYSIOLOGY

Epstein–Barr virus (EBV) is the causative agent of infectious mononucleosis and selectively infects B lymphocytes and epithelial cells.[135] Most adults have been infected with EBV by age 25 and harbor the latent virus in B cells. As immune function in HIV-infected individuals deteriorates, EBV reactivates and causes spectra of clinical diseases varying from benign lesions such as oral hairy leukoplakia (OHL) to malignant neoplasms such as EBV-associated large B cell lymphoma and Burkitt's lymphoma.[135] In addition, EBV may precipitate progression of HIV disease by enhancing the growth capabilities of the virus in lymphocytes.

OHL is a benign proliferation of squamous mucosa secondary to EBV infection of the oral epithelium[135] (27, 28). Considered one of the most specific cutaneous manifestions of HIV infection, OHL occurs almost exclusively in HIV-infected individuals with rare cases reported in organ transplant recipients and two cases in healthy individuals.[136–139]

OHL commonly affects all HIV-associated risk groups except HIV-positive pediatric patients in which it is rarely seen. OHL has not been reported in infants. The incidence of OHL among HIV-positive individuals is estimated as 25% (the estimation may not be very accurate, however, because of frequent confusion of OHL with oral candidiasis and *vice versa*) and has significantly decreased since HAART became the standard of care in HIV-infected patients. Appearance of OHL usually correlates with moderate to advanced immunodeficiency. The CD4 count is usually below $200 \times 10^6/l$ at time of presentation, but OHL can occur in association with any CD4 count level. In cases of OHL in which HIV seropositivity has not been established, OHL is considered a marker of HIV infection with 48% probability of developing AIDS within 16 months and 83% within 31 months of the diagnosis.[140]

CLINICAL FEATURES

OHL presents as one to multiple white to gray, well-demarcated, adherent verrucous plaques with a hairy surface texture that are most commonly localized on lateral borders of the tongue[135] (27, 28). In early stages of typical lesions, vertical fissures are seen running perpendicular to the long axis of the lateral tongue. When multiple lesions are present, they are usually distributed on the bilateral margins of the tongue with intervening normal mucosa. The next highest frequently involved site is the under-surface of the tongue, with rare cases reported affecting the dorsal tongue, buccal mucosa, and soft palate. The lesions wax and wane for an indefinite period of time, and unlike oral candidiasis, they do not rub off easily and exhibit poor response to antifungal therapy. OHL is generally asymptomatic, although some patients may complain about dysphagia.[141]

HISTOPATHOLOGY

The lesions of OHL are characterized by hyperkeratosis, parakeratosis, and acanthosis with irregular, hair-like keratin projections on the epithelial surface[135] (29). Neutrophils can be noted within the keratin layer. Underlying the keratin layer is a characteristic band of vacuolated and ballooned keratinocytes, which harbor viral inclusions in their nuclei. The nuclear features may resemble koilocytes seen in human papillomavirus (HPV) infection. In fact, HPV is not uncommonly present and is thought to play a role in the development of lesions of OHL. The other characteristic nuclear morphology observed in OHL is the Cowdry type A viral inclusions with beaded condensation of chromatin just beneath the nuclear membrane ('beaded effect'). Coexisting candidal hyphae are shown in 80% of biopsy specimens, within the epithelium without associated spongiotic vesicles. A mild, nonspecific inflammatory infiltrate is usually seen in the dermis. In cases that lack either typical clinical or histologic characteristics of OHL, *in situ* hybridization can be used as a more specific diagnostic method to confirm the presence of EBV DNA in tissue sections or scrapings.

DIAGNOSIS

Diagnosis of OHL is usually straightforward in HIV-positive patients with characteristic clinical presentations. Biopsy is undertaken only in cases in which the serologic status of HIV is unknown or negative. In those instances, confirmation of the presence of EBV by *in situ* hybridization is often necessary.

MANAGEMENT

OHL is a benign proliferation of squamous epithelium that has no malignant potential. Therefore, reassurance is often all that is needed to resolve patients' anxiety unless the lesions cause significant symptoms or cosmetic embarrassment. A variety of drugs including oral acyclovir (200–400 mg five times a day), oral zidovudine (300 mg three times a day), oral gancyclovir (1 g three times a day), and intravenous foscarnet (40 mg/kg every 8–12 hours) can achieve resolution of OHL.[59,65,68] However, the resolution is often temporary, and recurrent lesions usually appear 2 weeks to 2 months after the drugs are discontinued. Like systemic therapy, topical application of tretinoin, podophyllin resin, trichloroacetic acid, or glycolic acid is successful in removing the lesions, but meets with the problem of post-therapeutic recurrence.

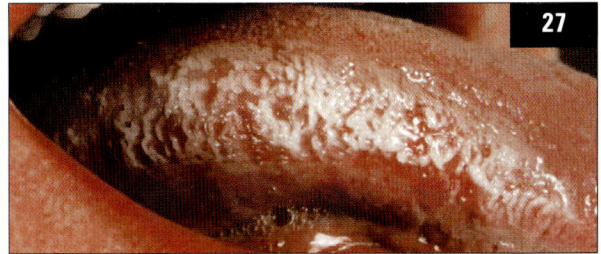

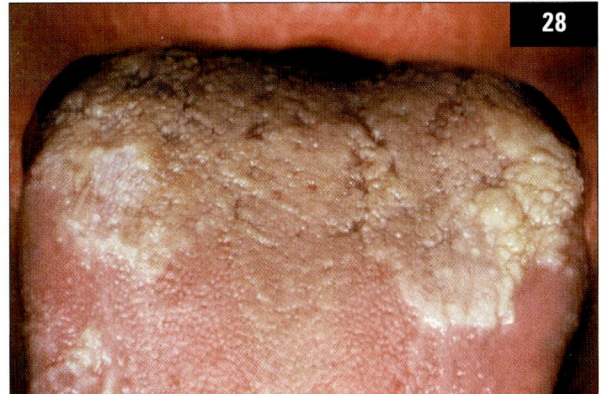

27, 28 Oral hairy leukoplakia of the tongue.

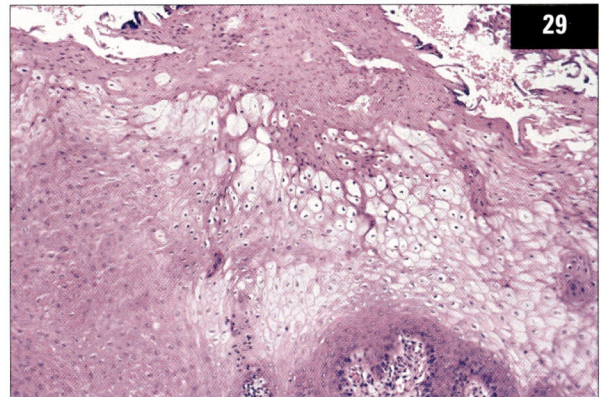

29 Oral hairy leukoplakia with characteristic ballooning degeneration of keratinocytes on histology.

CHAPTER 3

BACTERIAL AND ATYPICAL MYCOBACTERIAL INFECTIONS

Kumar Krishnan, Antoanella Calame, and Clay J. Cockerell

ERYTHRASMA

DEFINITION/OVERVIEW

Erythrasma is a cutaneous bacterial infection caused by *Corynebacterium minutissimum*, a gram-positive bacillus and part of the normal skin flora. It generally presents as a red, scaly plaque with well demarcated borders involving an intertriginous site (30). Progression of the lesion may cause the borders to advance and the color to change from red to brown with an area of central clearing. Infection by *C. minutissimum* occurs most commonly in the skin between the toes, in the axillae, inframammary skin folds and, in obese persons, the infrapannicular skin. Infection between the toes remains the most common site of erythrasma where it is often confused with localized fungal infections. The reason for this localization is due to the predilection of the organism for warm moist environments and explains why it is more common in warm, humid climates and in those with hyperhidrosis. Poor hygeine may also contribute to the development of the condition. Fungi also infect similar sites and up to 30% of patients with erythrasma are coinfected with *Candida albicans*.[1]

CLINICAL FEATURES

The findings are mainly aesthetic in nature although a percentage of patients may complain of mild to moderate pruritus. Erythrasma is not an entirely banal condition, however, as so-called disciform erythrasma has been associated with Type 2 diabetes mellitus. Severe forms of the infection include recurrent breast abscesses, cellulitis, and central line sepsis. One study reported *C. minutissimum* cellulitis

30 Erythrasma in the axilla. (Courtesy of St John's Institute of Dermatology (King's College), Guy's Hospital, London.)

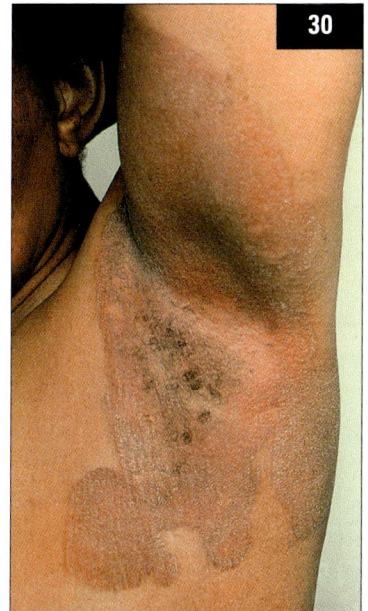

with subsequent bacteremia in an immunocompetent patient, although bacteremia is more commonly reported in immunocompromised individuals.[2] The condition is usually not self-limiting and may last from weeks to months.

DIAGNOSIS

The differential diagnosis includes candidal infection, which may be present concomitantly, dermatophyte infection, as well as psoriasis. The diagnosis can be made with examination using a Wood's lamp as it displays a characteristic coral-red fluorescence that distinguishes it from superficial mycotic infection as well as psoriasis. Direct scraping followed by gram stain reveals gram-positive rods. Other special stains including Ziehl–

Neelsen, methylene blue, and periodic acid-Schiff (PAS) may also reveal organisms. The organisms are present in the upper one-third of the stratum corneum and are present both within and between cornified cells.

C. minutissimum has recently been recognized as a significant infectious agent in immunocompromised individuals. One case report described chronic granulomata and abscesses of the leg which grew *C. minutissimum* in an HIV individual.[3] While the development of granulomas is rare, it is more common in HIV-positive patients. Most cases are sensitive to oral antibiotics, but there have been reports of multi-drug resistant *C. minutissimum* causing abscesses in HIV-positive individuals.[4]

MANAGEMENT

Antimicrobial treatment is usually effective for erythrasma. Erythromycin 250 mg orally four times a day for 14 days has been shown to be effective. If interdigital spaces are involved, the addition of a topical antibacterial such as 2% clindamycin is recommended to increase the overall success rate. In one study, 2% aqeuous clindamycin applied three times a day for 7 days resulted in complete eradication of the infection. Although antimicrobials are effective, erythrasma recurs commonly.[1] Recurrence may be lessened with adequate hygiene and preventative measures such as weight loss.

PITTED KERATOLYSIS

DEFINITION/OVERVIEW

Pitted keratolysis (PK) is a cutaneous infection commonly found on weight bearing areas such as the plantar aspect of the foot (**31, 32**), caused by one of several gram-positive organisms. While the etiological agent remains elusive, there is an association with *Corynebacterium* species, *Micrococcus* (*Kytococcus*) *sedentarius*, and *Dermatophilus congolensis*. The micro-organisms cause a characteristic crateriform lesion measuring 1–7 mm in size. The individual lesions may coalesce to form larger pits.

PATHOGENESIS/PATHOPHYSIOLOGY

PK has been associated with tight fitting shoes in military personnel and miners; however, it is most common in barefooted individuals living in tropical climates. In one study, 80% of participants with PK had involvement of pressure bearing areas of the foot including the ventral aspect of the large toe and heel.[5] It has been proposed that the development of the characteristic crateriform lesion results from the secretion of proteolytic enzymes by gram-positive cocci. *In vitro* studies of *Kytococcus* have shown high levels of protease activity of which there are two, P1 and P2.[6] These proteases have activity against extracted forms of keratin and may be responsible for ultrastructural damage to the stratum corneum.

Biopsies of the crateriform lesions reveal organisms in the upper stratum corneum. Deeper in the lesion, the organisms are filamentous bacteria while more superficially, small cocci are present.[5] Two distinct lesions have been described in patients with PK. One is a crater whose size was proportional to the size of the colony growing beneath that may be up to 7 mm in diameter. A second, smaller lesion, approximately 5 mm in size, is linear in configuration. It is possible that dirt trapped in these furrows facilitates the colonization of *K. sedentarius* and allows the development of the typical crateriform lesion under appropriate environmental conditions.

CLINICAL FEATURES

The main complaints associated with PK are aesthetic in nature and include malodor, hyperhidrosis, and sliminess of the affected region. In one study of 53 patients with PK, 96% reported hyperhidrosis of the affected area. Malodor was a complaint in 86% of patients and sliminess was reported by 69.8%. Pain and pruritus are relatively rare and were reported in 11.3 and 7.5% of patients respectively.[5]

Weight bearing areas are those most commonly affected and include the ventral aspect of the first toe, ball of the foot, and heel. Nonweight bearing areas may also be infected and are more common in barefooted individuals. These include the areas between the toes, the arches, and instep; however, PK in these areas is much less common. Two case reports described PK on nonweight bearing sites in individuals who were not habitual barefoot walkers. In one, it was identified on the arch and was confirmed by biopsy. The second report identified PK on the dorsum of the toes but it was also present on weight bearing areas of the same foot, suggesting that infection along weight bearing areas may lead to spread towards nonweight bearing areas.[7]

HISTOPATHOLOGY

A clinical study of 125 patients with PK revealed two histologically distinct subtypes. The most common form from the denuded pits reveals small dells in the upper portion of the stratum corneum of a dimorphic population of coccoid and filamentous bacteria seen on staining with gram or PAS. The less common type demonstrates only superficial colonization of the stratum corneum with clusters of bacteria found extracellularly.[8]

DIAGNOSIS

The diagnosis is made on the basis of clinical appearance as well as presenting complaints. If unclear, biopsy of the lesion will reveal causative organisms as well as alteration in the upper stratum corneum.

MANAGEMENT

Treatment involves local hygienic care such as keeping the area dry with frequent sock changes and the avoidance of occlusive footwear. Topical antibiotics such as erythromycin, clindamycin, tetracycline, as well as bactericidal soaps and benzoyl peroxide are also effective. Two cases of refractory PK were successfully treated by low-dose botulinum toxin injection, which reduces hyperhidrosis and thus the nidus for infection.[9]

31, 32 Pitted keratyolysis. (Courtesy of St John's Institute of Dermatology (King's College), Guy's Hospital, London.)

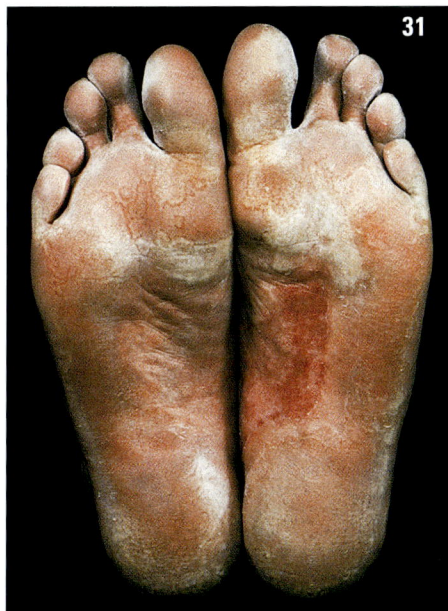

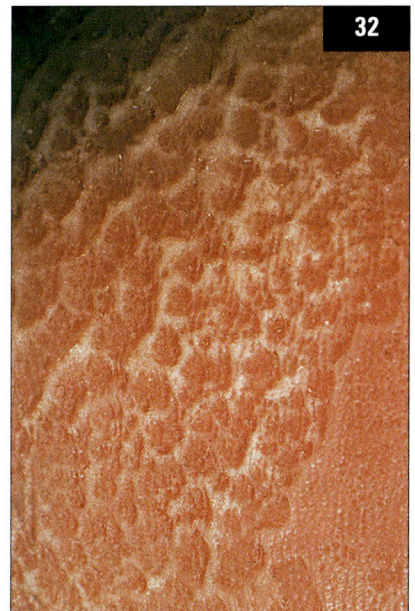

FOLLICULITIS

DEFINITION/OVERVIEW

Folliculitis is an inflammatory process involving the pilosebaceous unit of the hair follicle. It may be caused by a number of factors including bacterial, fungal, autoimmune, or chemical. The classic presentation is the presence of clusters of erythematous papules or pustules in hair bearing areas. Bacterial folliculitis is most common in children and in adults with predisposing conditions that increase the prevalence of cutaneous bacteria[10] such as those being treated with antibiotics as well as immunocompromised individuals. Exposure to poorly chlorinated swimming pools or hot tubs predisposes *Pseudomonas* folliculitis. While *Staphylococcal aureus* is the most common cause of folliculitis,[10–12] other organisms such *Micrococcus* sp. and *Acinetobacter baumannii* may cause widespread folliculitis in HIV-infected patients.

PATHOGENESIS/PATHOPHYSIOLOGY

The pathophysiology of folliculitis varies depending on the cause. Staphylococcal species are the most common cause of cutaneous bacterial infections in HIV patients which is likely due to the abundance of *S. aureus* on normal skin. Cutaneous infection with *Staphylococcus* can lead to both superficial and deep infections. Today, many of these strains are resistant to methicillin, even when they are community acquired. Streptococcal groups A, B, C, D, and G are also common pathogens associated with cutaneous bacterial infections.[12] Less commonly encountered organisms likely lead to infection as a consequence of altered immunity.

Two patients with chronic cutaneous micrococcal folliculitis in the absence of a prosthetic device and without associated bacteremia have been reported in HIV-infected patients. Micrococcal infections are exceedingly rare due to their low pathogenic potential, but *Micrococcus* sp. are, however, part of the normal skin flora and are ubiquitous. When *Micrococcus* sp. does produce an infection, it tends to cause a severe systemic illness and has a propensity to gain entry through catheters.[13] Another recently published report was that of *Acinetobacter baumannii* causing folliculitis in an AIDS patient. This is unusual as, unlike both staphylococcal and micrococcal species, *Acinetobacter* is not a part of the normal skin flora.

CLINICAL FEATURES

The classic presentation of infectious folliculitis is the development of small pustules with an area of surrounding erythema (33–35). Pustules tend to cluster and eventually begin to crust. Typical areas of distribution include the face, axillae, arms, and legs in adolescent girls and buttocks in children. Lesions may be tender to palpation and occasionally present with pruritus. The most common causative organism is *S. aureus*. The high rate of staphylococcal folliculitis in HIV patients is most likely due to the increased rate of nasal carriage of in these patients. Most patients have widespread lesions. Extension beyond the follicular infundibulum is not uncommon and may lead to furunculosis or carbuncle formation. Micrococcal folliculitis, unlike staphylococcal folliculitis, often presents with moderate to severe pruritus. Lesions tend to be more uniform than those caused by *Staphylococcus* and may have a central area of ulceration. Lesions are often present for several months.[13]

Acinetobacter baumannii is a gram-negative bacterium commonly associated with hospital acquired infections. It is most commonly isolated from burn and wound infections. One case has been reported of folliculitis in a severely ill, hospitalized HIV patient caused by this organism. There were multiple, erythematous pustules present on the face, neck, and back.[14]

HISTOPATHOLOGY

In acute folliculitis, there is an infiltrate of abundant neutrophils in involved hair follicles. In one study of folliculitis in HIV patients, it was found that bacteria tend to be located near the follicular ostium, whereas fungi tend to reside deeper within the base of the follicle. There is also usually a perifollicular and perivascular infiltrate of lymphocytes. Eosinophilic folliculitis, a common cause of folliculitis in HIV-infected patients, reveals an admixture of inflammatory cells with a predominance of eosinophils both

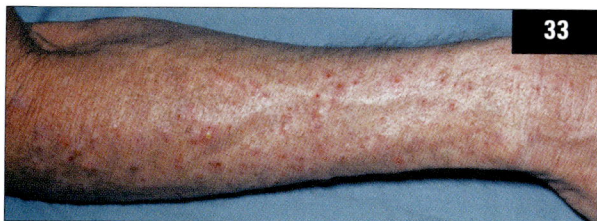

33 Folliculitis, perifollicular erythematous pustules on the forearm.

34 Close up view of follicular pustules in the same patient as **33**.

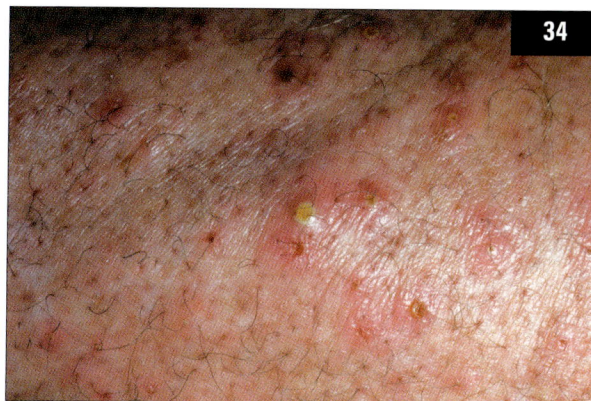

within and surrounding affected hair follicles.[15]

In microccocal folliculitis, histology reveals superficial ulceration and an abundance of gram-positive tetrads in perifollicular areas within abscesses. Organisms can be visualized using Brown–Hopps, Warthin–Starry, and Gomori methenamine silver (GMS) staining.[13] Chronic lesions of folliculitis often demonstrate suppurative and granulomatous inflammation and scarring in the interfollicular dermis with free hair shafts on occasion.

35 Folliculitis. Widespread follicular papules and pustules and older lesions with post-inflammatory hyperpigmentation.

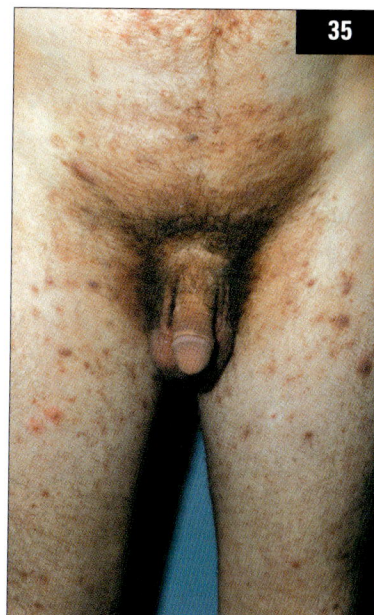

MANAGEMENT

Treatment of folliculitis in HIV-infected patients begins with delineating the specific cause. As stated earlier, folliculitis in an HIV-positive individual may be the result of infection with bacteria, viruses, or fungi or may be caused by nonspecific inflammatory reactions. In one study of 33 HIV-positive patients, examination of skin biopsy material failed to identify clear histopathologic characteristics that would guide presumptive therapy. This study, however, failed to include multiple biopsies from individual patients.[15]

Uncomplicated cases of staphylococcal folliculitis usually respond to topical antibiotics such as mupirocin, although this may not be as effective when the cause is a methicillin-resistant strain (MRSA). Oral antibiotics are also efficacious and the most commonly used ones include dicloxacillin and cephalexin. With the ever increasing incidence of MRSA, however, these antibiotics are of limited efficacy and cases require treatment with vancomycin. Washing with soap containing bactericidal agents and use of ethanol-based gel cleansers are also efficacious at decreasing the bacterial burden. The absence of clinical improve-ment with antistaphylococcal antibiotics along with negative culture may be indicative of either an atypical organism or a nonbacterial cause of the lesion. If *Micrococcus* folliculitis is suspected, treatment is with rifampicin 1200 mg daily by mouth for 4 weeks.[13] In one case report of folliculitis caused by *A. baumannii*, the patient responded well to IV ticarcillin–clavulanic acid 3 g/200 mg four times daily;[14] however, susceptibility studies ultimately guide definitive therapy. Folliculitis that is refractory to topical or oral antibiotics may indicate that the lesion represents either a fungal disease or a noninfectious condition such as eosinophilic folliculitis.

STAPHYLOCOCCAL SCALDED SKIN SYNDROME

DEFINITION/OVERVIEW

Staphylococcal scalded skin syndrome (SSSS) represents a systemic illness caused by an exfoliatoxin secreted by certain strains of *S. aureus*. There are three serologic forms of exfoliatoxin, ETA, ETB, and ETD. Local cutaneous infection with toxin-producing strains of *S. aureus* leads to the development of localized skin blisters of bullous impetigo. Systemic illness from toxin-producing *S. aureus* leads to a generalized desquamation, termed SSSS (**36**). This term was given because of the similarity of the condition to that of a widespread first-degree burn. While SSSS is most common in children, likely due to decreased renal clearance of the toxin in children,[16] cases have been reported in immunocompromised individuals. This is especially significant in the HIV-positive population due to the high prevalence of *S. aureus* infections in general.

PATHOGENESIS/PATHOPHYSIOLOGY

As noted above, the cutaneous blister formation in SSSS is due to a circulating toxin secreted by certain strains of *S. aureus*. Serological types ETA and ETB are the two most associated with blister formation.[17] ETA causes localized bullae in impetigo and ETB is more commonly associated with SSSS. Furthermore, circulating titers of exfoliatoxin are higher in SSSS than in impetigo. Since ETB is plasmid coded whereas ETA is chromosomal, there may be multiple copies of ETB within each bacterium, possibly leading to increased expression; however, this has not been proven *in vivo*.[17]

Recently, the mechanism of action of exfoliatoxins has been elucidated, and all bear structural homology to mammalian serine proteases. It was discovered a number of years ago that proteins readily cleaved by serine proteases were not affected by exfoliatoxins, suggesting that substrate specificity was important in exfoliatoxins' mode of action. The crystallographic structure of exfoliatoxin suggests that the protein is folded in an inactive form and requires the binding of a specific substrate to cause conformational modification to an active, catalytic

form.[18] This substrate was found to be desmoglein-1, a cell surface protein crucial to the adhesion of adjacent keratinocytes in the granular layer.[18,19] The exquisite specificity of this enzyme for desmoglein-1 was found to be in part due to the calcium-dependent binding of exfoliatoxins to desmoglein-1. Binding results in cleavage of desmoglein-1 at one peptide bond between the EC3 and EC4 domains. This cleavage results in inactivation of the desmoglein-1, and subsequently damages epidermal network structure.[18] Interestingly, this pattern is also observed in pemphigus foliaceus, an autoimmune disorder characterized by blister formation that is histologically identical to SSSS. This disorder is caused not by a bacterial-derived toxin, but rather by antibodies directed toward desmoglein-1.[20]

Proteolytic cleavage is the mechanism of epidermal damage in both impetigo and SSSS. In contrast to impetigo, in SSSS, culture of the skin blisters fails to reveal bacteria. This is due to the fact that SSSS is caused by circulating toxin produced by bacteria at a site distant from the skin lesion. The toxin is so specific for epidermal desmoglein that SSSS spares mucosal stratified squamous epithelium, distinguishing SSSS from toxic epidermal necrolysis (TEN).

CLINICAL FEATURES

SSSS most commonly affects children. There have been only about 50 cases reported in adults. Of these, three have been in HIV-positive individuals. Predisposing factors for adult SSSS include renal insufficiency and frank immunocompromise. The increased incidence associated with depressed immunity is thought to be due to increased bacterial proliferation and toxin release as opposed to increased skin sensitivity.[21] Though SSSS has a mortalitity of 4% in pediatric patients, the mortality in adults approaches 50%, necessitating early identification and treatment. Pediatric patients tend to present with a prodrome of sore throat and conjunctivitis, a culture of which frequently reveals *S. aureus*. The patient subsequently develops fever and tender erythematous patches on the face, neck, axilla, and perineum. These lesions progress to flaccid bullae with a positive Nikolsky's sign that is also often present in seemingly unaffected skin. Shearing of the superficial epidermal layer reveals a moist base resembling scalded skin.[22]

In one case report, a 38-year-old HIV-seropositive man presented with fever, hypotension, and a generalized desquamating rash involving the trunk and proximal limbs. He had no prior AIDS-defining illness and his CD4 count was 270×10^6/l. On physical examination, there was a skin eruption with a characteristic scalded appearance, with separation of the superficial epidermal layer. Chest radiography revealed wide areas of consolidation and culture of sputum grew *S. aureus* group II type 3c which released ETB. He had no other coexisting skin infections.[23]

HISTOPATHOLOGY

While there are several diseases causing intraepidermal bullae, such as bullous impetigo and pemphigous foliaceus, SSSS is distinct because of the marked absence of inflammatory cells either in the dermis or in the blister space due to the absence bacteria in the skin. There is acantholysis with a split between the stratum corneum and the granular layer which leads to blister formation. There is no significant epidermal necrosis and the basal cell layer is intact, two features that aid in distinguishing SSSS from TEN. Electron microscopy reveals widening of intracellular spaces and a loss of desmosomes. A split at the same location in the epidermis is also seen in pemphigus foliaceus, an autoimmune bullous disease, although the presence of inflammatory cells as well as positive immunofluorescence studies for deposits of IgG and C3 between keratinocytes distinguishes it from SSSS.[22]

MANAGEMENT

Although childhood mortality of SSSS is low at 4%, in adults, especially in HIV-infected hosts, the mortality can be as high as 50%. Early antibiotic therapy with antistaphylococcal drugs such as flucloxacillin has been found to be effective. While community acquired staphylococcal infections are frequently methicillin resistant, those strains that produce toxin are usually methicillin sensitive.

Close monitoring of these patients is strongly recommended, often in the setting of an intensive care unit. Skin blisters should be left intact and may be covered with petroleum gauze. As with burn patients, special consideration should be given to pain management, temperature regulation, fluid status, and infection precaution. As such, appropriate analgesics should be provided to the patient. In addition, room temperature, as well as the patient's temperature should be appropriately monitored. Increased insensible fluid losses in these patients should be accounted for when providing maintenance fluids. Lastly, with the compromise of the epidermal layer, secondary infections of the skin are a concern and standard precautions should be taken. It should be noted that corticosteroids are associated with worsening of SSSS and should not be administered.[22]

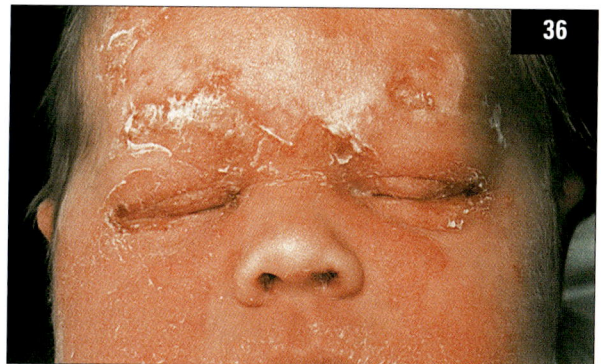

36 Staphyloccal scalded skin syndrome. (Courtesy of St John's Institute of Dermatology (King's College), Guy's Hospital, London.)

BACILLARY ANGIOMATOSIS

DEFINITON/OVERVIEW

First identified in 1983, bacillary angiomatosis (BA) is a vascular infection caused by *Bartonella* species. It is a rare cutaneous disease that presents most commonly in moderately immunocompromised HIV-positive patients, such as those with CD4 cell counts of less than 200×10^6/l. Some studies suggest that the incidence of BA within the HIV-positive population is approximately 0.1%. The etiological agents have been identified as both *Bartonella henselae*, the organism responsible for cat scratch disease, and *Bartonella quintana*, the causative organism of trench fever. The skin as well as many different visceral organs may be involved, but the most common extracutaneous site of involvement is the liver, with peliosis hepatis. Bacteremia and sepsis are also complications.[24]

PATHOGENESIS/PATHOPHYSIOLOGY

Culture studies have revealed that the causative agents favor microaerophilic environments.[25] *B. quintana* is usually transmitted by the human body louse and is common among homeless individuals. *B. henselae* is transmitted by cat fleas and thus is more common in those patients who have contact with cats. It is unclear as to why *B. henselae* causes cat scratch disease in some patients and BA in others. These two *Bartonella* species are equally likely to cause BA; however, there is some difference in visceral involvement depending on the organism. Subcutaneous infection, soft tissue involvement, and lytic bone disease are more closely associated with *B. quintana*, whereas peliosis and lymph node involvement are exclusive to *B. henselae*.[26]

CLINICAL FEATURES

There have been numerous case reports describing BA in the HIV-positive population since its identification in 1983. It is clearly a disease of the immunocompromised, although there have been several reports describing BA in immunocompetent individuals.[27] Most patients with BA have a CD4 count of less than 200×10^6/l. While cutaneous involvement is most common, visceral disease may also occur. The most common extracutaneous manifestation is peliosis hepatis involving the liver, although deep tissue and lytic bone disease may also occur.[26] Patients may complain of fever, chills, nausea, anorexia, and generalized malaise. Lymphadenopathy may also be present. The cutaneous lesions of BA are varied (37–39) and include violaceous papules similar to pyogenic granuloma, nodules similar to Kaposi's sarcoma that may be ulcerated or crusted, subcutaneous nodules, as well as widespread reddish papules. The lesions vary in size from millimeters to centimeters and may be surrounded by an area of scaling. They are occasionally painful and do not have a predilection for any particular body surface.[27] Although the disease was observed with some frequency in the late 1980s and early 1990s, because of the advent of highly active antiretroviral therapy (HAART), it is very rarely encountered today.

HISTOPATHOLOGY

Biopsies from representative lesions reveal a lobular capillary proliferation with cuboidal endothelial cells lining vessels and present in the interstitium (40, 41). An inflammatory infiltrate consisting of lymphocytes, abundant neutrophils, and histiocytes is also present. There is scattered, violaceous, granular debris throughout the interstitium.[25] Warthin–Starry staining of these areas reveals abundant argyrophylic bacteria that are highlighted black (42). Gram stain, acid-fast, and PAS stains fail to highlight the microorganisms. Immunohistochemical staining with antibodies directed against *Bartonella* will demonstrate the deposits of bacteria and may be used to confirm the diagnosis.[25,28]

37 Bacillary angiomatosis. Multiple dome-shaped deeply erythematous and hemorrhagic nodules on the face in an HIV-infected patient.

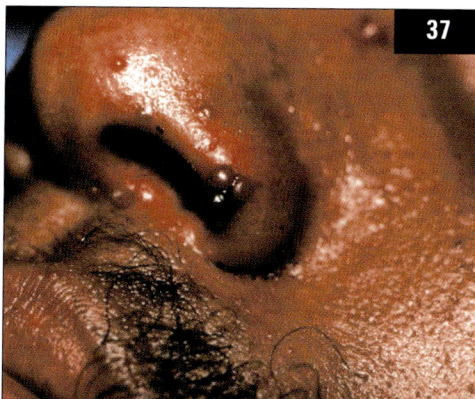

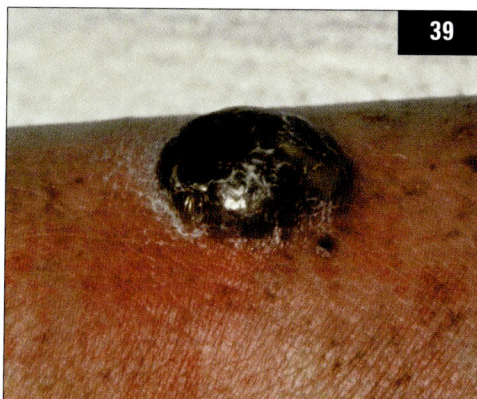

38 Erythematous nodule in the web space in a patient presenting with a single lesion of bacillary angiomatosis.

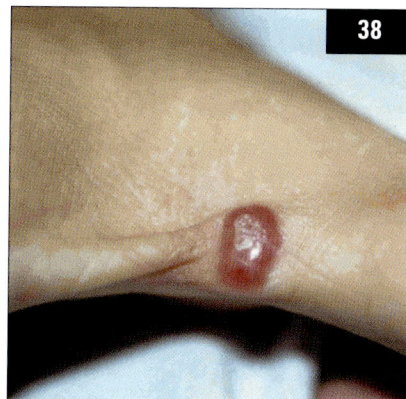

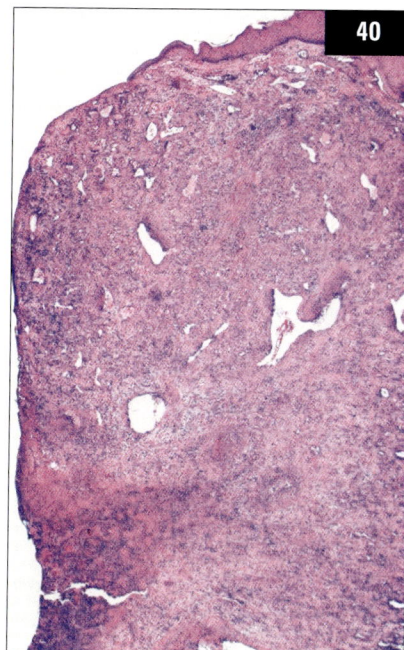

39 Large hemorrhagic nodule with a small satellite lesion on the forearm.

40 Bacillary angiomatosis. Histologic appearance of bacillary angiomatosis showing a diffuse infiltrate of neutrophils surrounding a vascular proliferation.

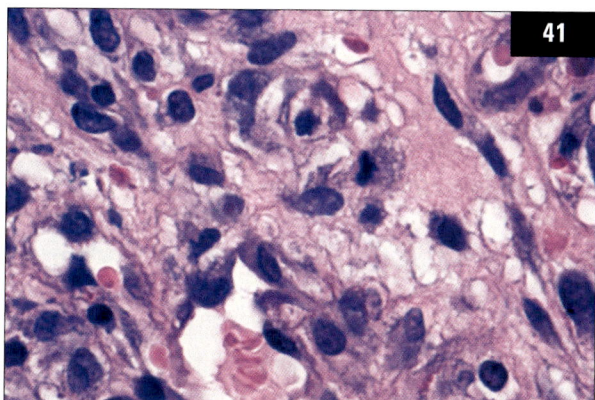

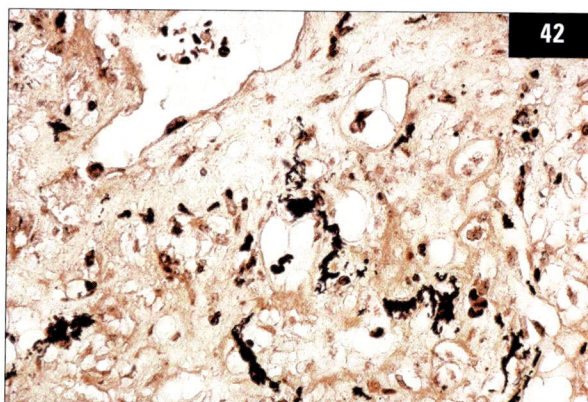

41 Higher power view of the vascular proliferation typical of bacillary angiomatosis, showing pale-staining cells and plump endothelial cells protruding in the lumen of the vascular channel (in the lower part of the photomicrograph).

42 Warthin–Starry stain demonstrating irregular masses of darkly-staining bacteria of the *Bartonella* species.

Culture of the organism reveals that it prefers a microaerophilic environment. In one report, scattered colonies on two slants of *Legionella*-buffered charcoal yeast extract agar were observed to grow after 8–10 days and were able to be propagated in 100% horse serum incubated at 30°C. Gram staining revealed only faintly staining gram-negative organisms, although Warthin–Starry stained smears revealed small ovoid bacilli similar to those identified on hematoxylin and eosin stained biopsy specimens.

MANAGEMENT

As BA is often a systemic illness, it should always be treated systemically despite the fact that some cases have resolved without treatment. BA responds to a number of different antibiotics including erythromycin at doses of 500 mg four times a day for 8–12 weeks. Patients with evidence of systemic disease may require longer courses of treatment. As an alternative, doxycycline 100 mg orally twice daily has also been shown to be efficacious. Patients may experience disseminated inflammatory reactions after administration of antibiotics although these symptoms can be diminished by administration of an anti-inflammatory agent.[29]

MYCOBACTERIAL INFECTIONS

DEFINITION/OVERVIEW

Cutaneous mycobacterial disease often represents a manifestation of systemic illness. Although it is relatively rare in developed countries, it is increased in incidence among immunocompromised patients, especially HIV-infected patients. The most common mycobacterial species to cause cutaneous infection include *Mycobacterium tuberculosis*, *M. bovis*, and bacillus Calmette–Guérin (BCG), an attenuated form of *M. bovis*. Other organisms such as *M. szulgai*, *M. marinum*, and *M. avium* complex may also present as cutaneous disease, more commonly in HIV-seropositive individuals.

Cutaneous mycobacterial infection is most commonly caused by *M. tuberculosis*. While the incidence of cutaneous infections has declined, much like that of pulmonary tuberculosis, disseminated infection remains a concern in the immunocompromised population. The morphologic appearance of cutaneous lesions caused by tuberculosis are protean and they may result from direct inoculation of the skin, cutaneous spread from an endogenous source, or an inflammatory response to mycobacteria. The manifestations may also differ depending on whether the host is naïve or sensitized towards tuberculosis. Although in the US there is a general decline in the prevalence of tuberculosis, it remains a serious problem for immunocompromised individuals including those who are infected with HIV.

CLINICAL FEATURES

The cutaneous manifestations of tuberculosis can be divided into three major categories: exogenous infection, endogenous infection, and tuberculid lesions. Exogenous infections occur when the organisms come in contact with broken skin and begin colonization. In a naïve host, *M. tuberculosis* infection presents as a tuberculous chancre which is a localized ulcerated papule or nodule. Common ports of entry include minor abrasions on the face and limbs as well as skin injuries due to tattoos, circumcision, and piercing. There has been one case report of a tuberculous chancre that developed in a patient with malignant melanoma treated with BCG vaccine.[30] Approximately 4 weeks after inoculation, a rust-colored papulonodular lesion developed. The lesion enlarged then ulcerated resulting in a painless ulcer with a well demarcated border. This appearance is similar to that of primary inoculation tuberculous chancres.[31,32] Regional lymphadenopathy is often present when the skin lesion develops and is generally considered to be the cutaneous counterpart to the ghon complex.

Exogenously derived mycobacterial infection

Cutaneous infection with M. tuberculosis in a previously sensitized individual results in a skin condition known as tuberculosis verrucosa cutis. This is more common among healthcare workers who come in contact with infected patients, especially when they are exposed to secretions or body fluids. It is also known as pathologist's warts or prosector's warts as it is often caused by autoinoculation.[33,34] It begins as one or more asymptomatic reddish-brown papules that develop a markedly verrucous surface with abundant crust. When diascopy is performed by pressing a glass slide on the lesion, there is a translucent 'apple jelly' appearance. Lesions may undergo necrosis and ulcerate although significant scarring is rare. Occasionally, pus may be expressed; however, in contrast to tuberculous chancre, lymphadenopathy is rare.[34] The diagnosis is made by finding acid-fast bacilli in smears or in biopsy specimens and confirmed by cultures.

Although lupus vulgaris is most commonly the result of endogenous infection, there have been reports of exogenously derived lupus vulgaris secondary to the administration of BCG vaccine. This is particularly significant in the immunocompromised population. One report described a patient with lupus vulgaris secondary to BCG vaccination and no other signs of endogenous mycobacterial infection elsewhere. This patient was a healthy 12-year-old Polish girl who was vaccinated with BCG vaccine at 3 days of life. Twelve years later she underwent a purified protein derivative (PPD) intradermal skin test and the next day, an erythematous eruption developed at the injection site. This was followed by the development of an enlarging, brown, nodular lesion that grew to 4 × 5 cm which underwent a central ulceration. There was neither lymphadenopathy nor other pulmonary findings on either physical examination or via chest radiography. Polymerase chain reaction (PCR) studies performed on the lesion identified Mycobacterium tuberculosis. On further workup, the patient was found to have a congenital defect in lymphocytic transformation.

Other mycobacteria have also been reported to cause primary cutaneous lesions (43–45).

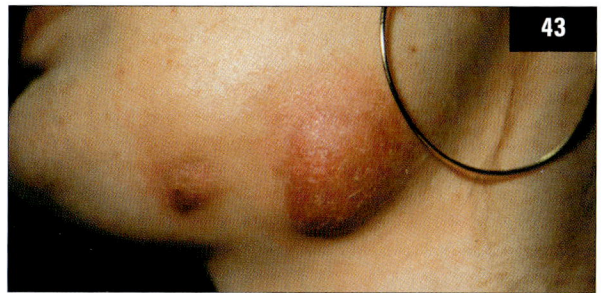

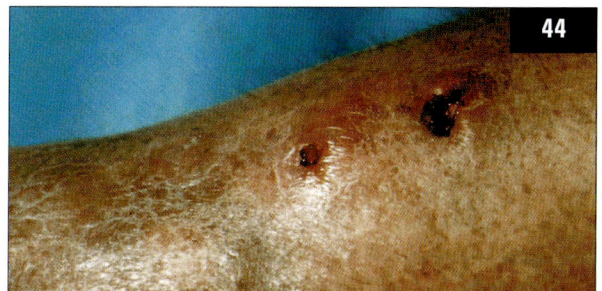

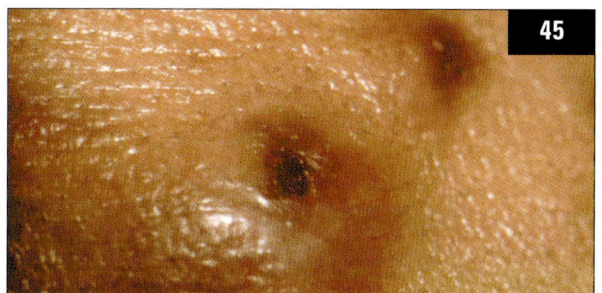

43 Mycobacterial infection. Large abscesses caused by acid-fast mycobacteria on the face of a young woman.

44 Ulcerated lesions on the forearm of an HIV-infected patient.

45 Close up of large, crusted nodules of cutaneous mycobacterial infection.

M. kansasii and *M. marinum* are among the more commonly seen atypical mycobacterial infections, although others have also been reported. A 56-year-old AIDS patient with a CD4 count of $4 \times 10^2/l$ developed an asymptomatic 1 cm ulcerative lesion of the right inguinal fold without inguinal lymphadenopathy. Histology of the lesion revealed numerous acid-fast bacilli and culture was positive for *M. kansasii*. The patient had no evidence of pulmonary or otherwise systemic infection. Clinical manifestations of *M. kansasii* are protean and include verrucous papules, ulcers, cellulitis-like plaques, and indurated 'granulomatous' plaques. *M. kansasii* is sensitive to typical antimycobacterial drug regimens.[35]

Endogenously derived mycobacterial infections

Lupus vulgaris may also present secondary to endogenous infection, either from hematogenous, lymphatic or direct extension. It is the most common form of cutaneous tuberculosis in Europe and Hong Kong. Lesions typically present in the head and neck region, although the distribution tends to involve the lower extremity in patients from east Asia. The clinical features are identical to those caused by BCG vaccination; however, patients will also have symptoms originating from the primary infection and are often pulmonary symptoms.[32]

Severe tuberculosis infections in HIV patients may lead to dissemination and subsequent miliary tuberculosis. Although at one point this infection was exceedingly rare, it has seen a reemergence with the increasing prevalence of AIDS. Much like other endogenously acquired mycobacterial infections, cutaneous spread occurs via a hematogenous route from an active primary pulmonary lesion. Miliary TB is characterized by the presence of small purpuric papulovesicular lesions. The lesions ultimately rupture leaving a crusting lesion with central umbilication. The lesions then heal over the next several weeks leaving a scar with a white colored halo.

Recent miliary tuberculosis has been described in two HIV-seropositive males. The first patient was a 39-year-old HIV-positive male who presented in respiratory distress with pneumonitis. In addition, the patient had approximately 20 punctate, erythematous, papulovesicular lesions located on the trunk and extremities. Many of the lesions had undergone a central area of necrosis. Skin and sputum cultures grew *M. tuberculosis*. The second patient was an 18-year-old woman who presented with productive cough, fever, weight loss, and pruritic skin lesions that were described as numerous 3–5 mm erythematous papules distributed over her face, neck, trunk, and arms. On close examination, the lesions were noted to be pustular, with central umbilication. At first, this patient was thought to have a zoster infection and varicella pneumonia; however, Tzank smears of the lesions failed to reveal multinucleated giant cells. Biopsy and sputum culture provided the diagnosis of miliary tuberculosis.[36]

While these organisms represent the most common primary cutaneous mycobacterial lesions among the HIV population, other rare mycobacterial species have been reported. One case of *M. szulgai* has been reported in an AIDS patient. This organism is found in water reservoirs such as fish tanks and swimming pools. Pulmonary infection is the most common presentation in immunocompromised hosts, especially those with underlying pulmonary disease. In this case report, the patient suffered comorbid hepatitis B, C, and D, and developed *M. szulgai* osteomyelitis and cutaneous mycobacterial infection of the chest and forearm. There were two ulcerating lesions, one of the distal forearm and the other on the lateral chest wall. There was no evidence of a primary pulmonary lesion, however.[37] Chest radiography revealed no abnormalities and sputum smears and bronchoalveolar lavage were negative for acid-fast organisms.

Mycobacterium avium-intracellulare (MAI) has also been shown to cause cutaneous lesions in HIV-positive patients. Typically, this is an infection of the severely immunocompromised and is essentially nonexistent in healthy, immunocompetent patients. In this case report, the patient was a 46-year-old male with numerous AIDS-defining illnesses, a CD4 count of $8 \times 10^6/l$, and a viral load of 56000. The patient presented with a 1.5 cm violaceous nodule on the right forearm. The cutaneous manifestations of MAI are variable and include papules, pustules, ulcers, nodules, verrucous lesions, and draining sinuses.[38] Cutaneous infection with MAI rarely occurs without disseminated primary infection and bacteremia. Diagnosis is usually made through histology and cultures.

PATHOGENESIS/PATHOPHYSIOLOGY/HISTOLOGY

Exogenously derived mycobacterial infection

None of the clinical lesions described above are diagnostic of mycobacterial infection. As such, the diagnosis is usually made based on the histologic presence of granulomatous inflammation, identification of acid-fast bacilli, and culture of the organism. In tuberculous chancre, histology reveals a diffuse infiltrate of neutrophils and histiocytes with extensive degeneration of collagen. There are numerous acid-fast bacilli visible with acid-fast stains. Several weeks after the intial lesion, there is a more granulomatous appearance with epithelioid histiocytes and giant cells with few demonstrable acid-fast bacilli.

Tuberculosis verrucosa cutis shows marked hyperkeratosis and papillomatosis of the epidermis with a diffuse infiltrate of histiocytes and neutrophils in the papillary and reticular dermis. There is also degeneration of collagen. More chronic lesions reveal fibrosis and scarring. Cutaneous infection caused by *M. kansasii* histology has been reported rarely and revealed an acute inflammatory reaction with neutrophils and minimal granulomatous inflammation. Numerous acid-fast bacilli were seen on Ziehl–Neelsen stain confirming the diagnosis of a mycobacterial infection.[35]

The histopathologic findings of lupus vulgaris reveal a diffuse granulomatous reaction with epithelioid giant cells mainly in the lower dermis. There may be caseation, especially of the upper dermis. Acid-fast bacilli may or may not be identified due to the scarcity of the organisms within the lesion.

Endogenously derived mycobacterial infections

Miliary tuberculosis, much like most cutaneous mycobacterial infections, requires biopsy and histologic characterization for the diagnosis. Histology typically reveals numerous acid-fast bacilli

as well as marked acute inflammatory cells and microabscesses. Of note, in HIV-infected patients, there may be minimal granulomatous inflammation secondary to the patient's immune suppression. There is also often degeneration of collagen in the dermis.[32,36] Fite stain usually reveals numerous acid-fast bacilli and cultures and/or PCR studies can definitively identify the organism.

Cutaneous MAI infection typically demonstrates a diffuse infiltrate of histiocytes with numerous organisms. There is usually diffuse involvement of the dermis and/or the subcutaneous fat. In one case report, 'pseudo-gaucher' cells were found on biopsy. There is also an inflammatory infiltrate of lymphocytes, neutrophils, and plasma cells. Classic granulomatous changes may or may not be seen although there may be vasculitis. One report has described an HIV-infected patient with cutaneous MAI that histologically resembled histoid leprosy with abundant spindle cells with foamy histiocytes that revealed abundant acid-fast bacilli with Fite staining.[38]

While infections in immunocompetent patients and immunocompromised patients usually have similar histology, the necessity of an intact immune system to produce granulomatous inflammation produces some variation on histology, specifically with regard to mycobacterial infections. In general, immunosuppressed patients have more diffuse infections that involve the subcutaneous tissue and fascia. There are also more prominent epidermal changes in immunocompetent patients such as acanthosis and pseudoepitheliomatous hyperplasia. This is especially true for those infected with *M. marinum* (fish tank granuloma).[39] Granulomatous inflammation was only observed in 60% of samples from immunocompromised patients, likely due to the impaired CD4 function and subsequent lack of cytokine production necessary for the formulation of granulomas. The granulomatous pattern was usually suppurative. In contrast, 83% of immunocompetent patients had evidence of granulomatous inflammation and many demonstrate a sarcoidal pattern although there may be tuberculoid, palisading, and suppurative granulomatous patterns as well.[39] Interestingly, only 11% of biopsy specimens from immunocompetent hosts were positive for acid-fast bacilli, whereas 90% of immunocompromised patients have identifiable acid-fast bacilli[39] (46, 47).

DIAGNOSIS

Diagnosis of cutaneous mycobacterial infection involves a careful history with attention to risk factors for contracting tuberculosis such as prolonged stays in close quarters, extended prison time, and homelessness. Since most lesions are the result of dissemination from a primary pulmonary source, evaluation for pulmonary involvement should be undertaken. Conversion of PPD skin testing to positive may or may not be helpful in making the diagnosis especially in the HIV/AIDS population as there may be anergy towards the tuberculin antigen. Biopsy provides important information although there are pitfalls in diagnosis due to the relative absence of granulomatous inflammation. Staining for acid-fast bacilli usually reveals a large number of organisms. Culture remains the most definitive measure for the diagnosis of these infections although it may prove to be difficult due to the relative paucity of viable mycobacterium. Using PCR is even more sensitive and may be especially useful when there is a limited number of viable organisms.

MANAGEMENT

The principles of treatment of cutaneous tuberculosis are the same as the treatment for pulmonary tuberculosis and involve a multidrug regimen for a duration that is long enough to eradicate the organism, to prevent recurrence, and to prevent the selection of resistant strains. The Centers for Disease Control (CDC) currently recommends a two phase approach in the treatment of tuberculosis. Initial treatment includes isoniazid, rifampin, pyrazinamide, and ethambutol (or streptomycin) for 8 weeks. Ethambutol may be discontinued once susceptibilities return and the organism is found to be susceptible to isoniazid and rifampin. The next phase of treatment consists of treatment with isoniazid and rifampin either daily or three times weekly for a duration of 16 weeks. Surgery or cryotherapy may be needed as an adjunct to antimicrobials for complete resolution of cutaneous lesions.[32]

The treatment of many of the nontuberculous mycobacteriae generally follows the same principle as that for *M. tuberculosis*, namely multidrug treatment for an extended period of time with a combination of rifampin, isoniazid, pyrazinamide, ethambutol, and streptomycin. Ciprofloxacin has been found to be efficacious in some studies. Treatment, of course, should be guided by culture and susceptibilities. Some organisms such as *M. marinum* may be treated more conservatively but in HIV infection, more aggressive therapy is often required.

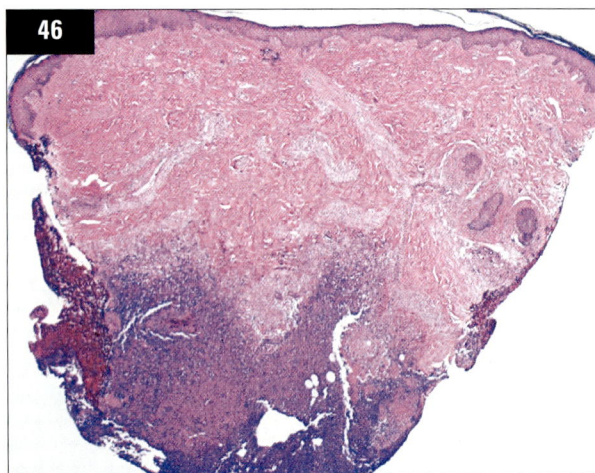

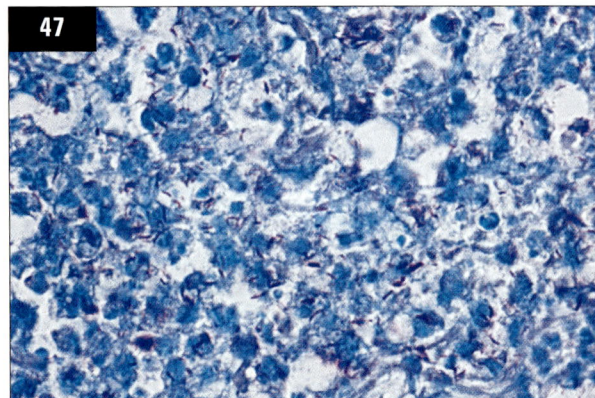

46, 47 Histology of cutaneous mycobacterial infection showing a dense, deep suppurative granulomatous infiltrate (**46**) with multiple acid-fast bacilli (**47**).

CHAPTER 4

CUTANEOUS MANIFESTATIONS OF DEEP FUNGAL INFECTIONS IN HIV DISEASE

Julia Kamalpour, Antoanella Calame, and Clay J. Cockerell

While the advent of highly active antiretroviral therapy (HAART) has led to a fall in the incidence of deep fungal infection in HIV patients in the US and Europe, no such decline has been witnessed in countries with limited funds and access to such therapy. In the HIV-infected population, the occurrence of fungal infections is largely dependent upon the degree of CD4+ T-lymphocyte depletion as well as exposure to endemic dimorphic fungi.[1] This chapter reviews the most frequently seen deep fungal infections in the HIV-infected population, and highlights their significance in light of their accompanying high mortality rates in the immunocompromised population.

CRYPTOCOCCOSIS

DEFINITION/OVERVIEW

Cryptococcus neoformans, an encapsulated yeast-like fungus, is the second most common opportunistic fungal infection in HIV-positive patients with *Candida albicans* being the most common. In 1987, Lynch and Naftolin were the first to report a case of cryptococcal infection in a patient with advanced acquired immunodeficiency syndrome (AIDS).[2] *C. neoformans* causes symptomatic cryptococcosis in 5–10% of HIV-infected individuals[3] and most often affects individuals with AIDS with CD4 lymphocyte cell counts below 100×10^6/l.[4]

Cryptococcus neoformans was first isolated from a fruit extract in San Felice in 1894.[5] The organism is approximately 5 μm in diameter, although the encapsulated form can be up to 30 μm in diameter.[6] The *Cryptococcus neoformans* species complex is

comprised of basidiomycetous yeasts that cause systemic infections in both immunocompetent and immunocompromised populations. There are two varieties of *C. neoformans* which encompass the five known serotypes. Serotype differences are based upon cell wall antigenic variability and mating conditions.

C. neoformans var. *neoformans* includes serotypes A and D and generally causes disease in immunocompromised patients. Found worldwide, the environmental source for *C. neoformans* var. *neoformans* is soil contaminated with excreta from certain birds including pigeons, canaries, and cockatoos.[5] *C. neoformans* var. *gattii* includes serotypes B and C and is a frequent cause of infection in HIV-negative hosts.[7] *C. neoformans* var. *gattii* is found predominantly in tropical and subtropical areas and has been associated with several species of eucalyptus trees. When compared with cases of cryptococcosis due to serotypes A and D, those resulting from serotypes B and C exhibit greater neurologic morbidity, an increased number of pulmonary and cerebral nodules, and slower response to antifungal therapy.[8]

Cryptococcal infection is an AIDS-defining illness in 3% of HIV-infected patients and has been identified as the cause of death in 5% of HIV-infected patients in a recent study.[9] Disseminated cryptococcosis is by far the most common life-threatening fungal infection in HIV-infected patients.[10]

Although there has been a decline in the incidence and severity of patients presenting with HIV-associated cryptococcal infection in the US, Australia, and western Europe, the disease remains a leading cause of meningitis in many African nations.[11] The decrease in incidence within the US has been attributed to the advent of HAART after 1996.[12] The use of HAART therapy reduces viremia and increases CD4 cell counts, resulting in an enhanced immunologic state that is associated with significantly decreased risk of cryptococcal infection.[12] Prior to HAART therapy, 2.9–23.3% of HIV-infected patients had a concomitant cryptococcal infection. With the introduction of HAART, the incidence has decreased to 1.7% and 6.6% in San Francisco and Atlanta, respectively.[13] Unfortunately, the high cost of HAART and complicated logistical infrastructure necessary for its administration have limited its use in less-developed countries of Africa and Asia where the prevalence of HIV infection and AIDS has increased dramatically along with that of cryptococcosis.[3]

PATHOGENESIS/PATHOPHYSIOLOGY

Infection with C. neoformans occurs via inhalation of small diameter organisms which go on to enter the respiratory passages.[14] Although the primary site of infection is generally the respiratory tract or the central nervous system (CNS), other primary sites of C. neoformans infection can include the skin, eyes, or genitourinary tract.[14]

Inside an immunocompetent host, C. neoformans is generally eliminated or controlled via an intact cell-mediated immune response. The macrophage is considered to be the central effector cell active against C. neoformans, and alveolar macrophages are likely to be the first immune effector cell encountered by inhaled cryptococcal cells.[15,16] The macrophage ingests and kills yeast cells and produces inflammatory cytokines. Chemokines, including MCP-2 and MIP-1α, are important in the recruitment of inflammatory cells to the site of cryptococcal infection. The role of T cells in host defense involves cytokine production that activates macrophage fungicidal activity, such as interferon-γ, and the promotion of alveolar macrophage transformation into giant cells capable of ingesting large encapsulated yeast cells.[17]

The cryptococcal cell wall evades destruction by these immune processes by making an antiphagocytic

virulence factor that enables the organism to survive within macrophages.[18] C. neoformans has a unique strategy of intracellular replication in macrophages, whereby capsular polysaccharide is secreted into vesicles. The consequent disruption of the macrophage vesicular network results in cytotoxicity.[18] The organism then prompts a continuous production of intracellular polysaccharide which eventually causes the macrophages to burst.[18] Should the organism survive the immune system, a granulomatous wall is formed that prevents its systemic spread. A lack of granulomatous reaction may be seen in HIV-positive and other immunocompromised hosts, resulting in localized symptomatic disease or disseminated infection. [18]

CLINICAL FEATURES

Clinical manifestations of infection can vary from asymptomatic colonization of the respiratory tract to widespread dissemination depending on the host immune response. Significant risk factors for the development of disseminated cryptococcosis include advanced HIV infection, systemic steroid therapy, lymphoproliferative disorders, and organ transplantation.[19] In HIV-infected patients, the incidence of cryptococcosis is inversely proportional to the CD4 lymphocyte count, and rises dramatically once the CD4 lymphocyte count drops below $100 \times 10^6/l$.[20]

The most common clinical presentation of cryptococcosis in HIV-positive patients is subacute meningitis or meningoencephalitis with brain and meningeal involvement occurring in 40–85% of patients.[21] Most patients present with fever, headache, and malaise and are symptomatic for 2–4 weeks prior to presentation.[22] Cryptococcal infection of the lungs is also common, with symptoms of pulmonary cryptococcosis including fever, cough, dyspnea, and hypoxemia. Unlike in the HIV-negative population, most patients with AIDS and pulmonary cryptococcosis have disseminated disease. Manifestations of extrapulmonary disseminated disease comprise hepatosplenomegaly, bone marrow suppression, or lesions in other tissues.[22]

Disseminated cryptococcosis demonstrates cutaneous involvement in 10–20% of cases.

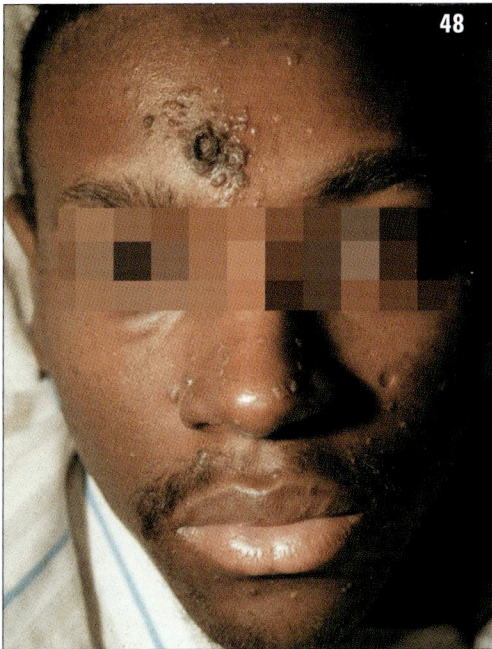

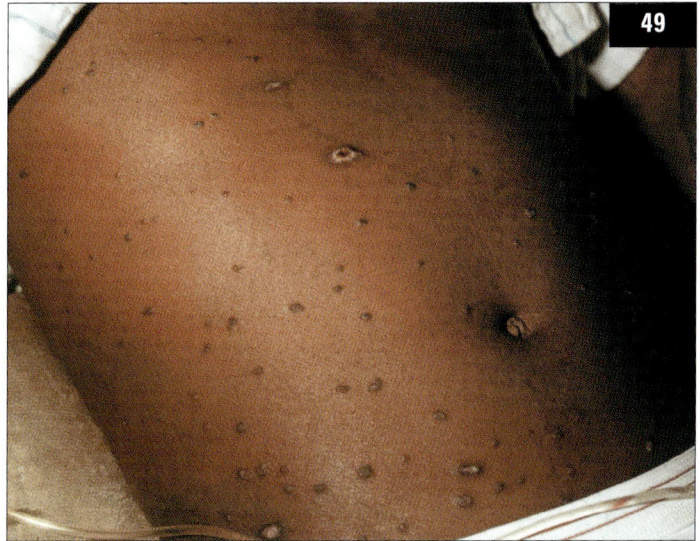

48, **49** Disseminated cryptococcosis with multiple verrucous lesions on the face and trunk in a patient with advanced HIV infection.

Cutaneous manifestations may present 2–6 weeks prior to the onset of signs of systemic disease.[10] As cutaneous signs may be the first manifestation of this potentially fatal disease, clinicians should have a high index of suspicion for cryptococcosis when a new rash develops in patients with a CD4 count below $10 \times 10^7/l$.[23]

The most common presentation of cutaneous cryptococcosis is umbilicated flesh-colored papules or nodules that are similar in appearance to lesions of molluscum contagiosum (MC).[5] Other possible morphologies include pustules, ulcers, subcutaneous abscesses, cellulitis, panniculitis, palpable purpura, and plaques[23] (48–50). Lesions frequently occur on the face, but can be widespread.[10] Oral nodules or ulcers may be seen along with the cutaneous lesions or as the sole presentation of disease.[10] When crusting or ulceration occurs, lesions resemble those of herpes simplex virus infection.[10] Cryptococcal cellulitis presents as red, warm, tender plaques and is seen most often in immunodeficient hosts. Of note, cutaneous cryptococcosis may occur in the absence of demonstrable fungal infection in the lung or meninges.[10]

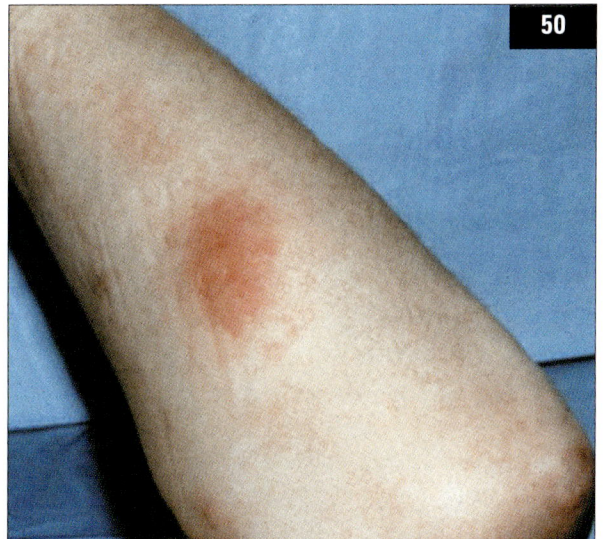

50 Cryptococcal abscess. Fluctuant nodule on the forearm.

DIAGNOSIS/HISTOPATHOLOGY

C. neoformans infection is diagnosed by culturing the organism from clinical specimens or by organism visualization on histopathologic exam. Diagnosis can be established by demonstrating cryptococcal yeast forms with hemotoxylin and eosin (H&E), periodic acid-Schiff (PAS), or methenamine silver stain of clinical biopsy specimens or of a touch preparation.[10] Tzanck smears which are performed by scraping the surface of a lesion, placing the material on a glass slide, fixing with methyl alcohol, and staining with rapid Giemsa technique, reveal multiple encapsulated and budding yeast forms. Alternatively, India ink preparation of skin scrapings can be used to show encapsulated and budding yeast forms.[10] For cultures, the organism should be grown on Sabouraud's agar or other selective fungal media, with plates incubated for up to 14 days.[24] Positive cultures of *C. neoformans* should be considered significant and are an indication for further evaluation and initiation of treatment.[24]

In immunocompetent hosts, histopathologic examination of tissue from infection sites shows typical granulomas with aggregates of histiocytes with epithelioid features and multinucleated giant cells of both foreign body and Langhans type, containing intracytoplasmic yeasts.[25] In patients with AIDS, histopathologic examination reveals loosely aggregated histiocytes and multinucleated giant cells of the foreign body type; Langhans giant cells are not typically seen.[25] In addition, cryptococci are seen as extra- and intracellular yeast forms with budding[25] (51–53).

Diagnosis of cryptococcosis can also be established via serum, cerebrospinal fluid (CSF), or urine antigen with latex agglutination which is highly sensitive, being positive in over 95% of cases.[26] Most AIDS patients (75%) have a large burden of organisms, evidenced by a heavily positive CSF India ink preparation and high titers of cryptococcal antigen in blood and CSF.[27]

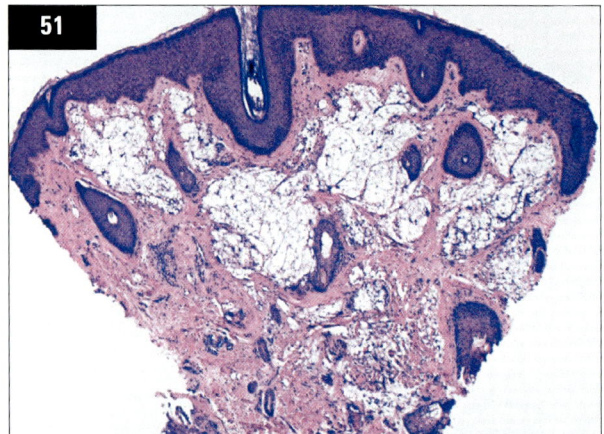

51 Histopathology of cutaneous cryptococcosis. Low power view of a skin biopsy reveals areas of clear-staining cells throughout the dermis.

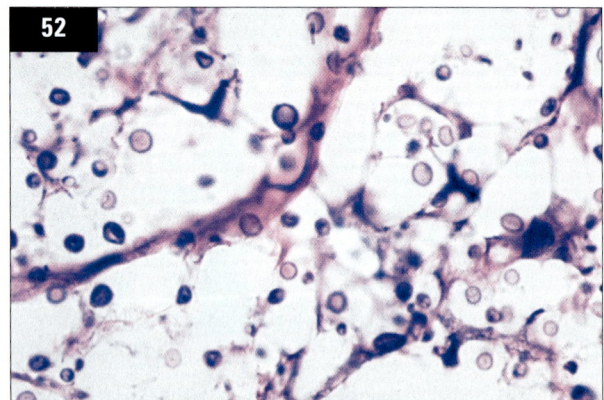

52 Higher magnification shows multiple organisms of *Cryptococcus neoformans* throughout the clear-staining areas.

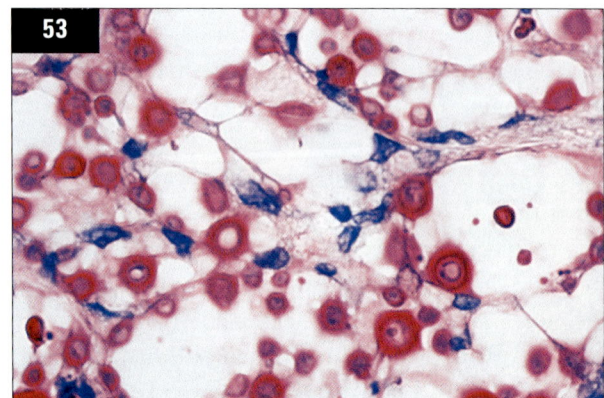

53 Mucicarmine stain highlights the mucinous capsule of *Cryptococcus* organisms.

MANAGEMENT

Clinical management of cryptococcosis is dependent upon the extent of disease and the underlying status of host immunity.[28] Cryptococcal disease that occurs in HIV-infected patients always requires therapy. For nonmeningeal cryptococcosis, an induction phase of amphotericin B (0.7–1 mg/kg/day for 2 weeks) followed by fluconazole (400 mg/day) for a minimum of 10 weeks is recommended.[28] The addition of 5-flucytosine during the induction phase reduces the risk of relapse.[29]

Untreated cryptococcal meningitis is uniformly fatal. The recommended initial treatment for acute cryptococcal meningitis is amphotericin B deoxycholate 0.7 mg/kg body weight/day IV with or without flucytosine 25 mg/kg PO QID for 2 weeks.[30] Aggressive treatment for elevated intracranial pressure via daily repeated lumbar punctures or CSF shunt placement in patients with meningoencephalitis may improve outcome.[31]

Chronic suppressive therapy has now become the standard of care in patients with HIV-associated cryptococcosis, with oral fluconazole (200 mg/day) being the most widely used drug. Alternatives include the use of either intravenous amphotericin B (50 mg weekly or biweekly) or itraconazole (400 mg/day).[29] While relapse rates of only 2–3% are seen with the use of fluconazole, rates of 18–25% are seen when weekly amphotericin B or itraconazole is used. Several studies have shown that it is acceptable to discontinue cryptococcal suppressive therapy after 6–12 months in patients who have a sustained immunologic response to HAART (with CD4 counts >150 × 10^6/l) if they have had adequate initial antifungal treatment.[32,33] Maintenance therapy should be resumed if the CD4 counts decrease to <100 × 10^6/l.[22]

The dramatic reduction in incidence of cryptococcal infections since the advent of potent antiretroviral therapy suggests that the best prophylaxis for cryptococcosis is effective treatment of HIV disease.[34] Using HAART, a rise in the CD4 lymphocyte count is seen along with an improvement in CD4 cell function, allowing the safe withdrawal of maintenance antifungal therapy once cryptococcosis has been successfully treated.

Institution of HAART in patients with AIDS-associated cryptococcosis may be complicated by immune reconstitution inflammatory syndrome (IRIS), a potentially fatal outcome.[35] IRIS is a result of an exuberant inflammatory response towards incubating opportunistic pathogens. Risk factors for cryptococcosis-associated IRIS include previously undiagnosed HIV infection, disseminated cryptococcosis, fungemia, lack of CSF sterilization after 2 weeks of antifungal treatment, and the introduction of HAART within 2 months after the diagnosis of cryptococcosis.[35] Patients with identified risk factors for IRIS should be watched carefully during the months following the introduction of HAART. The most frequent signs of cryptococcosis-associated IRIS are enlarged necrotic lymph nodes and acute CNS-related symptoms.[35] Treatment for IRIS includes continuation of the primary therapy against the fungal pathogen as well as continuation of effective HAART and other supportive measures.[1]

PROPHYLAXIS

Epidemiologic studies have shown exposure to cryptococcosis to be unavoidable. Prevention is thus dependent upon immunization or chemotherapy. Fluconazole is effective in the prevention of cryptococcal meningitis in patients with AIDS.[13] A randomized trial comparing fluconazole 200 mg daily with clotrimazole in the prevention of fungal infections in AIDS patients showed a 2 year rate of invasive fungal infection of 2.8% in the fluconazole group compared to 9.1% in the clotrimazole group, with a seven-fold reduction in the risk of cryptococcosis.[36]

HISTOPLASMOSIS

DEFINITION/OVERVIEW

Disseminated histoplasmosis is a progressive granulomatous disease caused by the intracellular dimorphic fungus, *Histoplasma capsulatum*. Samuel Darling, a pathologist, first identified *H. capsulatum* in the visceral tissues and bone marrow of an adult male presumed to have died of miliary tuberculosis in Panama (1905).[37] It was designated *H. capsulatum* based on its appearance in histiocytes, an archaic term for macrophages ('histo'), its resemblance to protozoan parasites ('plasma'), and the apparent presence of a surrounding capsule ('capsulatum').[38] Progressive disseminated histoplasmosis has been included among the AIDS-defining illnesses since 1987.

H. capsulatum causes a progressive disseminated disease in 2–5% HIV-positive individuals who have inhabited or traveled to endemic regions, including the river valleys of central and eastern US, South America, and the Caribbean.[39] Conditions favoring the growth of *H. capsulatum* in soil include a mean temperature between 22°C and 29°C, an annual precipitation of 35–50 inches (890–1270 mm), as well as a relative humidity of 67–87%.[40]

The two identified human pathogenic variants are *Histoplasma capsulatum* and *duboisii*. *H. capsulatum* is endemic to areas of North America (including the Mississippi and Ohio valleys), latin America, sub-Saharan Africa, and east Asia; *H. duboisii* is restricted to central Africa, from Senegal to Uganda.[40,41] Histoplasmosis occurs in 2–5% of AIDS patients from endemic areas, and usually occurs in patients with CD4 counts <150 × 10^6/l.[22]

PATHOGENESIS/PATHOPHYSIOLOGY

The environmental source for *H. capsulatum* is surface soil, especially in areas which abound with decaying guano (soil within the vicinity of chicken coops, roosting places of birds, and bat caves). Bird and bat excrement enhance the organism's growth in soil by accelerating sporulation. At soil temperatures, *H. capsulatum* exists in the mycelial form, harboring macroconidia and microconidia. Microconidia probably represent the major infection propagules due to their ready aerosolization and small size of

25 µm in diameter. Upon inhalation by a host, the organism converts from the mycelial phase into its parasitic morphotype, a budding yeast which survives and replicates rapidly within macrophages and monocytes.[39]

Fungal antigens are processed and presented to T cells during the development of cell-mediated immunity. Infected macrophages induce cytokine release in order to recruit additional macrophages and monocytes to help destroy the organism. The recruited immune cells coalesce to form granulomas. The activation of the T cell-mediated immune response is generally complete within a period of 2–3 weeks. Failure of the immune response allows the organism to disseminate.[38]

CLINICAL FEATURES

Histoplasmosis has a broad spectrum of clinical presentations, including asymptomatic infection, acute or chronic pulmonary infection, mediastinal fibrosis, granulomas, and disseminated histoplasmosis. The clinical presentation of histoplasmosis is determined by the magnitude of exposure and the host's immune status.[42] Low level exposure frequently results in asymptomatic infection. In endemic regions, over half of the population has been infected with *H. capsulatum* and yet most remain asymptomatic. Occasionally, low level exposure results in symptomatic pulmonary histoplasmosis manifest as a subacute flu-like illness with fever, dry cough, and fatigue. In such instances, ensuing antigen-specific T-lymphocyte-mediated immunity and fungistatic macrophage activation lead to containment of the infection and resolution of symptoms within a 1–2 week period.[39]

While self-limiting upper respiratory illness occurs with *H. capsulatum* exposure in normal hosts, symptomatic disseminated histoplasmosis may occur in immunodeficient patients and those at the extremes of age.[43] Patients with HIV-1 infection and histoplasmosis have reduced CD4 counts that correlate with depressed cellular immune responses to *H. capsulatum* antigens. Severity of histoplasmosis correlates with the degree of immunodeficiency. Such patients may present as a result of an exogenously acquired infection in endemic regions or due to

54 *Histoplasma capsulatum* infection. Multiple nodules with peripheral hyperpigmentation.

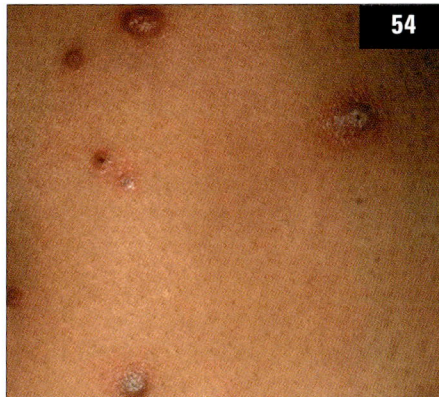

55 Close-up view of one the larger nodules.

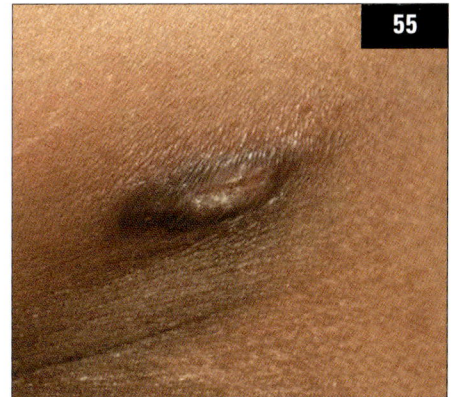

56 Numerous psoriasiform papules and plaques on the back in a patient with disseminated histoplasmosis.

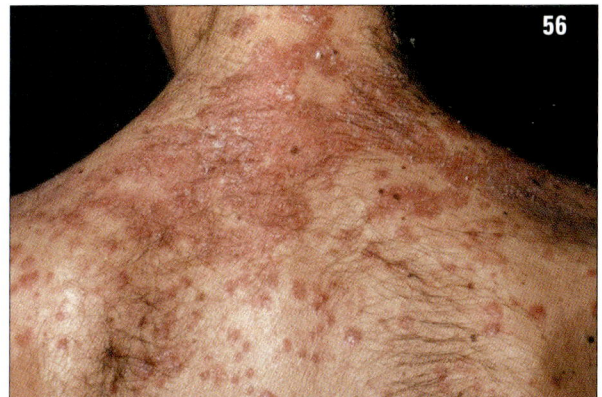

57 Confluent psoriasiform plaques on the buttocks.

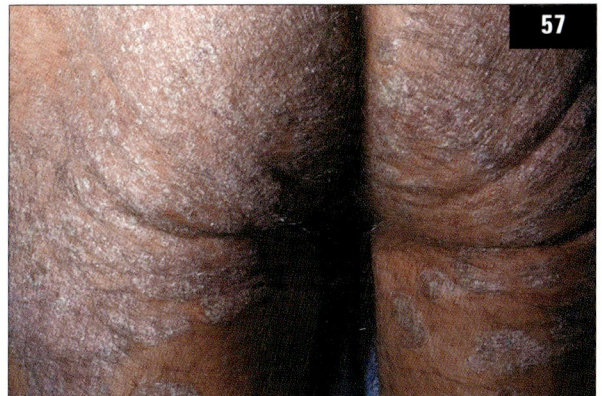

58 The plaques extend down on the lower extremities, where several violaceous nodules are also present.

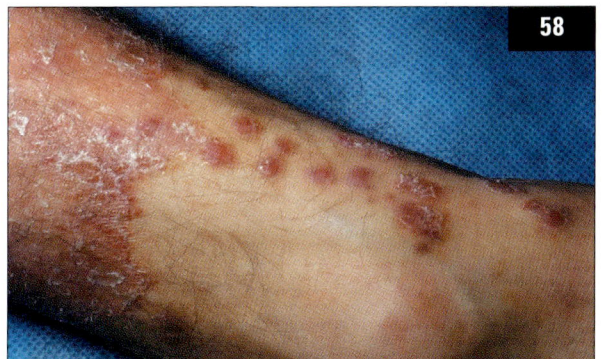

reactivation of latent fungal infection from calcified persisting granulomas in nonendemic regions.[44] In patients with AIDS, histoplasmosis presents as disseminated infection in 95% of cases. Those with severe disease may undergo an acute, rapidly fatal course with diffuse reticuloendothelial involvement. Such patients may present with fever, weight loss, pulmonary infiltrates, pancytopenia, hypergamma-globulinemia, respiratory distress, rhabdomyolysis, shock, hepatic and renal failure, obtundation, or coagulopathy.[45] Less than 10% of patients with disseminated disease present with a 'septic shock' syndrome.[46] Gastrointestinal, CNS, and cutaneous manifestations each occur in less than 10% of cases.[45]

A variety of skin lesions may be seen in histoplasmosis (54–58), including diffuse macules, papules, plaques, pustules, ulcers, subcutaneous nodules, and rosacea-like eruptions. The presentation can also appear disseminated in a folliculitis-like pattern, or with umbilicated papules, similar to MC. Lesions occur most often on the face, followed by the extremities and trunk.[10] Mucosal lesions can be seen at any point along the gastrointestinal tract, from the mouth to the colon. Oropharyngeal plaques, nodules, and ulcers are also common. Gastrointestinal involvement with masses or ulceration can result in pain, bleeding, perforation, or malabsorption.[42]

DIAGNOSIS

Diagnosis of histoplasmosis can be established via culture, fungal stain, antigen detection, or serologic testing for antibodies.[47] While fungal stains of clinical specimens can be used to diagnose rapidly patients with acute disseminated infection or those with severe pulmonary infection, sensitivity is less than 50%.[27] A silver (GMS) or PAS stain is done on tissue sections and Wright's stain is used on peripheral blood smears. Histopathologic examination of stained specimens reveals small, intracellular budding yeasts (**59–61**). Cultures are positive in 85% of cases with disseminated or chronic pulmonary histoplasmosis, although the cultures must be held for 4–6 weeks as it can take a long time for the culture to become positive.[47]

In patients with disseminated disease, serologic tests for antibodies to *H. capsulatum* are positive in over 80% of cases.[48] The standard serologic tests for antibodies to *H. capsulatum* are the complement fixation (CF) test and the immunodiffusion (ID) assay. Although CF testing is more sensitive than the ID assay, it is less specific.[47] An important limitation of serologic testing is its decreased sensitivity in immunosuppressed individuals. Furthermore, prior infection can result in positive serologic tests and thus inaccurately suggest a diagnosis of active histoplasmosis in a patient with other disease. Antibody titers will decrease following self-limited infection and reach undetectable levels within 2–5 years. Disease relapse results in a rise in antigen levels.[49] Persistent antigenemia or antigenuria indicate ongoing active infection and a need for chronic maintenance therapy.[49]

MANAGEMENT

In HIV-associated severe or disseminated histoplasmosis, amphotericin B is the drug of choice.[50] The recommended treatment regimen for such patients is liposomal amphotericin B for the first 3–10 days until clinical improvement is observed. Patients responding well following completion of initial amphotericin B treatment may be switched to oral treatment with itraconazole capsules to complete 12 weeks of treatment and then placed on maintenance therapy.[30]

Amphotericin B should also be used in the initial treatment of mild or moderately severe histoplasmosis.[30] Patients who cannot tolerate amphotericin B can be treated with IV itraconazole using a loading dosage of 400 mg daily with a goal concentration of >1 µg/ml.[51] Fluconazole 800 mg daily is no longer recommended, as disease relapse has been observed secondary to drug resistance.[52]

Suppressive therapy is necessary in all patients with AIDS given the high relapse rate (>50%) seen without suppression.[1] Maintenance therapy with itraconazole 200 mg twice daily is recommended in patients who remain immunosuppressed.[22,30] A reasonable, though comparatively less effective, alternative for chronic suppressive therapy is fluconazole 800 mg daily.[30,53] Amphotericin B 50 mg intravenously once weekly has been shown to be effective as suppressive therapy, but is generally considered second-line as it is poorly tolerated by most patients.[54]

PROPHYLAXIS

Itraconazole 200 mg daily has been used effectively as primary prophylaxis in AIDS patients with CD4 counts below $150 \times 10^6/l$.[55] A placebo-controlled trial showed a 70% reduction in the occurrence of histoplasmosis and cryptococcosis via itraconazole prophylaxis.[55] Although no survival benefit has been shown, itraconazole is recommended as primary prophylaxis in HIV-positive patients living in regions experiencing high rates of histoplasmosis (over 5 cases per 100 patient-years).[50]

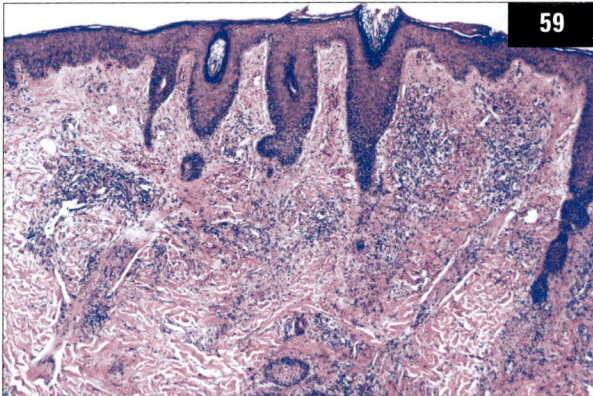

59 Histoplasmosis. Mild epidermal hyperplasia overlying a lymphohistiocytic infiltrate in the dermis.

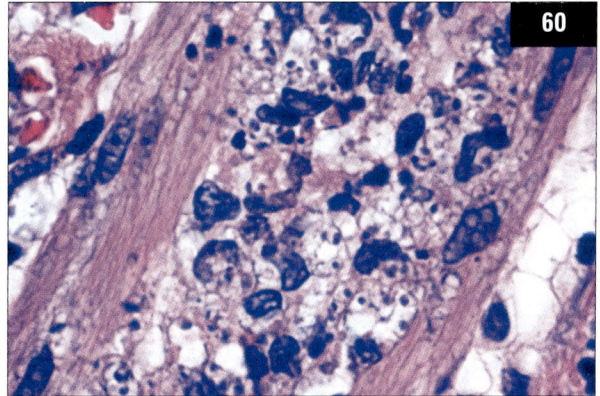

60 Higher power view reveals histiocytes filled with multiple *Histoplasma capsulatum* organisms.

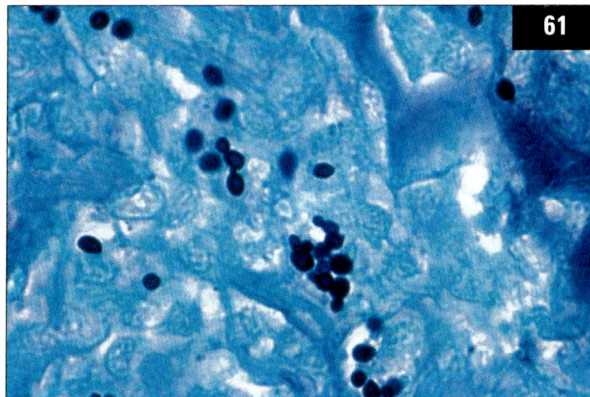

61 *Histoplasma capsulatum* organisms are highlighted with a GMS stain.

COCCIDIOIDOMYCOSIS

DEFINITION/OVERVIEW

Coccidioidomycosis was first reported in 1892 in an Argentine soldier who presented with skin lesions resembling mycosis fungoides.[56] Round organisms were found within the lesions that were thought to be a protozoan, and the name *Coccidioides* was given because it resembled a coccidian. In a separate case, similar skin lesions were seen on an immigrant in California.[56] The organism isolated from the lesions was named *immitis* (not mild) as an indication of its virulence, and the name *Coccidioides immitis* was coined.[56] Eight additional years passed before Ophüls and Moffitt determined the fungal nature of the organism and described its life cycle.[57] Valley fever (a self-limiting common illness of the San Joaquin Valley) was first linked to coccidioidomycosis 35 years later with the discovery of their common etiology.[58]

Coccidioidomycosis is endemic to certain regions within the western hemisphere, especially the lower Sonoran life zone, an area with hot summers, few winter freezes, 5–20 inches (127–508 mm) of rainfall each year, and alkaline soil.[59] Endemic portions of the US are mainly within the southwest, including parts of California, Nevada, Arizona, New Mexico, and Texas.[59] The highest endemicity is seen within southern Arizona and the southern San Joaquin Valley in California. Endemic regions are also seen in northern Mexico and scattered regions of Central and South America.[59]

PATHOGENESIS/PATHOPHYSIOLOGY

It is estimated today that over 100,000 new cases of coccidioidomycosis occur each year in the US.[60] Infection occurs upon inhalation of arthroconidia. Individuals exposed to soil and dust are at increased risk for infection; clusters of disease have been described in archeologists.[61]

C. *immitis* is a dimorphic fungus. The mycelial form represents the saprobic (environmental) phase which grows in soil of endemic regions. It forms the branching septate hyphae from which arthroconidia develop. Mature arthroconidia become stable and easily airborne. Once inhaled by humans or animals, the fungus changes into its parasitic (tissue)

phase. When it reaches the bronchiole, the arthroconidium converts into a multinucleate spherical structure (spherule). The spherule undergoes internal division to produce hundreds of uninucleate endospores. Endospores are released once the spherule matures; those that remain in tissue are each capable of forming new spherules. Once released into the environment, they develop into the mycelial form.[60]

The small size of the inhaled arthroconidia (<10 μm) allows for easy escape of first-line defenses of the respiratory tract which include filtration, mucoid chemical inhibitors, and mucociliary transport, and breach of the terminal bronchus. The host immune response initially targets the arthroconidia leading to complement activation with chemotaxin production. The chemotaxins result in an influx of polymorphonuclear leukocytes.[62] Once the arthroconidia convert to spherules, a mononuclear cell infiltration occurs which continues throughout infection and can lead to granuloma formation. The spherules' ability to resist host defenses has been seen by the *in vitro* inability of polymorphonuclear leukocytes to kill mature spherules.[60] The outcome and severity of infection are determined by the host's specific immune response. Cellular (TH1-type) immune response is associated with control of infection. The TH1 cytokine, interferon-γ, has been specifically linked to protective immunity in experimental murine infection, while TH-2 type immune responses with elevated levels of antibody and IgE have been associated with severe worsening disease and dissemination.[63] Patients with AIDS, those in late stages of pregnancy, or those undergoing cytotoxic chemotherapy have defective cellular immune responses and are consequently at higher risk of developing disseminated disease.[60]

CLINICAL FEATURES

The majority (60%) of individuals infected with C. *immitis* remain asymptomatic. The remaining individuals often present with a mild influenza-like illness, with symptoms of fever, drenching night sweats, cough, pleuritic chest pain, fatigue, and anorexia. The synonym 'desert rheumatism' arises from the fact that arthralgia and myalgia are usually prominent symptoms. Chest radiographic findings are seen in half of all cases and include peripneumonic pulmonary effusions and infiltrates with ipsilateral hilar adenopathy. The majority of symptoms clear within a 2–3 week period; however, the associated fatigue and residual symptoms may last for several weeks to months. Five percent of patients will have residual pulmonary lesions or complications, whereas less than 1% will go on to develop extrapulmonary disease.[60] Patients with progressive disease develop pulmonary nodules and cavities; a large inoculum can result in diffuse pulmonary involvement and pneumonia. Hematogenous spread of the fungus with dissemination leads to the extrapulmonary manifestations of coccidioidomycosis.[60]

Males are at higher risk for development of extrapulmonary dissemination from an initial primary pulmonary infection when compared to females. Of interest, pregnant females are also at higher risk for disseminated disease than the general population, particularly if infection is acquired in, or the disease reactivates in, the second or third trimester.[65] However, the frequency of disease has not been seen to be increased among pregnant women. These findings suggest that while infection occurs infrequently in pregnancy, it can generate serious complications when present.[60] Certain racial groups also appear to be at higher risk for disseminated disease, including individuals of Filipino ancestry.[66] Other high risk populations include immunocompromised patients, such as individuals with AIDS and those on immunosuppressive therapy. A prospective study has shown that 10% of HIV-infected individuals in endemic areas will develop disease each year either as a new manifestation or as a recurrence. Clinically significant infections are diagnosed more frequently in individuals with a previous AIDS-defining illness or CD4 count below 250×10^6/l.[67]

C. *immitis* infection in HIV patients most frequently affects the lungs and diffuse reticulonodular infiltrates are typical.[67] An earlier report found a 42% mortality rate in patients despite antifungal therapy.[67] Many AIDS patients will go on to develop disseminated disease involving extrapulmonary sites including the skin, soft tissue, bones, meninges, or peritoneum. The majority of patients have CD4+ cell counts below 250×10^6/l at the time progressive disease occurs.[67]

The most common site of disseminated disease is the skin, with papules and verrucous lesions forming the majority of skin manifestations (62). These lesions may evolve into pustules, plaques, or nodules with minimal surrounding erythema.

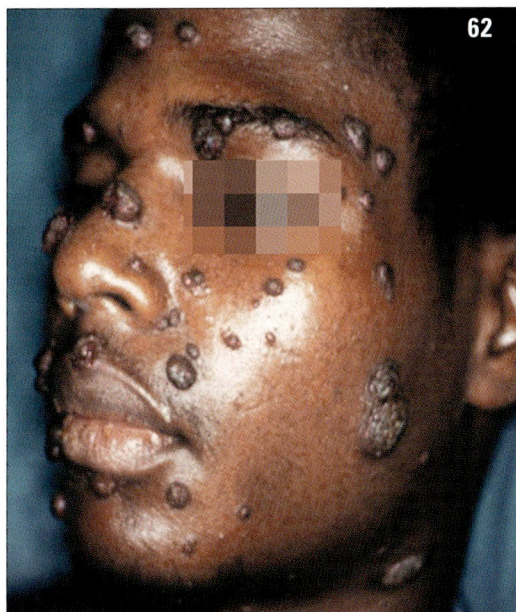

62 Coccidioidomycosis. Multiple exophytic nodules on the face of a patient with AIDS.

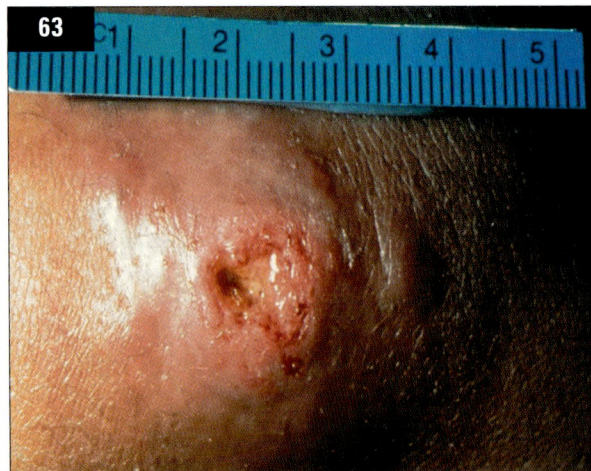

63 Close-up of a large, ulcerated nodular abscess in another patient with coccidioidomycosis.

In some cases, lesions will continue to enlarge and become confluent, with formation of abscesses (**63**), multiple draining sinus tracts, cellulitis, ulcers, or granulomatous nodules.[68] The finding of skin lesions necessitates a detailed investigation for other possible sites of dissemination.[68]

Other common manifestations of disseminated disease include osteomyelitis and synovitis. Coccidioidomycosis can infect practically any organ, and there have been reports of cases involving the eye, larynx, thyroid, peritoneum, prostate, kidney, and uterus.[60] The most severe and lethal form of *C. immitis* spread is that involving the CNS, a form which presents as chronic granulomatous meningitis with or without brain abscesses.[69]

DIAGNOSIS

Definitive diagnosis can be established if the organism is isolated from a clinical specimen. Tissue specimens can often be used for rapid diagnosis of coccidioidomycosis as detection of spherules with endospores from such specimens is pathognomonic[60] (**64, 65**). This technique can also be used on bronchoalveolar lavage fluid and sputum specimens.

Culture should always be done in addition to direct examination in order to increase test sensitivity. The fungus can be cultured on most culture media and will appear after incubation at a broad range of temperatures. Relatively rapid growth may be seen as early as 2 days postinoculation of media, but 5 or more days are generally required. Once growth is noted, a DNA (deoxyribonucleic acid)-specific probe is used to identify the organism quickly.[70] The clinical lab must be notified if *C. immitis* is suspected so as to minimize risk of accidental exposure of lab personnel to infection.[60]

Serologic testing involves the use of the tube precipitin-reacting antigen and the CF antigen. Antibodies of the IgM type to the tube precipitin-reacting antigen can be detected in the serum of 75% of patients with primary disease.[60] These antibodies eventually disappear and are not seen in chronic infections. In contrast, IgG antibodies against the CF antigen are found in chronic disease and persist for the duration of disease.[71] CF serology is generally positive in the CSF in coccidioidal meningitis.[30] Changes in antibody titer correlate with the course of the disease and can help determine whether the disease is worsening or improving. Early evidence suggests that polymerase chain reaction (PCR) amplification and hybridization techniques which target *C. immitis* ribosomal ribonucleic acid (RNA) may be helpful for diagnosis; however, further clinical evaluation is needed.[72]

MANAGEMENT

Although therapy of initial infection with *C. immitis* in the majority of the population is generally considered inadvisable,[60] therapy should be used in individuals who have received a high inoculum of fungus, exhibit elevated antibody titers or extensive pneumonia, and those with risk factors for extra-pulmonary disease (e.g. AIDS patients, immunosup-pressed transplant patients, and pregnant patients).[60]

HIV patients with nonmeningeal pulmonary and disseminated disease should be treated initially with amphotericin B 0.5–0.7 mg/kg/day until resolution of signs and symptoms of infection is achieved (a qualification usually requiring several weeks of therapy and administration of 500–1000 mg of amphotericin B).[30] Once clinical improvement is observed, patients may be switched to oral azole therapy. Diffuse pulmonary involvement in this patient population signifies a poor prognosis, as mortality approaches 60% despite appropriate therapy.[73] Coccidioidal meningitis should be treated with fluconazole, an approach which has an 80% success rate.[30] The most appropriate, though toxic, alternative treatment for *C. immitis* meningitis is intrathecal amphotericin B.[30]

AIDS patients and any patient with disseminated disease should be placed on lifelong azole therapy. Secondary prophylaxis with either fluconazole 400 mg/day (first-line) or itraconazole 200 mg twice daily is recommended as standard of care when patients respond to initial treatment.[30] Although patients who have achieved CD4 cell counts $>100 \times 10^6$/l in response to antiretroviral therapy may be at low risk for recurrent systemic mycosis, the number of patients who have been evaluated are insufficient to warrant a recommendation to discontinue secondary prophylaxis in this setting.[30]

An appropriate T cell (TH1) response is necessary for effective control of infection. This response requires the formation of both interferon-γ and interleukin-12 (IL-12). Use of these cytokines as adjunctive therapy in very ill or immunocom-promised patients has been proposed and warrants clinical study.[30]

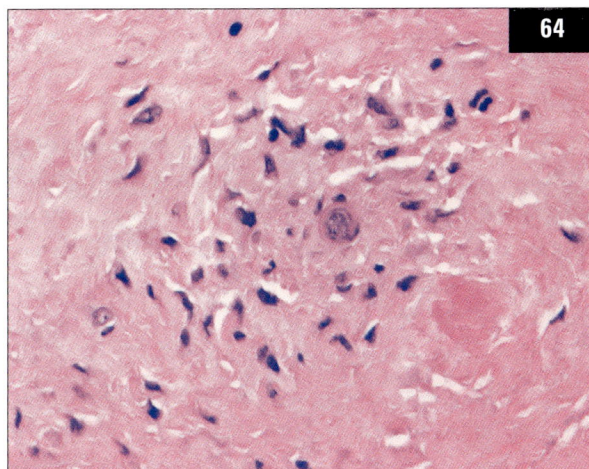

64 Histology of *Coccidioides immitis* infection. Skin biopsy showing a large, thick-walled *Coccidioides* spherules containing numerous endospores.

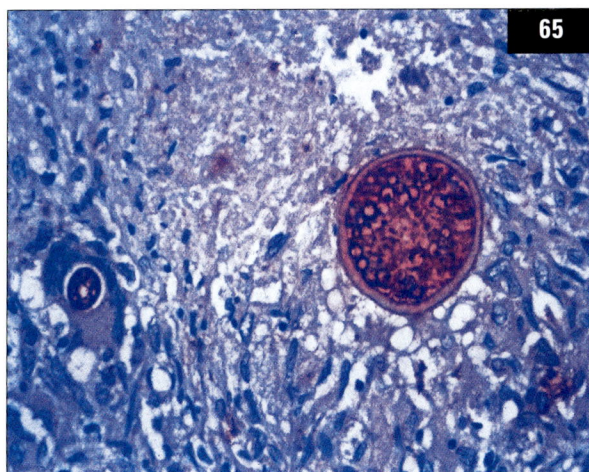

65 Higher power view of *Coccidioides* spherules stained with PAS.

ASPERGILLOSIS

DEFINITION/OVERVIEW

Over 250 species of *Aspergillus* have been recognized; however, only a few cause invasive human disease with any regularity. *A. fumigatus* is the most common etiologic agent and accounts for 80–90% of human infections.[74] Other pathogenic species include *A. flavus* (10–15%), *A. terreus* (2–5%), *A. niger* (1–2%), and *A. nidulans* (less than 1%).[75]

Invasive aspergillosis is rare in AIDS, but when present, has a very poor prognosis. It occurs predominantly in patients with advanced HIV disease in the setting of neutropenia, extended use of high-dose corticosteroids, exposure to broad spectrum antibacterial therapy, or previous underlying lung disease.[30,76] CD4 lymphopenia has been identified as an important risk factor for HIV-1-associated aspergillosis and CD4 cell counts below $50 \times 10^6/l$ are reported in the majority of cases.[30,77]

PATHOGENESIS/PATHOPHYSIOLOGY

The environmental source for *Aspergillus* is soil, decaying vegetation, and potted plants. Large amounts of *Aspergillus* spores are released into the air from these sources.[78] Also, building or demolition activities correlated with high concentrations of *Aspergillus* spores in the air. Air filtration is effective in reducing the number of airborne fungal spores in high-risk units.[79]

Aspergillosis is typically acquired via inhalation of fungal conidia. Conidia that are not cleared by alveolar macrophages germinate in the alveolar space and hyphal forms invade the pulmonary tissues.[74] Pulmonary disease is the most common manifestation, but concurrent sino-orbital infection and disseminated disease also occur. Vascular invasion is a prominent feature, leading to hematologic dissemination to other organs.

CLINICAL FEATURES

Noninvasive forms of aspergillosis include allergic bronchopulmonary aspergillosis (ABPA) and aspergilloma. ABPA occurs when patients with asthma are colonized with *Aspergillus*, leading to a hypersensitivity response, whereas aspergillomas are fungus balls which develop in pre-existing pulmonary cavities.[74] These forms of disease occur without tissue invasion and rarely require antifungal therapy. They are differentiated from invasive aspergillosis, in which the tissues of the lungs or sinus are invaded and dissemination occurs through the blood stream, often with a rapid course.[80]

HIV-related aspergillosis may present with various distinct clinical syndromes. Invasive pulmonary aspergillosis has been found to account for 71% of all cases of aspergillosis in AIDS patients in a review by Khoo *et al*.[81] The case fatality ratio of invasive aspergillosis for HIV-positive patients is 86%.[82] Obstructing bronchial aspergillosis is a separate clinical syndrome sometimes seen in HIV-infected patients, in which the characteristic feature is the expectoration of large mucoid casts containing *Aspergillus* organisms. These casts can lead to airway obstruction and atelectasis.[83] Although noninvasive in its early stages, obstructing bronchopulmonary aspergillosis can progress and invade tissue, leading to pseudomembranous or ulcerative tracheobronchitis.[1] At this stage, involvement of adjacent lung parenchyma may occur in 50% of cases, and extrapulmonary dissemination is seen in 25% of cases.[81]

Among reported cases of HIV-related cutaneous aspergillosis, the majority have had *A. fumigatus* infection.[84] The initial lesions of cutaneous aspergillosis may present as macules, papules, plaques, or nodules (**66**). Cutaneous lesions may also appear as skin-colored to pink umbilicated papules similar to those seen with MC.[10]

DIAGNOSIS

Diagnosis of aspergillosis is suspected when septate hyphae are seen in fungal stains of tissue. In some cases, a presumptive diagnosis of primary cutaneous aspergillosis can be made rapidly by staining the roof of a bulla or by examining a potassium hydroxide preparation of a biopsy specimen.[85] In general, however, diagnosis of cutaneous *Aspergillus* infections requires biopsy of a skin lesion taken for both culture and histopathology. Skin biopsy specimens for suspected fungal lesions should be taken from the center of the lesion and should reach the subcutaneous fat as *Aspergillus* tends to invade blood

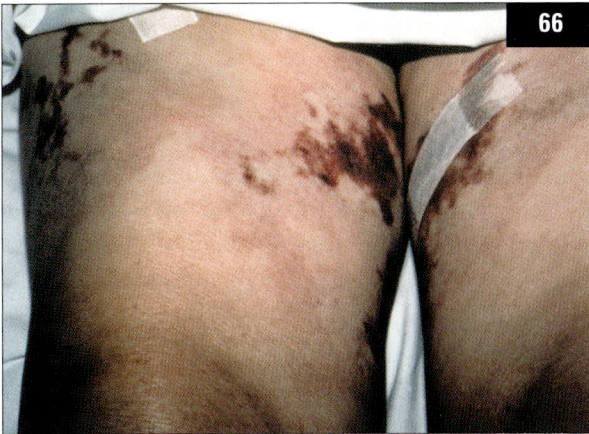

66 *Aspergillus* infection. Hemorrhagic plaques with incipient cutaneous necrosis on the thighs in a patient with aspergillosis.

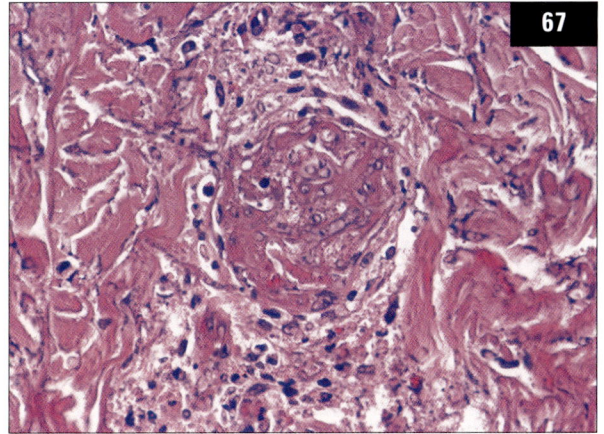

67 Histology of cutaneous aspergillosis shows numerous large hyphae throughout the dermis and invading thrombosed blood vessels.

68 Higher power view of multiple hyphal elements highlighted in this GMS-stained skin specimen.

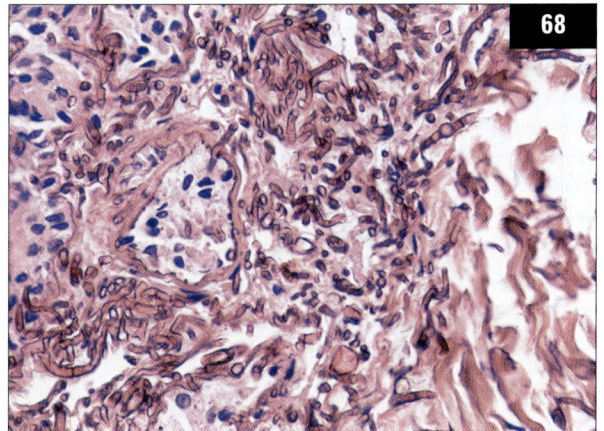

vessels of the dermis and subcutis, resulting in an overlying ischemic cone.[84]

In the microbiology laboratory, fungal hyphal structures can be stained directly from tissue specimens with the whitening agent calcofluor, which will fluoresce when exposed to UV light.[84] On histopathologic examination with routine stains (such as H&E), *Aspergillus* hyphae may be seen in consequence of either staining the nucleus and cytoplasm of the fungus or revealing the cell wall by a negatively staining shadow (67, 68). The Gomori methenamine silver (GMS) stain can clearly and reliably detect hyphae, as the hyphal cell wall stains black while the tissue background stains green. *Aspergillus* hyphae have acute angle branching with frequent septations.[76] Should aspergillosis be diagnosed, further efforts should then be aimed at determining whether the patient has a primary infection or whether there is secondary dissemination from a primary focus (such as the lung).[84]

Isolation of *Aspergillus* in respiratory secretions can be misleading as the organism may colonize airways. A study by Pursell *et al.* showed that while *Aspergillus* was isolated from respiratory secretions of 5% of patients, it was merely a colonizer in 90% of cases.[86] In cases of pulmonary disease, radiographic findings may include diffuse interstitial pneumonitis or a localized wedge-shaped dense infiltrate representing pulmonary infarction, related to the organism's predilection for invasion of vascular endothelium. [30,87]

MANAGEMENT

The recommended treatment for invasive asper-gillosis is voriconazole.[30] Amphotericin B (conventional or liposomal formulation) in doses equivalent to 1 mg/kg body weight/day can be used as an appropriate alternative in patients who cannot tolerate voriconazole.[30] In a small study of neutropenic patients, survival was seen to be better in patients treated with liposomal amphotericin B compared to standard formulation; however, the difference was not found to be statistically significant.[88] Caspofungin may be effective in cases that fail to respond to standard treatment; however, it has not yet been studied in this patient population.[30] There is insufficient data to make a recommendation for or against chronic maintenance or suppressive therapy in patients who have successfully completed an initial course of treatment.[30]

PARACOCCIDIOIDOMYCOSIS

DEFINITION/OVERVIEW

Paracoccidioidomycosis (PCM), caused by the thermally dimorphic fungus *Paracoccidioides brasiliensis*, is the most important endemic deep mycosis in South America. Lutz first described PCM in 1908 in two Brazilian patients with oral lesions and lymphadenopathy. Splendore named the fungus isolated by Lutz *Zymonema brasiliensis*.[89] In 1930, Floriano Almeida showed that the fungus was distinct from *Coccidioides immitis*, and named the genus *Paracoccidioides brasiliensis*.[90]

PCM is a chronic, progressive, and insidious systemic mycosis, causing predominantly pulmonary and lymph nodal infection, although mucocutaneous sites often become secondarily involved. The disease is restricted to countries of South and Central America, where it is the most widespread and serious systemic fungal infection.[91] Regions favoring fungal growth include those with acid types of soil, temperatures between 12°C and 30°C, altitudes between 150 and 2,000 meters, and pluviometric indices between 1000 and 4000 mm/year (39–157 inches).[92]

PATHOGENESIS/PATHOPHYSIOLOGY

The natural reservoir for *P. brasiliensis* is soil, where it exists in the mycelial phase.[93] Disease is most commonly acquired by inhalation of airborne propagules (conidia) produced in the mycelial phase.[94] Direct inoculation of the parasite in both skin and oral mucous membranes are alternate, but less common, routes of infection and can account for cases of cutaneous lesions without pulmonary involvement.[95]

Pathogenicity and invasiveness appear to be associated with X-1-3 glucan, in addition to proteases such as Gp43.[96] Cell wall glucans and chitins are not antigenic. The main known antigen is Gp43, a 43-kD glycoprotein of the fungus wall secreted extracellularly.[97] Gp43 appears to be capable of inhibiting some dermal dendrocyte functions and thus evading cellular immunity.[98]

Surprisingly, there is a rather low incidence of PCM in HIV-infected patients, probably explained by the higher prevalence of PCM but lower prevalence of HIV in rural regions, as well as the extensive antifungal use in HIV-infected patients.[90] Trimethoprim–sulfamethoxazole (TMP-SMX) prophylaxis for *Pneumocystis jiroveci* also appears to be effective in preventing clinical disease caused by *P. brasiliensis*.[30] There is a correlation of T cell depression with the severity of PCM, and patients with PCM show a decreased cellular immune response, with a decreased CD4+/CD8+ ratio in blood, likely mediated by increased IL-4 production. Patients with the acute juvenile form of PCM exhibit impaired response to *P. brasiliensis* culture filtrate antigen and a TH-2 response with lower IFN-γ levels and high levels of IL-4, IL-5, and IL-10.[99]

CLINICAL FEATURES

Subclinical infections have been detected by skin tests with paracoccidioidin antigen in up to 60% of the population in endemic regions. Humans seem to be fairly resistant to infection; hormonal, genetic, immunologic, and nutritional factors predispose to the development of the infection and clinical disease.

The acute form of disease is characterized by bone and skin lesions along with involvement of the mononuclear–phagocytic system (lymph node enlargement, hepatosplenomegaly). The acute form generally affects individuals below the age of 30 residing or traveling in endemic areas.[93] Chronic disease is characterized by mucosal involvement as well as involvement of the upper and lower respiratory tract.[93] Chronic disease generally affects individuals in the fourth decade of life. The chronic form of PCM predominantly affects men,[100] and while the acute form has no sexual predilection prior to puberty,[101] men are predominantly affected after puberty.[102] Women are thought to be relatively protected against PCM because estrogens appear to inhibit the transformation of yeast into conidia in the infected host, a crucial step for disease development.[103] The host's main defense against the fungus is cell-mediated immunity, which induces dense, compact granulomatous formations that are associated with low numbers of fungal cells in patients with less severe disease.[93]

Patients with the acute form of the disease mount a less effective immune response than those with the chronic form, evidenced by the ability of the latter to mount a response that restricts fungal proliferation for years or decades. Those with the acute form of the disease have a more conspicuous *in vitro* hypo-responsiveness to cell wall *P. brasiliensis* antigen, as well as decreased CD4+ cell counts.[104] Not surprisingly, given the acuity of their presentation, the vast majority of coinfected HIV–PCM patients had $<200 \times 10^6$/l CD4+ cells.[105]

With respect to clinical presentation of PCM, 56 patients (77%) had disseminated disease with many characteristics of the acute form: superficial lymph node enlargement was evident in 41 (73%); hepatomegaly in 24 (43%); splenomegaly in 16 (29%); osteoarticular lesions in 10 (18%); and deep lymph node enlargement in 9 (16%).[105]

Of note, a striking incidence of paracoccidioidal skin involvement was seen in HIV-infected patients (34 patients [61%])[105] in comparison with that in HIV-negative patients with the acute form of PCM (10–15%).[102] The majority of the lesions in these cases were described as ulcerated papular lesions, sometimes with a necrotic center. Biopsies or smears of the lesions often revealed the typical *P. brasiliensis* yeast cells.[93]

DIAGNOSIS

While the majority of fungal infections can be diagnosed by culture, serology, or histopathology (**69**), the diagnosis of PCM proves somewhat more challenging. *P. brasiliensis* may require weeks to grow, serology can be inconclusive, and histopathology does not always lead to a definitive diagnosis.[90]

Histology reveals pseudoepitheliomatous hyperplasia with intraepithelial microabscesses, and a granulomatous reaction with giant cells, interspersed with neutrophils, plasma cells, and eosinophils. The granuloma represents an immune response intended to neutralize and destroy the fungus; destruction occurs primarily within the multinucleated cells. In HIV-positive patients, multinucleated cells, macrophages, and lymphocytes do not form well-organized granulomas because of the depression of the cellular immune response in these patients.[106]

Yeast forms are found in tissues, frequently within multinucleate giant cells, but also in microabscesses. Although they can be observed in routine H&E sections, they are more readily seen with PAS or methenamine silver (GMS) stains.[90] Yeast forms in

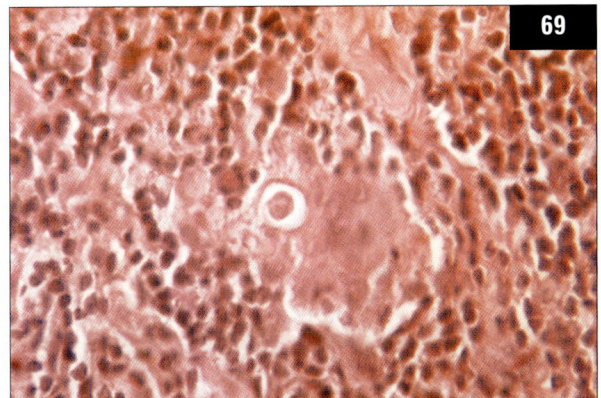

69 Histopathologic changes seen in paracoccidioidomycosis. A *Paracoccidioides brasiliensis* conidium is visible at center. (Courtesy of CDC/Dr. Lucille K. Georg.)

tissue form a wheel-house pattern due to the radial budding of daughter yeast from a mother cell (**70**).[30] In contrast to the other mycoses, there have been no reports of mycelia in tissue sections.

Culture can at times be useful for diagnosis, but *P. brasiliensis* grows very slowly. On Sabouraud agar, colonies begin to appear only after 20 days.[90] Serologic examination via immunodiffusion or complement fixation and skin tests with para-coccidioidin are mainly used for epidemiologic studies or as a parameter to monitor treatment rather than as diagnostic aids.[107] Alternatives for fungal detection include immunohistochemistry and *in situ* hybridization.[108]

The use of molecular techniques is promising due to their high specificity and sensitivity, especially with use of DNA probes. Molecular identification of *P. brasiliensis* has been successfully accomplished by immunohistochemistry and PCR amplification of ribosomal DNA.[109] However, at present, the diagnosis of PCM continues to be dependent upon the results of clinical evaluation and cytological diagnosis, along with supportive histopathology.[90]

MANAGEMENT

Amphotericin B is the recommended initial treatment for severe PCM, but other agents (e.g. TMP-SMX and azole antifungals) may also have comparable efficacy; single-arm studies of itraconazole 100–200 mg daily, ketoconazole 200–400 mg daily, and sulfonamides have demonstrated efficacy in immunocompetent hosts.[30] The use of fluconazole is not recommended as

it has been associated with high failure rates even when given at doses up to 600 mg daily.[30] Long-term secondary prophylaxis should be used in patients who respond to induction therapy and have CD4 counts of $<200 \times 10^6$/l. Azoles and cotrimoxazole[110] may be used for this indication; however, definite recommendations have yet to be established.[111]

OTHER MYCOSES

Several other endemic mycoses occur less frequently in AIDS patients but may be problematic in certain areas of the world. These include blastomycosis, sporotrichosis, African histoplasmosis, and peni-cilliosis.[22] *Blastomyces dermatidis*, the causative agent of blastomycosis, is confined to the midwestern and south-central US and has rarely caused disease in HIV-positive patients. Blastomycosis may present as localized pulmonary infection or as disseminated disease. In the disseminated form, crusted papular facial lesions may be seen.[10]

Penicilliosis is due to the dimorphic fungus *Penicillium marneffei*, and represents the third most common opportunistic infection in HIV-infected patients of countries of southeast Asia and southern part of China.[112] The majority of cases of penicilliosis are seen in patients with CD4 counts $<50 \times 10^6$/l.[30] A report of 92 patients found the most common clinical presentation to include fever, cough, weight loss, anemia, and disseminated papular skin lesions (71%).[113] The most frequent skin lesions were umbilicated papules (**71**) seen over the face, pinnae, extremities, and occasionally the genitalia.[30] Diagnosis can be established by fungal isolation from blood or other clinical specimens, or by histo-pathologic demonstration of organisms on biopsy material (**72**). Wright stained samples of skin scrapings reveal intracellular and extracellular basophilic, spherical, oval, and elliptical yeast-like

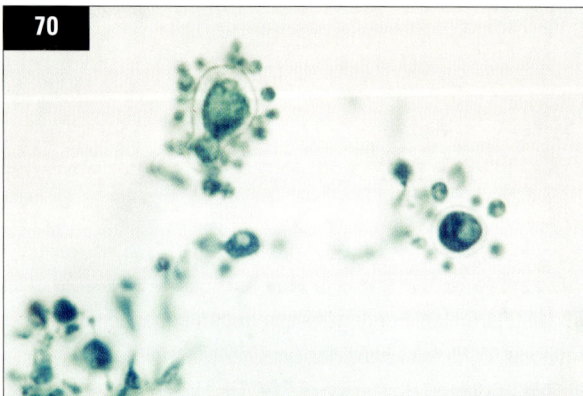

70 Photomicrograph of budding cells of the fungus *Paracoccidioides brasiliensis* during its yeast phase. (Courtesy of CDC/Dr. Lucille K. Georg.)

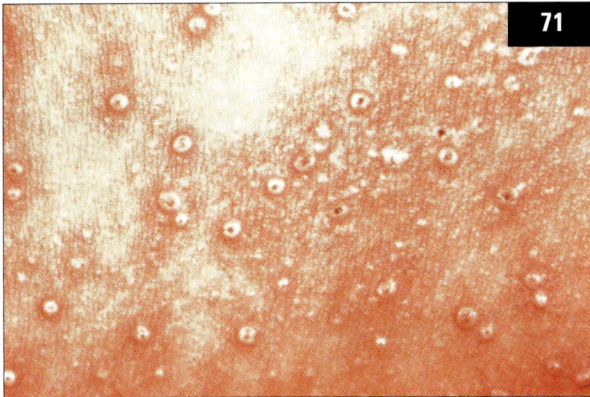

71 Penicilliosis. Multiple umbilicated, flesh-colored papules with surrounding erythema.

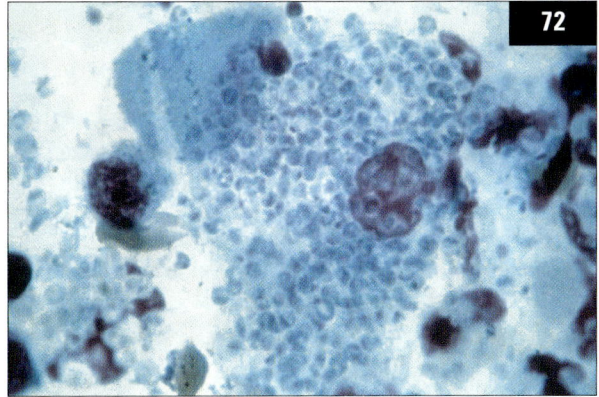

72 The organism, *Penicillium marneffei*, is easily visualized histologically with GMS staining.

73 Sporotrichosis. Large, scaly, ulcerated plaque on the forearm, with ulcerative nodules extending proximally along lymphatic channels.

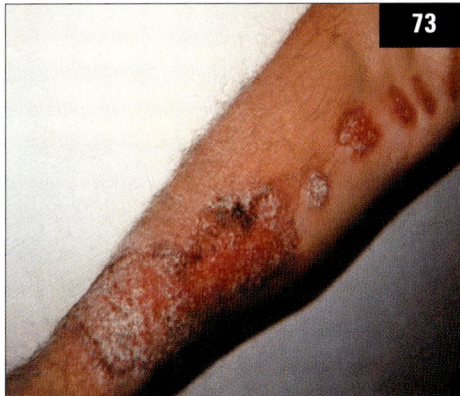

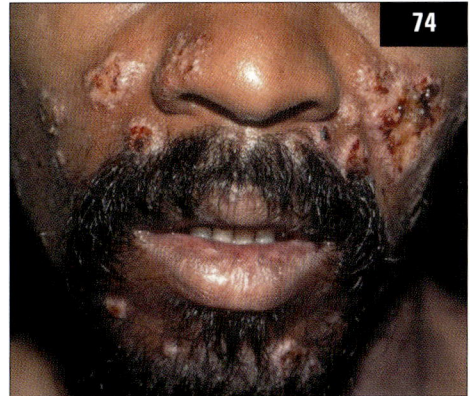

74, 75 Numerous suppurative, ulcerated nodules on the face, arms, and trunk of a HIV-infected patient with disseminated cutaneous disease.

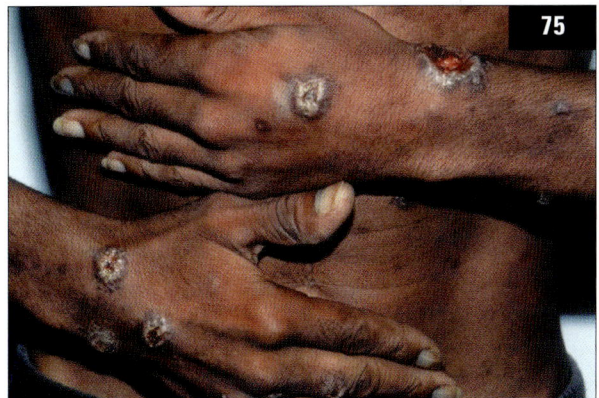

organisms, some with the characteristic clear central septations of *P. marneffei*.[30] Treatment is with amphotericin B 0.6 mg/kg/day IV for 2 weeks, followed by oral itraconazole solution in a dose of 400 mg daily for a subsequent duration of 10 weeks.[30] Simultaneous administration of treatment for penicilliosis and initiation of HAART may improve outcome. Upon completion of initial therapy, secondary prophylaxis with oral itraconazole 200 mg daily should be given for life.[30]

Sporotrichosis is caused by *Sporothrix schenckii*, a ubiquitous organism found predominantly in rotting organic matter. Percutaneous inoculation leads to limited forms of cutaneous sporotrichosis. In HIV-infected patients, dissemination of local infection to other organs can occur from the lungs or cutaneous foci. Skin findings may present as papules or nodules, and go on to become eroded, ulcerated, crusted, or hyperkeratotic (**73–75**).[114] Individual lesions may remain discrete or expand to become

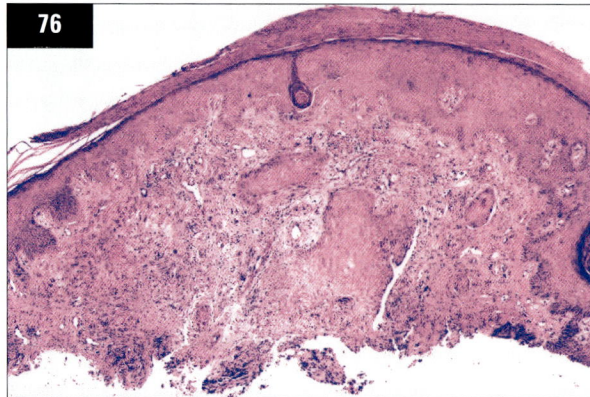

76 Histology of sporotrichosis. Low power view of a skin biopsy with pseudoepitheliomatous hyperplasia and a granulomatous infiltrate in the dermis.

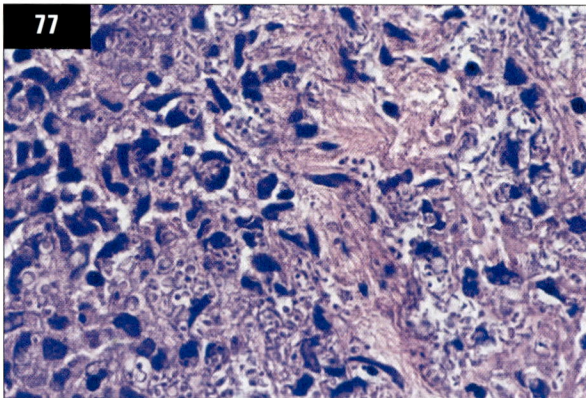

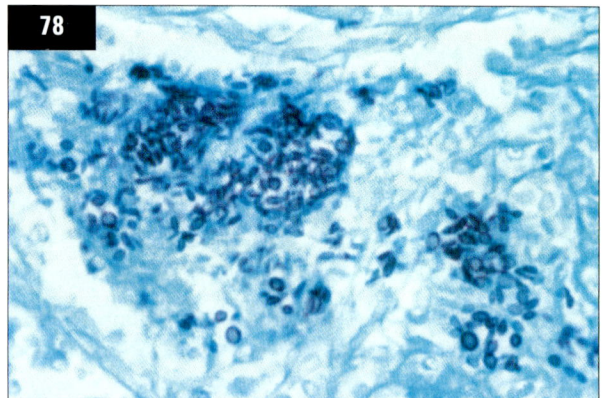

77, 78 Higher power showing numerous organisms (**77**), which are highlighted with a GMS stain (**78**).

confluent. Lesions commonly disseminate, but spare the palms, soles, and oral mucosa.[10] The HIV-associated disseminated form of sporotrichosis can also involve the eyes, joints, lungs, liver, spleen, intestines, and meninges. Definitive diagnosis at any site requires culture isolation of *S. schenckii* from a normally sterile body site. Biopsy of an immuno-compromised patient with sporotrichosis may reveal a great number of oval, cigar-shaped yeasts (**76–78**).

The drug of choice for cutaneous, lymphocutaneous, and osteoarticular sporotrichosis in immuno-competent hosts is itraconazole, while disseminated sporotrichosis in the immunocompetent host should be treated with amphotericin B.[115] However, therapy for disseminated sporotrichosis in HIV-infected patients remains unclear as there has been a variable response to therapy.[115]

CHAPTER 5
CUTANEOUS MANIFESTATIONS OF PARASITIC INFECTIONS IN HIV/AIDS

Molly V. Burns and Clay J. Cockerell

INTRODUCTION

In immunocompromised persons, parasitic diseases, like most infectious diseases, may present in typical or unusual fashion. The interactions between human immunodeficiency virus (HIV) and parasitic infections are important for several reasons. The natural history of parasitic infections in persons with HIV/acquired immunodeficiency syndrome (AIDS) may be altered due to incompetent immune response, at times leading to extraordinary manifestations of even the most common of infestations. Of interest, chronic parasitic infections may affect the natural history of infection with HIV itself. Furthermore, tropical parasitic infections are present in a great proportion of those in geographic regions that encompass the brunt of the HIV pandemic so that coinfection not uncommon. Finally, atypical presentations of common infestations may lead clinicians to suspect HIV infection in undiagnosed persons, facilitating diagnosis and management of a previously undetected infection.

SCABIES

DEFINITION/OVERVIEW

Sarcoptes scabiei var. *hominis* is an obligate human parasite that causes an intensely pruritic infestation. The World Health Organization (WHO) estimates 300 million cases of scabies worldwide each year. It is known that infestation is more likely to occur during winter months, in urban populations, and in women and children.[1] Infestation shows no predilection for ethnicity or socioeconomic groups. Scabies spreads rapidly in overcrowded conditions, especially when personal hygiene and access to clean water is poor. The incidence of scabies in the HIV-positive population is unknown, though one report indicated 6% of HIV-positive persons were diagnosed with scabies over a 38 month period, with a significantly increased frequency in more advanced HIV.[2] In general, scabies should be considered in any HIV-positive person with papular, crusted, or eczematous skin findings.

PATHOGENESIS/PATHOPHYSIOLOGY

Transmission of the scabies mite may be through direct contact or, less commonly, indirect contact via clothing, bedclothes, and shared items. Mites are capable of surviving 24–36 hours when away from a human host. The female mite burrows by secreting proteolytic enzymes to dissolve the stratum corneum of the epidermis. Infestation typically becomes clinically apparent after an incubation period of 3–6 weeks in primary infections and 1–3 weeks in reinfections. In classic scabies, 10–15 female mites are usually present; however, in immunocompromised individuals, this number can soar into the thousands or even millions.

CLINICAL FEATURES

Classic scabies is easily recognized as a generalized intensely pruritic eruption that may involve the finger webs, wrist flexor regions, elbows, axillae, buttocks, genitalia, and breasts in women. Burrows in the finger webs are characteristic physical signs (79). Inflamed papules and nodules may be present, as well as secondary changes such as excoriations, eczematous changes, and impetiginization.

In persons with HIV infection, the severity and atypicality of the presentation is correlated with the immune status and CD4 count. These persons are more likely to manifest nail, face, and scalp involvement, sites uncommonly involved in immunocompetent adults.[3] Crusted (Norwegian, hyperkeratotic) scabies (80, 81) occurs when thousands to millions of mites infest a person creating white-gray psoriasiform hyperkeratotic plaques that may be minimally or nonpruritic. This form of scabies may occur in a generalized or localized distribution and is highly contagious. These lesions are characteristically found on the extremities but may also involve the back, face, scalp, and nail folds. There has also been a report of a single isolated lesion involving the penis.[4] Atypical (exaggerated, papular) scabies, presenting as severely pruritic generalized papules with overlying burrows, is well reported in HIV-positive persons, even when the CD4 count is greater than $200 \times 10^6/l$.[5] Persons with AIDS and scabies may also present with septicemia, as they are at higher risk of developing secondary infection and bacteremia.[6,7]

HISTOPATHOLOGY

Superficial skin scrapings (82) and skin biopsies (83, 84) revealing mites, ova, or pellets are diagnostic of scabies infestation. In Norwegian scabies, hyperkeratosis and inflammatory response is observed as well as numerous mites. When biopsies are performed, there is a superficial and deep infiltrate of lymphocytes, some histiocytes, and numerous eosinophils, with variable degrees of overlying spongiosis and epidermal hyperplasia. Occasionally, a small dell which represents the burrow may be seen. Mites, ova, or scybala may be seen in the cornified layer although when the number of mites in an infestation is small, they may not be visualized. In crusted scabies, there are usually several or more mites seen in the thickened cornified layer.

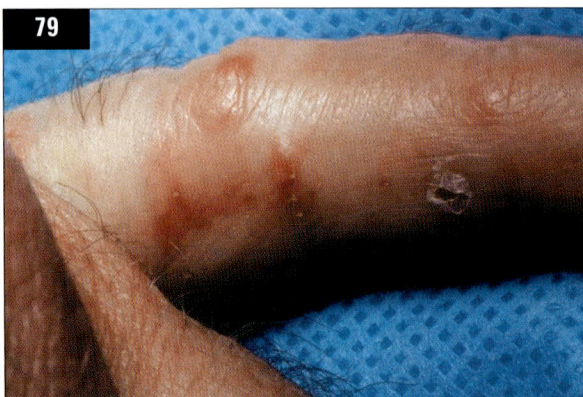

79 Scabies infestation. Erythematous papules, excoriated nodules and a characteristic burrow on the index finger of a patient with scabies infestation.

80 Crusted scabies. Confluent hyperkeratosis on the lateral face, neck, ear, and scalp in an immunocompromised patient.

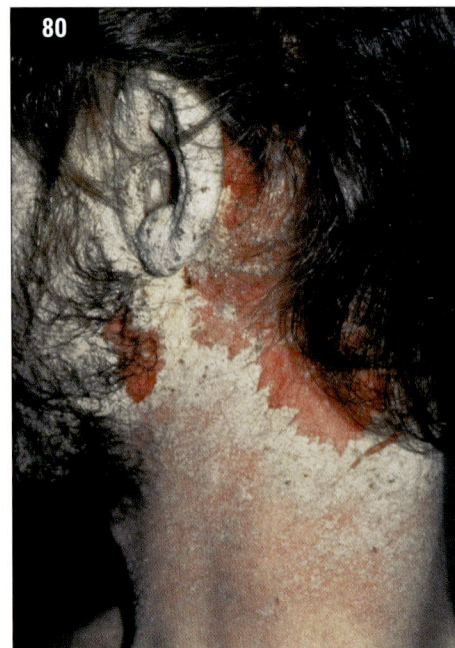

DIAGNOSIS

In immunocompetent persons, classic scabies is typically a clinical diagnosis after a supporting history and examination. Identifying mites, eggs, or pellets in superficial skin scrapings may further support the diagnosis. In Norwegian scabies, due the heavy infestation load, a superficial skin scraping from nonexcoriated lesions is often revealing. However, in atypical cases it may be necessary to obtain a skin biopsy to avoid misdiagnosis. Due to the highly variable presentation of scabies in persons with AIDS, the clinician must be aware of potential misdiagnoses, such as psoriasis, eczema, Darier's disease, contact dermatitis, icthyosis, seborrheic dermatitis, dermatophytosis, and adverse drug reactions. High clinical suspicion should be maintained in the HIV-positive person with an atypical or pruritic rash, as scabies is a common infestation and readily treated, even in immuno-suppressed persons. Alternatively, infection with HIV should be suspected in otherwise healthy appearing persons who present with severe or atypical scabies, as it rarely occurs if the immune system is competent.

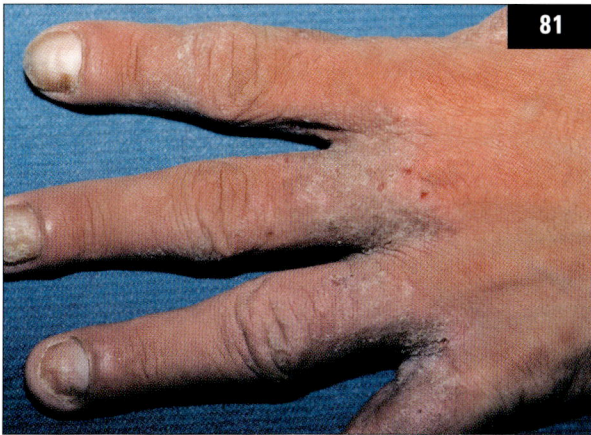

81 Hyperkeratosis of the web spaces with areas of excoriations.

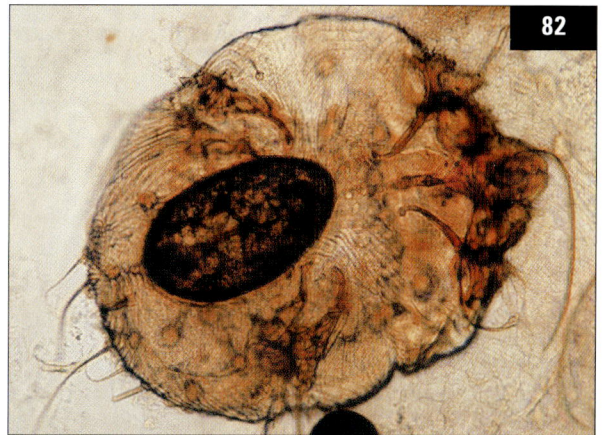

82 *Sarcoptes scabiei* mite with an ovum.

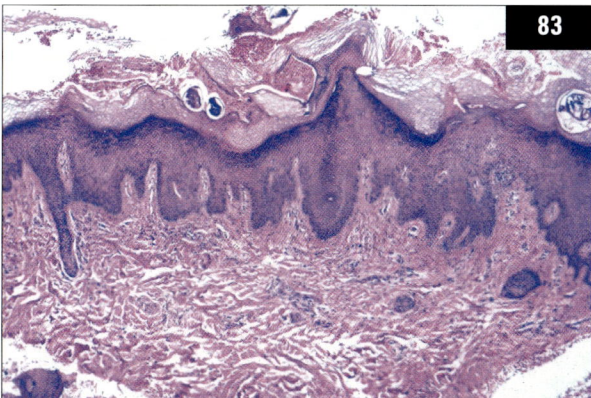

83 Histology of scabies infestation showing parts of scabies mites within burrows in a hyperkeratotic stratum corneum and a mild perivascular infiltrate with eosinophils in the dermis.

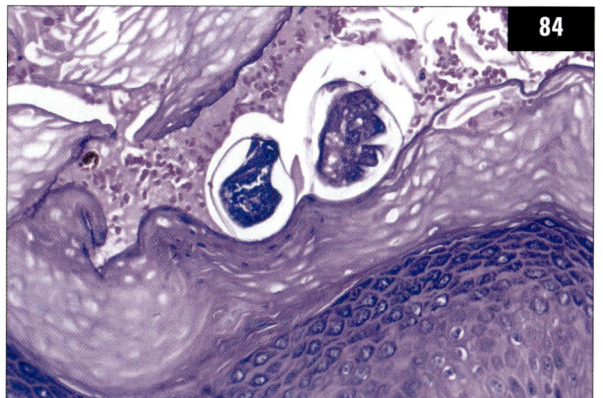

84 Higher power view of the scabies mites in the stratum corneum.

MANAGEMENT

Several topical and oral therapeutic options exist for the treatment of scabies. It should be noted that topical agents may poorly penetrate the hyperkeratotic epidermis in Norwegian scabies, necessitating the concomitant use of a keratolytic agent such as 6% salicylic acid or manual debridement. A standard treatment is permethrin 5% cream applied to the skin and washed off 8–14 hours later. This regimen may be repeated if the patient is still symptomatic and, in cases of Norwegian scabies, it may be necessary to prescribe treatments twice or thrice weekly for up to 6 weeks. Topical lindane has also been used; however, use of this agent is limited by potential neurotoxicity resulting in convulsions and death. In crusted scabies, topical therapies are often inadequate, as mentioned above. Oral ivermectin has proven to be a highly effective therapeutic agent in this scenario.[8,9] Despite some controversy, a regimen of two doses of 200 µg/kg given 2 weeks apart has proven to be an effective dosing schedule. Topical pimecrolimus twice daily has been reported as a useful agent in nodular scabies.[10] Other topical agents that have been used to treat scabies include malathion, benzyl benzoate, and sulfur.

It is advisable to have the patient machinewash recently worn clothes and used bedding. Vacuuming the affected person's living environment may be helpful. At this time, there is no supporting evidence for the use of environmental acaracides.

Due to the highly contagious nature of scabies, it is reasonable to consider offering treatment for cohabitants or close contacts of the affected person. Multiple cases of HIV-positive persons acting as a nidus for nosocomial outbreaks have been reported, as the diagnosis of scabies is often delayed due to atypical presentation.[5] In addition to prescribing treatment for scabies, prescribing prophylactic antibiotics for the immunocompromised person with scabies should be considered to prevent bacteremia and potentially fatal sepsis.

DEMODICIDOSIS

DEFINITION/OVERVIEW

Demodex folliculorum and D. brevis are the species of Demodex mites known to inhabit human hair follicles and pilosebaceous glands, obtaining sustenance from sebum. Demodex mites infest nearly 100% of the adult population, but may be pathogenic in HIV-positive patients. Though younger persons may not produce enough sebum to be adequate hosts, there are reported cases of demodicidosis in children. In one study of folliculitis in HIV-infected persons, Demodex mites were reported to be present in one-third of biopsies, with no correlation in distribution to the type of folliculitis.[11] However, it is reasonable to assume a similar rate of infestation among adults, regardless of HIV status. Worsening health status may simply increase susceptibility of developing clinical disease due to mite infestation.

PATHOGENESIS/PATHOPHYSIOLOGY

While most people harbor these mites, their role in cutaneous diseases has been less than clear. They have been implicated in contributing towards the pathogenesis of at least three dermatologic conditions: pityriasis folliculorum, rosacea-like demodicidosis, and demodicidosis gravis. Other conditions have been associated with these mites, including pustular folliculitis, papulo-pustular eruptions, perioral dermatitis, and hyperpigmented patches. Known factors influencing development of disease include degree of infestation, duration of disease, and patient age and health status. However, the pathogenesis of symptomatic infestation is largely unknown at this time.

CLINICAL FEATURES

As noted above, multiple skin disorders have been inconsistently associated with the Demodex mite. Pityriasis folliculorum is a condition characterized by diffuse facial erythema with pruritus and a burning sensation. Affected persons are most commonly female and may give a history of poor facial hygiene. Rosacea-like demodicidosis resembles the facial erythema, pustule, papules, and scaling of rosacea, as the name implies. In rosacea-like demodicidosis, the scaling is perifollicular and the lesions are typically small papulovesicles and vesicopustules. Rosacea-like demodicidosis is differentiated from classic acne rosacea by smaller more superficial papules and pustules and the lack of skin oiliness. Discriminating characteristics also include sudden onset with rapid progression, asymmetric distribution, and involvement of the eyelids (demodectic blepharitis). The patient may deny flushing and report burning and pruritus. Demodicidosis gravis is the most severe form of human reaction to *Demodex*, with development of dermal granulomas composed of giant cells engulfing mite remnants. There may also be caseation necrosis. In addition to the previously noted conditions, atypical presentations have been reported in HIV-positive persons such as papulonodular demodicidosis and hypopigmented indurated plaques.[12,13] There is also some speculation that *Demodex* mites may play a role in the papular pruritic eruption of AIDS.[14] Symptomatic disease has been reported to begin after initiation of anti-retroviral therapy, perhaps due to improvement in immune function allowing the body to mount a response to the mite antigens.[15]

HISTOPATHOLOGY

In pityriasis folliculorum, biopsy reveals diffuse and perivascular lymphocytic infiltrate in the dermis without granuloma formation. Biopsies of *Demodex* abscesses may also show spongiosis of the follicular epithelium, lymphohistiocytic follicular and perifollicular infiltrate, and mites (85).[16] There are often numerous *Demodex* mites seen in follicles and sometimes free in the dermis.

DIAGNOSIS

Diagnosis can be established in the above conditions by obtaining a supporting history and examining superficial skin scrapings after maceration of samples with 40% potassium hydroxide. Alternatively, a punch biopsy may also be used to establish the diagnosis. Presence of *Demodex* mites alone is not sufficient to declare infestation as the etiology of skin findings, as the mites are ubiquitous, although in the context of an appropriate clinical picture, a presumptive diagnosis can be made. Response to antimite therapy provides further confirmation of etiology.

MANAGEMENT

Treatment of conditions associated with the *Demodex* mites includes topical and oral agents. Good facial hygiene with regular cleansing and avoidance of occlusive agents, such as heavy creams and makeups, is essential to managing these problems. Topically, salicylic acid and retinoids may prove beneficial by promoting desquamation of epidermal cells, which allows quicker shedding of mites and the associated waste products. Topical 1% lindane lotion, 1% gamma benzene hexachloride lotion, 1% permethrin cream rinse, or sulfur has also been used to treat demodicidosis in AIDS patients. Orally, metronidazole may offer clinical benefit, though the exact mechanism is uncertain as mites can tolerate relatively high concentrations of this agent. Other treatments that have been used are similar to those implemented for eosinophilic folliculitis including UV light and retinoids.

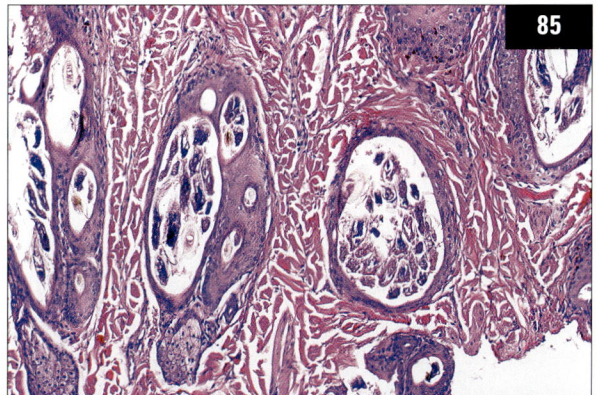

85 Cross-sections of skin showing *Demodex* mites (H&E).

AMEBIASIS

DEFINITION/OVERVIEW

Amebas are free living protozoa that can be contracted by sexual contact or by contaminated water or soil. Several different ameba species are capable of causing cutaneous disease in immunocompromised humans. Though relatively rare, detection and correct diagnosis of cutaneous lesions may allow prevention of potentially life-threatening dissemination. Cutaneous infection by *Acanthamoeba* has been reported more than 20 times in HIV-infected persons since Gonzalez *et al.* reported the first case in 1986.[17] All reported cases of cutaneous *Acanthamoeba* have occurred in persons with a CD4 counts below $250 \times 10^6/l$. There is no association with race or route of HIV acquisition.

Though more commonly associated with gastrointestinal disease, *Entamoeba histolytica* may also rarely produce cutaneous lesions, primarily involving the genitals, in both immunocompromised and immunocompetent persons. *E. histolytica* is estimated to infect nearly 500 million persons worldwide, with higher risk in travelers to tropical regions, immigrants, migrant workers, immunocompromised individuals, homosexual men, and institutionalized persons. A review of reported cases of genital amebiasis due to *E. histolytica* showed that 85% were adult females.[18] Countries of origin of infection included Mexico, New Guinea, Asia, and the US, with the majority of patients being of Hispanic ethnicity. Poor genital hygiene and concomitant intestinal or rectosigmoid amebic infections increase the risk of developing genital amebiasis. This ameba is common in tropical regions and is spread by fecal–oral contact, sexual transmission, or by contaminated food and water.

PATHOGENESIS/PATHOPHYSIOLOGY

Acanthamoeba exists in two forms, cyst and trophozoite. The cyst form allows the organism to tolerate unfavorable environmental conditions until favorable conditions are present at which time the trophozoite form develops, which is the infectious form of the organism. Infection may occur either by hematogenous spread from primary sites in the lungs or sinuses or directly through the skin.

CLINICAL FEATURES

Cutaneous infections with *Acanthamoeba* manifest as one or multiple hard erythematous skin nodules or nonhealing painful ulcerations with central eschars. These lesions are often located on the face, trunk, and extremities (86). Infestations may present as early firm papulonodules with purulent drainage that become indurated ulcerations or may present in the cutaneous disseminated form. At times, these lesions precede potentially lethal systemic dissemination and CNS involvement. However, due to the rare occurrence, diagnosis may be delayed until ineffective treatment for presumed bacterial infections warrants a biopsy. If wrongly treated with topical or intralesional steroids, the lesions tend to worsen in severity. Patients usually have advanced HIV disease and considerable immunodeficiency. Due to the poor health status of these patients, mortality after onset of lesions is reported at 73% when CNS involvement is not detected; if CNS involvement is present the mortality rate is virtually 100%.[19]

Infection with *E. histolytica* has been reported to produce genital lesions, independent of immune status. Female genital amebiasis often manifests as a malodorous bloody vaginal discharge and occasionally is the cause of deep genital ulceration that may be mistaken for cervical carcinoma. If neglected, infection may lead to necrotizing vulvitis requiring radical vulvectomy.[20] Vigilence should be maintained for concurrent cancer, as one study reported 7.4% of patients with genital amebiasis also had concomitant genital squamous cell cancer. The majority of men with genital amebiasis present with a painful discharging ulcer, which also may be mistaken for carcinoma. There is no reported difference in the manifestation of this infestation with concurrent HIV/AIDS infection.

HISTOPATHOLOGY

Biopsy of cutaneous lesions typically reveals a dermal lymphohistiocytic perivascular infiltrate, neutrophilic panniculitis with variable necrosis, and suppurative or granulomatous inflammation. *Acanthamoeba* organisms in cyst or trophozoite form may be identified in biopsies taken from the lesion margins.[21] Cysts can be visualized with periodic acid-Schiff

(PAS) and Gomori methenamine silver (GMS) stains. Trophozoites are relatively large (15–35 μm), stain PAS-positive, and have surface projections called acanthopodia.

Histologic findings in *E. histolytica* infections are nonspecific, such as ulceration with acute and chronic inflammation and granulomas with pseudo-epitheliomatous hyperplasia. *Entamoeba* organisms may be identified in biopsies taken from the base of the ulceration. Cysts stain negatively with GMS, differentiating them from *Acanthamoeba* cysts. Trophozoites are 15–25 μm in size with a small nucleus and may contain phagocytized erythrocytes, which *Acanthamoeba* typically do not demonstrate.

DIAGNOSIS

In any AIDS patient with a nonhealing cutaneous lesion, evaluation should include cultures for bacteria, mycobacteria, fungi, and *Bartonella*. Cultures for trophozoites in ameba growth medium, onto mammalian cell cultures, or onto non-nutrient agar plates seeded with *E. coli* or *E. aerogenes* will allow definitive diagnosis. Serologic testing is not useful due to the ubiquitous nature of these organisms. Histologic findings from biopsies may mimic fungi, viruses, mycobacteria, or foreign body inflammation; mistaken diagnosis is commonly reported. Therefore, if clinical suspicion is high and the first biopsy is unrevealing of trophozoites, a second biopsy may be indicated.

Diagnosis of genital amebiasis due to *E. histolytica* can be obtained in females by Papanicolaou smear in the majority of cases, with biopsy necessary in less than 10%. In males, however, biopsy is necessary in more than 90% in order to derive the correct diagnosis. Other diagnostic tools include culture, direct smear, and wet prep of discharge fluid. Serologic tests, such as immuno-fluorescent antibody tests, radioimmunoassays, enzyme-linked immunosorbent assays, and counter-current immunoelectrophoresis are also available; however, tests may remain positive for over 10 years after infection.

MANAGEMENT

Many agents have been used to treat cutaneous *Acanthamoeba* infections, including pentamidine, fluconazole, ketoconazole, neomycin, polymyxin B, rifampicin, sulfadiazine, 5-flucytosine, azithromycin, topical econazole, and chlorhexidine. Only three cases of successful treatment have been reported. One patient was treated with 5-flucytosine, one with both pentamidine and 5-flucytosine, and one with a combination of fluconazole, 5-flucytosine, and sulfadiazine.[22–24]

Genital amebiasis is often successfully treated with antibiotics, including metronidazole. In women, puromycin or iodoquinol vaginal suppositories may be used in combination with antibiotics. If metronidazole therapy fails, a biopsy is warranted to investigate for carcinoma. Treatment is independent of HIV status.

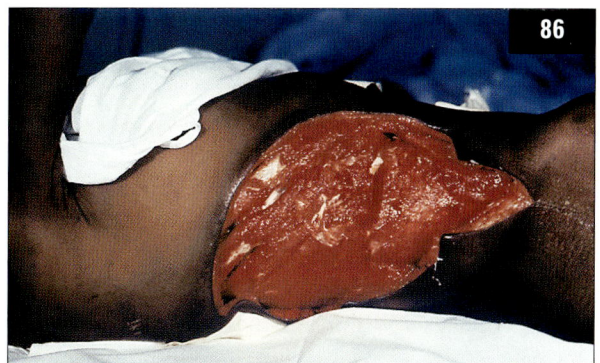

86 Invasive extraintestinal amebiasis affecting the cutaneous region of the right flank causing severe tissue necrosis. (Courtesy of CDC.)

LEISHMANIASIS

DEFINITION/OVERVIEW

An estimated 15 million people are infected with leishmaniasis, with 2 million new cases occurring each year. Leishmaniasis is primarily a disease of warmer climates, as the spread of disease is largely limited by the geographic range of its vector, the sandfly. To date, leishmaniasis has been reported in 88 countries and five continents. Both the number of cases annually and the geographic distribution of this disease have been increasing in recent years due largely to environmental changes and human development. Approximately 90% of muco-cutaneous leishmaniasis cases are from the South American countries Bolivia, Brazil, and Peru. Approximately 90% of cutaneous leishmaniasis cases are from Afghanistan, Brazil, Iran, Peru, Saudi Arabia, and Syria.

All persons living within endemic regions are at risk of developing leishmaniasis. This disease is more common in rural areas, especially in persons likely to be outdoors at night time hours, during peak sandfly activity. In the US, cases are primarily limited to those cases originating in rural southern Texas and cases contracted abroad in immigrants, travelers, and military personnel.

PATHOGENESIS/PATHOPHYSIOLOGY

Leishmania spp. are bloodborne protozoan parasites responsible for a spectrum of human diseases from self-healing ulcers to disseminated and potentially fatal infections. Clinically, manifestation and severity depend upon both host immune status and which of the more than 20 species is the responsible parasite. This parasite is spread by a sandfly vector, genus *Phlebotomus* in the Old World and *Lutzomyia* in the New World. Within the vector, they develop into the promastigote form, which is motile via anterior flagella. The protozoa are transmitted to humans by the bite of the sandfly, whereupon it is phagocytosed by macrophages. Within the macrophage lysosomes, the parasite develops into an immobile amastigote form, the obligate intracellular form responsible for human disease. The lifecycle is repeated when another sandfly feeds upon an infected person, allowing the amastigote to enter the vector and develop into the promastigote form. Persons with HIV are more susceptible to developing infection after inoculation of the parasite by the vector, tend to develop more severe disease, and have more recurrences after treatment than immunocompetent persons.

CLINICAL FEATURES

As previously mentioned, leishmaniasis is responsible for a wide spectrum of human disease. This chapter will discuss mucocutaneous and cutaneous leishmaniasis.

Cutaneous leishmaniasis is caused when one of several different *Leishmania* spp. is transmitted to a human. In the Old World, *Leishmania tropica* and *L. major* are the most commonly contracted species. In the New World, responsible species include *L. leishmania* (e.g. *L. mexicana*, *L. amazonensis*, *L. chagasi*) and *L. viannia* (e.g. *L. panamensis*, *L. braziliensis*, *L. guyanensis*). Disease becomes evident 2–6 weeks after initial infection when an erythematous papule develops at the site of inoculation. This papule increases in size, becoming a nodule that undergoes central ulceration and crusting (87, 88).

The ulcer can be large in size with raised distinct borders and is painless unless secondarily infected. Multiple lesions may be present if more than one bite occurred and nodular lymphangitis has been described.[25] With no intervention, the ulceration will spontaneously heal in months to years, depending upon the infecting species, leaving a depressed scar. It should be noted that leishmaniasis has been reported as a source of genital ulcers in tropical regions.[26]

Mucocutaneous leishmaniasis typically develops in the nose or palate after an initial cutaneous infection. These lesions are progressively destructive to mucosa and cartilage, ultimately leading to severe scarring and disfigurement.

In persons with immunocompromise due to HIV, several atypical forms may develop, perhaps due to the fact that both agents infect monocytes and macrophages. HIV-infected persons may be unable to mount a sufficient TH-1 response to control the parasitic infection. Coinfection with HIV and

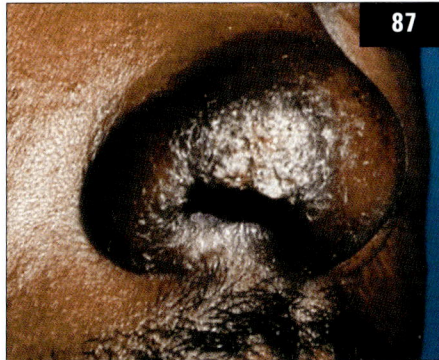

87 Leishmaniasis. Crusted nodule on the alar rim.

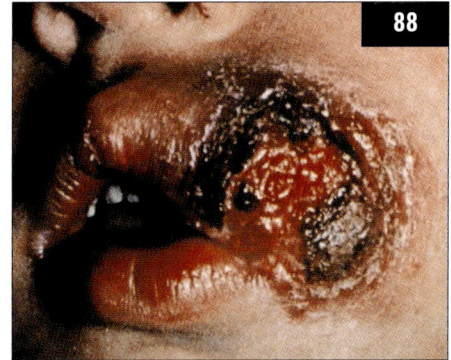

88 Large ulcerative, crusted nodule on the lip.

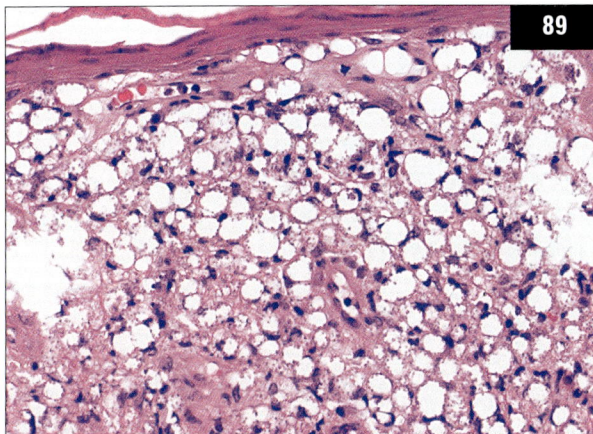

89 Histology of leishmaniasis. Skin biopsy showing numerous organisms contained in clear vacuoles within macrophages.

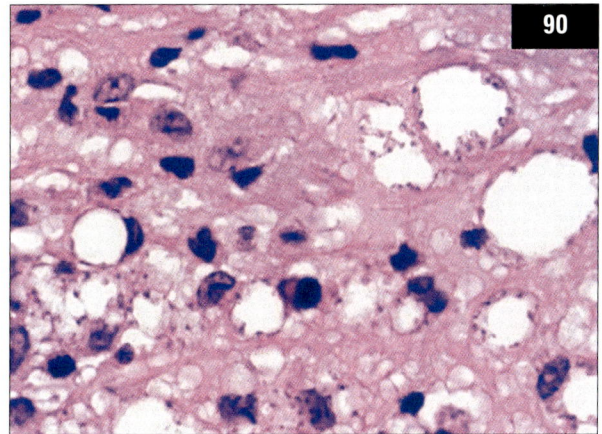

90 Higher power view of the *Leishmania* organisms arranged peripherally in clear vacuoles within macrophages.

Leishmania also increases the risk of developing visceral leishmaniasis and, due to frequent parasitemia, efficiency of transmission to other persons is increased. Diffuse cutaneous leishmaniasis is a form of infection that persists for years with no spontaneous resolution. Leishmaniasis recidivans has been reported in approximately 10% of cases. It is characterized by papules and nodules with an 'apple jelly' appearance upon diascopic pressure. Postkala-azar dermal leishmaniasis (PKDL) occurs 6 months to 5 years after an episode of untreated or undertreated visceral leishmaniasis, due to *L. donovani*. PKDL manifests in three different morphologies which may be present singularly or simultaneously: hypopigmented macules, nodules and plaques, and erythema of the face. *L. donovani* is identified in the lesions of less than 50% of patients.[27]

HISTOPATHOLOGY

The characteristic findings microscopically include a dense diffuse infiltrate of histiocytes, lymphocytes, and plasma cells with variable overlying epidermal hyperplasia that may be frankly pseudocarcinomatous. Many of the histiocytes have abundant pale-staining cytoplasm and within them, characteristic *Leishmania* organisms are often readily visualized. The organisms tend to be situated at the periphery of these cells giving an appearance similar to a ferris wheel (89, 90). In some cases, the number of organisms may be small and, as such, they may not be visible. Histopathologic findings in PKDL include epidermal atrophy, follicular plugging, and an inflammatory infiltrate composed of plasma cells, lymphocytes, and histiocytes.

DIAGNOSIS

Obtaining a history of recent travel to endemic regions should increase suspicion for a diagnosis of leishmaniasis in patients with cutaneous ulcerations. Superficial skin scrapings may be used as a diagnostic test, but yield a sensitivity of only 70–75%. The affected area should be cleaned of any existing crust and scraping should be obtained from the center and margin of the ulceration, keeping in mind that parasites are less likely to be detected in lesions older than 4 months. Slides should be fixed, stained with Giemsa stain, and examined thoroughly under oil emersion. The amastigotes may be identified inside monocytes or extracellularly. In order to differentiate *Leishmania* from other infectious organisms, it is necessary to identify both the nucleus and the kinetoplast, a rod-shaped structure of extranuclear DNA. Alternatively, a 2–3 mm punch biopsy from the active ulcer border may also be used for diagnosis. In papular and nodular lesions, diagnosis may be obtained with a culture of needle aspirate after injecting a small amount of sterile saline into the affected area. *Leishmania* will grow on blood agar Nicolle–Novy–MacNeal media. Immunologic tests, such as antibody detection and PCR, are highly sensitive but not standardized and are species specific.

MANAGEMENT

Several therapeutic agents are available for treatment of leishmaniasis. It has been reported that pretreatment HIV viral load correlates with therapeutic response in persons with visceral leishmaniasis, though no studies have looked at treatment response and HIV in those with cutaneous or mucocutaneous lesions.[28] Pentavalent antimonials, including meglumine antimoniate and sodium stibogluconate, administered intravenously for 20 days have a cure rate of 94% in immunocompetent patients. Therapeutic success is determined by evidence of healing at 2 months following treatment, no evidence of recurrence at 12 months, and no occurrence of mucosal disease. Care must be taken in patients with HIV nephropathy or other renal disease as this drug class is renally excreted. Recently, there have been reports of antimonial-resistant strains of leishmaniasis, leading to increased investigation of

treatment with amphotericin B in both regular and liposomal forms. Liposomal amphotericin B is known to be less toxic than the conventional form and there have been reports that it is more rapidly effective in visceral leishmaniasis. However, reports of amphotericin use in cutaneous leishmaniasis have been conflicting and no definitive randomized studies have been reported to date. There has been one reported case of intralesional ampotericin B injections resulting in clinical resolution in leishmaniasis recidivans. Recently, there has been some speculation on the possibility of resistance developing to amphotericin B. Pentamidine isethionate is another alternative, administered as intramuscular injections every other day for a week, though this drug may induce diabetes and the toxic effects to the pancreas, bone marrow, and kidney may be irreversible. Topical paromomycin is effective with *L. major* and *L. mexicana* and can be combined with antimonials. Oral antifungals have demonstrated conflicting results, but may be effective for infection with *L. mexicana* and *L. major*. Allopurinol also has demonstrated conflicting results and it is not recommended as a lone agent, though if used in conjunction with antimonials, a synergistic effect has been reported. Physical destruction with heat or cryotherapy may be effective, though reported trials failed to compare destructive therapy with standard treatment controls.

OTHER PARASITES

FILIARIASIS

In tropical regions of Africa, Asia, South America, the Caribbean, and the Pacific, *Wuchereria bancrofti* is the most common filarial worm causing disease in humans, infecting 100 million people. Mosquitoes are responsible for transmitting the larvae, which develop into adult worms in the human host. When adult worms die, the immune system manifests an acute inflammatory reaction with lymphatic dysfunction leading to classic symptoms of lymphangiectasis, hydroceles, and elephantiasis. The diagnosis may be made early by detecting microfilaria released into the blood stream or later by ultrasound. Antibody and antigen detection is also available, though limited. Treatment of infestation is with diethylcarbamazine 6 mg/kg/day in three doses for 12 days. Ivermectin is effective for killing microfilariae but is ineffective in adult worms. However, manifestations of the damaged lymphatic system may necessitate surgery, even after resolution of the infestation. Skin overlaying involved areas may develop bacterial skin infections due to poor lymphatic drainage and severe edema. There is no reported case of HIV/AIDS altering the natural history of this parasitic disease. However, it has been reported that persons with untreated lymphatic filariasis show enhanced HIV replication that may lead to rapid progression to AIDS.[29]

SCHISTOSOMIASIS

Schistosomiasis is the second most prevalent tropical disease after malaria, with an estimated 193 million people currently infected, 85% of whom are in Africa. This parasite is transmitted through exposure to water shared by certain snail species, which are natural hosts. The motile parasite form, the miracidium, penetrates human skin and initiates the disease process. Infestation by one of three helminthic parasites causes human disease involving the bladder (*Schistosoma haematobium*) and rectum (*S. mansoni, S. japonicum*). Less commonly known, these parasites may also cause genital lesions in both men and women.

Female genital schistosomiasis develops in 6–60% of females with intestinal schistosomiasis, depending on the infecting species. This condition occurs at all sites of the genital tract and may be confused with cervical carcinoma or genital warts. Affected areas show thinning, erosion, and ulceration of the epithelium as an inflammatory response mounts around ova, leading to granulomata formation near the basal layer of the epithelium.[30,31] Vulvar manifestations include swelling, ulceration, pruritus, and verrucous growths. Vaginal 'sandy patches' are distinctive; other vaginal manifestations include ulcers, growths, and rectovaginal or vesicovaginal fistulas. There is concern that genital schistosomiasis may accelerate the development and spread of cervical cancer from human papillomavirus infection. The mucosal lesions and inflammation may increase

HIV transmission more so than other sexually transmitted infections that disrupt the mucosal barrier.[30,32] This is due to the high percentage of CD4+ cells present in the granulomata, leading to numerous ports of entry for the virus after it crosses the friable and eroded epithelium.[33]

Male genital schistosomiasis manifests primarily as changes in semen volume or consistency, or as hemospermia. Inflammation of the prostate and seminal vesicles may also increase susceptibility to infection with HIV in afflicted males.[34] Additionally, this inflammation may also increase viral shedding in males coinfected with HIV and genital schistosomiasis.

Though there has been speculation that antihelminthic therapy is less effective in immunodeficient persons, this has not proved true to date.[35]

TRYPANOSOMIASIS

Trypanosomiasis has not been reported to produce cutaneous lesions and coinfection with trypanosomosomes and HIV is poorly characterized.

CHAGAS' DISEASE

Asides from an ulcer at the initial site of inoculation and the potential development of Romana's sign (periorbital edema), there are no reported cutaneous manifestations of Chagas' disease, regardless of immunocompetence.

ONCHOCERCIASIS

Onchocerciasis has not been reported to produce cutaneous lesions and coinfection with onchocerciasis and HIV is poorly characterized, though it has been noted that coinfected persons have impaired cellular immune response of unknown significance.[36]

CHAPTER 6

CUTANEOUS MANIFESTATIONS OF HIGHLY ACTIVE ANTIRETROVIRAL THERAPY

Deborah B. Henderson and Clay J. Cockerell

INTRODUCTION

The introduction of combination antiretroviral drug therapy in the mid 1990s resulted in a dramatic decrease in morbidity and mortality among patients infected with human the immunodeficiency virus (HIV).[1] These drug combinations, referred to as highly active antiretroviral therapy (HAART), have been shown to reduce viral replication significantly and reconstitute CD4+ lymphocyte counts in HIV-positive patients.[2] The drugs that comprise HAART regimens are categorized by their distinct mechanisms of action into four main groups: non-nucleoside reverse transcriptase inhibitors (NNRTIs), nucleoside reverse transcriptase inhibitors (NRTIs), protease inhibitors (PIs), and fusion or entry inhibitors. Since their implementation, the overall utility of these medications has been complicated by an increasing number of adverse drug reactions that have become recognized. Documented cutaneous side-effects such as pigmentation disorders, urticarial eruptions, and hypersensitivity reactions have all been associated with HAART therapy. In addition, a common adverse effect is a syndrome of hyperlipidemia, abnormal fat distribution, and glucose intolerance known as the lipodystrophy syndrome.[3] Such side-effects have substantially diminished compliance with antiretroviral medications and pose a problem for their continued use.[4]

NON-NUCLEOSIDE REVERSE TRANSCRIPTASE INHIBITORS

Overall, the non-nucleoside analogs have less associated toxicity than other antiretroviral agents. Cutaneous complications, however, comprise a substantial proportion of the side-effects that are encountered. These medications selectively bind the active site of the viral reverse transcriptase enzyme and block the HIV replication cycle at the point of ribonucleic acid (RNA)-dependent deoxyribonucleic acid (DNA) synthesis. This binding triggers a conformational change in the enzyme thus rendering it inactive. NNRTIs have specific antagonism against the HIV-1 (and not HIV-2) reverse transcriptase enzyme, a characteristic that explains in part the lower incidence of side-effects associated with this class of antiretrovirals. Currently, there are three drugs in this category: nevirapine, delavirdine, and efavirenz (*Table 2*).

Previous studies have documented a morbilliform eruption as a major clinical toxicity in patients receiving nevirapine and delavirdine. Skin findings range from mild to severe and generally occur within the first few weeks of therapy. Overall, the incidence of developing drug hypersensitivity is higher with nevirapine than with delavirdine and efavirenz, ranging from 9% to 32% in recent studies.[5,6] Roughly 4% of patients on nevirapine must discontinue the agent because of toxicity. In a smaller percentage of cases, severe and potentially life-threatening eruptions such as Stevens–Johnson syndrome (SJS)[7]and 'drug rash with eosinophilia and systemic symptoms' (DRESS)[8] result from continued nevirapine use. Patients receiving this treatment may also

Table 2 Antiretroviral agents currently approved in the US and/or UK

	MUCOCUTANEOUS ADVERSE DRUG REACTIONS	OTHER ADVERSE EFFECTS
Non-nucleoside reverse transcriptase inhibitors	Morbilliform eruption, EM, SJS	Hepatotoxicity, lactic acidosis
Delavirdine		
Efavirenz	Gynecomastia, leukocytoclastic vasculitis, hypersensitivity	CNS effects (i.e. dizziness, psychosis)
Nevirapine	DRESS/hypersensitivity syndrome, SJS	
Nucleoside reverse transcriptase inhibitors	Hypersensitivity	Lactic acidosis, hepatomegaly with steatosis
Abacavir	Hypersensitivity syndrome	Gastrointestinal upset
Abacavir/lamivudine/zidovudine		
Didanosine	Xerostomia, alopecia, peripheral neuropathy, SJS, leukocytoclastic vasculitis	Pancreatitis, optic neuritis, retinal changes
Emtricitabine	Dry skin, rash, palmoplantar hyperpigmentation	
Lamivudine	Paronychia, rash, alopecia	Pancreatitis
Lamivudine/zidovudine		
Stavudine	Peripheral neuropathy, lipodystrophy syndrome	
Tenofovir DF		
Zalcitabine	Macular rash, urticaria, peripheral neuropathy, oral/esophageal ulceration	Pancreatitis
Zidovudine	Blue-black pigmentation of nails and mucosa, urticaria, morbilliform eruption, leukocytoclastic vasculitis, anaphylaxis, lipoatrophy, acral/periarticular reticulate erythema	Bone marrow suppression, increased mean corpuscular volume, thrombocytopenia, nausea, dilated cardiomyopathy, myalgia
Protease inhibitors	Morbilliform eruption, generalized erythema, SJS, lipodystrophy syndrome, striae formation, pruritus, paronychia, ingrown toenails, xerosis, desquamative chelitis	Hyperlipidemia, insulin resistance, hepatotoxicity, lactic acidosis
Amprenavir		Hyperbilirubinemia
Atazanavir		
Fosamprenavir		

(Continued overleaf)

Table 2 Antiretroviral agents currently approved in the US and/or UK (*continued*)

	MUCOCUTANEOUS ADVERSE DRUG REACTIONS	OTHER ADVERSE EFFECTS
Indinavir	Paronychia, alopecia, gynecomastia, acute porphyria, SJS, xanthomas/striae/angiolipoma formation, lipodystrophy	
Lopinavir/ritonavir		
Nelfinavir		
Ritonavir	Perioral numbness, subcutaneous granuloma formation	Spontaneous bleeding
Saquinavir	Fixed drug reaction	
Fusion inhibitors	Injection site reaction	
Enfuvirtide		

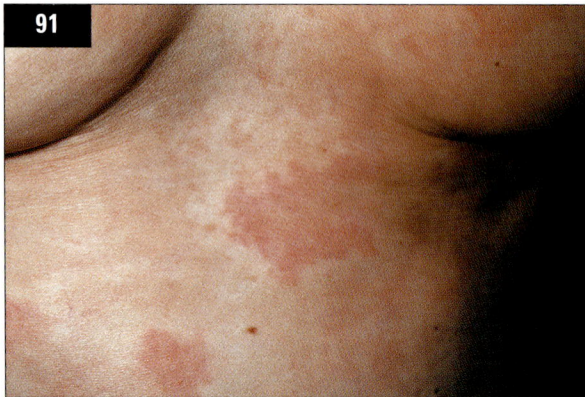

91 Urticarial vasculitis. Erythematous, slightly edematous irregular plaques with peripheral pallor on the chest and abdomen.

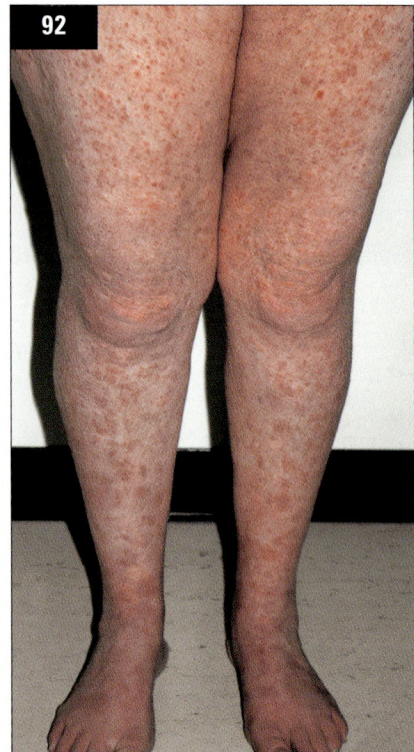

92 Extensive erythematous and purpuric coalescing papules on the legs.

exhibit signs of a systemic hypersensitivity syndrome with fever and abnormal liver function. Progressive lead-in dosing and cessation of drug use at the onset of the eruption can significantly reduce the severity of this side-effect.[9] In contrast, although delavirdine has been associated with isolated cases of severe morbilliform eruptions, patients on this NNRTI frequently have resolution of the eruption without discontinuation of the drug. On average, only 18% of patients taking delavirdine manifest a morbilliform eruption and it is seen more commonly in patients with low CD4+ counts.[10] In patients taking either medication, systemic antihistamines and corticosteroids are often used to provide symptomatic relief.

While central nervous system (CNS) adverse effects such as dizziness or psychosis are among the most important toxicities associated with efavirenz, cutaneous reactions are also quite common and develop in up to 34% of patients within the first 2 weeks of therapy. Patients generally develop a cutaneous hypersensitivity eruption that may take several forms including urticarial and morbilliform eruptions (**91, 92**). It also may induce gynecomastia[11] and leukocytoclastic vasculitis.[12] Fortunately, none of these commonly require drug discontinuation[13] and patients may successfully be desensitized using a short 14-day desensitization protocol in a controlled environment.[14]

In most cases, the clinical appearance of a cutaneous eruption along with a thorough medication history is sufficient to determine the etiology. Occasionally, however, identification of the specific offending agent is complicated by the multiplicity of drugs routinely being administered to HIV-positive patients. In these cases, skin biopsy and rechallenge with the suspected agent can be utilized to assist with the diagnosis. The histopathology of a typical NNRTI-related urticarial allergic eruption is distinguished by mixed infiltrates of interstitial inflammatory cells in the dermis with minimal change of the overlying epidermis. Eosinophilia may also be observed. In contrast, SJS is characterized histologically by prominent vacuolar interface changes with extensive keratinocyte necrosis in the epidermis.

MANAGEMENT

Essential to the treatment of a cutaneous drug eruption is withdrawal of the offending agent. This action lessens the likelihood of progression to dangerous life-threatening complications such as hepatic or renal toxicity, SJS, or toxic epidermal necrolysis (TEN). Adjunctive therapies used for symptomatic relief of pruritus include systemic antihistamines and corticosteroids. As noted above, desensitization has also been shown to be effective in some cases.

NUCLEOSIDE REVERSE TRANSCRIPTASE INHIBITORS

NRTIs also inhibit the HIV reverse transcription process. These drugs incorporate themselves into the viral DNA chain thereby impeding further DNA elongation and terminating the viral replication process. The list of currently approved NRTIs includes zidovudine, abacavir, didanosine, emtricitabine, lamivudine, stavudine, tenofovir, and zalcitabine (*Table 2*). Each of these medications has characteristic associated adverse effects. The toxicity profile of this group is best known for the hyperpigmentation disorder seen with zidovudine along with hypersensitivity reactions to abacavir. Similar to the PIs, certain NRTIs are also thought to produce the metabolic abnormalities and fat redistribution seen in lipodystrophy patients.

Nail and mucocutaneous hyperpigmentation are well established skin complications of zidovudine (93–96). Nail dyschromia is most commonly characterized by blue, brown, or black pigmented longitudinal bands beginning in the proximal nail fold and extending throughout the length of the nail

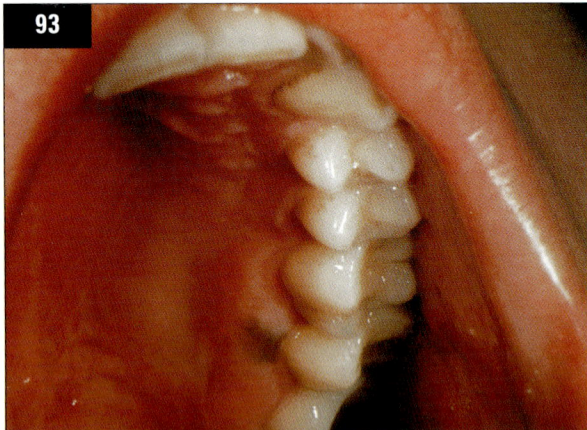

93 Hyperpigmentation of the palatal gingiva secondary to zidovudine.

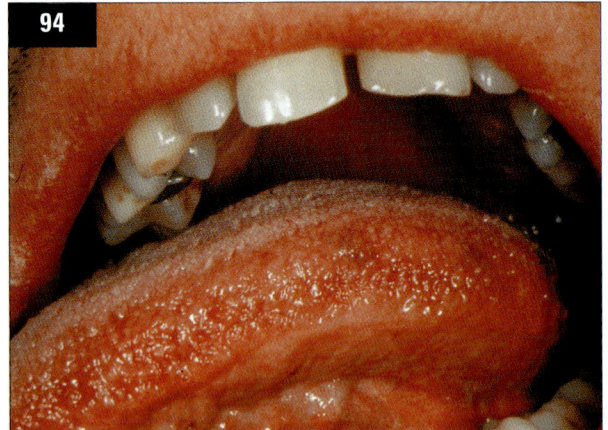

94 Subtle tongue hyperpigmentation in an HIV-infected patient treated with zidovudine.

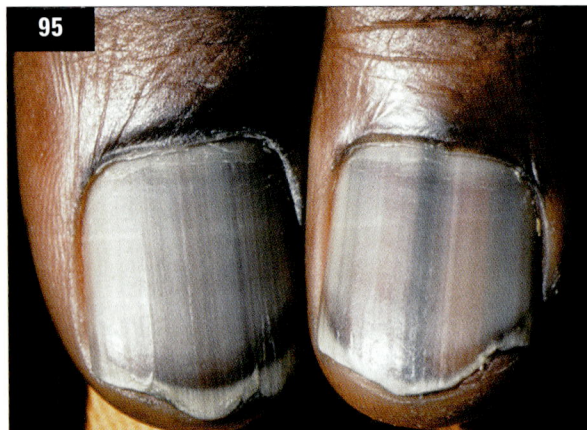

95 Longitudinal hyperpigmentation of the thumbnails characteristic of zidovudine hyperpigmentation.

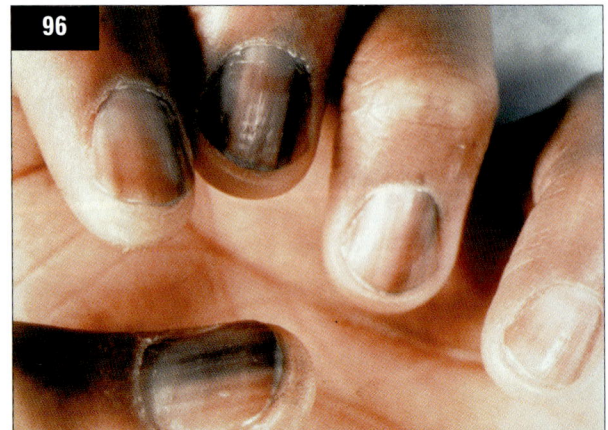

96 Extensive nail hyperpigmentation caused by zidovudine.

plate. They are usually multiple and begin within 8 weeks of treatment initiation.[15] Transverse or diffuse banding is seen less commonly. Histologically, zidovudine-induced nail pigmentation demonstrates increased melanin in the epidermis with scattered melanophages in the subepithelial connective tissue. Zidovudine may also produce skin or mucosal hyperpigmentation that mimics that seen with adrenal insufficiency.[16] These are dose-dependent and reversible, resolving with discontinuation of the drug. In addition to pigmentation abnormalities, pruritus, urticaria, morbilliform eruptions,[17] leukocytoclastic vasculitis,[18] SJS, and TEN[19] can rarely occur as side-effects of zidovudine therapy. Lichenoid drug-induced reactions that appear very similar to lichen planus, including white plaques of the oral mucosa and polygonal papules of the glabrous skin, have also been reported.[20]

Side-effects of abacavir include gastrointestinal upset and a cutaneous eruption. In 2–3% of cases, a multisystem hypersensitivity reaction may be observed within 6 weeks. The symptoms of this phenomenon include fever, morbilliform cutaneous eruption, nausea, diarrhea, hypotension, and respiratory or musculoskeletal dysfunction.[21] In general, the characteristic skin finding is a mild to moderately severe eruption that is generally less severe than that seen with the NNRTIs.[22] However, continued use of abacavir in the setting of hypersensitivity may lead to fatal complications; thus, current clinical guidelines recommend discontinuation of the abacavir with the appearance of a systemic allergic reaction. Similarly, rechallenge with abacavir after such a reaction is not advised as there have been rare cases of severe erythema multiforme (EM) developing as a consequence.[23] Patch testing with abacavir has been utilized in attempts to confirm the medication as the causal agent of cutaneous hypersensitivity and it may be useful in some cases.[24]

Various other cutaneous complications may arise from the use of other NRTIs. Emtricitabine has been shown to induce dry skin and a cutaneous eruption in up to one-third of patients. Palmoplantar hyperpigmentation is also rarely seen.[25] Cutaneous effects of didanosine, zalcitabine, and lamivudine are infrequent although rare cases of SJS[26] and leukocytoclastic vasculitis[27] have been reported with didanosine administration.

Changes in body fat are commonly inducted with NRTIs. NRTI-related lipoatrophy is proposed to involve drug-induced mitochondrial DNA depletion and overall mitochondrial dysfunction.[28] Histologically, fine needle or surgical biopsies of fat demonstrate nonencapsulated subcutaneous mature adipose tissue with occasional sclerotic changes.[29] Objective measurements of the body fat in lipodystrophic patients with dual energy X-ray absorptiometry, computed tomography (CT) and magnetic resonance imaging (MRI) scans confirm peripheral subcutaneous fat loss with intra-abdominal rather than subcutaneous increases in abdominal fat.[30] While all NRTIs can induce lipodystrophy, some do so more frequently than others[31] and switching from either stavudine or zidovudine to abacavir has been shown to reverse it.[32]

MANAGEMENT

As with other hypersensitivity reactions, those caused by zidovudine and abacavir are best managed by discontinuing administration of the offending agent. Resolution of a hypersensitivity eruption generally occurs once this is done although some eruptions may last for weeks or longer after the offending agent is removed from the therapeutic regimen. Additional supportive care is utilized as needed. A discussion of the treatment of lipodystrophy is included later.

PROTEASE INHIBITORS

PIs are the most recently approved agents used for treatment of HIV infection. Current treatment guidelines recommend the use of one PI in combination with nucleoside analogs to suppress viral load maximally. PIs function by binding the HIV-1 viral protease and inactivating it. This enzyme cleaves nascent virions from the infected CD4+ cell and inhibition of this protein arrests viral maturation and thwarts further production of infectious viral progeny. When used in combination with reverse transcriptase inhibitors, PIs have shown unparalleled efficacy in the suppression of viral replication as well as augmentation of CD4+ lymphocyte levels. For this reason, they are used extensively in antiretroviral treatment protocols. Unfortunately, obstacles to the regular use of these medications include a number of drug–drug interactions, increasing viral resistance, and frequent cutaneous complications.

Currently approved PIs include indinavir, ritonavir, saquinavir, nelfinavir, lopinavir, amprenavir, fosamprenavir, and atazanavir (*Table 2*). Each of these has its own distinct toxicities. Of the PIs, indinavir has the greatest number of reported cutaneous complications which include gynecomastia,[33] acute porphyria,[34] hypersensitivity eruptions,[35] and SJS.[36] Two nonhypersensitivity toxicities that are seen quite commonly include progressive alopecia and painful inflammation of the fingernails and toenails. Indinavir-related hair loss is diffuse or patchy and it involves the scalp, lower extremities, axilla, thorax, and genital areas. It is usually first noticed during the first 6 months of treatment. Similarly, indinavir-associated paronychia typically develops within 1–9 months after initiation of the PI therapy. Patients with paronychia often exhibit concurrent granulomatous lesions and granulation tissue in their nail sulci.[37,38] These adverse effects have been shown to resolve completely upon discontinuation of the medication. A higher incidence of lipodystrophy is seen with indinavir than any other PI and includes other manifestations of abnormal lipid metabolism such as xanthomas.[39] Striae[40] and angiolipomas[41] may also be seen.

While neither amprenavir nor its prodrug, fosamprenavir, cause the metabolic disturbances seen with indinavir, cutaneous hypersensitivity reactions are a common side-effect of both. Approximately 20% of patients taking amprenavir are reported to develop an eruption soon after starting treatment. Generally, the eruption is mild and fewer than 5% of patients discontinue their therapy because of it. In rare cases, it may be more severe.[42] An isolated cutaneous eruption occurs in 7% of patients receiving fosamprenavir. Most of these eruptions are mild although SJS has been reported.[43] Atazanavir, an azapeptide PI with convenient single day dosing, may cause hyperbilirubinemia and a mild eruption comparable to that of fosamprenavir; as with amprenavir and fosamprenavir, it does not alter lipid levels.[44]

Of the remaining PIs, ritonavir, nelfinavir, and saquinavir all may cause a number of cutaneous side-effects. Ritonavir induces spontaneous bleeding with purpura in both hemophiliacs and patients with normal hemostasis.[45] It can also cause perioral numbness, subcutaneous granulomas,[46] and hypersensitivity reactions that are refractory to steroid suppression.[47] Nelfinavir causes urticarial and morbilliform eruptions in up to 25% of patients.[48] Fixed drug eruptions associated with saquinavir have also been reported.[49] Several other adverse events common to PIs as a group include hypersensitivity reactions,[50] acute generalized eruptive pustulosis (AGEP),[51] and altered gustatory sensation.[52] Previous studies have documented 4–12.5% of PI recipients developing morbilliform or urticarial hypersensitivity reactions.[53] A much higher proportion of patients identify taste disturbances to bitter, salt, citrus, and sweet flavors.[4] Other rare cutaneous adverse events associated with PI use include generalized pruritus, xerosis, desquamative chelitis,[54] striae formation, angiolipomatosis,[55] and ingrown toenails.[56]

In general, PIs are thought to induce skin complications via several different mechanisms. These drugs are known to inhibit the P-450 3A cytochromes, an action that leads to diminished retinoic acid oxidative metabolism, with subsequent increase in effects associated with elevated retinoic acid levels such as alopecia, paronychia, and xerosis. Other suggested mechanisms to explain cutaneous side-effects specific to PIs include alterations in retinoic acid signaling, autoimmune destruction of hair follicles, and immunoglobulin (Ig)A/IgE-mediated hypersensitivities. In patients taking ritonavir therapy, biopsies of drug-induced hypersensitivity reactions have demonstrated normal C3 and C4 levels, a sign suggestive of an IgA-mediated etiology since it does not activate complement by the classical pathway.[13] Alternatively, successful desensitization in patients suffering from nelfinavir-induced urticaria suggests an underlying IgE-mediated mechanism.[57] Finally, a large number of PI-related cutaneous complications are attributed to an immune reconstitution phenomenon. Research is still ongoing to determine more specific mechanisms through which these drugs exert their clinical effects.

MANAGEMENT

As mentioned before, many of the PI-related toxicities demonstrate complete resolution without treatment following discontinuation of the PI. Steroid coadministration has varying success at improving cutaneous eruptions and hypersensitivity syndromes,[58] and systemic antihistamines are administered for symptomatic improvement of accompanying pruritus. Desensitization is also utilized to prevent additional cases of nelfinavir-associated urticarial eruptions. Diet, exercise, and weight loss are simple, first-line therapies for PI-associated fat redistribution and metabolic derangement. Other more invasive treatment modalities for lipodystrophy are discussed below.

FUSION INHIBITORS

Fusion inhibitors (FIs) are the newest class of antiretrovirals. This group of drugs exerts its effect through specific inhibition of gp41, a CD4+ trans-membrane glycoprotein. This action successfully blocks the binding between the host and virus cells, and prevents structural changes necessary for membrane fusion between virus and host. Of this drug class, only enfuvirtide/T-20 is currently approved for use in patients with poor response to other antiretroviral agents. Enfuvirtide is administered via subcutaneous injection and is most commonly associated with injection site reactions. These are characterized by induration, erythema, nodules, cysts, and tenderness at and around the injection site. Up to 98% of patients experienced this complication in Phase III trials.[59] Biopsies of involved areas reveal a localized hypersensitivity reaction with changes suggestive of an interstitial granulomatous drug reaction.[58] Mixed lymphocytic infiltrates with neutrophils and with or without eosinophils are also seen histologically. Some authors have proposed that rotating injection sites, smaller injection volumes, and specific peptide use may help to minimize the number of enfuvirtide-induced injection reactions.[60]

LIPODYSTROPHY

Perhaps the most feared adverse effect associated with HAART therapy is lipodystrophy syndrome (97, 98). This condition is characterized by a constellation of findings that include fat redistribution with disturbed lipid and glucose metabolism. It is most commonly observed with the PI and NRTI antiretrovirals. Within 2–12 months of drug initiation, up to 60% of HIV-positive patients develop symmetric lipomatosis, buccal and parotid fat pad atrophy, and peripheral fat wasting with prominence of their superficial vasculature. Additionally, these individuals exhibit increased central and visceral adiposity ('protease paunch' or 'crixbelly'), supraclavicular adiposity ('buffalo hump'), and gynecomastia. Finally, metabolic changes such as insulin resistance, hyperglycemia, hypertriglyceridemia, and hypercholesterolemia are commonly present.[61]

Much remains unknown about the underlying pathogenesis of this condition. Notably, while PI or NNRTI use was initially felt to be solely responsible for this pattern of symptoms, lipodystrophic changes have now been reported in patients naïve to antiretrovirals.[62] Among the PIs, this abnormal fat distribution tends to occur irrespective of specific protease exposure, although its clinical onset is observed most rapidly after initiation of ritonavir and saquinavir. Of the NNRTIs, lipodystrophic changes are most commonly seen in patients taking zidovudine and stavudine. Recent studies have proposed a multifactorial etiology to explain this constellation of symptoms, with risk factors such as older age, lower CD4+ count, greater duration of HIV disease and treatment duration, and specific PI type all contributing to its development. In addition, a significant homology exists between the HIV protease and regions of two proteins that regulate lipid metabolism: low-density lipoprotein-related proteins (LRP) and cytoplasmic retinoic acid binding protein-1 (CRABP-1).[63] The cross reaction between PIs and these proteins is presumed to increase apoptosis of adipose cells, increase lipid release, and diminish the differentiation of peripheral adipocytes. Antagonism of LRP may also cause a decreased uptake of circulating fatty acids and chylomicrons, which in turn contributes to the metabolic disturbances that are seen in the lipodystrophy syndrome. Finally, drug-related inhibition of mitochondrial DNA replication and subsequent mitochondrial impairment may also play an etiologic role in this syndrome. Several congenital lipodystrophy syndromes known to be caused by mitochondrial dysfunction support this assumption.

MANAGEMENT

Treatment of the lipodystrophy syndrome initially involves medical management of hyperlipidemia and withdrawal of the offending agent. A complete reversal of body habitus is not always observed following discontinuation of drug administration. Furthermore, successful reversal of fat redistribution has been observed after changing drugs from zidovudine or stavudine to abacavir. However, switching among antiretrovirals generally does not significantly resolve fat redistribution.[29] Alternative treatments include diet, exercise, weight loss, liposuction, appetite stimulants, anabolic agents, recombinant human growth factor administration, and autologous fat transplantation to wasted areas. Injection of nonpermanent soft tissue augmentation with bovine or allogenic collagen and hyaluronic acid has also been reported. All of these modalities have had limited and varied success. A recently approved product for facial wasting is Sculptra (Dermik, Berwyn, PA), an injectable form of polylactic acid.[64] High-grade silicone, which can give permanent improvement of facial wasting, is currently under investigation by the Food and Drug Administration. Finally, some studies report that ketoconazole, known for its potent inhibition on adrenal steroidogenesis, can lead to partial resolution of enlarged cervical fat pads.[65] Unfortunately, recurrences are common.

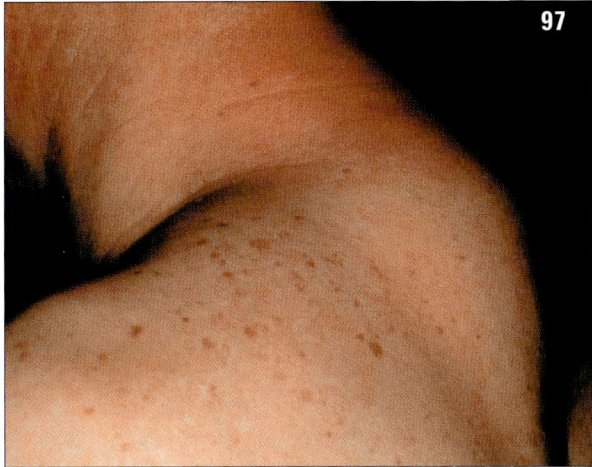

97 Lipohypertrophy of the dorsocervical fat pad ('buffalo hump').

98 Lipoatrophy with resulting nodularity of the forearm.

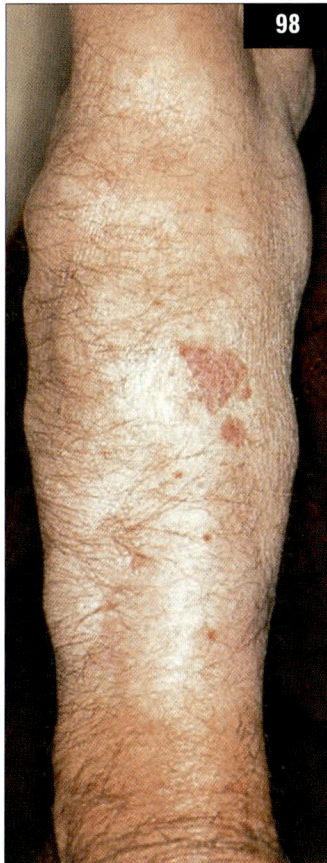

SUMMARY

Advances in HIV treatment have resulted in promising HAARTs that reduce patient morbidity, prolong survival, and improve quality of life. However, as new drugs are introduced and more patients are maintained on long-term antiretroviral treatment regimens, other systemic and cutaneous effects of antiretroviral therapy will likely be identified. Systemic corticosteroid administration during the period of immune reconstitution (generally, the initial 8 weeks of HAART therapy)[66] can potentially prevent undesirable drug reactions and other forms of hypersensitivity. Those who treat HIV-positive patients must be cognizant of these drug-related toxicities to tailor treatment for each patient, thus improving compliance and preventing potentially grave complications.

CHAPTER 7

PAPULOSQUAMOUS SKIN DISORDERS IN HIV INFECTION

Peter Morrell, Antoanella Calame, and Clay J. Cockerell

INTRODUCTION

Papulosquamous cutaneous diseases are a loosely defined category of dermatoses bound together by the fact that they all present clinically with scaly plaques and papules. In many cases, their exact etiologies are unknown. The major disease entities falling into this category include psoriasis, 'parapsoriasis', pityriasis lichenoides et varioliformis acuta (PLEVA), pityriasis lichenoides chronica (PLC), lymphomatoid papulosis, pityriasis rosea (PR), pityriasis rubra pilaris (PRP), pityriasis alba (PA), lichen planus (LP), lichen striatus (LS), lichen nitidus (LN), and seborrheic dermatitis (SD). Some clinicians also include xerosis, acquired icthyosis, and asteatotic dermatitis, especially in human immunodeficiency virus (HIV)-positive patients.

Many of the aforementioned conditions, in addition to being more prevalent, may display a fulminant or unusual clinical presentation in the setting of HIV infection. This is an important point to remember as it may serve as an important clue to the diagnosis of HIV infection where it might not otherwise be suspected. This is especially true of older individuals in whom HIV infection is less often considered and thus may be diagnosed at advanced stages.[1] As most of these conditions develop unusual characteristics when T cell counts fall below 150×10^6/l, they may guide prognosis and their severity often mirrors immunologic collapse.[2] The fact that these conditions change with the immune status of the host suggests an important role of the immune system in their pathogenesis.[3]

PSORIASIS

DEFINITION/OVERVIEW

Psoriasis is a chronic relapsing-remitting cutaneous disease that affects approximately 1–3% of the world's population. Along with SD and xerosis generalisata, it is by far one of the most commonly seen papulosquamous diseases in the HIV-infected population. Although its cause remains unknown, it is clear that both genetic and environmental factors play a role in pathogenesis. Psoriasis shows a wide heterogeneity of clinical expression. The characteristic sharply demarcated erythematous plaques with silver scale on the extensor surfaces tend to follow a bimodal distribution in terms of age of onset, but can appear at any age. Similarly, this disease, though it affects men and women equally, displays a wide range of severity. One patient may have 30% body surface area involvement while the next may simply show one localized plaque of disease.

Psoriasis in HIV-infected patients has the potential to be quite severe, often presenting in an explosive, even erythrodermic manner. For most patients, however, psoriasis is more emotionally and psychologically scarring than physically disabling.[4] Self-consciousness and depression are major causes of morbidity in psoriasis, resulting in higher rates of suicide in these patients.[5]

PATHOGENESIS/PATHOPHYSIOLOGY

Psoriasis is a complicated and multifactorial disease. Though research has shown it to have a predominately immune-mediated pathogenesis, its exact trigger remains unknown. Current theories revolve around the idea of a genetically susceptible individual being exposed to a critical initial antigen. Years of anecdotal evidence as well as concordance rates amongst monozygotic and dizygotic twins have proven this genetic susceptibility to be a fact.[5,6] Although the exact polygenic inheritance pattern has yet to be discovered, human leucocyte antigen (HLA) and linkage analysis may yet find it (*Table 3*).[6–9]

These histocompatibility antigens seem to be important not only in determining the psoriatic phenotype but also its clinical onset. Psoriatic patients have been subdivided into two subtypes, type I and type II. Type I patients have an early onset (less than 40 years of age), a positive family history, and express HLA-Cw6. Type II patients have a later onset and no family history or HLA-Cw6 expression.[5–7,10] Using polymerase chain reaction (PCR) typing with sequence specific primers, it has been shown that HLA-Cw 0602 is strongly associated with the development of HIV-associated psoriasis.[7]

Linkage studies have revealed the genetic loci PSOR1–PSOR7 to be fundamentally important in psoriasis (*Table 4*).[5,6] The S (corneodesmosin) gene that produces a protein found in terminally differentiated keratinocytes, and which is located only 160 kb from HLA-C is another target that is currently being investigated.[5,8]

It is on this background of genetic susceptibility that the immune dysregulatory process of psoriasis takes place.[10] TH-1 cells and the cytokines they elaborate appear to be the central effectors.[10] The most current theory proposes the initial event to be an (as yet to be determined) antigen being exposed to antigen-presenting cells (APCs) in the skin which in turn interact with subpopulations of T cells. Costimulation occurs and these activated T cells release a cascade of mediators such as tumor necrosis factor (TNF)-α and interferon (IFN)-γ. It is this cytokine milieu, in the end, which induces the secondary hyperproliferation of epidermal, vascular, and synovial cells that is characteristic of psoriasis.[4]

Although the precise antigenic stimulus for psoriasis remains unknown, a number of directly observable triggers are well recognized. One of the first described is the Koebner phenomenon which refers to physical trauma such as a sunburn inducing psoriatic lesions in previously healthy skin. Hypocalcemia, psychogenic stress, and drugs such as lithium or beta-blockers have all been found to induce psoriasis.[5,6] Infections caused by *Staphylococcus* sp. or *Streptococcus* sp. especially, may lead to flares of pre-existing disease as well as the appearance of guttate psoriasis.[5,9] Indeed, infection by group A, beta-hemolytic *Streptococcus* is recognized as one of the most repeatable triggers for the development of guttate psoriasis.[8] Current understanding hinges on the observation that there is sequence homology between keratin 14, a 50 kDa type I keratin, and the M6 protein of group A, beta-hemolytic *Streptococcus*.[7] Consequently, it is thought that a T cell directed response to this type of pathogen leads to a cross reaction with keratin

Table 3 HLA types associated with psoriasis	
HLA-Cw6	
HLA-Cw7	Japanese patients
HLA-Cw4	Chinese patients
HLA-DR7	
HLA-DR8	Kuwaiti children with (+) family history
HLA-B13	
HLA-B17	
HLA-B37	
HLA-Bw16	

Table 4 Genes linked to psoriasis[5,6,10]	
GENE	**CHROMOSOMAL LOCATION**
PSOR1	6p21.3
PSOR2	17q
PSOR3	4q
PSOR4	1q
PSOR5	3q
PSOR6	19p
PSOR7	1p

epitopes in the skin, producing the guttate psoriasis phenotype.[7]

One of the most important and repeatable inducers of psoriasis is HIV. The frequency of psoriasis is increased in HIV-infected patients as is aggravation of pre-existing disease. Furthermore, the severity of psoriasis is greater in these patients.[7,11–13] How HIV induces or exacerbates psoriasis is not known. In general, up until the terminal stages of HIV infection, psoriasis tends to worsen as immunodeficiency increases.[7] HIV virions have been detected in both keratinocytes and dendritic cells in psoriatic plaques[2,13] and *in situ* hybridization studies have found virions in dermal dendrocytes of lesional but not normal appearing skin.[13,14] It is still unknown whether it is the heightened immune response to HIV or the HIV itself that causes psoriasis, however. The direct causation theory points to the fact that transgenic mice with whole proviral sequences of HIV develop psoriasiform epidermal hyperplasia and acral scarring spontaneously.[7,14] Furthermore, the tat gene of HIV has been shown to stimulate epidermal and endothelial cell proliferation directly.[7] HIV has also been associated with the overexpression of TNF and INF-γ, as is found in psoriasis of the general population.[12,15,16] Another possibility is that HIV destroys the immune system to the point that other opportunistic infections or latent viruses trigger psoriasis.[7,13,15,17] Indeed, there have been multiple case reports of psoriasis in aquired immunodeficiency syndrome (AIDS) patients being cleared by nothing more than simple antibiotics.[18] Finally, the critical factor may not be that the immune system in general is destroyed but that the T cell population is skewed toward CD8 cells, which are thought to be the predominant effector cells in psoriasis.[13] More research needs to be done to elucidate the exact mechanism of the complex disease that is HIV-associated psoriasis.

CLINICAL FEATURES
Chronic plaque-type psoriasis
As with the general population, the most common form of psoriasis seen in HIV-infected individuals is chronic plaque-type psoriasis. This variant is characterized by sharply demarcated erythematous plaques covered by thick silvery scale classically on the extensor surfaces of the body (**99, 100**). The size of lesions can vary significantly from patient to patient. Other classic findings that can sometimes be observed are the pinpoint bleeding of Auspitz sign when scale is removed and the pale blanching of Woronoff's ring.[6] Plaques are usually fairly symmetrically distributed throughout the body with a predilection for the following sites: scalp, elbows, knees, presacrum, hands, and feet.[6] Pruritus may be an important symptom in up to 30% of patients and seronegative erosive arthritis develops in some patients. HIV-induced or exacerbated chronic plaque psoriasis tends to have all these same characteristics, but its onset has the potential to be more rapid and it can be more severe. Thus, any patient who presents with acute severe eruptive psoriasis or a sudden

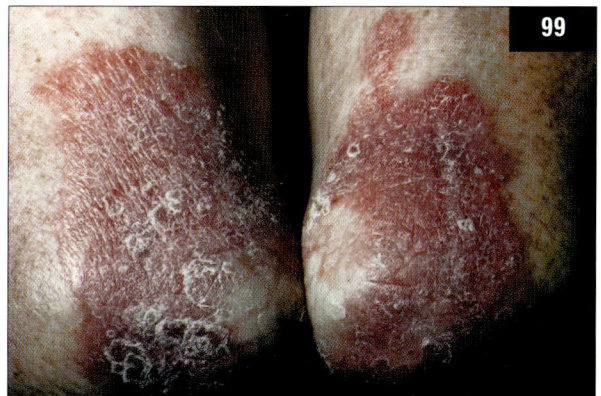

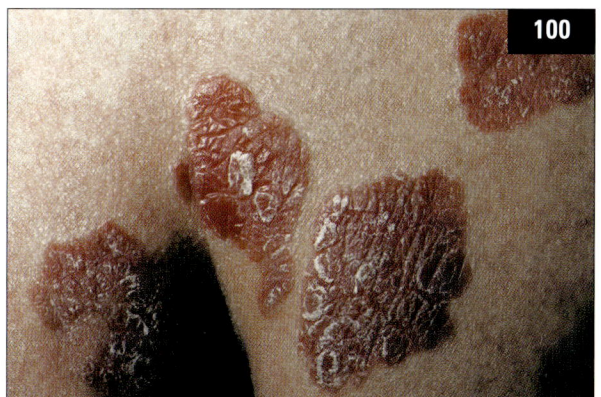

99, 100 Psoriasis. Sharply demarcated, erythematous plaques with silvery scale on elbows (**99**) and trunk (**100**).

exacerbation of previously chronic stable plaque psoriasis should be evaluated for the possibility of underlying HIV infection if they have any risk factors.[2]

Guttate psoriasis

Guttate psoriasis, though far less common than the chronic plaque type, is another important variant. This form is seen most commonly in children, usually after an upper respiratory infection. Streptococcal infection has also been known to trigger an outbreak.[9] In HIV/AIDS patients, guttate psoriasis is commonly seen without any evidence of streptococcal disease.[2] As described in the name, this form appears as small discrete papules and plaques (**101**). Usually, compared to the chronic plaque type, the scale is finer and sites such as the face and intertriginous areas like the genital region are more commonly affected, especially in children.[9] The prognosis is usually excellent in children and many do not develop psoriasis later in life. This is less commonly the case in HIV-infected patients, however.

Pustular psoriasis

Pustular psoriasis is a relatively unusual manifestation of psoriasis that may be seen in HIV infection. It may present in either a localized or generalized form. The chronic localized variety presents clinically as bilaterally symmetric involvement of the palms and soles both with and without accompanying psoriatic plaques elsewhere.[19] The acute localized form is seen on the palms, soles, and the dorsal aspects of the hands and feet.[19] Similar clinical manifestations, as well as palmoplantar keratoderma, have been reported in AIDS patients (**102, 103**).[2]

There are several generalized subtypes of pustular psoriasis. The Von Zumbusch form begins with severe generalized erythema and extensive pustule formation that may be painful. Patients often have fever and are ill-appearing for several days until the pustules resolve and extensive crusting is observed.[6,7] This subtype may be seen in pregnancy in which case it usually lasts until delivery.[19] Another form is widespread annular psoriasis which, as the name implies, has centrifugally expanding erythema, scale and pustulation with central healing.[6,19] This form may

be accompanied with fever.[6] Finally, the exanthematic type refers to an acute eruption of pustules that disappears soon thereafter without systemic symptoms. This type is often related to infections or associated drug hypersensitivity, but may also be seen after solar irradiation or irritation from topical therapies.[19]

Reiter's syndrome-like pattern

A form of psoriasis that demonstrates features virtually identical to Reiter's syndrome in immunocompetent individuals is seen in some AIDS patients.[16] Most often, it arises in the nonterminal phase of AIDS when the CD4+ T cell count remains $>200 \times 10^6$/l. It has been speculated that this form may be fundamentally similar to psoriasis in AIDS patients but manifests itself in different way due to the presence of genetic factors such as HLA-B27.[16] Clinical findings include: 1) arthritis, most commonly of the interphalangic and ankle joints (**104**); 2) pustulosis of the palms and soles (**105**); 3) nail dystrophy; 4) facial SD; and 5) psoriasiform plaques in an acral, inverse, and flexural distribution (**106**).[16] Urethritis and conjunctivitis are sometimes present.[2,16]

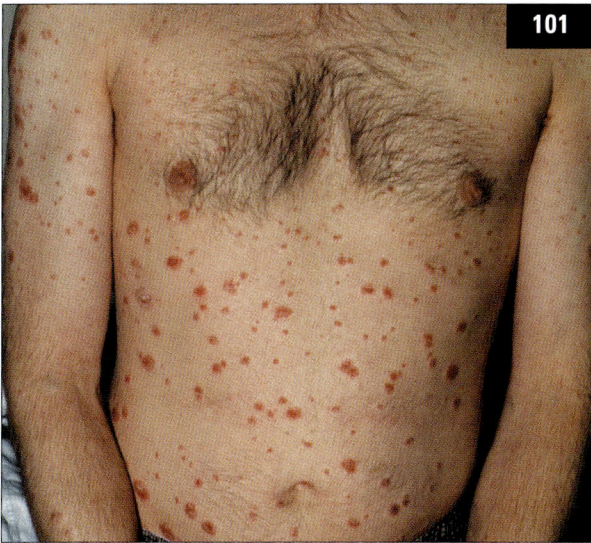

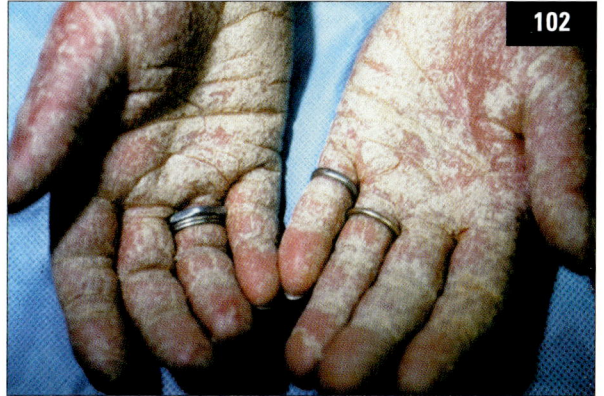

101 Guttate psoriasis. Widespread scaly, erythematous papules and plaques.

102, 103 Psoriasis. Severe palmoplantar keratoderma in an HIV-positive patient with psoriasis.

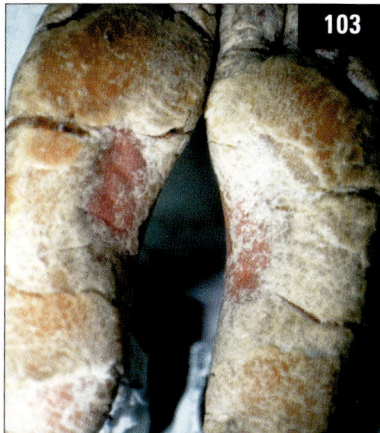

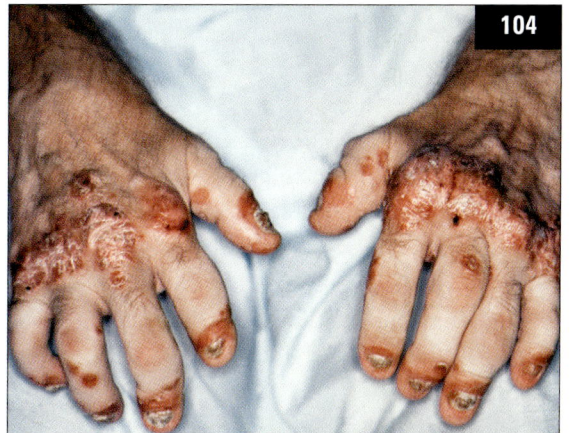

104 Arthritis of the hands in Reiter's syndrome.

105 Reiter's syndrome. Extensive pustulosis with secondary erosions on the palms.

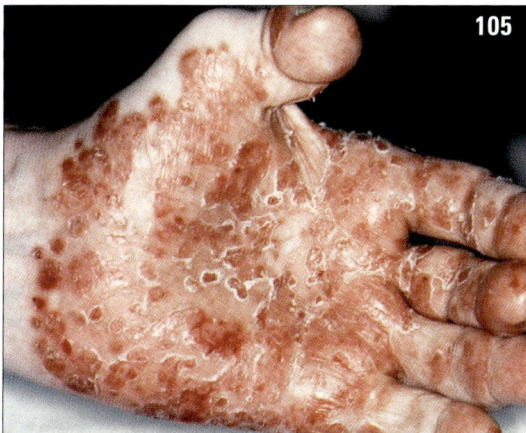

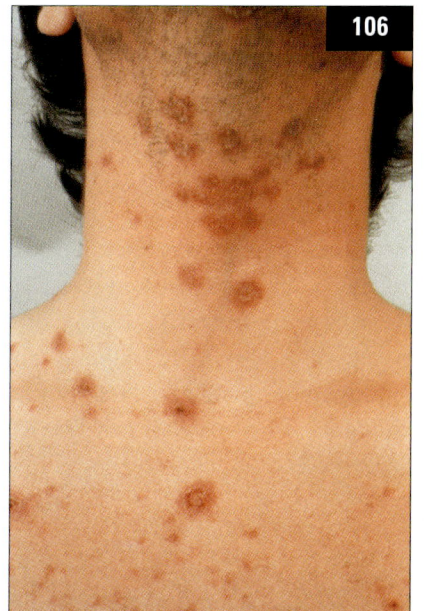

106 Psoriasiform plaques in an HIV-infected patient with Reiter's syndrome-like psoriasis.

Histopathology

The histopathology of psoriasis varies depending on the type of lesion biopsied and the presence or absence of pustular lesions. Characteristic features of an active lesion include marked regular psoriasiform hyperplasia of the epidermis and increased number, length, and tortuosity of papillary dermal capillaries.[5,6,11] There is a mixed perivascular infiltrate of leukocytes.[5,6] There is acanthosis and focal collections of neutrophils (spongiform pustules of Kogoj) in the superficial part of the epidermis. Additionally, there are mounds of parakeratosis-containing neutrophils and a diminished or absent granular layer.

A stable lesion differs in that it shows only a modest perivascular infiltrate but displays full and classic hyperproliferation of the epidermis. Thus, the pathologist will see the classic elongated rete ridges that coalesce at the base but the micropustules and microabscesses may not be seen.[6]

In a biopsy of pustular psoriasis, on the other hand, the most notable feature is the presence of neutrophils.[11] They accumulate between keratinocytes as well as in the stratum corneum to form the classic Kogoj and Munro microabscesses.[6] Reiter's disease is indistinguishable from pustular psoriasis histologically.[11]

Psoriasis in the HIV/AIDS population may have a number of different appearances microscopically. In some cases, it may appear histologically indistinguishable from psoriasis in uninfected persons.[2] Another form that has been termed 'AIDS-associated psoriasiform dermatitis', however, is histologically distinct. The characteristic features of this disorder include psoriasiform hyperplasia of the epidermis which is more irregular than ordinary psoriasis, relatively fewer Munro's abscesses, slight spongiosis, keratinocyte necrosis, and lymphocyte karyorrhexis.[2,20] Additionally, there is no thinning of the suprapapillar plate and there is a relative increase in the ratio of plasma cells to CD45RO+ T cells.[20]

Diagnosis

Diagnosis is made predominantly on clinical grounds, with biopsies and cultures performed as necessary to rule out other possible conditions in select cases. In the HIV-positive population in particular, the clinical diagnosis may be difficult due to the fact that many entities such as fulminant SD or disseminated cutaneous histoplasmosis can mimic the disease.[21] Even histologic features may overlap with SD, particularly after psoriasis has been partially treated.[2]

Management

Above all else, when treating psoriasis, it is imperative that the physician show empathy, concern, and understanding. Time must be taken, especially in the first visit, to establish a rapport with the patient through education about the chronic nature of the disease. There are many excellent support organizations for patients with the disease, especially the National Psoriasis Foundation, that can be very helpful.

There is a wide range of agents available for treatment (*Table 5*). Even carbamazepine has been shown sometimes to improve psoriasis, possibly by controlling the release of neuropeptides in the skin.[22] H2 antagonists such as ranitidine are sometimes effective.[23] Whichever therapeutic route the clinician may choose, he or she should be aware of side-effects that will inevitably be encountered and that may be unique to HIV-infected patients.[17,24]

Treating HIV-associated psoriasis is often a difficult task due in large part to the fact that the disease is often refractory to therapy in severely immunocompromised individuals.[2] Although there are many options for treating psoriasis in HIV-positive patients, a few general observations should be noted. First, due to the nature of HIV-associated psoriasis, it is advisable, if at all possible, to avoid immunosuppressive drugs, or use them with extreme caution. For instance, even though cyclosporine can be used to treat psoriatic erythroderma and it directly inhibits HIV replication, its immunosuppressive effects are rightly regarded as a profound risk factor for opportunistic infection.[22] Second, it has been observed that controlling and treating the HIV itself may have a marked impact on the course and severity of psoriasis.[13,15] In one case, HIV-associated psoriasis underwent complete resolution after 8 weeks of combination antiretroviral therapy and promptly recurred when therapy was interrupted.[15] These clinical improvements occurred in parallel with the viral load and CD4 count but also may have been due to a decrease in the fraction of activated T-lymphocytes or a decrease in cytokines such as TNF-α associated with HIV replication.[15]

Another study has shown that oral zidovudine alone can result in dramatic improvement of HIV-associated psoriasis even as T cell counts continue to fall.[2,25] Interestingly, zidovudine has been shown to clear psoriasis in patients without HIV infection.[25,26] Thus, aggressive HAART therapy should be an integral part of treatment for any HIV-associated psoriasis patient. However, the so-called immune reconstitution syndrome in which psoriasis is exacerbated or flares after the initiation of HAART therapy may be encountered.[12]

Beyond effective control of HIV itself, many other systemic and topical drugs may be tried with varying efficacy. Initial treatment of HIV-associated psoriasis is often phototherapy with ultraviolet light, either in the form of UVB, narrow band (nb) UVB, or psoralen with ultraviolet A light (PUVA).[26] Importantly, studies have reported no decrease in CD4 T cells with ultraviolet therapy.[26] Phototherapy without antiretroviral therapy may cause viral load to rise, however.[26,27] Clinicians should also be aware that long-term UVB or PUVA increases the risk for the development of skin cancers.[27,28]

The newer biologic agents such as the LFA-3 antibody alefacept, cytokines such as IL-10, the anti IL-12/23 monoclonal antibody ustekimumab, the CD11a compound efalizumab, and anti-TNF-α drugs such as etanercept, adalimumab, and infliximab have also been used in these patients.[5] In many instances, these agents have been found to be effective in particularly recalcitrant cases where older more traditional therapies have failed.[12]

Table 5 Treatment options for psoriasis

Highly active antiretroviral treatment (HAART) or combination antiretroviral therapy

Zidovudine	Hydroxyurea
Calcipotriol	Carbamazepine
Calcitriol	H2 antagonists: ranitidine
Tacalcitol	LFA-3 antibody: alefacept
Narrow band UVB	IL-10
Topical corticosteroids	CD11a efalizumab (withdrawn from US market)
Dithranol	Etanercept
Topical retinoids	Infliximab
Photochemotherapy (PUVA, rePUVA)	Adalimumab
Methotrexate	Ustekimumab
Cyclosporine	

'PARAPSORIASIS' (PITYRIASIS LICHENOIDES AND PATCH STAGE MYCOSIS FUNGOIDES)

DEFINITION/OVERVIEW

Parapsoriasis is a term that refers to many different unrelated conditions that are largely of historical interest. However, it is discussed here because it still appears in the literature and may be confusing to clinicians. It has traditionally been categorized into small (SPP) and large (LPP) plaque parapsoriasis but also includes acute and chronic variants of pityriasis lichenoides (**107**) and even lymphomatoid papulosis (LyP).[6,29] SPP is generally synonymous with pityriasis lichenoides chronica (PLC), and LPP with patch stage of mycosis fungoides (MF).[6,29] They all appear in a worldwide distribution and in every ethnic group, but males do seem to be disproportionately affected.[6,29] There have only been a handful of HIV-associated PLEVA cases reported in the literature.[30] Of these, all presented with PLEVA while still having CD4 T cell counts greater than 200×10^6/l.[30] This leads researchers to conclude that PLEVA is most likely a marker of early to mid HIV infection.[30] HIV-associated PLC is similar.[31]

PATHOGENESIS/PATHOPHYSIOLOGY

The etiology of all these diseases is unknown. All show CD4+ lymphoid infiltrates and they may demonstrate clonal populations.[6,29] So-called LPP is a clonal process that is thought by most to represent patch stage cutaneous T cell lymphoma that may progress to more severe disease over time at a rate of around 10% per decade.[6] Studies have been done to try and implicate viruses such as human herpesvirus (HHV)-8 in the pathogenesis of parapsoriasis en plaque and cutaneous lymphomas but they have been unsuccessful.[32]

In lesions of PLC, the pathogenesis centers around an influx of CD4+ cells. PLEVA, on the other hand, demonstrates a CD8+ T cell infiltrate.[6,31] These conditions are thought to be a response to infectious disease and drugs in some cases, although in others the cause is unknown.[6,30,31] Though rare, the most frequently reported of these infectious triggers for pityriasis lichenoides is Epstein–Barr virus (EBV), *Toxoplasma gondii*, and HIV itself.[33] Perhaps this mechanism stems from superantigen formation and binding of MHCII cells which produce clones of T cells, or, in the case of HIV, immunologic dysregulation may play a role.[30,33] In HIV-associated PLEVA, this response to superantigen formation is only possible in the early to middle stages of HIV infection when the body is still capable of being induced by HIV to produce a TH-1 cytokine response and increase IFN-γ.[30] Since we know that increased IFN-γ upregulates HLA-DR expression on keratinocytes, this theory would predict PLEVA to reflect this in HLA-DR staining – which it does.[30]

CLINICAL FEATURES

Both SPP and LPP present clinically as chronic generally asymptomatic patches which may be mildly pruritic.[6,29] These lesions can appear anywhere on the trunk or extremities but they appear to favor sun-protected areas.[6] The patches of LPP are sometimes well marginated, but are just as frequently found to have borders which blend into the surrounding skin.[29] SPP patches are usually round to oval, less than 5 cm in diameter and sometimes have a digitate contour, while LPP is round or irregular and greater than 5 cm.[6,34] In both cases, the lesions are a variably erythematous and covered in a fine scale reminiscent of 'cigarette paper', while those of LPP may or may not be poikilodermatous.[6,29]

This clinical picture is in stark contrast to that of

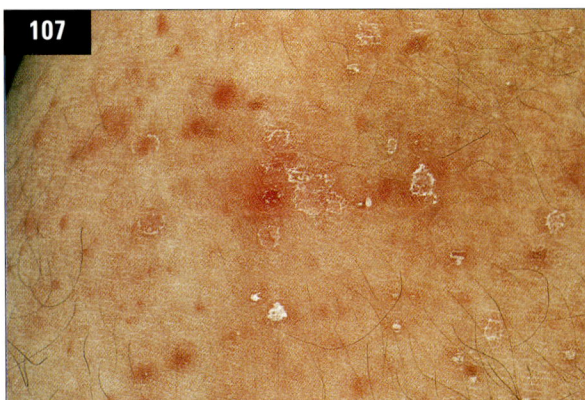

107 Chronic pityriasis lichenoides. (Courtesy of St John's Institute of Dermatology (King's College), Guy's Hospital, London.)

pityriasis lichenoides with its recurrent erythematous to purpuric papules.[6,29] In the acute form, PLEVA, these lesions develop crusts and pseudovesicles which commonly ulcerate with central necrosis but usually resolve in a few weeks to months.[6,30,33] Only rarely are systemic symptoms such as malaise, fever, or lymphadenopathy experienced.[6] It must be noted, however, that there is a wide range of possible systemic symptoms that one might encounter when dealing with PLEVA, including interstitial pneumonitis and central nervous system (CNS) and rheumatic manifestations may be seen prior to the onset of the cutaneous eruption.[30] In the few reported cases of HIV-associated PLEVA, most patients had only mild constitutional symptoms, if any.[30]

In PLC erythematous and scaly papules develop and do not regress until months later, often leaving hypopigmented macules.[6] When PLC is associated with HIV, the clinical presentation is reported to improve with increasing CD4+ T cell counts.[33] As in many other HIV-associated papulosquamous diseases, its clinical presentation can be severe and atypical.[31]

LyP usually presents clinically as red papules that progress to papulovesicles or papulopustules which eventually necrose and heal weeks later.[35] This clinical picture bears a striking similarity to PLEVA, but the course is usually more chronic.[35] The prognosis, though, is by no means identical. While the vast majority of these cases are benign and self-limited, a significant portion of approximately 10–15% eventually progress to malignant lymphoma.[35] In the literature, there has been at least one case of LyP reported in a male with a CD4+ cell count of 4×10^6/l and CD4/CD8 ratio of 0.03.[35] This patient had multiple, pruritic, slightly violaceous nodules about 1 cm in diameter distributed haphazardly on the upper extremities, which waxed and waned over time.[35]

HISTOPATHOLOGY

The histopathologic findings of what has been referred to as SPP are nonspecific and reveal focal hyperkeratosis, scale crust, slight exocytosis, and a sparse perivascular lymphohistiocytic infiltrate.[29,34] LPP demonstrates changes of patch stage MF with a band-like infiltrate of lymphocytes with epidermotropism.[6,29] Lesions of LPP will often show a

predominance of CD4+ T cells, CD7 antigen deficiency, and positive HLA-DR staining when analyzed immunohistologically.[29] Finally, if the lesion of LPP biopsied displays poikilodermatous features there will be thinning of the epidermis, telangiectases, and pigment incontinence.[6]

In pityriasis lichenoides, the characteristic finding is a wedge-shaped lesion with a superficial perivascular lymphocytic interface dermatitis.[6,30] There is also interface involvement, dykeratosis, extravasation of erythrocytes, and variable dermal edema.[30] In both acute and chronic forms, parakeratosis will be observed, but in the chronic variant the erythrocyte extravasation and lymphocytic infiltrate tends to be milder in comparison with the acute variety.[6] As for immunohistochemical findings, HIV-associated PLEVA shows an inflammatory infiltrate which stains positively for CD3, CD29, and CD8.[30] Likewise, the mononuclear and dendritic cells stain for HLA-DR.[30]

Finally, in LyP the histologic picture can be divided into type A, in which there are large atypical lymphoid cells similar to Reed–Sternberg cells, and type B, in which there are large pleomorphic cerebriform cells similar to those seen in MF admixed with smaller lymphocytic cells.[35] CD30 staining of lymphocytes is seen in both, although surprisingly, the large cells often are not highlighted. Both types typically display a superficial or deep lymphocytic infiltrate that may or may not show epidermotropism. T cell clonal rearrangements may be demonstrated in about 40% of cases.[35] The individual case of LyP in a HIV-infected patient had a histologic picture consistent with type B classification. One significant difference that was reported, however, was that the lymphocytic infiltrate in this case was mostly CD8+ as opposed to the more common CD4+ type. The authors speculate this may be due to the inherent immune dysregulation of HIV which preferentially depletes CD4+ cells.[35]

DIAGNOSIS

For SPP, LPP, PLC, and PLEVA, clinicohistopathologic correlation is more valuable than any ancillary test. Both SPP and LPP can be differentiated from MF and other similar appearing entities largely based on histologic criteria.[6] Other than immunopathologic studies to show increased CD8+ T cells in

PLEVA, or CD30+ cells to rule out pityriasis lichenoides, few tests other than for infectious diseases are useful.[6] In a study of HIV-associated PLEVA patients, tests for hepatitis B, hepatitis C, EBV, cytomegalovirus (CMV), and toxoplasmosis were performed to exclude these disorders although none were found.[30] Other studies that might be considered include serologic studies for varicella or syphilis.[30]

LyP may often be confused clinically with PLEVA, but histologically it most resembles cutaneous anaplastic T cell lymphoma and Hodgkin's disease.[35] Once again, this underscores the importance of clinicohistopathologic correlation.

MANAGEMENT

Treatment of these conditions varies depending on the disorder (*Table 6*). For SPP, the standard treatment consists of emollients, topical corticosteroids, tar, or narrow band UVB and PUVA phototherapy.[6,29,33] LPP should be treated as patch stage MF initially similar to SPP, with the same modalities and close follow-up. If it is more advanced, topical mechlorethamine, carmustine, bexarotene, IFN-α and IL-12 may be required.[6]

Treatment for pityriasis lichenoides centers around removing any suspicious drugs and instituting trials of topical or oral corticosteroids, coal tar, tetracycline, erythromycin, or phototherapy.[6,29] Indeed, a case report of a HIV-positive patient with PLC required only topical dipropionate betamethasone and antiretroviral therapy to induce complete remission with no relapse after 1 year.[36] Methotrexate, PUVA and intravenous gamma-globulin have also been reported to be effective.[29,33] Of all these it should be noted that UVB, PUVA, and methotrexate are considered the most consistently effective treatments.[29]

There has been one case reported in the literature of cyclosporine A being used to treat refractory life-threatening HIV-associated PLC and PLEVA.[31] The authors speculate that perhaps the cyclosporine worked by inhibiting the cyclophilin-related virion maturation of HIV, thus decreasing HIV replication, or by inhibiting T cell activation and the production of IL-2.[31] Once the PLC was brought under control, combination antiretroviral therapy was able to bring the patient into complete remission, once again highlighting the necessity of HAART in HIV-associated papulosquamous diseases.

For the one case of LyP in the setting of HIV, treatment consisted of clobetasol 0.05% applied twice daily and all lesions promptly cleared within several weeks.[35]

Table 6 Treatment options for parapsoriasis

SPP	LPP	PLC	PLEVA
(Reassurance)	(Close follow-up)	Topical and oral corticosteroids	Topical and oral corticosteroids
Emollients	Emollients	Tar	Tar
Topical corticosteroids	Topical corticosteroids	Tetracycline	Tetracycline
Tar	Tar	Erythromycin	Erythromycin
nbUVB	nbUVB	Phototherapy	Phototherapy
PUVA	PUVA	Methotrexate	Methotrexate
		PUVA	PUVA
		Cyclosporine A	Cyclosporine A
		Combination antiretroviral therapy	Combination antiretroviral therapy

SEBORRHEIC DERMATITIS

DEFINITION/OVERVIEW

Seborrheic dermatitis (SD) is by far one of the most common cutaneous diseases to manifest itself in the HIV population. Epidemiologic studies demonstrate its prevalence to be approximately 85% or more in HIV-infected individuals.[2,11,37] The severity of the disease in this population correlates with the extent of clinical deterioration and decline of helper T cell numbers, but it can be seen at any stage of HIV infection and is not exclusively linked to a poor prognosis.[2,38,39] Most patients in one study with HIV and SD, however, were demonstrated to have helper T cell counts $<100 \times 10^6/l$.[2] A different analysis of African HIV patients showed that SD had a 48% positive predictive value (PPV) for HIV and manifested itself early in the occurrence of HIV.[38] Given the higher prevalence of SD in western industrialized countries, the PPV of SD for HIV would not be nearly so high, but this study does serve to highlight the strong association between these two diseases.

PATHOGENESIS/PATHOPHYSIOLOGY

Like almost all of the diseases in the papulosquamous category, the exact etiology of SD remains a mystery. Many theories have been put forward from infectious etiologies to altered sebum, neurologic, and endocrine regulation.[3,37] Up to this date though, it appears that the strongest evidence is in the favor of yeasts being a major causative factor. Yeasts from the genus *Malassezia* have been linked to SD for many years and they have been regularly isolated from lesions.[2,6] Although the number of *Malassezia* in normal controls does not differ significantly from those with the disease, it is clear that decreased numbers of the yeasts correlate with increasingly efficacious treatment.[6,39] This insignificant difference in the skin flora of patients with SD as compared to normal controls has been confirmed and corroborated in the HIV-positive population as well.[39] The exact mechanism by which they cause or exacerbate SD has remained elusive. This may be due to an immune response to *Malassezia*.[6,39] The frequency and recalcitrance of SD in the HIV

population has bolstered this idea, but again, no studies have been definitive.[40] In the past, some believed SD might be linked to changes in skin surface lipids. Multiple studies in both HIV-positive and negative patients, however, have not verified this.[39]

CLINICAL FEATURES

SD consists of slightly indurated, erythematous patches usually with abundant greasy scale (**108**).[6,11,40] In the general population, it is usually found in the first few months of life, disappears in childhood and redevelops in the postpubertal period when the sebaceous glands are active. It displays a preference for the scalp, eyebrows, nasolabial folds, ears, presternal and intertriginous areas.[6,11,37,40,41] Most often, it causes only moderate discomfort, but in HIV-infected patients it has a propensity to be more severe with thicker scale that can become generalized, and, rarely, even erythrodermic.[2,3,11,37,42] Five further characteristics that characterize AIDS-related SD include: (1) a greater degree of inflammation of lesions; (2) more indurated plaques reminiscent of psoriasis; (3) involvement of unusual

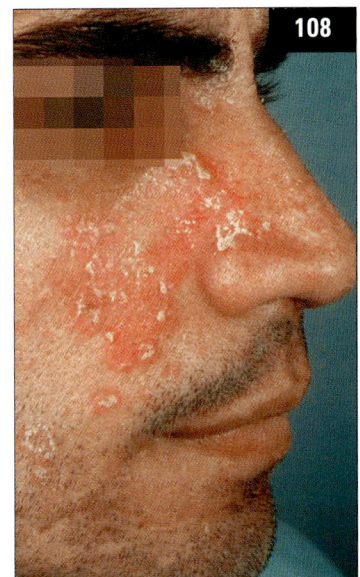

108 Seborrheic dermatitis. Erythematous plaques with seborrheic scale in the glabellar area and spreading from the nasolabial folds onto the cheeks and nose.

areas such as the trunk, groin, and extremities; (4) 'cradle cap' of the scalp with nonscarring alopecia; and (5) hypo- or hyperpigmentation within the inflammatory lesions.[2,3,42,43] Patients may develop these manifestations either *de novo* or as an exacerbation of pre-existing disease.[42] In either case AIDS-associated SD tends to develop as the patient becomes more immunocompromised, and its severity often correlates with lower helper T cell subset numbers.[3,42] Finally, there is an association between HIV-infected patients with severe SD, xerosis, erythroderma, and the future development of dementia.[3] This parallels closely with the finding that SD and neurologic disorders such as Parkinson's disease and epilepsy are often linked.[2] When one takes into consideration the known neurotropism of HIV-1, there may be a common etiologic link here that remains to be elucidated.[2]

HISTOPATHOLOGY

The histology of SD remains mostly unchanged whether the patient is HIV positive or not. In both cases, it consists of epidermal psoriasiform hyperplasia with parakaratosis and neutrophils near follicular ostia.[11] Typically, mounds of parakeratosis with neutrophils and serum are seen near the ostia of follicles (109).[44] In addition, the dermis will contain an infiltrate of lymphocytes and plasma cells.[11] There

are a few differences, however. Most notable is the presence of scattered individually necrotic keratinocytes, along with a relatively more dense inflammatory infiltrate, focal leukocytoclasis, greater parakaratosis, and more plasma cells in the HIV-associated cases (110).[2,3,11,42,43]

DIAGNOSIS

Generally speaking, the diagnosis of SD can be made upon clinical inspection alone. Usually, this can be done quite easily, with scrapings and microscopic examination reserved for excluding fungal infections and scabies.[11]

MANAGEMENT

Therapy for SD centers around the use of topical antifungal and corticosteroid preparations. Treatment of the HIV-associated SD tends to mirror that of ordinary SD.[42] One such regimen that has been advocated is 2.5% topical hydrocortisone cream applied twice daily or topical ketoconazole cream applied twice daily.[2,11] Other adjunctive options to be considered are UVB phototherapy, or coal, tar, sulfur, salicylic acid shampoos and, most recently, application of pimecrolimus cream.[2,11,42] Some cases, however, seem to be refractory to all treatments.[42] Fortunately, HAART therapy has been known to help even these cases sometimes.[11]

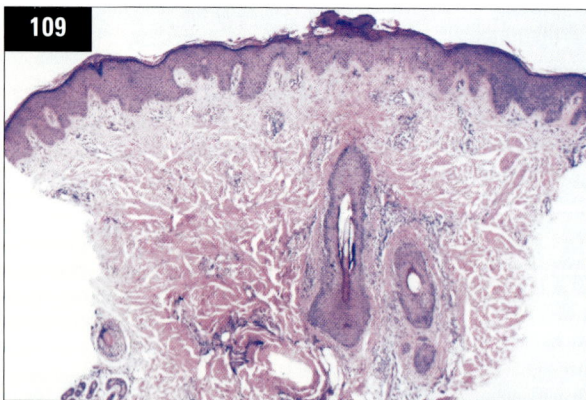

109 Histology of seborrheic dermatitis. Psoriasiform hyperplasia with a mound of parakeratosis overlying the follicular ostium and dermal perifollicular inflammation.

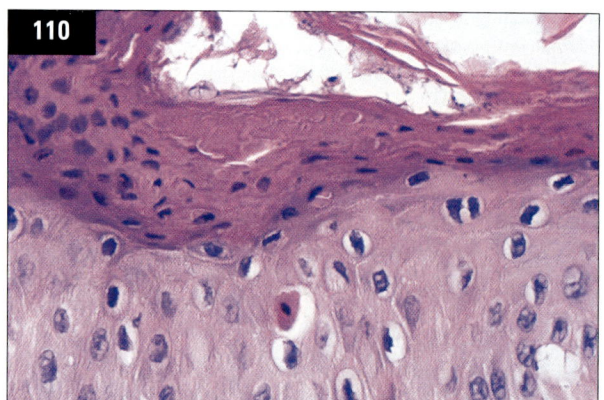

110 Close-up view of the thick mound of parakeratosis with a necrotic keratinocyte in the epidermis.

PITYRIASIS RUBRA PILARIS

DEFINITION/OVERVIEW

Pityriasis rubra pilaris (PRP) has been a well known entity since the 19th century and manifests itself most often as an acquired disorder which affects men and women equally.[6,29] Both autosomal dominant and recessive familial forms have been described, but they are rare. People in the HIV-infected population fall into PRP type VI. Of these, there have been less than 20 reported in the literature with most patients being 27–45 years old.[45]

PATHOGENESIS/PATHOPHYSIOLOGY

The exact pathologic cause of PRP is unknown. Everything from abnormal keratinization due to incorrect vitamin A metabolism, physical triggers, and infection to autoimmune pathogeneses have been suggested, but nothing has been proven.[6,29,45] Interestingly, due to the observed therapeutic response to zidovudine and its association with HIV, even this virus has been implicated in its pathogenesis.[45] It is theorized that perhaps the HIV infects the follicle hair bulge and causes follicular inflammation.[45]

CLINICAL FEATURES

PRP is characterized by scaly orange-red plaques involving the scalp, trunk, extremities, palms, and soles.[6,11] The general pattern witnessed is follicular involvement with islands of skin unaffected.[11,29] Indeed, it is this symmetric follicular hyperkeratosis on an erythematous base and palmoplantar keratoderma that are key findings (**111–113**).[6,45] Clinically, individual lesions consist of rough papules that coalesce into plaques with varying degrees of erythroderma, exfoliation, and desquamation.[6,45] In classic cases of PRP, the disease usually demonstrates

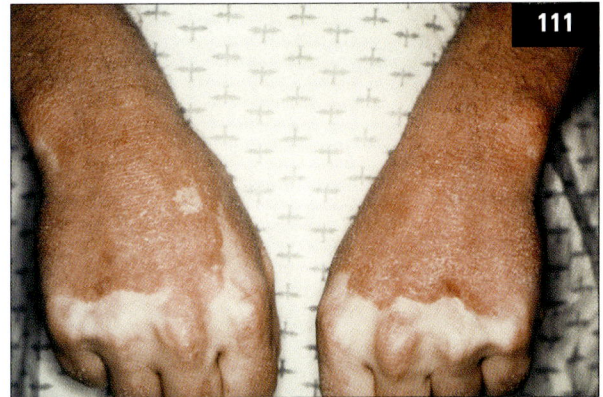

111 Pityriasis rubra pilaris. Symmetrical orange-red, confluent, hyperkeratotic, scaly plaques with islands of uninvolved skin.

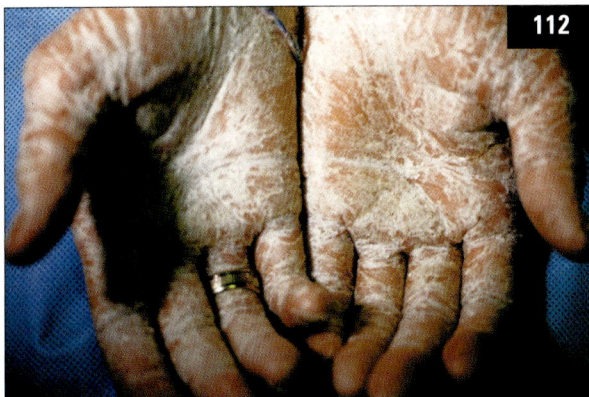

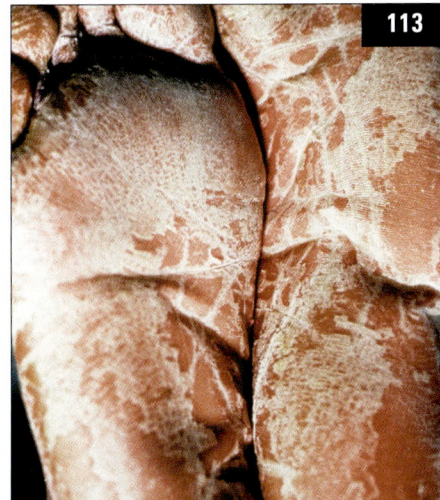

112, 113 Pityriasis rubra pilaris. Severe palmoplantar keratoderma.

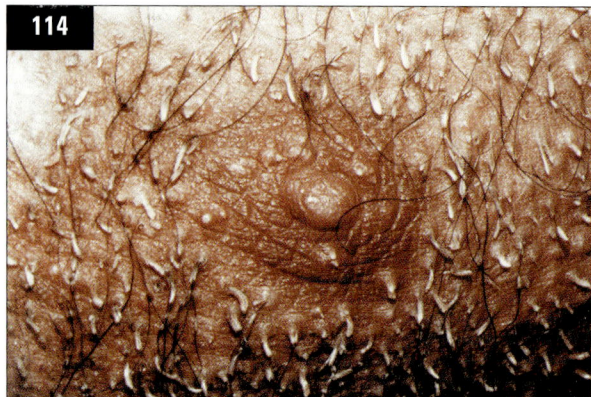

114 Elongated hyperkeratotic follicular spines.

a caudal spread with varying amounts of burning and pruritus.[6] New cases of PRP are customarily grouped into six different categories, types I–VI with HIV-associated PRP in type VI. There have been reported cases of explosive cystic acne and elongated follicular spines (**114**) associated with PRP in these HIV-infected patients.[6,11,45] In fact, this prominent follicular plugging and formation of spicules seems to be one of the hallmark features of HIV-associated PRP.[45] PRP may be the first sign of HIV infection, but more often develops in patients with already established HIV disease.[45] Similarly, CD4 counts at the onset of HIV-associated PRP tend to vary. Of the patients reported in the literature, most had CD4 counts $<500 \times 10^6$/l, but a significant minority did not.[45] A striking feature to note is that those patients with higher T cell counts and no opportunistic infections often exhibited much more serious PRP manifestations.[45] PRP is often associated with acne

conglobata, but nail, palm/sole, and scalp involvement is extremely variable from patient to patient.[45] Patients will, however, frequently become erythrodermic.[45]

HISTOPATHOLOGY

The distinctive histopathologic feature of PRP is the so called 'checkerboard pattern' of alternating vertical and horizontal ortho- and parakeratosis.[6,29,45] This also holds true for HIV-associated PRP. In addition to this, other signs that may or may not be present include: follicular dilation, shortened rete, lymphohistiocytic perivascular infiltrate, and focal acantholysis.[6,45] Features such as psoriasiform epidermal hyperplasia and a prominent granular cell layer can sometimes be seen.[45]

DIAGNOSIS

The diagnosis can usually be made on a purely clinical basis. Observation, careful questioning, and histopathology should be able to differentiate PRP from the few other entities such as psoriasis and SD which it can sometimes be confused with.[29] Some cases may overlap with psoriasis histologically, especially early in the course of the condition, so that repeat biopsies may be required to confirm the diagnosis in questionable cases.

MANAGEMENT

Partly because the pathogenesis of PRP is not known, there is no perfect consensus on appropriate treatment. Even if untreated, many patients may undergo spontaneous resolution. In the case of AIDS-associated PRP, therapies that have been tried with some success include isotretinoin, 13-cis-retinoic acid, topical vitamin D analogs, PUVA, and UVB phototherapy.[6,11,45] Effective delivery of HAART has also proven efficacious.[11] There is at least one case report of zidovudine 250 mg/12 hr, lamivudine 150 mg/12 hr, and saquinavir 600 mg/8 hr greatly improving the cutaneous lesions of PRP in as little as 2 months, with complete resolution in 7 months.[45] Even zidovudine alone has proven effective. In almost all cases, however, it has been found that PRP type VI relapses if therapy was stopped or when the underlying AIDS progressed.[45]

PITYRIASIS ROSEA

DEFINITION/OVERVIEW

Pityriasis rosea (PR) is a self-limited pink scaly cutaneous disease which commonly affects young adults.[6] It is found worldwide with equal sex distribution and, in most cases, arising in healthy persons aged approximately 10–40 years old.[6,29] This disease has been reported in the HIV-positive population but only rarely have cases been documented in the literature.

PATHOGENESIS/PATHOPHYSIOLOGY

For a variety of reasons, an infectious or viral etiology for PR has long been suspected.[6,29,46] Chief among these include seasonal outbreaks in the spring and fall, prodromal symptoms in some patients, clustering of cases in families or among those in close contact, and sometimes successful experiments at transmitting PR from one person to another.[6,29] Many studies have been undertaken to find the infectious agent to no avail but two viruses that seem to be the most likely candidates are HHV-7 and HHV-6.[29,46,47] Both of these viruses are ubiquitous in the population and become latent after taking up residence in mononuclear cells and saliva.[46] PCR studies have shown HHV-7 DNA in lesional skin of PR patients but not in healthy controls or people with a past history of the disease.[48] Thus, it has been proposed that perhaps reactivation of HHV-6 and HHV-7, sometimes demonstrable by viremia, may result in the outbreak of PR. If this is true, the severe immunosuppression seen in HIV/AIDS patients may help explain the so-called 'persistent' PR documented in this population.[3] Nevertheless, there have been no definitive results published which would fully explain the etiology of PR at this time.

CLINICAL FEATURES

Classic PR usually first becomes apparent with a solitary 'herald patch' that usually appears on the trunk, neck, or extremities (115). Mild prodromal symptoms may or may not be present. This initial solitary pink scaly lesion enlarges over the next few days with its size ranging from a few centimeters to as large as 10 cm.[6,29] Usually within a few days after the appearance of the 'herald patch', numerous other similar lesions begin to appear. Just as with the initial lesion, these smaller ones are usually oval in shape, have the classic collarette of scale, and an advancing border.[6,29] Most patients experience at least mild pruritus. Another distinguishing characteristic of these lesions is the fact that their long axis follows Langer's lines of cleavage, producing the classic 'Christmas tree' pattern on the back (116).[6,29] As with most diseases however, there are atypical forms of PR that deviate from this classic picture in a multitude of ways.[29] In patients with HIV, PR may occur in a widespread fashion[11] and usually lasts 6–12 weeks before spontaneous resolution.[6] There has been at least one report, however, of so-called 'persistent' PR that presented in an AIDS patient.[3] This person had lesions which appeared to be PR both clinically and by histopathologic evaluation.

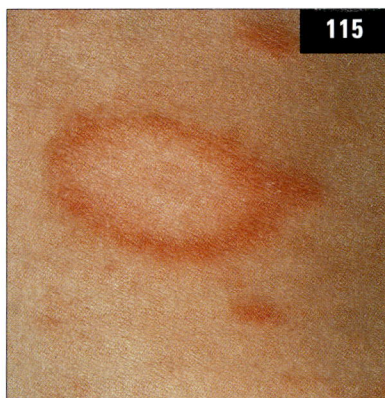

115 'Herald patch' in pityriasis rosea. (Courtesy of St John's Institute of Dermatology (King's College), Guy's Hospital, London.)

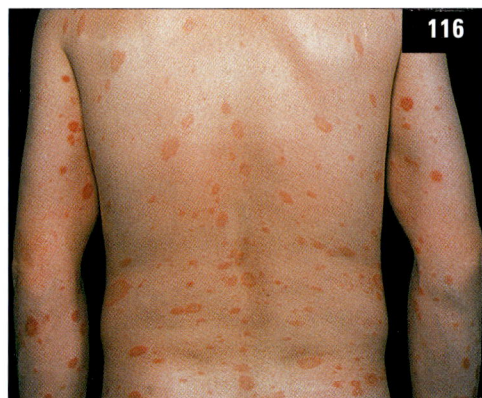

116 'Christmas tree' pattern in pityriasis rosea. (Courtesy of St John's Institute of Dermatology (King's College), Guy's Hospital, London.)

There was no herald patch reported, but lesions did follow the characteristic cleavage lines of Langer. Unlike typical PR, this case did not resolve but persisted for 12 months until the patient's death.

HISTOPATHOLOGY

Usually biopsy and histopathologic evaluation are not necessary as there is usually a classic and distinctive presentation. Microscopically, there is slight spongiosis, parakeratosis, and a sparse lymphohistiocytic infiltrate.[6] The findings are not pathognomonic as other conditions such as drug eruptions and viral exanthems may give similar histologic findings.[29]

DIAGNOSIS

Classic PR is usually not difficult to diagnose clinically. Some entities that may be confused with PR include secondary syphilis, drug eruptions, erythema annulare centrifugum, lichen planus (LP), some forms of pityriasis lichenoides, and nummular dermatitis.[29] In any case, serologic tests, careful history, and histologic evidence may be necessary if the diagnosis is in question.

MANAGEMENT

Usually, since PR is a self-limited disease, treatment is unnecessary or is directed towards symptomatic relief. To this end, topical corticosteroid preparations and antihistamines can be prescribed as needed. In one study, however, erythromycin was shown to cause resolution of PR in 14 days, although this finding has not been reproduced to date. Acyclovir has also been shown more recently to be effective for PR in a small study from Italy.[6,29] In the acute phase, water, soap, wool, and sweating should be avoided as they all have been reported to cause irritation.[29] UVB phototherapy has been described as having some efficacy but may accentuate postinflammatory pigmentation in some cases.[29]

LICHEN NITIDUS

DEFINITION/OVERVIEW

Lichen nitidus (LN) is an uncommon cutaneous eruption with little reliable epidemiologic data. One study of a black population determined the incidence to be approximately 3.4 cases per 10,000.[29] Little data have been published concerning its presentation in the HIV-infected population.

PATHOGENESIS/PATHOPHYSIOLOGY

Little is known about the pathogenesis of LN, although initially it was thought to be related to tuberculosis although no infectious etiology has ever been demonstrated conclusively.[6,49] It has been considered by some that LN truly represents a variant of LP and the fact that they may coexist and may appear indistinguishable from LN clinically bolster this view.[49] LN has been linked to certain viruses and antigens, especially the recombinant hepatitis B vaccine.[49] As with other papulosquamous diseases, it is likely that this vaccine or some similar stimulus serves to activate an autoimmune inflammatory cascade against keratinocytes in a genetically susceptible individual. Obviously, to discover the exact details of the mechanism, however, much more research is needed.

CLINICAL FEATURES

The classic presentation of LN is multiple discrete firm skin-colored papules that are very small, pinhead sized, and uniform but asymptomatic (**117**).[6,49] Other colors such as pink or yellow have been reported and can sometimes be hypo- or hyperpigmented compared to the surrounding skin and display a minimal amount of scale.[6,49] Lesions may be found on multiple sites ranging from the dorsal aspects of the hands, to the flexor aspects of the upper extremities, genitalia, and trunk.[6,49] The mucous membranes may be involved in some cases. Like LS, LN exhibits koebnerization. The condition is self-limited and usually resolves in 1 year.[6,49] There is little, if any, information in the literature on the presentation of LN in the HIV-positive population. One presumed case presented as a slightly pruritic skin-colored papular eruption that demonstrated histologic changes similar to those of LN.[50]

HISTOPATHOLOGY

The histology of LN shows an atrophic epidermis with parakeratosis overlying a well circumscribed lymphocytic infiltrate with epithelioid and Langhans giant cells (**118**).[6,49] A 'ball and claw' configuration is often described in which this infiltrate is nestled in between two to three hyperplastic rete ridges.[6,49] As in LS, degeneration of the basal layer may be seen and there may be scattered colloid bodies, Max–Joseph spaces, and melanin incontinence.[6]

DIAGNOSIS

Usually the clinical features are characteristic although a skin biopsy will be confirmatory in most cases.

MANAGEMENT

Due to spontaneous resolution, treatment is often not undertaken. Topical corticosteroid creams, topical tacrolimus and pimecrolimus, PUVA, etretinate, itraconazole, and astemizole have all been used with varying success.[6] In one case of a lymphopenic patient with LN and possible HIV infection, topical dinitrochlorobenzene (DNCB) showed impressive results.[51]

LICHEN PLANUS

DEFINITION/OVERVIEW

LP, like most papulosquamous diseases, is poorly understood. It generally tends to present in patients aged 30–60 years old, has no clear sexual preponderance, and a prevalence of <1% worldwide.[29] Statistics of prevalence in the HIV/AIDS population are rare but one study has shown that oral LP occured in roughly 0.5% of its HIV-infected participants.[52]

PATHOGENESIS/PATHOPHYSIOLOGY

Little, if anything, is known about the exact pathogenesis of LP. Most current theories and research center around the thought that LP is due to a T cell-mediated autoimmune phenomenon. For many years, dermatologists have suspected that exposure to things like viruses, medication, or contact allergens could precipitate an outbreak of LP. Researchers have hypothesized that these cause a critical antigen to be presented to T cells, thus stimulating apoptosis and a cytokine cascade that leads to LP.[6]

Viruses have been associated with LP and the one most closely associated is the hepatitis C virus (HCV), especially with oral LP.[6,53,54] HCV has been documented to replicate actively in lichenoid lesions.[53] HHV-6, herpes simplex-1 (HSV-1), EBV, and CMV are also thought by some to be potential

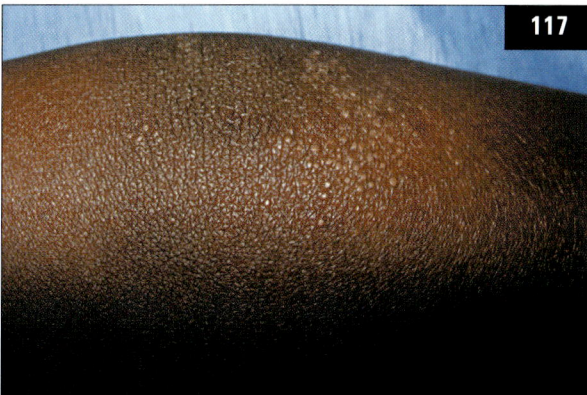

117 Lichen nitidus.

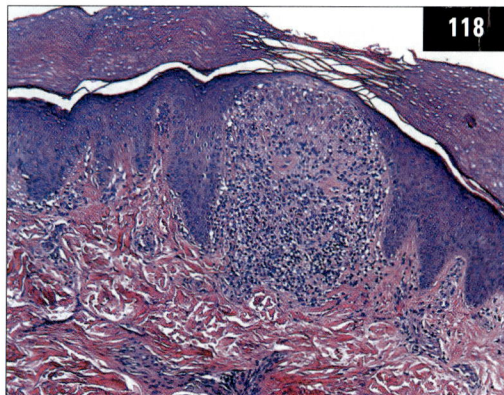

118 Histopathology of lichen nitidus.

causes of LP.[6,54] A few scattered reports in the literature document an association between HIV and mostly oral LP.[54] In most cases though, these have been attributed to drug reactions to zidovudine or ketoconazole and not to the HIV itself. One study found the mean time to develop oral LP after initiating these drugs was 14.5 weeks.[55] Another variant of LP that may be seen in HIV-infected patients is a photodistributed hypertrophic form. While unclear, the pathogenesis may be due to altered keratinocyte antigenicity due to the HIV infection and UV light exposure.[56,57]

It has been suggested that at least in the case of oral LP, HIV may have a protective effect towards developing the disease.[53] Some researchers have hypothesized that this may be due to immuno-suppression and CD4+ T cell deficiency not allowing the requisite self-cytotoxic mechanisms necessary to establish LP.[53]

Other exogenous agents have been associated with LP or at least a lichenoid dermatitis and/or stomatitis. Contact allergens, especially mercury, copper, and gold, may cause or exacerbate oral LP.[6] A long list of drugs may initiate LP or cause a lichenoid dermatitis. Some of these include antimalarials, beta-blockers, gold salts, penicillamine, spironolactone, and thiazide diuretics.[41] Seemingly innocuous agents such as nonsteroidal anti-inflammatory drugs (NSAIDs), ketoconazole, and tetracyclines may also cause this eruption.[41] Finally, in addition to viruses, metals, and drugs, occasionally LP may be caused by an underlying neoplasm.[6]

As with psoriasis, most of these triggers probably have to be combined with a genetically susceptible individual before LP will manifest. In support of this idea, a number of different HLA antigens have been found to be associated with LP (*Table 7*).

Through whichever mechanism, once this initial antigen is exposed, an infiltrate of CD8 T cells occurs at the epidermal–dermal interface.[6,54] These are the cells that demonstrate cytotoxic activity towards basal keratinocytes, causing apoptotic death.[6,54] This action, along with secretion of IFN-γ and TNF-α by CD4+ and CD8+ T cells, appear to be the critical factors involved in generating the LP lesion.[6,54]

CLINICAL FEATURES

Classic LP is often, if not always, described as cutaneous pruritic, purple (violaceous), polygonal, flat-topped papules (**119, 120**) and mucosal milky white reticulated lesions.[41] Koebnerization is commonly seen, and upon close examination, Wickham's striae, lace-like reticulated areas on the surface of the lesion, are usually evident. These lesions may be closely grouped in localized plaques or dispersed throughout the skin and mucous membranes.[6,41]

The most common locations for LP include the flexor surfaces, especially wrists and forearms, dorsal aspect of the hands, oral mucosa, glans penis, anterior lower legs, neck, and presacral area.[6,41,57] Untreated, the prognosis depends largely on the variant of LP. Unfortunately, most hypertrophic, oral, and nail lesions (**121**) are chronic, sometimes lasting decades, with remission being the exception to the rule.[6,41]

To aid in diagnosis and prognosis, LP has classically been divided into multiple variants. Actinic, acute, annular, atrophic, bullous, LP pemphigoides, hypertrophic, lichen planopilaris, linear, nail, oral, and ulcerative forms have all been described in the literature.[6] While a complete review of these different manifestations is beyond the scope of this chapter, their expression in the HIV-infected patient population is of special concern.

Although there are only a few reports in the literature of LP-like dermatoses in HIV-positive patients, one that has been described is a lichenoid photoexacerbated drug eruption. Most often, this eruption of violaceous plaques appears in a photodistributed pattern in HIV-positive patients after using NSAIDs or trimethoprim–sulfamethoxazole.[58] This highlights the importance of garnering a complete drug history, including over the counter and herbal medicines. Fortunately, avoidance of the sun, sunscreens, and discontinuation of the drug will, more often than not, result in resolution of symptoms.[58]

Another form of LP that has been described in AIDS patients is hypertrophic LP.[56] This entity has been documented in various case reports and seems to evolve from a pre-existing photosensitivity dermatitis. It has been reported to respond to treatment with etretinate.[56]

Table 7 HLA markers for lichen planus[6,29]

NONFAMILIAL LP	FAMILIAL LP
HLA-A3	HLA-B7
HLA-A5	HLA-Aw19
HLA-A28	HLA-B18
HLA-B8 (oral only)	HLA-Cw8
HLA-B16	
HLA-Bw35 (cutaneous)	
HLA-B27 (oral in British patients)	
HLA-B51 (oral in British patients)	
HLA-Bw57 (oral in British patients)	
HLA-DR1	
HLA-DR9 (oral in Japanese and Chinese patients)	
HLA-DQ1	

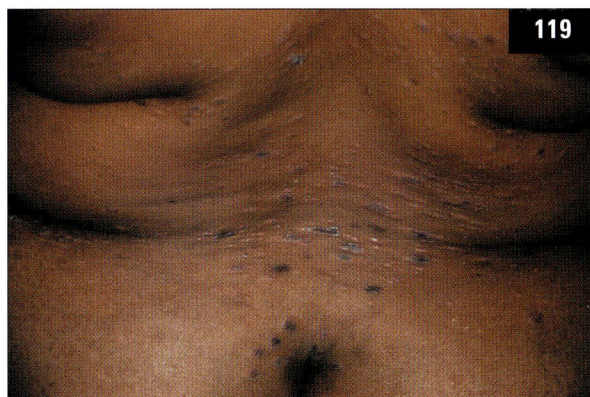

119 Lichen planus. Flat-topped, purple, polygonal, scaly papules on the lower back.

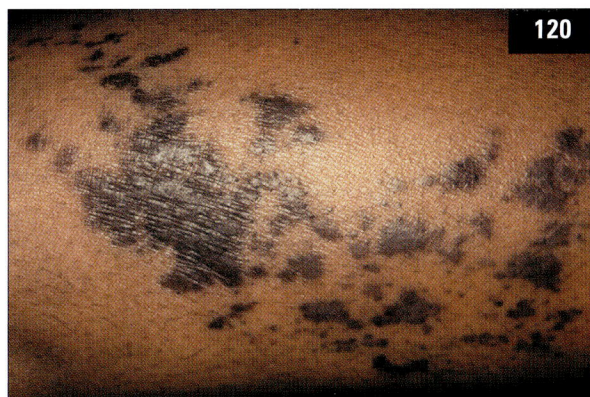

120 Lichen planus. Similar, more coalescent lesions with less prominent Wickham's striae.

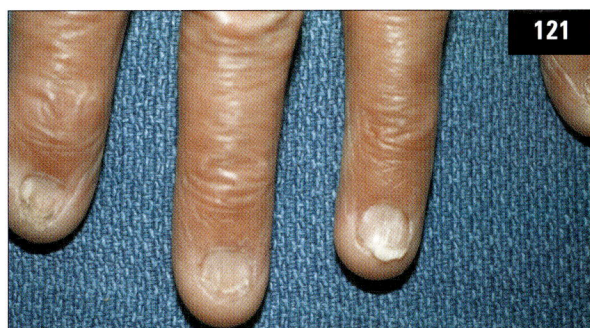

121 Lichen planus. Nail involvement with nail thinning, longitudinal ridging, pterygium formation and nail splitting.

Finally, there is at least one report of linear LP occurring in the HIV/AIDS population. This patient presented with three pruritic linear papular bands approximately 7 cm long distributed in the lines of Blaschko, that appeared clinically and histologically identical to LP.[59] The authors presume that HIV may have played a direct role in its pathogenesis due to the fact that other possible triggers such as HCV and metal dental amalgams were absent.[59]

HISTOPATHOLOGY

The characteristic histopathologic features of LP include hyperkeratosis, 'sawtooth' acanthosis, degenerative liquefactive necrosis of the basal cell layer with colloid bodies (necrotic keratinocytes), and a band-like lymphocytic interface at the dermo-epidermal junction.[6,41] This so called 'interface dermatitis' is classic for LP and will often be seen along with 'Max–Joseph spaces' and pigment incontinence.[6] As might be expected, HIV-associated LP may often not display this classic lymphocytic band-like infiltrate due to the virus' inherent T-lymphocyte depleting activity.[55] Direct immuno-fluorescence may show junctional fibrin deposits and IgM, and occasionally IgA, IgG, and C3 on colloid bodies.[41]

DIAGNOSIS

Clinical examination, history, and histologic evaluation are usually all that is necessary to differentiate LP from its main imitators. When trying to discern between LP and lupus erythematosus (LE), however, immunofluorescence studies may be helpful. A positive finding of immunoglobin deposition in the basement membrane zone is characteristic in LE.[6] It may be more difficult to distinguish between true LP and a lichenoid drug reaction, so history is often the most important element of the diagnosis.

MANAGEMENT

Treatment of LP may be difficult and there are many different agents that have been used with variable success.[57] Therapy depends in large part not only on the type and extent of the lesions but also on the personal experience of the dermatologist. Treatment is generally directed at suppressing inflammation and pruritus while preventing ulceration.[57] For symptomatic control of relatively mild cases, usually topical corticosteroid preparations and antihistamines are used. Other options that have been used include cryosurgery, intralesional and systemic corticosteroids, systemic retinoids, PUVA, gold, dapsone, azathioprine, mycophenelate mofetil, cyclophosphamide, methotrexate, cyclosporine, and alefacept.[6,37,41,60,61] PUVA, like cyclosporine and the other more dangerous treatment modalities, however, is often only employed as a last resort in long-standing resistant cases.[6] Finally, there are reports of griseofulvin, metronidazole, topical tacrolimus and pimecrolimus, and thalidomide being useful.[6,41,62] A study of refractory lichenoid photodrug eruptions in HIV-infected patients and hypertrophic LP has shown at least modest efficacy of etretinate therapy.[58]

LICHEN STRIATUS

DEFINITION/OVERVIEW

Lichen striatus (LS) is a rare, self-limited entity that is most commonly seen in children around the age of 3 years old.[29] This acquired linear skin eruption has a female predilection and is rarely seen in adults. To date, it has not been reported in the HIV-infected population.[29]

PATHOGENESIS/PATHOPHYSIOLOGY

There are several theories about the pathogenesis of LS, but almost nothing is known for certain. Genetic components, triggering factors, and viral associations have all been sought but never proven. Current theories suggest that genetically abnormal epidermal cells in the lines of Blaschko are subsequently triggered by an unknown infectious process coupled with environmental factors.[6,29] Others believe that LS is possibly a sequela of atopic dermatitis, although this seems unlikely given the prevalence of the latter.[6] At least one study has shown that many patients with LS also have a family history of atopic dermatitis, asthma, or allergic rhinitis, however.[6]

CLINICAL FEATURES

Clinically, there are pink to tan, flat-topped, smooth to scaly papules that are a few millimeters in diameter distributed in a linear fashion.[6,29] Papules coalesce to form a 1–3 cm band located unilaterally on an extremity and always along a line of Blaschko (**122**).[6,29] LS usually appears quickly over the course of days to weeks and spontaneously resolves by 1 year.[6,29] Most often, the condition is asymptomatic, but mild pruritus has been variably reported.[29]

HISTOPATHOLOGY

LS may demonstrate a number of different histologic reactions patterns (**123**). The most common is a lichenoid infiltrate with some spongiosis, exocytosis, parakeratosis, and dyskeratosis.[6] There is also a very characteristic infiltrate surrounding eccrine sweat glands. Immunohistochemistry reveals a CD3+ T cell infiltrate with CD8+ T cells surrounding necrotic keratinocytes.[6]

DIAGNOSIS

The main entities in the differential diagnosis include linear LP, linear graft versus host disease, and Blaschkitis.[6] In one AIDS patient, however, a case of herpes zoster was at first misdiagnosed as lichen striatus.[63]

MANAGEMENT

Due to spontaneous resolution and few if any symptoms, treatment is usually not needed. Topical corticosteroid preparations have sometimes been used, mainly in those with mild pruritus.[29]

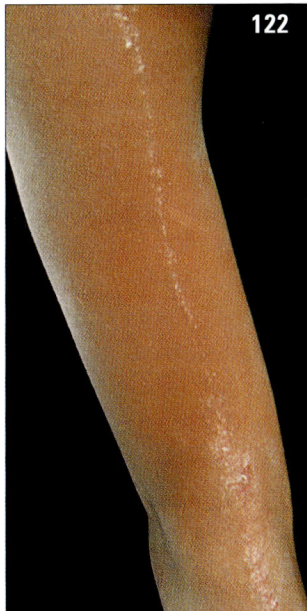

122 Lichen striatus.

123 Histology of lichen striatus.

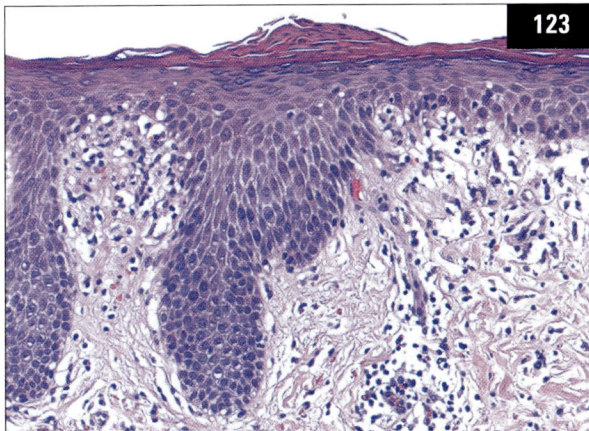

PITYRIASIS ALBA

DEFINITION/OVERVIEW

This common benign papulosquamous disease occurs in all races and is seen equally in both sexes.[29] Though it seems reasonable to suppose that cases of pityriasis alba (PA) should be present in HIV-positive patients, to our knowledge, it has not been observed to be increased in incidence.

PATHOGENESIS/PATHOPHYSIOLOGY

Although the exact etiology of PA has never been proven, it is thought to fall within the spectrum of atopic dermatitis.[6] There is a high incidence of PA in the atopic population and a reduced number of melanosomes has been documented in both conditions.[6]

CLINICAL FEATURES

The condition is most common in children and is characterized by patches of pale pink to light brown hypopigmentation (**124**) in a facial or maxillary distribution with vague borders.[6,29] Though PA is generally asymptomatic, in some patients a variable

124 Pityriasis alba.

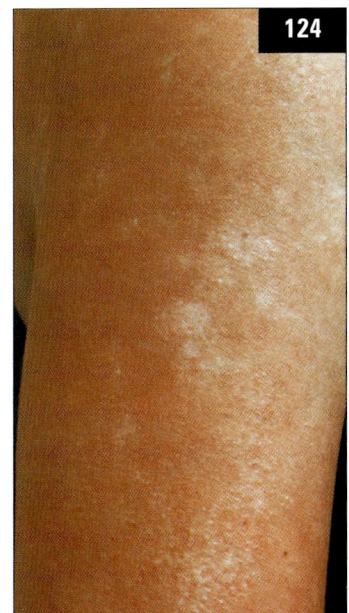

degree of burning or itching is reported.[29] The lesions are usually a few centimeters in diameter, have light powdery scale, and are accentuated in the summer months.[6] More uncommonly, PA can be found in other locations such as the shoulders, but regardless of location, will universally undergo spontaneous resolution with time.[6]

HISTOPATHOLOGY

The histology of PA demonstrates a sparse perivascular dermatitis with slight spongiosis. There is decreased epidermal melanin although it is usually not appreciable on examination of routine hematoxylin and eosin stained sections.[6]

DIAGNOSIS

The main entities in the differential diagnosis include vitiligo, tinea versicolor, and psoriatic leukoderma. These can ususlly be excluded on the basis of clinical examination, potassium hydroxide preparations, and Wood's light examination.[6,29]

MANAGEMENT

No treatment is advocated for PA other than emollients to reduce dryness. Topical corticosteroid preparations may also be beneficial.[29]

ACQUIRED ICHTHYOSIS

DEFINITION/OVERVIEW

Ichthyosis is a disorder of cornification with abnormal desquamation of the epidermis.[6] This disease, characterized by generalized scaling of the skin, may be either inherited or acquired.[6] Only the acquired form of ichthyosis has been associated with HIV infection. It may be associated with other conditions such as endocrine and metabolic disorders, as well as autoimmune conditions, some of which may develop in HIV-infected patients and may subsequently lead to its appearance.[29] The acquired icthyosis of HIV-positive patients is usually correlated with advanced AIDS,[64] developing when the T cell count is $<50 \times 10^6/l$ CD4+ cells.[6] At least one analysis has found icthyotic or xerotic skin in up to 30% of AIDS patients with severe helper T cell depletion.[29] Icthyosis is also more frequent in patients coinfected with human T cell lymphotrophic virus type 2 (HTLV-II) and HIV-1.[29]

PATHOGENESIS/PATHOPHYSIOLOGY

Icthyosis occurs as a result of increased cell to cell adhesion causing abnormal desquamation and scale formation.[44] Odland bodies are the responsible adhesive organelles hindering the desquamation process.[44] In X-linked variants there is a demonstrable deficiency in steroid sulfatase.[44] This leads to accumulation of nondegraded cholesterol sulfate and continued cell to cell adhesion, resulting in a compacted stratum corneum with loss of normal basket weave pattern.[44]

CLINICAL FEATURES

In comparison with the other icthyoses, acquired icthyosis tends to be mild and resemble icthyosis vulgaris.[29] As with many other conditions, it may be more severe in HIV-infected patients.[3] There is dryness of the skin with plates of fish-like scales that are often hyperpigmented (**125, 126**). It usually begins on the lower extremities and becomes generalized.[2,3] There is often palmoplantar keratoderma.[2,3] Most affected patients are profoundly immunocompromised with T cell counts of $<5 \times 10^4/l$. It is associated with a poor prognosis and usually relatively rapid deterioration.[2]

HISTOPATHOLOGY

The histopathology is similar to that of icthyosis vulgaris with minimal changes in the epidermis other than an absent or diminished granular layer, dense compact orthokeratosis, and little inflammation (**127**).[2,3,29]

DIAGNOSIS

The diagnosis is usually made on the basis of a distinct clinical appearance of icthyosis that first presents in adulthood. Once new-onset icthyosis is suspected, patients should be evaluated for underlying conditions such as malignancy, medications, AIDS, or sarcoidosis.[29]

MANAGEMENT

Usually, symptomatic therapy is centered around controlling scaling. Lactic acid- and urea-containing emollients are effective and commonly used preparations. Any underlying disorders should be addressed and following their treatment, the condition may improve.

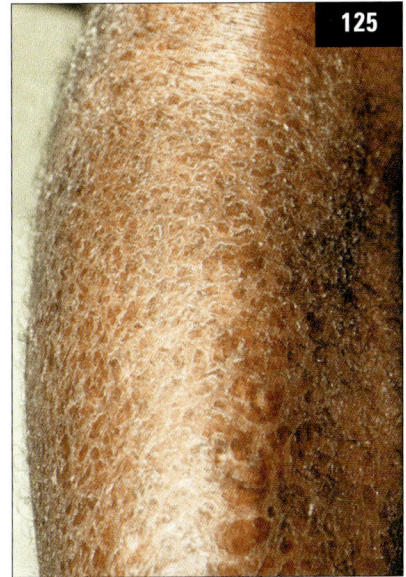

125 Acquired ichthyosis. Severe xerosis with plate-like, hyperpigmented scales on the leg.

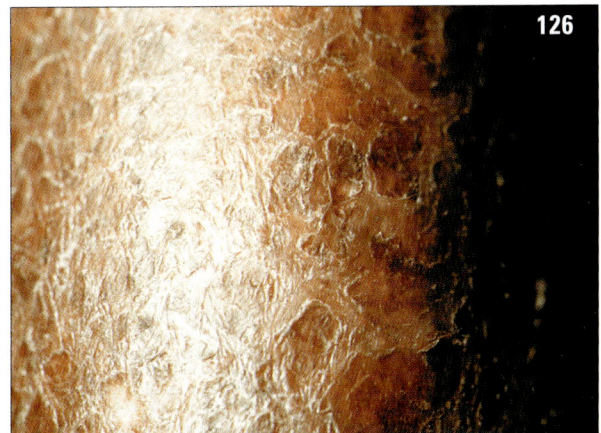

126 Acquired ichthyosis. Closer view of the plate-like scaling.

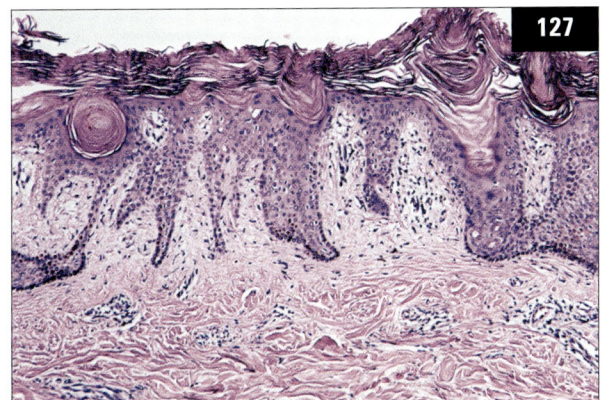

127 Histology of acquired ichthyosis. Compact orthokeratosis with diminished and focally absent granular cell layer and minimal inflammation.

XEROSIS GENERALISATA/ASTEATOTIC ECZEMA

DEFINITION/OVERVIEW

In some AIDS patient populations, xerosis generalisata has the highest prevalence of all papulosquamous diseases at around 4.5%.[2] It tends to arise before most other papulosquamous diseases when the helper T cell count is still >400 × 10^6/l,[2] thus can be recognized as an early harbinger of HIV infection. By the time the CD4+ cell count has dropped to <50 × 10^6/l, the generalized xerosis often transforms into a more severe generalized acquired icthyosis.[6]

PATHOGENESIS/PATHOPHYSIOLOGY

Xerosis is due, in large part, to decreased synthesis of 'natural moisturizing factor'.[6] Because of the lack of this compound, along with a general deficiency of intercellular lipids, corneocytes are retained in the stratum corneum and its water binding capacity is greatly reduced.[6] Thus, this top layer of the epidermis dries out, forms cracks, and becomes scaly.[6] Generally speaking, this is an almost universal problem of aging but is made worse by other factors such as chronic sun exposure, excessive bathing, low humidity, and low temperature.[6] In HIV-positive patients, the severe xerosis that is observed may be due to many factors such as abnormal nutrition and diminished autonomic nervous functions such as sweating and sebaceous gland secretion.[11]

CLINICAL FEATURES

Xerosis usually presents as dry, dull, flaky, scaling skin which, in advanced cases, can appear as the superficial cracks of a 'dried river bed' (**128**).[6] Asteatotic eczema in its advanced stages can also show erythema, oozing, crusting, and excoriations.[6] In the general population, the anterior tibial area is the region most often affected.[6] In AIDS patients, as might be expected, the xerosis can be quite extensive and is sometimes referred to as a 'generalized dry skin' syndrome.[2] This diffuse fine scaling is often so pruritic that it is refractory to all conventional methods of treatment.[2]

HISTOPATHOLOGY

Histologic examination reveals focal parakeratosis, slight spongiosis, a sparse superficial perivascular lymphocytic infiltrate, and a compact stratum corneum.[2,6] There is often only slight hyperkeratosis and parakeratosis that can be influenced by how much the patient scratches.[2]

DIAGNOSIS

The main entities to exclude in differential diagnosis include stasis dermatitis and contact dermatitis. Of course, in pruritic cases, scabies and other diseases such as dermatophytosis should also be excluded.[2]

MANAGEMENT

Usually, only topical corticosteroids, regular emollient use with urea- and 12% lactic acid-containing products and avoidance of aggravating factors are all that are necessary to treat this condition.[2,6,11] For the associated pruritus, H1 antihistamines such as hydroxyzine and super-saturated fatty acid soaps are recommended.[2]

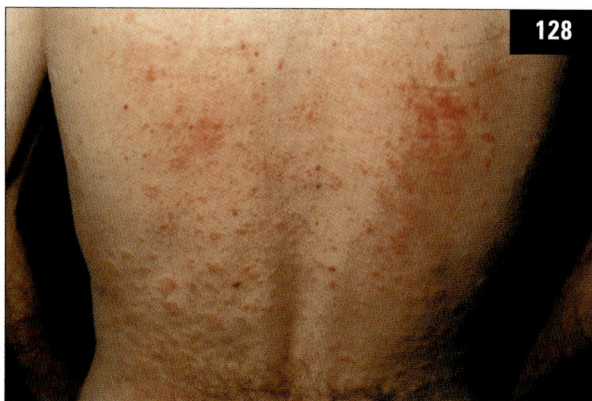

128 Xerosis generalisata.

CHAPTER 8

NON-NEOPLASTIC DISORDERS OF VASCULATURE IN HIV INFECTION

Benjamin K. Stoff, Antoanella Calame, and Clay J. Cockerell

INTRODUCTION

Human immunodeficiency virus (HIV)-related vascular diseases with skin manifestations are varied. The most common and well-studied disorder in this group, Kaposi's sarcoma (KS), is discussed in Chapter 12, as are the so-called angiocentric lymphoproliferative disorders. What remains is a broad array of rare disorders, often with bizarre clinical manifestations. As demonstrated below, the breadth of vascular disease results, in part, from the direct effects of HIV infection and, more commonly, from indirect consequences, such as immune suppression.

VASCULITIS

DEFINITION/OVERVIEW

Even as the most common non-KS vasculocutaneous lesion in HIV patients, vasculitis is nonetheless rare in this population, affecting roughly 1% of patients according to a recent review.[1] A variety of mechanisms for inflammation, as well as caliber of vessel affected, has been reported in the literature. Although sometimes similar in appearance, vasculitis in HIV-infected patients appears to bear no relation to the presence of KS.[2]

PATHOGENESIS/PATHOPHYSIOLOGY

Infectious

The pathophysiology of HIV-related vasculitis depends entirely on the mediator of inflammation. Infection appears to be most common, usually affecting small vessels.[3] Of the myriad of opportunistic agents reported to cause vasculitis in HIV-infected patients (e.g. *Toxoplasma gondii*, *Pneumocystis carinii*, *Salmonella* sp., Epstein–Barr virus [EBV], among others), cytomegalovirus (CMV) and *Mycobacterium tuberculosis* are the most common. Microbial invasion of the vessel wall is one of the mechanisms of inflammation in these cases. Indeed, HIV virions themselves have been demonstrated in perivascular cells of patients with vasculitis but no evidence of other infection.[4] In any case, damaged vessels allow red blood cells to extravasate, leading to characteristic purpura clinically.

Another mechanism of inflammation in infectious vasculitis affecting HIV patients is immune complex-mediated vasculitis. An example is presented in a recent case report, which documents nodular vasculitis of the lower extremities in an HIV patient with active pulmonary tuberculosis (TB), the so-called nodular tuberculid reaction.[5]

Hypersensitivity

Immune-mediated vasculitis in HIV-infected patients may also occur outside the setting of opportunistic infection. Indeed, some speculate that HIV infection predisposes to hypersensitivity.[6] Examples of causative factors include drugs, especially antiretrovirals such as abacavir, and cryoglobulins.[7] In these cases, vessel inflammation is triggered by immune complex deposition. Some have argued that low numbers of CD4+ T cells stimulate overcompensation by the humoral arm of the immune system, resulting in a relative abundance of antibodies.[8] Antibodies couple with haptens, evoked either by drugs or prior exposure to pathogens,[9] which subsequently deposit in vessel walls promoting an inflammatory response. The inflammatory cascade is carried out as immune complexes activate complement, attracting neutrophils that adhere to endothelial cells. This adherence promotes the release of cytokines, attracting other inflammatory cells to the site. Leukocytes subsequently release enzymes that mediate vessel wall damage. As described above, erythrocytes extravasate through inflamed vessels resulting in purpura.

CLINICAL FEATURES

Small vessel (arterioles, venules, and capillaries)

Small vessel vasculitic lesions usually begin as urticarial and/or petechial papules and develop into characteristic palpable purpura (i.e. red papules that do not blanch upon application of direct pressure) in dependent areas and areas of trauma (**129**). HIV-positive patients tend to have more diffuse cutaneous involvement than seronegative counterparts and lesions can be more severe, evolving into bullae or ulcers in some cases (**130**).[10] Occasionally, the palpable purpura of small vessel vasculitis in an HIV-positive patient may be a component of a larger symptom complex, such as that seen with Henoch–Schönlein purpura (HSP) (i.e. palpable purpura with abdominal pain, arthritis, and hematuria)[11] and Behçet's disease (i.e. palpable purpura with recurrent oral ulcers, ocular lesions, and arthritis).[12] Isolated case reports of HIV-positive patients with Wegner's granulomatosis, a necrotizing, granulomatous vasculitis affecting small vessels, are also present in the literature.[13]

Medium vessel (small/medium sized arteries and veins)

Although less common, medium vessel vasculitis with cutaneous manifestations has been documented in patients with HIV. Most often, this occurs in the setting of a polyarteritis nodosa-like syndrome that is analogous to cutaneous polyarteritis nodosa (c-PAN) in which nodules manifest as a result of medium vessel inflammation in the deep dermis.[14] Foci of punched-out ulceration ensue and lesions become tender. The lacy erythema of livedo reticularis often occurs concomitantly. HIV-infected patients with this syndrome can present with neurologic complaints, which may or may not precede cutaneous findings. While PAN is more common among HIV-positive patients than in seronegative individuals, other characteristic systemic involvement, such as gastrointestinal, renal, and musculoskeletal manifestations, tends to be less frequent. HIV-infected patients with the PAN-like syndrome experience more constant symptoms, not waxing and waning as classically described for PAN, and serology for hepatitis B virus (HBV) tends to be negative.

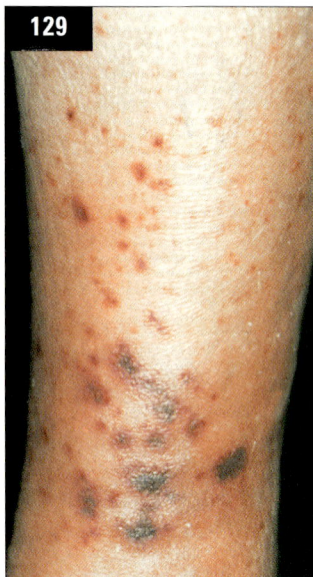

129 Small vessel vasculitis. Multiple erythematous to violaceous, nonblanching papules (palpable purpura) on the leg.

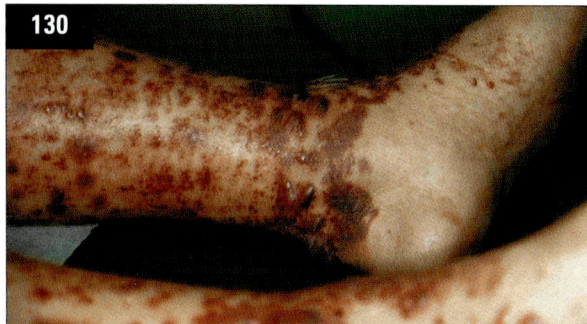

130 Small vessel vasculitis. Extensive violaceous papules and plaques with vesicles and bullae on the lower extremities.

Another medium vessel vasculitis with cutaneous association that affects HIV-positive patients is Kawasaki's disease.[15] Normally regarded as a pediatric entity, Kawasaki's disease is a poorly understood symptom complex, which includes fever of greater than 5 days, cervical lymphadenopathy, bilateral conjunctivitis, polymorphous rash (macular, morbilliform and/or urticarial), mucous membrane involvement (erythema/fissuring of lips, 'strawberry' tongue, and/or generalized erythema of pharyngeal mucous membranes), and cutaneous changes of the distal extremities (erythema of palms and soles, induration, and/or membranous desquamation of finger tips). Unlike PAN, however, the skin changes of Kawasaki's disease are not related to vasculitis. Further, the relative contribution of each symptom and natural course of disease appear to be different in HIV-positive patients when compared to seronegative children.

Large vessel

Inflammation affecting large vessels has been demonstrated in HIV-infected patients, particularly involving the central nervous system (CNS). However, these disorders fail to show cutaneous signs and thus are not discussed here.

HISTOLOGY

Small vessel

The cutaneous histology of small vessel vasculitis, either in isolation or as a part of a larger symptom complex, follows a characteristic evolution. Lesions begin with perivascular infiltrate composed of lymphocytes, eosinophils, and polymorphonuclear cells, which corresponds to urticaria clinically.[2] The onset of purpura correlates with inflammatory cells and fibrin deposition within the vessel walls, which allows leakage of red blood cells into the dermis. There is also fibrin deposition within vessel walls as well as vascular wall degeneration. There is prominent leukocytoclasia with fragments of neutrophils in the infiltrate (**131**). Finally, microthrombi are a late finding in affected vessels. Aneurysm formation has also been documented in HIV-infected patients.[3]

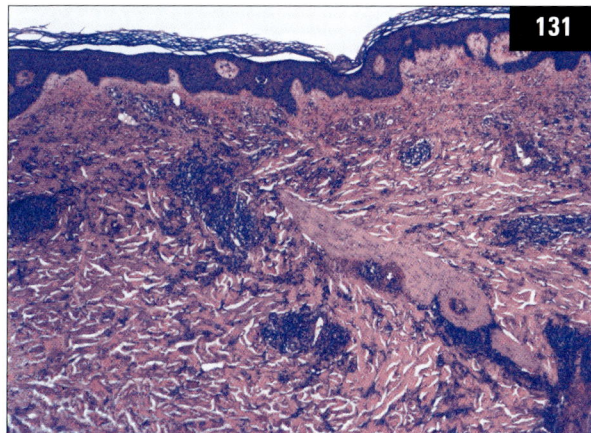

131 Histology of small vessel vasculitis. Dense perivascular infiltrate composed of neutrophils and lymphocytes with destruction of small dermal blood vessels, fibrin deposition in blood vessel walls, neutrophilic debris (leukocytoclasia), and extravasated red blood cells.

Medium vessel

The dermatopathology of PAN-like lesions includes necrotizing vasculitis of deep dermal vessels, corresponding to the clinical presentation of nodules, with a mixed infiltrate of polymorphonuclear cells, monocytes, and eosinophils. With disease progression, microthrombi can be seen. In the resolution phase, fibroblasts proliferate leaving perivascular scarring.[16] Leukocytoclastic vasculitis (LCV) of the superficial dermal vessels, with characteristic neutrophilic infiltration of vessel walls and accompanying nuclear debris from fragmented leukocytes, has been demonstrated in association with these lesions.

As mentioned above, the cutaneous manifestations of Kawasaki's disease are not related to vasculitis. Common histologic findings are nonspecific and include papillary dermal edema, dilated blood vessels with endothelial swelling, and mild perivascular infiltrate.[16]

DIAGNOSIS

Biopsy is the standard for diagnosing cutaneous vasculitis. Ideally, specimens from the lesion should be obtained within 48 hours of onset, as samples taken after that point may reveal healing rather than the original injury.[17] Supporting laboratory data may be useful as well, particularly if the vasculitis is suspected to be an element of a larger disease process. When considering HSP, for instance, blood urea nitrogen and creatinine levels as well as urinalysis should be pursued to assess renal involvement. Serologic markers classically used in the work-up of vasculitis, such as C-reactive protein and complement levels, may also be of use. In the rare HIV-infected patient in whom Wegener's disease is suspected, a positive antineutrophilic antibody (ANA) finding should be interpreted with caution, as false-positives are reportedly common.[18] It is important to note that the development of vasculitis in the HIV-positive patient has not been tightly correlated with CD4+ T cell count.[2]

MANAGEMENT

The treatment of HIV-related vasculitis, indeed vasculitis in any setting, revolves around identification and reversal of the underlying inflammatory process. Removal of the offending drug or antimicrobials targeted at infectious culprits should be pursued when appropriate. Nonsteroidal anti-inflammatory drugs (NSAIDs) are considered first-line therapy for small vessel vasculitides, although caution should be exercised in the face of renal dysfunction as in HSP.[19] Colchicine or dapsone is next on the therapeutic ladder for cutaneous small vessel vasculitis. Of note, no therapy has proven consistently effective for HSP, with the possible exception of dapsone and intravenous immunoglobulin (IVIG).[20] Medium vessel cutaneous vasculitis, as in the PAN-like syndrome seen in HIV-infected patients, is also treated first with NSAIDs. Methotrexate and cyclosporine are generally considered second-line agents but their use should be guarded in patients with background immunosuppression. Again, IVIG has been effective in some cases.[19]

ERYTHEMA ELEVATUM DIUTINUM

DEFINITION/OVERVIEW

Closely related to vasculitis, erythema elevatum diutinum (EED) is often regarded as a chronic, fibrosing form of LCV.[2] On the spectrum of neutrophilic dermatoses, the condition maintains a rare but documented association with HIV, with only 33 cases reported in the literature.[2,21–26] Although unrelated pathophysiologically, EED should be considered in the differential diagnosis of KS due to a similar clinical appearance.[27] EED also has an association with a number of systemic diseases other than HIV, including inflammatory bowel disease[28] and rheumatoid arthritis.[29]

PATHOGENESIS/PATHOPHYSIOLOGY

EED is a hypersensitivity phenomenon.[2] There is evidence to suggest that preceding streptococcal exposure may trigger the formation of immune complexes, which subsequently deposit in dermal blood vessels.[23] Complement fixation ensues which results in inflammation, damage to vessel walls, and extravasation of erythrocytes, as described in the preceding section.

CLINICAL FEATURES

Cutaneous lesions begin as palpable purpura but, unlike classic small vessel cutaneous vasculitis, evolve into violaceous or yellowish-brown, firm plaques or nodules distributed on the periarticular areas, buttocks, and torso (132).[2,16] As is often the case, HIV-infected patients can have more extensive involvement, including painful lesions on the palms and soles (133).[23]

HISTOLOGY

Early lesions reveal LCV with extensive infiltrate of neutrophils and histiocytes.[2] Of note, the presence of large numbers of neutrophils with paucity of eosinophils is a quality that distinguishes EED from granuloma faciale, histologically.[30] Lesions progress, developing perivascular fibrosis with persistence of neutrophils and occasional eosinophils in the mid-dermis (134). Ultimately, granulation occurs with proliferation of dermal spindle cells and development of intracellular lipid deposits.[31] Sections may stain positive for MAC-387 indicating a histiocytic infiltrate.[32]

DIAGNOSIS

Biopsy is diagnostic of EED.[2] Other laboratory studies to consider include antistreptolysin O titer, to document prior exposure to *Streptococcus*, and complement levels, which may be low due to immune complex formation with subsequent complement fixation. Also of note, EED tends to be associated with CD4+ counts of <200 × 10⁶/l.[25]

MANAGEMENT

There is documented response of EED in HIV-positive patients to both dapsone and antiretrovirals, although the effect is lessened when lesions are fibrotic histologically.[26] In cases refractory to medical treatment, surgical excision may be required.[2]

BACILLARY ANGIOMATOSIS

DEFINITION/OVERVIEW

Bacillary angiomatosis (BA) is an infectious vasculopathy affecting, by some estimates, 1 in 1000 HIV-infected individuals.[33] The disease is caused by either of two closely related species of *Bartonella*: *B. henselae*, acquired from cat exposure, and *B. quintana*, associated with poor living conditions. It is another condition to be considered in the differential diagnosis of KS. While relatively common in the early years of the HIV pandemic, it is much less common since the advent of highly active antiretroviral therapy (HAART).

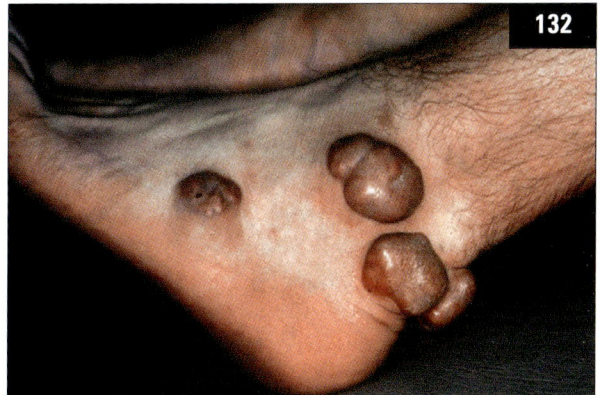

132 Erythema elevatum diutinum. Firm, violaceous nodules on the distal leg.

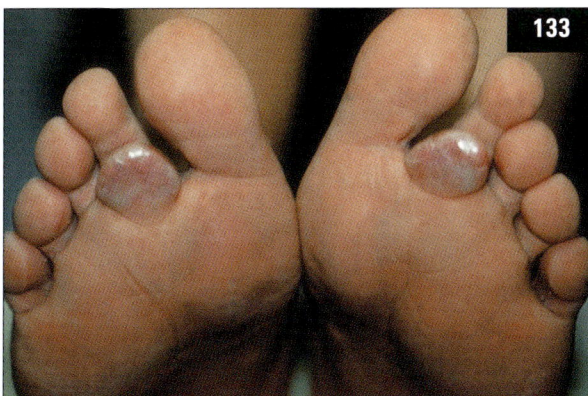

133 Erythema elevatum diutinum. Firm, flesh-colored to violaceous nodules on the soles.

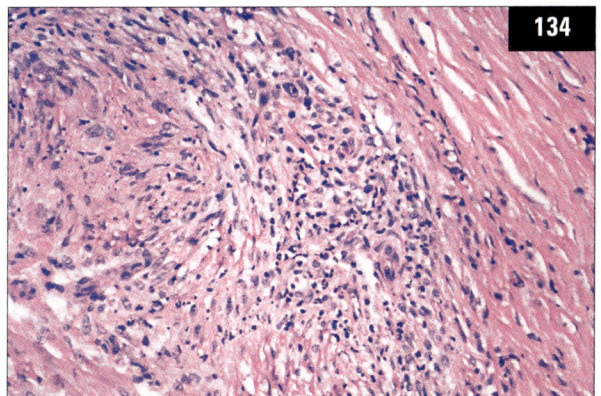

134 Histology of erythema elevatum diutinum. Leukocytoclastic vasculitis showing an infiltrate composed of neutrophils and some histiocytes, with leukocytoclasia, and destruction of a small blood vessel.

PATHOGENESIS/PATHOPHYSIOLOGY

The pathologic sequence of BA is triggered by infection of capillary endothelial cells in the dermis. It has been suggested that infected endothelial cells, in turn, release vascular endothelial growth factor (VEGF), which stimulates characteristic proliferation of small cutaneous vessels seen on histology.[34]

CLINICAL FEATURES

Typical lesions of BA begin as purple papules and evolve into red, friable, dome-shaped nodules ranging in size from 1 mm to 2 cm (see **37–39**).[35] Distribution can be limited or widespread, typically involving the face, trunk, and extremities. HIV-infected patients who develop this condition have often progressed to advanced aquired immunodeficiency syndrome (AIDS).

HISTOLOGY

Dermatopathologic analysis of BA reveals lobular proliferation of small dermal blood vessels with characteristic epithelial cell protrusion into the lumen. The surrounding infiltrate is predominantly polymorphonuclear. Warthin–Starry silver staining reveals the bacteria in the form of fine granular material in close proximity to the affected vessels (see **40–42**).[36]

DIAGNOSIS

Histology coupled with clinical features is usually required for the diagnosis of BA. Special blood and skin cultures may also be of use.[37,38] BA is associated with CD4+ counts of $<200 \times 10^6$/l.

MANAGEMENT

Erythromycin 500 mg given four times per day is the treatment of choice for BA.[39] Reports of resistance to other antibiotics, including vancomycin, penicillin, and sulfanomides, support the use of erythromycin. Relapse is common.

HIV-RELATED THROMBOCYTOPENIA

DEFINITION/OVERVIEW

Although not a vasculopathy, HIV-related thrombocytopenia is nonetheless included in this section, as skin manifestations of this condition involve incidental, microscopic vessel injury coupled with aberrant homeostasis associated with low platelet counts. It is a relatively common finding in HIV-infected individuals, with a prevalence of 16–30% in one study.[40] Indeed, many advocate HIV testing in patients with thrombocytopenia of unknown origin. The disorder is closely related to idiopathic thrombocytopenic purpura (ITP) clinically but remains a distinct entity. The cause is thought to be multifactorial in HIV-infected patients and there are differences in the nature of autoantibodies, as well as in correlation between antibodies and platelet count when compared to ITP.[41]

PATHOGENESIS/PATHOPHYSIOLOGY

As suggested above, HIV-related thrombocytopenia is a disease with multiple causes. In contrast to ITP, thrombocytopenia related to HIV is based, in part, on decreased platelet production.[42] This may be due to viral infection itself or the use of various therapeutic drugs which supress megakaryocytes. Like ITP, antibody-mediated destruction of platelets also plays a role. Studies have demonstrated that molecular mimicry may be involved, with the demonstration of shared epitopes among platelet surface proteins and viral peptides.[43] Antibody-bound platelets are cleared by tissue macrophages, particularly in the spleen. However, antibody quantity does not correlate as well with platelet count as in ITP, thought to be due to reticuloendothelial dysfunction associated with HIV.[44] In any case, low platelet counts disrupt primary homeostasis, as incidental microinjury to cutaneous vessels results in extravasation of erythrocytes, with petechiae, purpura, or ecchymoses.

CLINICAL FEATURES

Cutaneous lesions are nonblanching, red (fresh) to brown (older), and small, ranging in size from less than 2 mm (petechiae) to 2 mm–1 cm (purpura) to greater than 1 cm (ecchymoses) in rare cases. The severity of lesions depends on platelet count. Skin lesions typically develop with platelet counts between 5,000 and 20,000.[41] Counts below 10,000 can result in bleeding from mucosal sites, most commonly epistaxis. Patients with platelet levels from 50,000 to 100,000 typically display only easy bruising. In contrast to vasculitis, most lesions associated with thrombocytopenia are macular. Unlike ITP patients, splenomegaly is common with HIV-related thrombocytopenia.[44] Also of note, the degree of thrombocytopenia does not seem to correlate with HIV disease progression, in terms of viral load or CD4+ T cell count.[45]

HISTOLOGY

The histology of HIV-related thrombocytopenic skin lesions is nonspecific, demonstrating extravasated erythrocytes in the dermis. A biopsy is not necessary for diagnosis and, if performed, great caution should be exercised due to bleeding risks.

DIAGNOSIS

In the diagnosis of HIV-related thrombocytopenia, exclusion of other causes of low platelets is paramount. Patients will demonstrate a low platelet count with an otherwise normal complete blood count and normal coagulation studies. Peripheral blood smear shows normal-sized or slightly enlarged platelets. Bone marrow aspiration, which is often necessary to rule out malignant or infectious infiltration, shows a nonspecific increase in megakaryocytes.[46]

MANAGEMENT

The mainstay of treatment for HIV-related thrombocytopenia is antiretroviral therapy. For severe cases, short courses of systemic corticosteroids may be used but long-term therapy is unwise due to exacerbated risk of infection and malignancy.[47] Weekly doses of IVIG have also proven effective.[48] Splenectomy may be pursued in refractory cases without effect on HIV disease progression.[49]

DIFFUSE/FACIAL TELANGIECTASIA

DEFINITION/OVERVIEW

Relatively benign lesions, telangiectasias are more a cosmetic than medical problem for HIV-infected patients. As demonstrated time and again, a lesion or condition common in the general population is encountered in a more severe form in the setting of HIV infection. The finding of diffuse/facial telangiectasia without an obvious source may warrant testing for HIV.

PATHOGENESIS/PATHOPHYSIOLOGY

The pathogenesis of this condition is not well understood, although some have speculated that patients may have increased vascular endothelial growth factor (VEGF) in their circulation.[2]

CLINICAL FEATURES

The lesions are classically described as single or grouped erythematous strands with a central punctum, presenting on the upper chest in a crescentic pattern between the clavicles.[50] They may also appear on the cheeks and neck (135).[2]

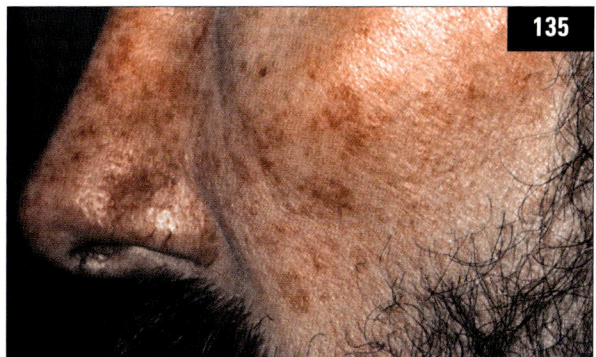

135 Extensive telangiectasias on the face in a patient infected with HIV.

HISTOLOGY

Histologic analysis reveals dilated dermal vessels with, according to one account, a perivascular infiltrate of plasma cells.[51] No endothelial proliferation has been demonstrated.[50,51]

DIAGNOSIS

Diagnosis is made solely by physical examination. While the differential diagnosis of diseases with telangiectasias is broad, the typical distribution in an HIV-positive patient should prompt suspicion for this condition.

MANAGEMENT

Cosmetic treatments such as laser ablation are effective for telangiectasias.[2] There is also a reported response to tetracycline.[52]

HYPERALGESIC PSEUDOTHROMBOPHLEBITIS

DEFINITION/OVERVIEW

The epitome of a bizarre, HIV-related abnormality of the vasculature, hyperalgesic pseudothrombophlebitis (HP) is a poorly understood, exceedingly rare phenomenon, with only six reports in the HIV literature.[53,54]

PATHOGENESIS/PATHOPHYSIOLOGY

Some have speculated that this lesion is a deeply-seated KS, as four of the five patients in whom the condition was originally described also had KS.[2] Otherwise, the mechanism of pathology is unknown.

CLINICAL FEATURES

Patients with this condition typically present with generalized swelling and tenderness of an extremity.[53] No chords are palpable and venous ultrasonography demonstrates patent vessels.

HISTOLOGY

No specific histologic pattern has been identified.

DIAGNOSIS

Doppler ultrasonography and/or venography can be performed to rule out true thrombophlebitis.[2] No laboratory abnormalities are associated with HP.

MANAGEMENT

The condition appears to be self-limiting, according to the cases in the literature.[53,54] Treatment is supportive with analgesics, warm compresses, bed rest, and extremity elevation.[2]

CHAPTER 9

PAPULOPRURITIC SKIN DISORDERS

Antoanella Calame and Clay J. Cockerell

INTRODUCTION

Papulopruritic dermatoses are a frequent initial manifestations of human immunodeficiency virus (HIV) and acquired immunodeficiency syndrome (AIDS) and are a cause of distress for many patients. Accurate and timely recognition of these conditions will lead to more rapid diagnoses, better targeted therapy, and most importantly, lessening of symptoms.

PRURITIC PAPULAR ERUPTION

DEFINITION/OVERVIEW

Pruritic papular eruption (PPE) of HIV infection is defined as a chronic pruritic papular eruption of unknown cause with a symmetric distribution on the head, neck, trunk, and extremities.[1] The prevalence is 11–46% so it is a relatively common skin disorder affecting HIV-positive patients.[2–6] HIV-infected individuals in warm tropical climates are more commonly affected and it is less common in patients in North America and Europe.[2]

PPE is frequently the initial manifestation of HIV infection and may occur months to even years before a serologic diagnosis of HIV is made.[2,7] However, it is also commonly found in patients with CD4 T cell counts $<100 \times 10^6$/l so that it is also a manifestation of late-stage HIV disease.[7,8]

PATHOGENESIS/PATHOPHYSIOLOGY

To date, the etiology is unknown, although many theories exist. One theory, supported by the fact that the condition is more prevalent in hot tropical environments, is that it is a reaction to arthropod assaults.[9] In fact, Eisman has even suggested calling this condition 'arthropod-induced prurigo of HIV'. Others believe that patients with PPE are exhibiting a hypersensitivity reaction to arthropod antigens to which the patient was previously exposed that in the past have not caused lasting discomfort.[10]

Although many causes such as scabies, *Demodex folliculorum*, and *Staphylococcus aureus* have been suggested,[11] they have not been confirmed.[4]

Another theory is that PPE may be related to drug hypersensitivity as many patients with HIV are receiving one or more therapeutic drugs. However, this is less likely to be valid as PPE occurs in a number of patients who are not receiving any medication.[9] No specific agent has been suggested and none has been proven to be causal.[2,12]

The histologic findings of PPE feature a folliculitis with a mononuclear cell infiltrate around hair follicles and follicular spongiosis of the external root sheath.[12] Because of this, it has been postulated that an immune reaction to sebum, one of the proposed causes of eosinophilic folliculitis,[13] may be at play in this entity as well. However, other studies have reported no infiltrates associated with hair follicles in biopsy specimens suggesting that this is a variable finding.[10]

Finally, there are two additional theories about the cause of PPE. In a study by Kinloch-de Loes *et al.*, antibodies to bullous pemphigoid antigen were detected in 75% of patients with PPE suggesting an autoimmune basis.[14] The second, which notes that PPE can arise in patients without HIV but who have an idiopathic decrease in CD4 T cells, suggests that the disorder is caused by an altered immune response associated with CD4 lymphopenia.[15]

Given these diverse possible causes, some have suggested that the condition is not one process but may represent a manifestation of several different disorders.

CLINICAL FEATURES

Patients with PPE have skin-colored to erythematous papules distributed in a symmetric distribution on the face, trunk, and extremities (136, 137). Most of the lesions are on the arms and legs, especially the extensor surfaces and the back of the hands.[2] Mucosal surfaces are spared as are the palms and soles, including the webbed spaces between the digits. Additionally, confluence of the papules is not seen and the lesions may involve hair follicles.[2] As lesions develop, they are accompanied by intense pruritus and, as such, are excoriated soon after they appear. Constant scratching often results in postinflammatory pigmentary changes, scarring, and prurigo nodules.[9]

HISTOPATHOLOGY

There have been no consistent microscopic findings reported. The epidermis may show hyperkeratosis, acanthosis, and focal dyskeratosis with numerous necrotic cells as well fibrosis of the dermis.[15] There is often an inflammatory infiltrate composed of neutrophils, lymphocytes, and eosinophils involving the superficial, interstitial, and deep perivascular tissue, with the inflammation often extending into the subcutis, a pattern quite similar to that seen in arthropod assault reactions.[10] Some specimens may demonstrate a central punctum. As noted above, in some cases there may be involvement of hair follicles with spongiosis and a mixed infiltrate of lymphocytes, histiocytes, and occasional eosinophils.[12] There is also an increase in CD8+ lymphocytes, as well as histiocytes and mast cells in the infiltrate. It is thought that these CD8+ lymphocytes are responsible for the inflammatory mediators that attract other inflammatory cells to the area.[16]

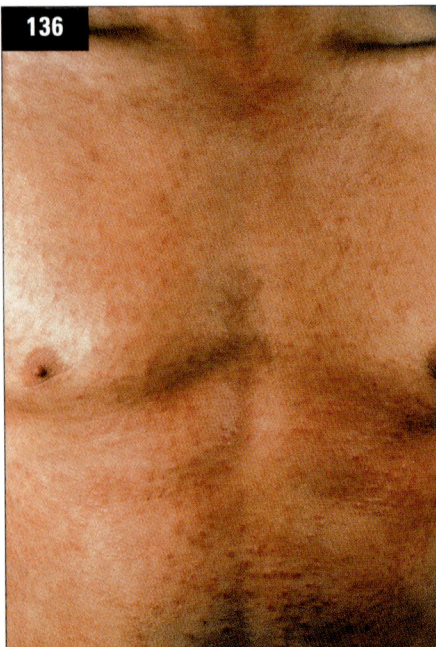
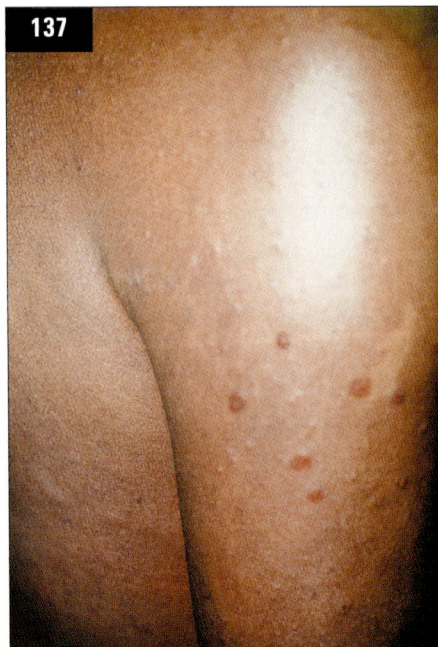

136, 137 Pruritic papular eruption of HIV. Multiple erythematous papules on the trunk (136) and arm (137) with several lesions showing evidence of excoriation and scarring.

DIAGNOSIS

The diagnosis is made on the clinical presentation and history. Histologic findings may be useful in the context of the clinical appearance, although there is no consensus on the pathologic findings.[9]

MANAGEMENT

Treatment of all papulopruritic skin disorders in HIV is difficult, PPE being no exception. Some of the methods of treatment include application of topical corticosteroid preparations, antifungal agents, oral antihistamines, oral antibiotics, anti-itch creams and lotions, as well as scabicides.[5,12] Few useful studies have been done to evaluate the efficacy of these,[9] although there are studies that have been done to evaluate a number of other modalities.

Ultraviolet (UV) light

A study involving eight patients with PPE reported that after 4 weeks of treatment with UVB therapy, seven of eight had a decrease in pruritus and the number of papules.[17] A concern was voiced that UVB may boost the transcription of HIV, making it unsafe for use in HIV-positive individuals.[18,19] It was also found that UV-induced cellular stress may be conducive to viral replication and growth. In spite of this, UVB exposure has not been associated with any short-term changes in immune function in these patients.[20]

Pentoxifylline

Pentoxifylline, a tumor necrosis factor (TNF)-α inhibitor, has proven useful in some cases. Berman *et al.* (1998)[21] demonstrated that 400 mg, three times a day for 8 weeks, led to a major decline in the pruritus. Unfortunately, the patients in this study were being concurrently treated with antiretroviral therapy, and this could not be excluded as the underlying cause of their improvement.

Antiretroviral agents

PPE has also been shown to improve with the use of antiretroviral agents and some have advocated that PPE is an indication for the institution of therapy.[9,10]

PRURIGO NODULARIS

DEFINITION/OVERVIEW

Prurigo nodularis is a chronic, nodular, pruritic skin eruption primarily affecting the extensor surfaces of distal extremities, characteristically seen in middle-aged women, although both sexes may be affected.[22] It may be a sign of systemic disease so it is important to exclude underlying disorders such as liver disease, renal disease, and anemia.[23] The condition is characterized by multiple, intensely pruritic nodular lesions that arise secondary to chronic rubbing and scratching. Pruritus may be severe and lesions can result in cosmetic disfigurement.[24] As prurigo nodularis is one of the cutaneous manifestations of HIV infection, it is important to assess the risk of HIV infection in patients presenting with this condition. Two studies have shown that 1.8–6.5% of individuals infected with HIV have prurigo nodularis.[25,26]

PATHOGENESIS/PATHOPHYSIOLOGY

The fundamental cause and pathogenesis for prurigo nodularis are to date unknown. It is likely that the causes are multifactorial with a combination of genetic factors, a damaged immune system, and a precipitatory incident or factor, either primary or secondary, leading to the development of lesions.[24] There has also been an association with human leucocyte antigen (HLA)-A19 which suggests that genetics plays a role in pathogenesis.[24]

It is not always clear whether the precipitating event for prurigo nodularis is a primary skin condition or simply a pathologic reaction to scratching without an underlying disorder.[27] Because there are myriad causes of pruritus in HIV-positive individuals, prurigo nodularis developing secondary to one or more of these is quite likely.[24] Patients with HIV often have exaggerated reactions to arthropod assaults,[24,28] and increased antibody titers to antigens found in the salivary glands of mosquitoes in patients with AIDS have been well documented.[29] Thus, this may be an important underlying source of pruritus that could lead to prurigo. However, not all lesions are found on the areas of the body most susceptible to arthropod bites.[4]

Other pruritic conditions which may lead to repetitive excoriations such as scabies and eosinophilic folliculitis may be precipitating factors for the development of prurigo nodularis.[30] In up to 50% of HIV-negative patients, systemic causes of pruritus were the core factor in the development of prurigo nodularis. It is likely that these may also be important in the HIV-positive population.[24]

Other factors may also be important in causing prurigo nodularis. One or more circulating pruritogenic factors that react with receptors of the cutaneous nerves may lead to pruritus and subsequent excoriation.[24] Emotional stress as well as the malnutrition suffered by patients living and coping with HIV may lead them to develop the disease.[24] Substance P, which is released in stressful situations, leads to the degranulation of mast cells and causes an itch response.[31]

It has also been suggested that prurigo nodularis may be a primary disease caused by immunologic abnormality in the skin itself.[24] One patient diagnosed with idiopathic CD4 leukopenia subsequently developed a number of skin disorders including prurigo nodularis.[32] In addition, there is an abnormally low number and function of Langerhans cells in the skin of persons suffering from AIDS.[33] The fact that treatment with thalidomide is effective, which works through immunodulation,[34,35] further corroborates a role for the immune system in causing prurigo nodularis.[24]

Finally, immune complex deposition has been suggested as a potential cause of prurigo nodularis. HIV leads to polyclonal activation of B cells which results in the formation of immune complexes which may be deposited in the skin. However, vasculitis with or without vacuolar interface changes would likely be seen if this were the case, but this has not been described.[24]

CLINICAL FEATURES

Patients presenting with prurigo nodularis report intense, chronic pruritus. Lesions are distributed in symmetric fashion on the extremities with the anterior surfaces of the thighs and legs and periarticular skin most severely affected, while the scalp and face are usually spared.[22,23] The lesions themselves are multi-

ple, grouped pink firm papules and nodules that are often hyperkeratotic. They often number over 100 but in some cases, only 1–2 nodules may be present.[22,23] Excoriations from constant scratching and the resulting crusting are virtually always prominent features, as are areas of hyper- and hypopigmentation (**138**).[23] The skin between lesions is commonly xerotic and lichenified with a thick and leathery feel.[22]

HISTOPATHOLOGY

Hyperkeratosis, acanthosis, papillomatosis, and a claw-like downward proliferation of the epidermis are the most prominent features seen on light microscopy.[23,36] There is also marked hypergranulosis and hyperkeratosis (**139**). In some cases the epidermis appears eosinophilic, which indicates premature cornification and epithelial hyperproliferation. The dermis shows marked fibrosis with thickened collagen bundles oriented parallel to elongated epidermal retia.[23] The superficial blood vessels appear tortuous with a superficial perivascular or dense superficial and deep infiltrate of lymphocytes, eosinophils, and neutrophils.[23,36,37] The number of eosinophils is not consistently increased, while an increased number of mast cells and basophils has been reported in both the epidermis and dermis. Additionally, there is extensive deposition of eosinophil granule proteins due to the degranulation of eosinophils.[38] Although electron microscopy is rarely utilized in skin biopsies, there is a proliferation of both Schwann cells and axons, as well as vacuolization and degeneration of nerves in the dermis.[39–41]

DIAGNOSIS

The diagnosis of prurigo nodularis is usually established using the clinical history and the appearance of the lesions alone; however, a skin biopsy may be needed to rule out other conditions associated with epidermal hyperplasia.[24]

MANAGEMENT

Immediate action should be taken to stop the excoriation of the lesions, with use of mittens or occlusive dressings. The fingernails should also be cut short.[24] A number of treatments have been tried with varying success. First-line agents include topical

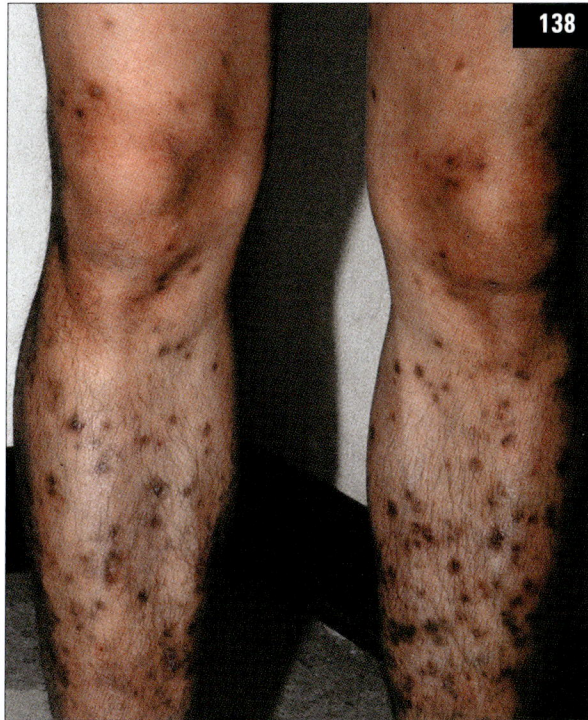

138 Prurigo nodularis. papules and nodules symmetrically distributed on the lower extremities with most lesions showing evidence of excoriation and postinflammatory pigmentary changes.

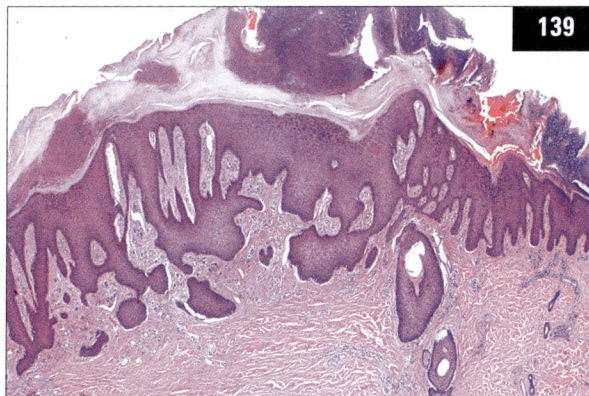

139 Histology of prurigo nodularis. Hyperkeratosis and epidermal acanthosis with elongated rete ridges; vertically oriented collagen fibers and tortuous capillaries in the dermal papillae. x40.

antipruritics, oral antihistamines, oral antidepressants, and topical and intralesional corticosteroid preparations.[27] If these are ineffective, thalidomide has been shown to be of benefit.[34,35,42]

Topical agents

Lotions containing menthol, phenol, or pramoxine provide relief from itching and may be used frequently although effects are temporary. A cream or lotion base with 1% menthol and/or phenol may also provide some relief.[24,27] Capsaicin, the ingredient in red pepper, has also been used with some success.[43] Capsaicin provides relief by exciting local cutaneous nerves, leading to the release of substance P, which in turn causes desensitization of the unmyelinated C-type neurons innervating the skin. Unfortunately, capsaicin is associated with mild to moderate burning of the treated area and, for best results, continual application is required.

Topical corticosteroid preparations such as betamethasone valerate and triamcinolone acetonide may reduce inflammation and decrease epidermal hyperplasia.[24] Betamethasone dipropionate at 0.5 mg/g is recommended. Injecting triamcinolone acetonide 10 mg/ml into the lesions itself is also effective,[27] but the sheer number of papules usually makes this difficult.[44]

Topical analgesics and antihistamines such as lidocaine ointment and 4% doxepin cream may provide some relief; however, their use is limited when the affected area is large.[24]

Systemic antihistamines

Systemic antihistamines such as hydroxyzine and promethazine hydrochloride also may provide some relief but are limited because of their tendency to induce somnolence. They are often administered at night because of this.[24,27] The antidepressant doxepin at 10–75 mg is also used in the evening as a sleep aid.[27]

Ultraviolet (UV) light

UV light treatments have been used with varied success in prurigo nodularis, with some suggesting only limited benefit.[45] However, others have shown it to be effective in breaking the itch–scratch cycle.[27]

There had been concern that UV irradiation in HIV patients would decrease the number and effectiveness of the skin's Langerhans and CD4 T cells; however, no adverse effects have been reported.[24]

Systemic corticosteroids

The risk of increased immunosuppression usually outweighs the benefit with regard to the use of systemic corticosteroids. If utilized, these agents should only be used for a short time.[24]

Thalidomide

Thalidomide has been used with success in treating prurigo nodularis in HIV-seronegative individuals,[46] and later in patients with AIDS.[34] Thalidomide has well known devastating teratogenic effects as well as neurotoxic side-effects.[47] Because of this, females of child bearing age must be instructed to use diligent contraception. The neurotoxic side-effect of diminished sensation is thought to be the way the drug decreases itching.[24] However, in a study published in 2004, one-third of patients treated with thalidomide developed peripheral neuropathy, emphasizing the importance of careful neurologic evaluations in these patients before and during therapy.[35]

Two other risks with use of thalidomide are the potential for immunosuppression, and an increased risk of a hypersensitivity reaction.[48] Despite these concerns, thalidomide is often chosen because of the great benefit it can afford.[24] It has been shown that thalidomide can be used safely in patients with AIDS and a low CD4 count.[34] However, if thalidomide leads to improvement, the dose should be tapered to lessen potential long-term side-effects.[48] Guidelines for the treatment of prurigo nodularis with thalidomide have been published.[35]

EOSINOPHILIC FOLLICULITIS

DEFINITION/OVERVIEW

Eosinophilic pustular folliculitis (EPF) (Ofuji's disease) was first identified in 1970 in three Japanese patients.[49] Recurrent crops of pruritic, follicular papules and pustules that coalesce into plaques with central clearing were initially described.[49] In 1986 a similar condition was described in HIV-infected patients,[50] and has been reported many times since.[51–53] The term HIV-associated eosinophilic folliculitis (EF) was not used to describe this entity until Rosenthal *et al.* introduced this idea in 1991.[53] He and his colleagues felt the condition was a separate entity from classic EPF because the clinical presentation differs from that of Ofuji's patients.[53] Notable differences have been established between classic Ofuji's disease and HIV-associated EF with reference to its distribution, appearance of lesions, disease course, and symptomatology.

HIV-associated EF arises in both males and females, and may be a presenting sign of HIV infection.[54] One study reported that it seemed to occur in HIV-positive individuals with CD4 counts less than 250×10^6/l with an incidence of 9%.[55] However, since the initiation of highly active antiretroviral therapy (HAART), there has been subjective evidence of a reduction in HIV-associated EF which is thought to be due to the ability of the treatment to keep CD4 T cell counts higher.[56]

PATHOGENESIS/PATHOPHYSIOLOGY

Not much is known about the cause of this condition; however, the fact that the inflammation centers in and around the hair follicle has led to the suggestion that an opportunistic infection may be the cause.[56] In the majority of patients, cultures are negative for micro-organisms, including bacteria, mycobacteria, fungi, and yeasts.[54] This was supported by a study of 52 carefully examined biopsies only one of which had yeast.[57] However, Ferrandiz *et al.* in 1992 described two cases of HIV-associated EF where profuse *Pityrosporum* yeast was identified, and treatment with topical ketoconazole resulted in recovery, supporting micro-organisms as a legitimate cause.[58] Berger *et al.* (1995) confirmed that treatment with itraconazole had been valuable in some patients, also supporting

Pityrosporum as a cause.[59] It is also believed that because HIV-positive patients suffer from immune dysregulation, a hypersensitivity response to the commensal yeast in the hair follicle may develop.[13] Finally, there have been additional cases reported of fungal infections imitating the clinical and histologic appearance of EF. Haupt *et al.* (1990) reported a case of an individual with a histologic appearance identical to that of EF; however, fungal hyphae were identified in one of the involved follicles and treatment with griseofulvin resulted in resolution of the lesion.[60]

Infestation with *Demodex* mites has also been suggested to be a cause of HIV-associated EF.[13] In nine of 52 biopsies examined, evidence of mite fragments suggestive of *Demodex* within the infundibulum of follicles was found.[57] Bacterial infection has also been suggested as a possible cause[13] and in support of this theory gram-negative bacilli have been identified in hair follicles, even within hair shafts, in one patient with HIV-associated EF. The patient was treated successfully with metronidazole. However, most cultures are typically negative, and treatment with antibiotics produces no definite results.[53]

Fearfield *et al.* (1999) have proposed that HIV-associated EF is an autoimmune disease with the sebocyte or another element of sebum acting as a target antigen.[13] This process may begin with the follicle being disturbed followed by an influx of inflammatory cells and inflammatory mediators, leading to the clinical expression of EF. Treatment with isotretinoin is effective,[61] which adds support to the theory that sebum may be at least partially to blame.[13]

Finally, it is thought that AIDS may cause an immune dysregulation with a shift toward TH-2 cytokines leading to the systemic eosinophilia seen in these patients. This theory suggests that triggering by an unknown agent in the skin may induce the same process leading to HIV-associated EF. Increased expression of two TH-2 cytokines, interleukin (IL)-4 and IL-5, and two chemokines, RANTES and eotaxin, has been found in the skin of patients with HIV-associated EF.[62]

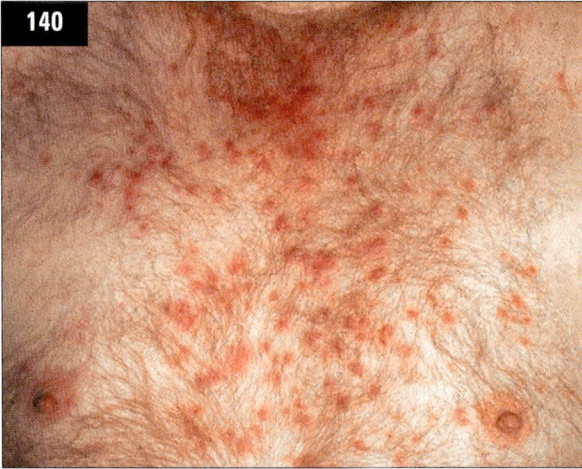

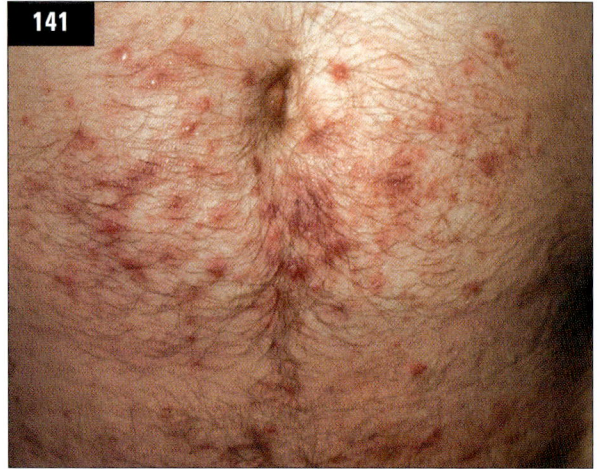

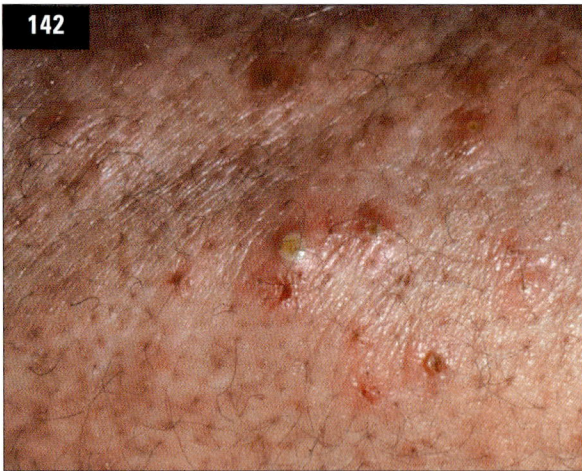

140–142 Eosinophilic folliculitis. Multiple follicular papules and pustules with evidence of excoriations on the chest (**140**) and abdomen (**141**). Close-up of follicular pustule surrounded by numerous smaller pustules and excoriations (**142**).

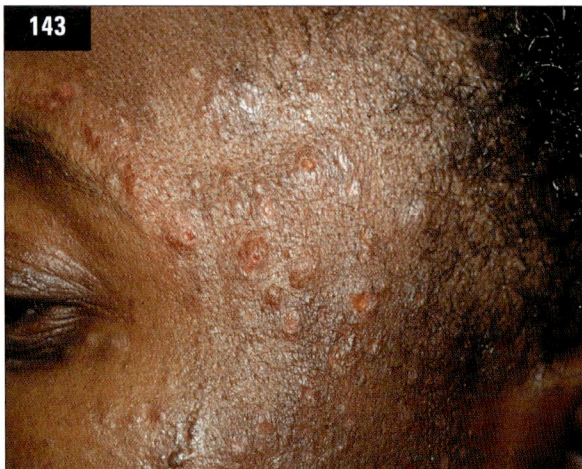

143 Facial papules and pustules.

CLINICAL FEATURES

Patients with HIV-associated EF may present in much the same way as those with classic Ofuji's disease; however, the clinical picture is often quite different.[63] Patients affected with HIV-associated EF classically complain of a persistent, erythematous, pruritic eruption with an intensity similar to that of scabies. This leads to excoriation so that it is often not possible to identify any of the primary lesions.[56] In contrast, in Ofuji's disease, pruritis affects less than 50% of patients and when it is present, it tends to be intermittent.[53] Clinically, in HIV-associated EF, follicular and non-follicular erythematous papules or pustules (140–142), urticarial lesions, and large erythematous plaques have all been reported.[50,51,53,56,64] In Ofuji's disease, papules coalesce into plaques with a central clearing.[53] Eruptions have been reported on the face (143), trunk, shoulders, upper arms, and neck, like Ofuji's disease; however, patients with HIV-associated disease may also develop disseminated or generalized lesions.[51,56,65] The palms and soles are usually spared in HIV-associated EF, while these areas are involved in up to one-fifth of patients with Ofuji's disease.[66]

HISTOPATHOLOGY

Histologically, HIV-associated EF appears similar to Ofuji's disease (144, 145). Spongiosis of the follicular epithelium with infiltration of the outer root sheath and perifollicular dermis with an inflammatory infiltrate of eosinophils, neutrophils, and mononuclear cells is seen in both entities.[49,57] There are also often mast cells, many of which have degranulated.[67] In time, the hair follicle may eventually be destroyed and formation of an eosinophilic abscess may be identified.[49] The intrafollicular inflammation is distinct from that seen in infectious causes of folliculitis.[56]

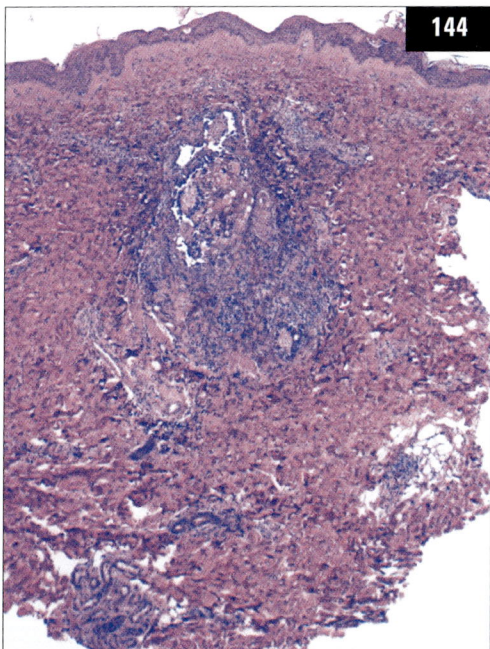

144 Histology of eosinophilic follicultis. Perifollicular inflammation with destruction of the follicular unit.

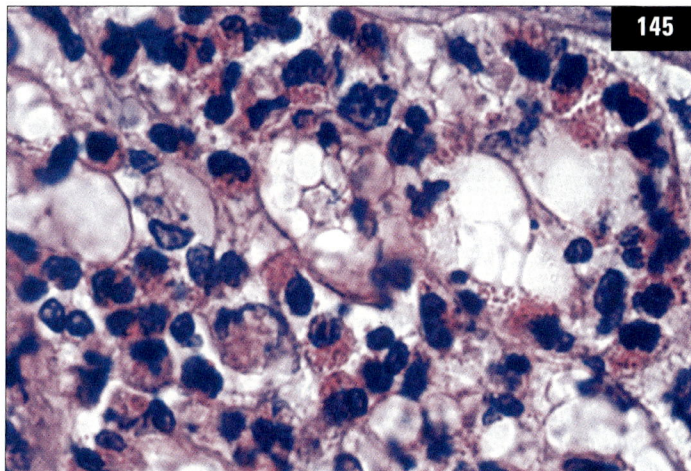

145 High power (x400) of the infiltrate showing numerous eosinophils.

Although the two conditions appear histologically similar in many respects, there are some significant differences between HIV-associated EF and Ofuji's disease. In HIV-associated EF, eosinophilic-rich pustules are not seen as often. Rosenthal *et al.* (1991) studied 13 patients with HIV-associated EF and found a large eosinophilic abscess in only one,[53] and McCalmont *et al.* (1995) found eosinophilic pustule formation in less than half of biopsies studied.[57] Furthermore, immunofluorescence studies are rarely positive in HIV-associated EF although there may be positive binding of immunoreactants in follicles in Ofuji's disease.[67]

DIAGNOSIS

While the diagnosis may be clinically apparent, a skin biopsy for microscopic evaluation may be helpful in excluding other conditions if the diagnosis is in question. The biopsy should be taken from an unexcoriated fresh lesion if possible, and serially sectioned by the histopathologist as the affected follicle may be missed. Special stains must be performed to rule out fungal, bacterial, and viral conditions.[56]

Additional work-up that may be done include cellophane tape stripping of the skin to search for *Demodex* mites and scrapings for scabies.[56] Although Ofuji's disease may appear clinically similar, the context of background HIV disease will easily allow the distinction between this and HIV-associated EF. Furthermore, in HIV infection, there will usually be a low white cell count found compared to the leukocytosis seen in Ofuji's disease.[50,53,63] In one study of 12 HIV-positive patients with EF whose CD4 counts were evaluated, all had $<300 \times 10^6$/l, while 10 out of the 12 had levels below 250×10^6/l.[53]

An absolute or relative eosinophilia is found in both entities and elevated IgE levels have been reported in patients with HIV-associated EF.[53,56]

MANAGEMENT

Treatment of EF is difficult and varied because the underlying pathogenesis remains unclear. Numerous treatments have been used with varying success, including application of topical corticosteroid preparations, administration of systemic steroids, phototherapy (UVA and B light), antihistamines, itraconazole, isotretinoin, and metronidazole;[56] however, there is no consistently effective treatment. First-line therapy is usually application of topical corticosteroids coupled with UVB phototherapy.[68]

Topical corticosteroids

The low cost and ease of application of topical corticosteroid preparations generally makes them the first line of treatment. Grange *et al.* (1996) reported remission with application of potent topical corticosteroid preparations in several patients.[69] However, others report only partial and temporary relief. Nevertheless, a dose of 0.1% betamethasone valerate can be utilized as a first-line and as adjunctive therapy.[56]

Ultraviolet B phototherapy

UVB light has also been used successfully.[17,51] Patients have responded to treatment with broad band UVB light three times a week for 3–6 weeks. Frequent relapses occur, however, and weekly maintenance therapy may be needed.[56]

These positive effects are thought to be a result of a local immunosuppressive effect on the skin.[56] There were early fears that this might accelerate the progression of HIV; however, that has not been experienced.[20,56]

Antihistamines

In some cases, either complete or partial resolution has been observed with administration of cetirizine, an H1 antagonist with specific antieosinophilic effects.[56,63] This is most effective when higher dosages of 20–40 mg are used, and may be divided into multiple doses.[56] Even at higher doses, there are still relatively minimal side-effects.[68]

Itraconazole

Because *Pityrosporum ovale* may be involved in the pathogenesis of HIV-associated EF, treatment with itraconazole has been employed. In a study by Berger *et al.* (1995), of 28 patients treated, 61% recovered completely and 14% had partial recovery.[59] At 3 months, 60% were still taking itraconazole with good results and 35% no longer needed any therapy or were controlled with application of topical corticosteroids alone. The authors suggested a starting dose of 200 mg daily with the expectation that a response should be appreciated within the first 2 weeks of therapy. If there is no response or it is inadequate, the dose may be increased to 300–400 mg daily. Of interest, fluconazole is not an appropriate substitute for itraconazole, as patients treated with this agent quickly relapsed. This suggests that at least some of itraconazole's activity in EF is due to anti-inflammatory action rather than antibiotic properties.[59]

Metronidazole

Metronidazole at a dose of 250 mg three times a day for 3–4 weeks was reported effective in clearing HIV-associated EF in five out of five patients, and resulted in long-term remissions in some. In those patients who do not respond initially, the dose may be increased up to 500 mg three times a day.

Isotretinoin

A study in 1995 reported complete response within 1–4 weeks of starting isotretinoin in seven patients.[61] A starting dose of 40–80 mg/day was administered, with higher doses given to those more severely affected. Patients who relapsed following treatment responded promptly to retreatment.[61] Simpson-Dent et al. (1996) reported that the lower dose of 20 mg daily for 6–8 weeks was also very effective and well tolerated.[56] The mechanism of action is thought to be a reduction in intra- and perifollicular inflammation, but it also leads to reduction in sebum production. Sebum reduction may result in secondary sterilization of follicles which may also account for at least part of its action.

Permethrin

As *Demodex* mites may be a trigger for HIV-associated EF, it stands to reason that agents directed at their destruction might be beneficial as therapy. One study published in 1995 reported that patients treated daily with 5% topical permethrin cream were able to control symptoms, eventually needing just one to two applications per week as a maintenance dose. However, when treatment was stopped, lesions promptly recurred.[70]

Antiretroviral therapy

Since the introduction of HAART, there have been anecdotal reports of a decrease in the number of patients suffering from HIV-associated EF. This is thought to be a consequence of the elevated CD4 count that often results.[56] In some cases, HIV-associated EF may appear at the time of initiation of antiretroviral therapy as a manifestation of the so-called immune reconstitution syndrome.[71,72]

Other treatments have been reported with varying success. These include topical antibiotics, astemizole, dapsone, and prednisolone.[50,53,56,64] Cromolyn sodium solution, which has an antimast cell effect, has been used successfully in a few patients.[56,67]

CHAPTER 10

CUTANEOUS MANIFESTATIONS OF NONANTIRETROVIRAL THERAPY

Saira B. Momin and Clay J. Cockerell

INTRODUCTION

A drug-induced symptom complex characterized by fever and an eruption with or without internal organ involvement has been termed acute drug hypersensitivity syndrome reaction. This syndrome typically develops within 1 to 2 weeks after the initiation of drug therapy.[1] It has been estimated that cutaneous drug reactions are 10–100 times more common in human immunodeficiency virus (HIV)-positive patients than in the general population,[2] and one study revealed that the frequency of drug hypersensitivity in HIV-positive patients ranges from 3% to 20%.[3] The most common group of drugs responsible for cutaneous hypersensitivity eruptions are antimicrobials used to treat or protect against opportunistic infections.[4] Allergic reactions have been reported with trimethoprim–sulfamethoxazole (TMP-SMX), clindamycin, dapsone, pyrimethamine/sulfadoxine, aminopenicillins, clavulanate, thalidomide, atovaquone, rifampin, probenecid, primaquine, isoniazid, and thioacetazone.[4,5] The incidence of reactions to these agents ranges between 18% and 64%[6–11] compared with only a 3.3% incidence in a general hospital population treated with TMP-SMX.[12] Cutaneous drug reactions are usually mild although severe eruptions such as erythema multiforme (EM), Stevens–Johnson syndrome (SJS), and toxic epidermal necrolysis (TEN) can occur.[1] Conjunctivitis is common and hepatic and hematologic abnormalities may develop and stem from immune-mediated injury or direct toxicity.[5]

There are four classic hypersensitivity reactions described by Coombs and Gel. Immediate hypersensitivity mediated by immunoglobulin (Ig)E may lead to urticarial and anaphylactoid reactions characterized by fever, urticarial papules and plaques associated with angioedema, shortness of breath, and bronchospasm. IgG and IgM antibody in type 2 reactions may induce hemolytic anemia and thrombocytopenia. Type 3 immune complex mediated-reactions may produce serum sickness-like eruptions, drug-induced lupus erythematosus, or morbilliform eruptions. However, cell-mediated, type 4 immune reactions may also result in morbilliform eruptions.[13]

A number of different factors have been associated with an increase in the risk of cutaneous adverse drug reactions (ADR) in HIV/acquired immunodeficiency syndrome (AIDS) patients including female sex,[14,15] history of cutaneous ADR,[16] CD4+ cell count lower than $200 \times 10^6/1$ but higher than $25 \times 10^6/l$, slow acetylation phenotype, and glutathione (GSH) deficiency.[15,17–22] In contrast, factors associated with a decreased risk of ADR include dark complexion[23] and simultaneous intake of systemic corticosteroids.[20,24,25] Most reports have been based on retrospective studies and, at times, the results have been inconsistent.[26]

There are a number of reasons why HIV infection may be associated with an increased likelihood for the development of an ADR. Many patients are receiving chronic and multiple drugs which is a known predisposing factor. High drug dose, administration of novel agents, many with unknown biological effects, perturbation of drug metabolism, increased oxidative stress, and immune hyperactivation are other important reasons.[27] HIV infection is characterized by immunodeficiency but it is also associated with chronic immune hyper-activation[28] and interferon (IFN)-γ and other cytokines are elevated.[29] IFN-γ increases the expression of different pro-inflammatory cytokines which plays a part in the oxidative stress seen in HIV disease.[30] This may be a significant factor in the alteration in metabolism[31] that in turn may lead to a shift in the balance between bioactivation and bioinactivation of drugs.[4] The secretion of TNF-α, interleukin (IL)-1, IL-6 and other cytokines is induced by HIV infection. Alteration of these cytokines could contribute in enhancing susceptibility because they are critical in the activation of keratinocytes, migration of Langerhans cells to lymph nodes, and stimulation of T cell responses.[32]

TRIMETHOPRIM–SULFAMETHAXAZOLE

There is a quite high incidence of eruptions caused by TMP–SMX in HIV-seropositive patients.[3] Virtually all patients with late stage HIV disease and low CD4 cell counts receive TMP–SMX as prophylaxis and treatment for *Pneumocystis carinii* pneumonia (PCP).[33] In most cases, SMX, not TMP, is responsible for the hypersensitivity reaction.[4] It has been demonstrated that the likelihood of developing an eruption is associated with the level of hydroxylamine, a major metabolite of SMX. A patient who develops a reaction to high doses of TMP–SMX used to treat PCP may not necessarily develop an eruption when doses to prevent PCP are administered, as that dose is about one-eighth of the treatment dose.[33] In *vitro* hydroxylamine SMX is not toxic to control lymphocytes from SMX-tolerant patients but it is toxic to those patients with adverse reactions to SMX.[34]

PATHOGENESIS/PATHOPHYSIOLOGY

SMX can be metabolized in two ways. The primary way is by acetylation and production of N-acetyl-sulfamethoxazole, a nontoxic metabolite excreted in the urine.[33] AIDS patients are predisposed to developing hypersensitivity reactions to TMP–SMX because they have a slow acetylator phenotype, having slow hepatic N-acetyltransferase activity

which results in higher levels of the toxic hydroxylamine metabolite.[35] The incidence of slow acetylation increases with disease progression among HIV-positive patients.[36] HIV-positive patients also have lower levels of circulating GSH which is required to metabolize the hydroxylamine metabolite.[37]

An alternate pathway of SMX metabolism is via the hepatic cytochrome P450 system that produces the toxic metabolite, hydroxylamine.[33] This is then auto-oxidized to the toxin nitroso-SMX, the actual toxin that mediates the hypersensitivity reaction.[38] This hydroxylamine metabolite can be detected in the urine of HIV-positive patients.[4,39] Keratinocytes, which are the site of attack in cutaneous eruptions, can bioactivate SMX to hydroxylamine,[4,40] which is consistent with findings that keratinocytes express multiple P450 isoforms and drug transporters.[4,41] The toxin nitroso-SMX can bind covalently to thiol residues in proteins and on surfaces of lymphocytes[4,42] and keratinocytes.[4,40] CD8+ dermal T cells proliferate more vigorously in response to microsome-generated SMX metabolites when compared with the parent compound alone.[4,43] All of these findings support the hypothesis that the toxin nitroso-SMX plays a significant role in the development of the hypersensitivity reaction.[4]

CLINICAL FEATURES AND HISTOPATHOLOGY

Morbilliform eruption (**146**) is the most common type of drug-related eruption in HIV-positive patients, as in the general population. The second most common type of eruption seen in HIV-infected patients is the urticarial eruption (**147**).[44] The histopathology of morbilliform drug eruptions is usually characterized by a superficial perivascular infiltrate of lymphocytes with scattered eosinophils. There may be scattered histiocytes and vacuolar alteration of dermoepidermal junction with slight spongiosis. Slight parakeratosis may be noted and scattered plasma cells and individually necrotic keratinocytes may be seen.[13,45] Mixed infiltrates of lymphocytes, eosinophils, and variable numbers of neutrophils interstitially in the dermis with minimal epidermal change characterizes urticarial drug eruption.[13] In patients with drug reactions, associated signs and symptoms include fever, neutropenia, thrombo-

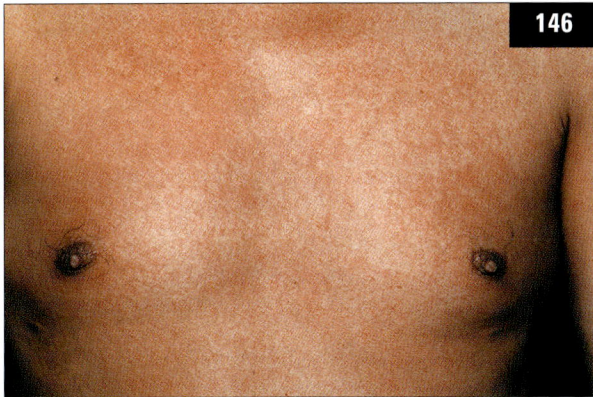

146 Morbilliform eruption secondary to sulfamethoxazole.

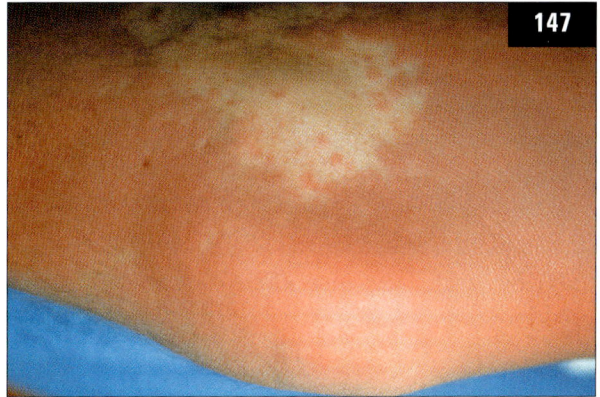

147 Urticarial drug eruption. Confluent erythematous wheals with an island of uninvolved skin.

cytopenia, abnormal liver function tests, and anemia.[13,45] Hypoglycemia may also develop. IgE levels are usually elevated and rise with diminishing CD4+ cell numbers.[13]

Porteous and Berger described patients with AIDS or AIDS-related complex (ARC) who experienced severe cutaneous drug reactions including EM, SJS, and TEN. In a number of these cases, patients had a history of hypersensitivity to multiple drug therapies.[46] SJS and TEN occur relatively frequently in AIDS patients, with sulfonamides as the main cause for the majority of documented cases. Nonsulfa drugs are also associated with higher incidence of SJS and TEN.[45] A study in Zambia of 1124 HIV-positive patients found that 22 patients had drug reactions and, of these, 15 received isoniazid, thiacetazone, rifampicin, and streptomycin for treatment of pulmonary tuberculosis. SJS developed in seven of these patients and the suspected drugs were thiacetazone and streptomycin.[47] Also, several case reports reveal that severe reactions such as TEN occurred during PCP prophylaxis with pyrimethamine and sulfadoxine.[48,49] In HIV-positive patients with central nervous system toxoplasmosis, the incidence of SJS or TEN is higher as the treatment of choice, pyrimethamine and sulfadiazine (along with anticonvulsants if seizures occur) are common

causes of SJS or TEN.[50] Patients with small blisters on purpuric macules with prominent involvement of the trunk and face and epidermal detachment of less than 10% of body surface most likely have SJS. In TEN, individual lesions are seen like those noted with SJS with confluent erythema and total epidermal detachment of greater than 30% of body surface area. Raised flaccid blisters that spread with sheet-like loss of epidermis are characteristic of TEN and patients demonstrate a positive Nikolsky's sign, detachment of the epidermis by lateral pressure.[2]

The histopathology of SJS and TEN is character-ized by extensive keratinocyte necrosis of the epidermis and prominent vacuolar interface changes. In TEN, there are minimal inflammatory cells in the dermis even though there is confluent epidermal necrosis with no parakeratosis.[13] Massive transepidermal fluid losses with associated electrolyte imbalance and prerenal azotemia are common complications. The likelihood of sepsis is also increased due to the bacterial colonization of the skin and decreased immune responsiveness. Sepsis is the main cause of death with mortality rates below 5% for SJS but around 30% for TEN.[2] Advanced age and greater surface area of epidermal involvement are associated with a worse prognosis.[51]

OTHER MEDICATIONS

Infection with Epstein–Barr virus (EBV), hepatitis B virus, herpes simplex virus (HSV), human herpesvirus-6, cytomegalovirus (CMV), and HIV has been shown to increase the risk for the development of allergic drug reactions.[4,5,27] The immune system may be stimulated by these infections which predisposes patients to drug reactions in a fashion similar to that noted with EBV and aminopenicillins. There is a strikingly increased incidence of drug eruptions that develop in patients with EBV infection who receive aminopenicillins, and it has been suggested that the increased risk for cutaneous adverse drug reactions in patients with AIDS is due to the reactivation of lymphotropic viruses.[20,52] In one retrospective study, HIV-positive patients with drug eruptions were shown to have significantly increased serologic evidence of acute or reactivated EBV or CMV infection.[19] In one study, having a CD8+ cell count above 460×10^6/l was identified as a risk factor for the development of an adverse drug reaction,[20] and it has been documented that CD8+ cell counts are elevated in acute EBV infection.[26]

Dapsone is used as an alternative for the prevention of *Toxoplasma* encephalitis and for the prevention and treatment of PCP. There is an approximately 30% incidence of cutaneous eruptions in HIV-seropositive patients receiving dapsone. This is most likely due to its toxic metabolite which is similar to sulfamethoxazole.[33] Many patients who are sensitive to TMP-SMX are also sensitive to dapsone.[13] In addition to drug eruptions, the sulfone syndrome has been observed in patients taking dapsone for PCP prophylaxis.[13] This is a severe disorder associated with fever, hepatic abnormalities, and lymphadenopathy among other symptoms.

Morbilliform eruptions may be seen in patients treated with amoxicillin–clavulanic acid (augmentin), fusidate sodium, and a combination of clindamycin and primaquine. In one study, patients developed exanthema when receiving intravenous clindamycin for *Toxoplasma* encephalitis.[13]

Pyrimethamine is a folate antagonist used in AIDS patients for prophylaxis and treatment of toxoplasmic encephalitis. When used for prophylaxis, it is combined with dapsone. It is combined with either sulfadiazine or clindamycin when used for treatment.[33] When administered as monotherapy in a large multicenter trial, 8.1% of patients on pyrimethamine developed an urticarial or morbilliform eruption. Patients who developed a drug eruption while on pyrimethamine had a higher incidence of toxoplasmic encephalitis than those patients who were on placebo. This similar observation was also seen in patients who developed eruptions to TMP-SMX.[33] One possible explanation could be that the development of a drug eruption leads to a more rapid detorioration in CD4+ lymphocyte count which would increase the risk of toxoplasmosis reactivation.[33] A combination of sulfadoxine and pyrimethamine was widely used in the early days of the AIDS epidemic because it was very effective for prevention and treatment of opportunistic infections, but is now rarely used because of the many reported cases of SJS associated with administration of this medication.[33]

Parenteral pentamidine may cause morbilliform to urticarial eruptions in 20% of AIDS patients.[53] A widespread pruritic erythematous morbilliform eruption may be caused by aerosolized pentamidine.[54,55] A 5-year retrospective study revealed that nephrotoxicity, dysglycemia, hepatotoxicity, hyperkalemia, and hyperamylasemia accounted for 80% of adverse drug reactions that occurred in HIV-positive patients who were receiving intravenous pentamidine treatment for PCP.[56]

Tuberculosis is a common infectious complication of HIV infection and 10% of patients on antituberculous regimens may develop morbilliform eruptions.[13,57] In a study of 59 patients with pulmonary tuberculosis in Kampala, Uganda, two-thirds of whom were HIV-positive, cutaneous drug reactions were seen in close to one-third of patients receiving thiacetazone.[58] There was also a higher incidence of recurrence of tuberculosis in patients who developed drug eruptions while being treated for tuberculosis with thiacetazone.[59]

Foscarnet (trisodium phosphonoformate) is indicated for acyclovir-resistant mucocutaneous HSV infections and is also used for the treatment of CMV disease, varicella zoster virus, and even HIV itself. Foscarnet has many serious side-effects and therefore, many physicians are reluctant to administer this medication. The most frequently reported serious side-effects are nephrotoxicity, electrolyte disturbances, and seizures. Genital ulceration develops in 5–30% of patients and is most commonly located on the periurethral glans penis. This represents a contact irritant dermatitis and is thought to be secondary to urine concentration of the drug as it is excreted through the kidneys. Due to the direct caustic effect of the drug, patients may develop ulceration at the urethral meatus.[60–63] Penile ulcers usually develop 11–16 days after start of therapy. The lesions are typically 1–5 cm in diameter, range from two to five in number, and consist of erosive, bullous, tender ulcerations.[64] Frequently, on the anterior scrotum where the meatus may be lying, there will also be a 'kissing' area of irritation. Uncircumcised men who take foscarnet may be at higher risk.[65] In women, vulval ulcerations have also been reported.[66] Oral and esophageal ulcers may also develop and a generalized cutaneous eruption has also been reported due to foscarnet.[67] Ulcerations may be avoided or the risk may be minimized by drying the meatus or vulva thoroughly and by providing increased hydration.[33,60,63]

Disseminated *Mycobacterium avium* complex infection may be treated with clofazimine, an aniline dye. Yellow brawny discoloration of the skin occurs because the drug accumulates in the skin and this does not represent a hypersensitivity reaction. For many patients, this discoloration is not bothersome, however.[33]

Hypericin, a substance isolated from the herb St. John's wort (*Hypericum perforatum*), has an extremely potent *in vitro* activity against HIV when photoactivated. An investigation of purified intravenously administered hypericin as treatment for HIV was halted when patients developed severe cutaneous photosensitivity reactions. The use of sunblocking agents could not prevent these photosensitivity reactions.[33]

Systemic therapy with immunosuppressive therapy such as methotrexate for psoriasis and systemic corticosteroids for non-Hodgkin's lymphoma or vasculitis has lead to the sudden appearance and rapid proliferation of Kaposi's sarcoma (KS) in some

patients.[68] Patients who developed this complication were typically receiving high-dose prednisone in the setting of advanced HIV disease and were not being treated simultaneously with antiretroviral therapy.[69] Corticosteroid use has also been shown to increase the risk of avascular necrosis of bone in HIV-positive patients.[70]

Anticonvulsant hypersensitivity syndrome is serious adverse cutaneous and systemic reactions to the arene oxide-producing anticonvulsants such as phenytoin, carbamazepine, and phenobarbital.[71] Many HIV-positive patients receive anticonvulsants due to opportunistic infections such as cryptococcosis and toxoplasmosis causing central nervous system disease.

MANAGEMENT

In most cases, drug eruptions in HIV-positive individuals are mild to moderate in severity. If the patient has mucous membrane involvement, mental status changes, meningitis, fever >103°F (39.4°C), signs of nephritis or hypersensitivity pneumonitis, the drug should be discontinued and subsequent administration is contraindicated. If the drug eruption is mild or moderate and has resolved after withdrawal of the offending agent, it is generally safe to rechallenge the patient if necessary.[33] The process of converting a patient from a state of sensitivity to one in which a therapeutic dose of the drug may be readministered safely is referred to as desensitization.[72] Desensitization has been successful in HIV-seropositive patients with TMP-SMX, clindamycin, sulfadiazine, and other agents.[5] There is a lower likelihood of developing an eruption upon rechallenge if it is administered in a gradually escalating dose.[33,73] Desensitization acts by temporarily reducing the ability of the body to react to the drug so that successive doses may be given to complete the course of therapy. The protocol must be repeated if subsequent courses of therapy are necessary as desensitization does not result in long-lived tolerance to the allergen.[73]

Severe ADRs such as SJS and TEN cause destruction of cutaneous tissue as a result of immune complex-mediated or cell-mediated immune damage, and as a result can respond to anti-inflammatory agents. Intravenous immunoglobulin (IVIG) has potent anti-inflammatory activity. When successful, treatment with IVIG results in prompt improvement of skin and mucosal lesions with resolution of constitutional symptoms.[74] IVIG infusion also restores protein and fluid that is lost in TEN patients and may help limit the extent of fluid loss that occurs through the denuded skin.[51] In a multicenter retrospective study, 48 patients with TEN were treated with supportive care and infusions of IVIG following diagnosis and/or admission to a study center. IVIG was given over a period of 1–5 days and 42 of the 43 patients who initially responded to IVIG achieved complete healing of the skin and mucous membrane lesions within an average of 15 days. These 42 patients also survived TEN for a survival rate at 45 days of 88%. One patient who died responded well to IVIG but suffered a coincidental myocardial infarction. No serious adverse events were reported. A reduction in the dose of IVIG is recommended in patients with renal insufficiency to minimize the risk of transient acute renal insufficiency due to proximal tubular dysfunction.[51] Fas-mediated apoptosis of keratinocytes is thought to be involved in the pathogenesis of TEN which occurs when keratinocytes induce expression of FasL, a cytolytic molecule.[75] IVIG inhibits Fas-mediated cell death; variability in the response of patients with TEN to IVIG is thought to be due to the differences in anti-Fas antibody content within IVIG batches. Analysis of clinical and therapeutic parameters of the group of patients who survived after IVIG infusion and those who did not respond, revealed that IVIG infusion was initiated later in those patients who did not respond and the total dose was lower. Furthermore, the coexistence of an underlying chronic disease may adversely affect the outcome of TEN patients treated with IVIG.[51]

SUMMARY

There is a higher incidence of adverse cutaneous drug reactions in HIV/AIDS patients than in the general population, which usually results in the cessation of treatment further increasing the challenge to treat these patients appropriately. The use of antimicrobials has diminished with the advent of highly active antiretroviral therapy (HAART) so that the frequency of these hypersensitivity reactions will likely fall. The majority of cutaneous reactions are morbilliform eruptions that are usually mild, although severe reactions such as TEN and SJS may be encountered.

CHAPTER 11

PHOTOSENSITIVE MANIFESTATIONS OF HIV DISEASE

Shadi Kourosh, Mary Feldman, and Clay J. Cockerell

HIV AND PHOTOSENSITIVITY

Cutaneous photosensitivity refers to an inflammatory skin reaction arising from an abnormal response to nonionizing radiation. Its association with human immunodeficiency virus (HIV) disease has become increasingly recognized and has served as a useful marker in the diagnosis and monitoring of disease progression. It is important for health professionals to understand this relationship to ensure accurate diagnosis of patients presenting with photosensitive symptoms, and the timely diagnosis of HIV infection if it is present. It is also necessary because sunlight as a pathogen cannot be avoided as one might avoid cats or penicillin. To go through life, as many of these patients do, with an 'allergy' to ultraviolet (UV) radiation and to attempt to avoid it, is a marginalizing experience that often cannot be realistically maintained. Thus, to improve longevity and quality of life for these individuals, it is incumbent that clinicians recognize and offer a sustainable way of managing the various photo-induced reactions seen with HIV infection. Furthermore, as the population of those infected with HIV increases, and more patients actually require phototherapy for treatment of the myriad dermatoses associated with the disease, it is imperative to determine whether light may contribute to the underlying pathogeneses in any way, and whether it benefits patients sufficiently to justify its employment.

EPIDEMIOLOGY OF HIV PHOTOERUPTIONS

In general, most of the photoeruptions reported in conjunction with HIV infection have been classified into the following categories: chronic actinic dermatitis (CAD), lichenoid photoeruption and erythroderma, porphyria cutanea tarda (PCT), photosensitive and nonphotosensitive hyperpigmentation, and photosensitive granuloma annulare (GA). Among these, CAD and lichenoid eruptions are the most common in HIV-infected patients.[1] The significant variation in the clinical presentation of HIV-related photodermatoses has posed a challenge to interpretation of findings; however, a few trends are important to note. First, there is a pronounced ethnic predominance of HIV-photosensitivity in African-American patients who manifest these photoeruptions at nearly seven times the frequency of all other ethnic groups combined.[1] While it is still unclear to what extent this may be a genetic versus a behavioral bias, several studies support African-American ethnicity as independent predictor of HIV-related skin disease.[1]

Second, there is some evidence of a dose-response role of immunosuppression, in that while patients often develop the first signs of photosensitivity in early stages of disease, patients in later stages with the greatest depletion of immune cells (in particular CD4+ cell counts) have seen the most chronic and severe eruptions. The degree of immunosuppression and viral load also correlates with the morphology of photo-induced lesions, delineating a partition between lichenoid and nonlichenoid eruptions. That is, nonlichenoid eruptions, which include acute and chronic spongiotic and hyperpigmentation reactions, are more common in patients with higher levels of viral load ($\geq 5.5 \times 10^7$/l) and lower T cell counts than lichenoid eruptions. This suggests that nonlichenoid eruptions are more characteristic of advanced disease than lichenoid types. Interestingly, this morphologic distinction carries through with respect to mode of HIV transmission, as sexual acquisition of the disease correlates with nonlichenoid forms of presentation.[1] The reason why this mode of transmission rather than IV drug use or maternal–fetal transmission is associated with a lower incidence of lichenoid eruptions is unclear. Contributing factors may include differences in viral strains or characteristic behaviors of different patient risk groups.

Beyond this, distinctions in submorphologies of the nonlichenoid group tend to be based on estimated UV exposure and immunologic profiles of patients, with chronic spongiotic lesions corresponding to highest mean HIV viral load ($\geq 5.5 \times 10^7$/l) and low CD4+ cell counts ($<350 \times 10^6$/l), followed by hyperpigmented lesions, and then acute spongiotic photodermatitis, which represents the least severe disease state of the three. As one might expect, patients in the lichenoid group exhibit the longest time intervals from peak HIV viral load and CD4+ nadir until their next visit to a physician, while those with spongiotic lesions have the shortest mean times.

UV LIGHT AND HIV GENE ACTIVATION

Reminiscent of the classic experiment of bacteriophage lambda in which UV light triggered stress-induced damage to the cell and activated the virus, there is evidence of a similar reaction caused by UV light in the case of HIV. It has been demonstrated that UVB light can directly activate latent HIV in cultures of chronically infected monocytes.[2] Also, UVB (wavelength 280–315 nm) and UVC radiation (wavelength 200–290 nm), at a dose of 10 J/m² have the capability to activate the HIV promoter, the gene sequence responsible for controlling viral gene expression;[3] UVB has additionally been demonstrated to stimulate the growth of HIV *in vitro*. Exposure of cell lines to the photosensitizing agent psoralen with ultraviolet A light (PUVA), a treatment used for a variety of skin lesions including psoriasis,

seborrheic dermatitis, folliculitis, and chronic urticaria, may also stimulate HIV expression. However, this must be a tandem effect of the combination, as neither UVA nor psolaren alone have demonstrated this effect.[4,5]

While the mechanisms by which UV light activates HIV are not completely known, the majority of studies support that, as in the classic lambda phage experiment, UV light most likely serves as a source of stress-induced damage to host cell deoxyribonucleic acid (DNA). Cellular DNA repair processes then cause viral genes, dormant but already incorporated into host genome, to become activated to replicate and destroy the cell.[3]

HIV AND OXIDATIVE STRESS

With perpetual infection, complicated drug regimens, poor absorption of nutrients, and failing organs, the immune system of an HIV-infected patient faces stress and injury on many fronts. In addition to this burden, the progression of HIV disease itself contributes significantly to the strain on the body by serving as a source of oxidative damage and by diminishing the natural mechanisms for coping with that stress.

Normal cellular respiration produces a baseline level of reactive oxygen species (ROS), including superoxides, hydrogen peroxide, hydroxyl radicals, and nitric oxide. The immune system adds to these free radicals in the form of reactive oxygen bursts as a response whenever something stimulates polymorphonuclear cells, monocytes/macrophages, or T cells. In an HIV-infected patient, the HIV infection itself and the numerous opportunistic infections secondary to it generate a state of chronic immune activation that is exacerbated by often misdirected reactions to other antigenic substances. This worsens as CD4+ helper T cells that normally regulate and direct immune activity fall to pathologically low levels and immune regulation breaks down, creating a state of constant oxidative stress.[6]

HIV directly alters the balance of the immune system toward an inflammatory state via dysregulation of cytokines, the signaling molecules of the immune system. Tumor necrosis factor alpha (TNF-α), the principle immune mediator of inflammation, is in particular up-regulated by HIV-1 itself. HIV-1, TNF-α, and ROS activate NF-kb, the transcription factor that induces expression of a host of proinflammatory genes. This further increases the production of TNF and ROS, creating an amplification loop that potentiates inflammation. In addition to TNF-α, HIV disease up-regulates interleukin (IL)-1 and IL-6, all three of which are among a subset of inflammatory cytokines known as pyrogens, as they induce fever when the body is fighting infection. This proinflammatory cascade of cytokines in turn up-regulates adhesion molecules for immune cells, enabling these cells to assemble in certain regions such as the skin, and may thereby lower the threshold for the development of clinical cutaneous disease in the face of a simultaneously increased stimulus for it.[6]

The normal mechanisms that allow an individual to manage physiologic sources of stress become increasingly critical under the pathologic levels of stress that challenge HIV-infected patients; these include a host of reducing agents and free radical scavenging pathways that compose the endogenous antioxidant system of the body. A fundamental purpose of these scavenger systems is to maintain the balance of redox (oxidation–reduction) potential within cells and thereby protect them from damage by ROS and electrophilic species. What is likely more important than the intensity of stress that a healthy or immunocompromised person may encounter is the individual's capacity to cope with that stress, which is represented by efficiency of these systems. As with most biological processes, there is considerable variation between individuals in this capacity, based on genetic polymorphisms, ethnic prevalence, and environmental factors such as nutrition.

HIV-infected patients have decreased levels of some major components of these antioxidant systems, notably potent endogenous thiol-reducing agents such as glutathione (GSH) and thioredoxin, involved in scavenger systems for electrophiles and ROS, as well as key enzymes such as catalase and superoxide dismutase. This may be due to an exhaustion of these scavengers caused by the overall increased state of oxidative stress. However, several

other factors could be contributing to this depletion. Alterations in bowel mucosa reduce the host's ability to absorb certain nutrients that play a direct role as free radical scavengers or key metabolites in their pathways, such as vitamins, flavonoids, quinones, minerals, and sulfur-containing amino acids.[6] As the liver is a major source of scavengers like GSH,[7] liver damage secondary to drugs and hepatotoxic viruses common in HIV disease may also limit production of these scavengers. Decreased levels of cystathionase, an enzyme necessary for GSH synthesis, and increased glutamate, which prevents intracellular transport of necessary substrates such as cysteine, further impede the patient's ability to replenish these defenses. In addition, the HIV-1 tat protein represses superoxide dismutase, depriving the body of yet another defense against free radical damage.[6]

Light presents another exacerbating factor. Electromagnetic radiation, both ionizing and non-ionizing, generates free radicals that are intrinsically unstable and impart oxidative stress. This impacts on macromolecules like DNA, and also incites many cellular disturbances that cause lipid peroxide and protease production and abnormalities of calcium homeostasis, which can lead to apoptosis of epithelial cells, endothelial cells, melanocytes, and stromal cells. Furthermore, UV radiation has been found to up-regulate the same inflammatory cytokines (IL-1, IL-6, and TNF-α) that are elevated in HIV, and both ionizing and nonionizing radiation are known to deplete thiol-reducing agents among other free radical scavengers.[7] Thus, UV radiation accelerates oxidative damage, and also drains the same natural defenses that are already depleted by HIV disease. Consequently sunlight potentiates the inflammatory and eruptive reactions to which the skin of an HIV-infected patient is already vulnerable.

MINIMAL ERYTHEMA DOSE (MED) DETERMINATION

In diagnosing the photosensitivity disorders of HIV patients, it is necessary first to exclude other conditions that may simulate these conditions such as photocontact dermatitis or a photosensitive drug eruption. Diagnosis of these conditions requires negative results of patch testing for airborne or contact allergens in tandem with photo-testing showing lowered minimal erythema dose (MED) values for UV and possibly also visible light, isolating light alone as the pathogen.

MED, which corresponds to the maximum UV radiation exposure endured without the development of erythema, is a measure of photosensitivity and values markedly lower than normal are considered a defining feature of photosensitivity disorders. Photosensitivity is generally tested on skin sites that are not normally exposed to the sun and is measured 24 hours after irradiation since UV erythema (particularly UVB) peaks within 24 hours of exposure. There is also variation of the normal threshold depending on skin type, with the lightest skin types (types I–III) generally having lower MED values reflecting higher sensitivity to UV radiation and darker skin types having higher MED values and lower sensitivity (*Table 8*). It should be noted that the MED of UVA is measured in joules while the MED of UVB is measured in millijoules. As UVA radiation is far less erythemogenic than UVB, the skin can absorb and sustain UVA radiation without erythema by orders of magnitude more than UVB.

Table 8 Skin phototype and UV sensitivity

SKIN PHOTOTYPE	MED OF UVA (J/cm^2)	MED OF UVB (mJ/cm^2)
I	20–35	15–30
II	30–45	25–40
III	40–55	30–50
IV	50–80	45–60
V	70–100	60–90
VI	>100	90–150

CHRONIC ACTINIC DERMATITIS

DEFINITION/OVERVIEW

CAD is a rare photosensitivity dermatitis that preferentially affects older men.[8] The term is currently used to describe a group of photosensitive disorders, including photosensitive 'eczema' (PD), actinic reticuloid (AR), and persistent light reaction (PLR), though only PD and AR were included when Hawke and Magnus originally introduced the term in 1979.[8,9] Common usage reflects the original definition, with CAD being used interchangeably with 'the photosensitivity dermatitis and actinic reticuloid syndrome' (PD/AR) in reference to light- sensitive patients who often demonstrate contact sensitivity to photoactive airborne allergens such as fragrances and plant resins (e.g. oleoresins, colophony, and sesquiterpene lactone).

CAD is distinct from the clinically similar PLR disorder, in that PLR implies photosensitivity secondary to a drug or chemical that persists in spite of it being discontinued. CAD (PD/AR) by definition excludes conditions with known primary etiologic agents such as drugs or chemicals, and while CAD patients may display increased susceptibility to exogenous allergens, these agents are not the primary cause of the persistent light sensitivity of the skin.[10]

As with several previously rare skin diseases, CAD has been observed with increased incidence in patients with HIV infection. In some cases, the presentation of photosensitivity has led to the diagnosis of HIV infection,[8] especially in patients who did not report HIV risk factors or display aquired immunodeficiency syndrome (AIDS)-defining illnesses.[11] Clinicians must be familiar with the typical clinical presentations of these diseases and recognize certain unusual features that can raise suspicion for infection with HIV. Some indicators for HIV-associated CAD include: male gender, decreased mean age of onset, and pronounced immune suppression, particularly in the form of diminished helper T cell (CD4+) counts.

PATHOGENESIS/PATHOPHYSIOLOGY

While many etiologic aspects of CAD and its link with HIV remain uncertain, multiple theories poin to immune dysregulation. HIV-induced abnormalities may include faulty regulation in antigen presentation, heightened or hypersensitive immune response to certain stimuli, e.g. UV radiation, and possibly also visible light and/or contact allergens. The efficacy of immune suppression in treating the disease supports the pathologic role of immune mechanisms in this process. Moreover, genetic abnormalities affecting enzymes involved in immune regulation have been shown to cause similar photosensitive eczematous eruptions, for example in α1-antitrypsin deficiency. This enzyme, a protease inhibitor synthesized in the liver, is an 'acute phase protein' involved in the suppression of cytokine-mediated inflammation responses. It limits the action of activated neutrophils by inhibiting elastase (a serine protease that degrades connective tissue elastin during immune and inflammatory responses) and thereby dampens immune responses. A homozygous genotype for the mutation, found in 10% of the European population, renders affected individuals more predisposed to inflammatory and immune-mediated diseases.

Abnormalities in the regulation of the immune response, often in the form of chronic and marked inflammatory conditions, arise from protease–antiprotease imbalances such as in the case of this enzyme deficiency. These include a number of dermatologic diseases such as persistent cutaneous vasculitis, cold-contact urticaria, acquired angioedema, psoriasis, Ehlers–Danlos-like syndrome, and some forms of panniculitis.[9] Drugs such as danazol restore balance to the protease–antiprotease system via increasing α1-antitrypsin, thereby strengthening the immune suppressive side of the balance and ameliorating the inflammatory responses, which may take the form of abnormal helper T cell and polyclonal B cell activation.[9]

While the linking mechanisms remain unclear, the critical role of T cells remains a central theme in hypotheses regarding the etiology of CAD. HIV and CAD separately manifest the common feature of markedly suppressed CD4+ T cell counts and strikingly low CD4+/CD8+ T cell ratios.[11,12] (The T cell ratio is used as an overall indicator of the level of immune suppression and a measure of advancement of the disease, lower ratios reflecting more advanced

stages.) Hence it is low for patients who are HIV-positive and have CAD. Decreased CD4+/CD8+ ratios have also been found in skin lesions and blood of CAD patients who do not have HIV, particularly in severe cases of CAD.[11,12] Furthermore, low CD4+ cell counts are associated with several cutaneous conditions, including atopic dermatitis, cutaneous T cell lymphoma (CTCL), and photoaccentuated erythroderma, all of which occur independently of HIV infection. The link between HIV and photosensitivity may not necessarily reflect a causal relationship,[11] but rather a correlation of both with CD4+ suppression. It may not be a coincidence that with the advent of improved antiretroviral therapies there has been decreased incidence in the photosensitive disorders associated with HIV infection.

Several hypotheses regarding CAD involve the immune system reacting against some kind of photoproduct arising from the interaction of light and a photoabsorbing substance in the skin.[13] One of these suggests that cytotoxic (CD8+) T cells react to a photoinduced self-antigen, and that control of the antiself response is lost because of the diminished CD4+ T cells that usually regulate and direct the actions of cytotoxic T cells.[11] In HIV seronegative patients, the CAD response might still involve this T cell ratio but it could also arise from another selective immune defect. There is current speculation, for example, as to whether the underlying pathology of AR reflects a cell membrane defect with heightened sensitivity to UV light, where the persistent inflammatory reaction is caused by continued antigen presentation from damaged membranes. This could occur either appropriately, because membranes continue to sustain damage, or inappropriately, because of an inherent defect in the Langerhans cells themselves.[10]

CLINICAL FEATURES

The manifestations of CAD range from photosensitive eczema, appearing in light exposed areas with UVB sensitivity only, to AR where there is marked lymphoma-like induration and infiltration with both UVB and UVA sensitivity. Patients with the latter usually have more severe disease and are usually more difficult to manage than those with

UVB sensitivity only.[10] Photosensitivity is a defining feature of the disease and determined by MED values markedly below normal.

Extreme sensitivity to both types of UV radiation without a known photosensitizer has been termed 'severe chronic photosensitivity', CAD, and AR with normal cellular infiltrate.[13] It is important for proper identification of the disease to rule out any possibly contributing photosensitizing agents or drugs. Some more common examples of these include trime-thoprim–sulfamethoxazole, dapsone, and non-steroidal anti-inflammatory drugs (NSAIDs) which have been associated in particular with the lichenoid eruptions.[11]

CAD has a characteristically photodistributed pattern affecting predominantly the face, neck, upper V-portion portion of the chest, and areas of limbs commonly exposed to sunlight such as the extensor portions of the arms (**148**), while sparing areas that are relatively shaded such as the eyelids, submental, and retroauricular regions. Patients commonly present with erythema and eczematous plaques and papules, often of an erythematous or violaceous, lichenified, or scaly nature and associated with some-times severe pruritus. Eruptions may be accompanied by edema of the scalp, dorsa of hands, and the other commonly photoexposed regions mentioned,[13] and may in some cases progress to erythroderma.[8]

The disease is usually severe and longstanding, persisting for months to years without continued exposure to known photosensitizers, and is extremely resistant to treatment. While rare spontaneous improvements or gradual remittance over years have been reported, relapse is common especially upon discontinuation of treatment and may occur on re-exposure even to fluorescent light, although tungsten bulbs are generally not problematic.[10]

A guiding factor in recognition of HIV-related disease can be age of onset. Though there are rare reports of CAD presenting in young patients, it is characteristically a disease of individuals above the age of 60, while the mean age for HIV patients with CAD is approximately 50 years, with a range of 36–58 years, on average at least 10 years younger than the HIV-negative population.[8,11] There is also gender distributed pattern for both HIV and CAD, as both diseases affect males with marked pre-dominance. Additionally, there appears to be a higher occurrence of CAD in skin types V and VI (African-Americans), and III and IV (Chinese-Americans), which is unusual considering these skin types should be less photosensitive in general.

HISTOPATHOLOGY

The histology of CAD varies from a spongiotic dermatitis that may resemble chronic eczema to a dense dermal infiltrate with epidermotropism and cellular atypia that simulates mycosis fungoides.[10] The most common pattern is a psoriasiform lichenoid dermatitis with epidermal hyperplasia, often with focal necrotic keratinocytes, spongiosis, hyper-granulosis, and ortho- and parakeratosis. The infiltrate consists mostly of lymphocytes but there may be eosinophils.

Direct immunofluorescence testing in HIV-seronegative patients has revealed deposits of immunoglobulin (Ig)G, C3, and fibrinogen in the walls of superficial blood vessels in the dermis, with focal granular deposits of IgM at the dermoepidermal junction in some cases. Similar findings have been reported in HIV-infected patients and antibodies to HIV have been found 1 week after onset.[8]

Sézary cells, large atypical T cells exhibiting abnormal convoluted nuclei, have been found in the peripheral blood of patients with CAD (as up to 10% of the total number of circulating lymphocytes).

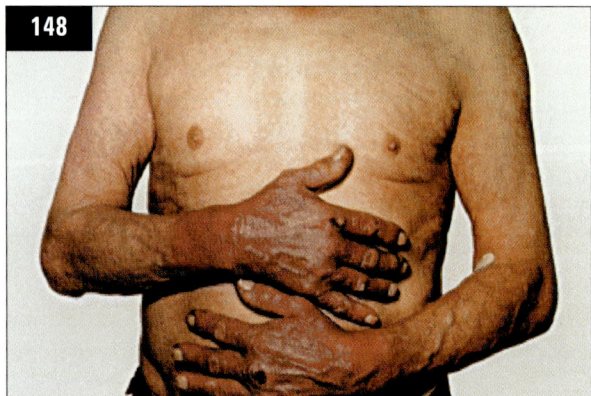

148 Chronic actinic dermatitis.

However, CAD can be distinguished from erythrodermic CTCL by the very low CD4+/CD8+ T cell ratio in circulating blood.[14]

DIAGNOSIS

For diagnosis, patients must present with a chronic photodermatitis that persists without continued exposure to photosensitizing agents, must have abnormal responses to photo-testing, and should demonstrate characteristic features microscopically.[8] Patients with CAD, whether associated with HIV and α1-antitrypsin deficiency or not, show markedly decreased MED to UVB and most also show decreased tolerance to UVA.[8,9] Laboratory studies should be performed for antineutrophilic antibody (ANA) titers and anti-Ro/La antibodies to rule out lupus erythematosus and similar autoimmune conditions as potential causes or contributing factors to the eruption. Photo-patch testing should be done to exclude the diagnosis of photoallergic contact dermatitis, which could resemble CAD and might be caused by many different allergens. Organic sunscreens should be included in the panel of allergens, as they can serve as contact allergens and would otherwise be recommended in the treatment regimen for the condition.

MANAGEMENT

Sunscreens, topical corticosteroid preparations, and high-dose systemic corticosteroids are first-line treatment (*Table 9*), and have ameliorating effects; however, are rarely sufficient to suppress the disease entirely. Thus immunosuppressive therapy is often required. Some experts are reluctant to use immunosuppressive treatment, for fear of worsening the patient's HIV disease. Meola *et al.* (1997), for example, recommend only first-line therapies for HIV patients with the rationale that CAD photoeruptions are a byproduct of a compromised immune system, and would be worsened by further suppression.[8] Others have reported improvement of CAD using immunosuppressive medications such as azathioprine and cyclosporine. While often effective, these should be used with caution in HIV patients as they do have the potential to leave the patient more vulnerable to other illnesses and complications of

Table 9 Treatment of CAD

First-line

Photoprotection (restricted exposure to UV and visible light if necessary)
- Virtual avoidance of sunlight between 10 am and 4 pm
- Protective clothing: long-sleeved shirts, long pants
- of dark colors and close weave materials (e.g. blue denim)
- Broad-brimmed hats
- Use of filtering window films whenever possible

Sunscreen
- Liberal application of broad-spectrum, high-factor hypoallergenic sunscreens every 2–3 hours

Avoidance of relevant contact allergens

Topical emollients

Corticosteroids
- Topical
- Systemic: intermittent courses of 30–60 mg daily, tapered over several weeks to bring acute flares under control

Desensitization to radiation and contact allergens (sunscreen can be a contact allergen)

Antihistamines

Second-line

Azathioprine (100 mg daily)

Cyclosporine (2.5–4 mg/kg daily)

Phototherapy (desensitization)
- PUVA
- UVB

Topical tacrolimus (0.1 %)

Third-line

Hydroxychloroquine (200 mg once or twice daily)

Oral retinoids (etretinate 0.8–0.25 mg/kg daily, used with PUVA)

Danazol (600 mg daily)

Topical mechlorethamine (nitrogen mustard, 10 mg dissolved in 50 ml water)

Mycophenolate (immunosuppressant used with PUVA)

their disease. Short-term administration of azathio-prine, 50 mg three times daily taken orally for 6 months, has been shown to cause remission, defined as complete subsidence of rash and itching, for the majority of patients. It has relatively few side-effects and has not been shown to cause biochemical or hematologic abnormalities in HIV-infected patients, although a rare case of gastrointestinal sensitivity or intolerance has been noted.[10]

While the mechanism of azathioprine in CAD is not clearly established, its metabolites, 6-mercapto-purine and 6-thioguanine, are implicated in its immunosuppressive action. Replacement of purine bases with purine analogs increases the sensitivity of cells to killing by UV radiation, especially wavelengths of 320–360 nm. If the eczematic reaction of CAD is in fact due to continued antigen presentation by the Langerhans cells, the remission achieved by this therapy could be explained by the reduction in their number, as topical application of azathioprine reduces Langerhans cell numbers in mice. Furthermore, PUVA, another Langerhans cell suppressing treatment, is also effective in treating CAD. Azathioprine may also exert its effect on the bone marrow, with cutaneous depletion of Langerhans cells developing as a consequence of a marrow suppressive effect, and may additionally have a nonspecific anti-inflammatory action.

While it may seem counterintuitive to consider phototherapy as a treatment for a photo-induced eruption, phototherapy itself may be useful in CAD in that it may lead to 'desensitization'. PUVA, as noted above, decreases Langerhans cells in the skin and is also useful in some patients.

Third-line therapies are used when other treatments are not effective or their side-effects are so troublesome that they minimize patient compliance; topical nitrogen mustard, for example, is highly irritating and may cause anemia in addition to worsened immunosuppression. Other agents such as mycophenolate mofetil have not been sufficiently studied and other regimens are often too complex or expensive to be practically maintained. Antihistamines can be a helpful addition to thera-peutic regimens to ease pruritus.

LICHENOID PHOTODERMATITIS OF HIV INFECTION

DEFINITION/OVERVIEW

Lichenoid dermatitis refers to a cutaneous eruption that bears similarity to lichen planus (LP), namely flat-topped, polygonal, hyperpigmented, violaceous papules and plaques (**149**). These may be induced by drugs or other allergens and may be induced by or exacerbated by UV irradiation. In the HIV-infected population, it predominantly affects African-American patients with advanced stage infection. The clinical manifestations are often nonclassical for LP, and eruptions may be persistent and generalized, or become exacerbated despite long periods without exposure to photosensitizing agents. In some cases, UV light alone may be the perpetuating, if not initial, trigger of this condition in the setting of HIV disease.

PATHOGENESIS/PATHOPHYSIOLOGY

Lichenoid eruptions in HIV-infected patients are more frequently seen as CD4+ T cell counts decrease (generally below $50 \times 10^6/l$) and are more common in African-American patients. Some of the potentially photosensitizing drugs that may incite the condition include NSAIDs, trimethoprim–sulfamethoxazole, and dapsone.[3,15]

The morphology of drug-induced and photo-induced eruptions in these patients is often similar and may represent a common underlying pathology, related to the intensified state of oxidative stress in HIV infection. Many medications impart oxidative stress and consume endogenous free radical scavengers as they are metabolized in the body. UV radiation, likewise, has been found to up-regulate the same inflammatory cytokines elevated in HIV infection, perpetuating a state of oxidative damage, and also to deplete thiol-reducing agents and other free radical scavengers.[7] It is possible, therefore, that one reason certain drugs are observed to be 'photosensitizing' is that they affect the same inflammatory immune pathways and exhaust the same antioxidant systems triggered by UV radiation. Thus, these medications and UV light, by converging to cause the same biochemical imbalances, render a patient more sensitive to develop a cutaneous

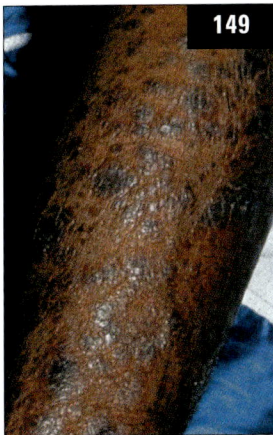

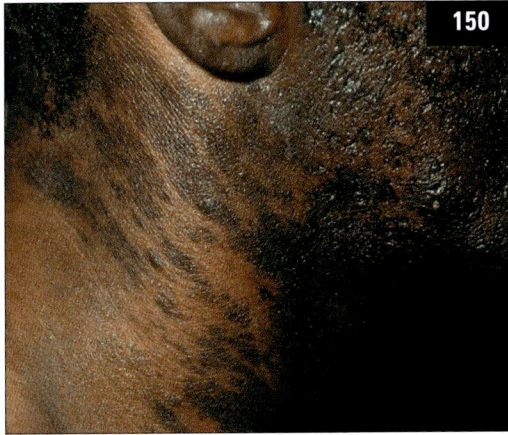

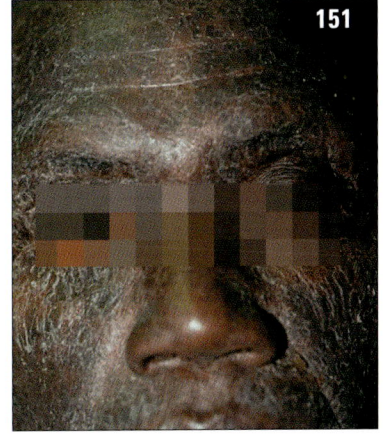

149 Lichenoid photodermatitis. Flat-topped, polygonal, hyperpigmented, violaceous papules and plaques on the forearm.

150 Lichenoid photodermatitis. Extensive hyperpigmentation with areas of lichenification on the lateral neck and face.

151 Long-standing lichenoid photodermatitis changes on the face with extensive ichthyosiform dermatitis and incipient ectropion formation.

eruption when faced with either stimulus.

The lack of mucosal involvement in the lichenoid eruptions of HIV-infected patients is one feature that distinguishes these lesions from idiopathic LP. Lower lip involvement reported HIV lichenoid eruptions is an exception; however, this could be considered an example of a sun exposed mucosal area and, therefore, another illustration of HIV-associated photosensitivity. Classic idiopathic LP in HIV-positive patients has yet to be reported.[15]

CLINICAL FEATURES

Lichenoid photodermatoses in HIV patients are characterized by violaceous, flat-topped papules that coalesce into plaques with increased skin markings[1] distributed primarily on the face, neck (**150, 151**), and dorsa of the hands and forearms (**149**).[15] Mucosal involvement is not seen except for the lower lip on occasion. Pruritus is a common feature and most patients display excoriations. The eruption is usually chronic, lasting in excess of several months. Postinflammatory hyperpigmentation is extremely common, especially in African-American patients, although occasionally depigmentation may be seen. Depigmentation may be more extensive involving the nail folds, upper lip, and scalp, including loss of pigment in the hair. Gradual repigmentation has been observed with treatment.[15]

Most affected patients are between 35 and 75 years with the mean age being approximately 55 years. It is associated with advanced stage disease as all patients that have been reported had AIDS, many having either Kaposi's sarcoma (KS) or AIDS-defining opportunistic infections.[15] Helper T cell counts in affected patients are usually $<50 \times 10^6$/l with a mean of 20×10^6/l. In a few patients, the absolute eosinophil count has been elevated.[16]

HISTOPATHOLOGY

Biopsy specimens of lichenoid photoeruptions in these patients are characterized by a lichenoid infiltrate of lymphocytes primarily with marked hyperkeratosis, focal parakeratosis, acanthosis, and scattered necrotic keratinocytes. Hydropic degeneration and incontinence of pigment into the dermis,[15] and 'sawtoothing' of the rete ridges are also common (152, 153). In some cases, eosinophils and plasma cells are present in addition to lymphocytes.[15]

While a lichenoid pattern of inflammation is seen in most lesions of this type, in some cases features include diffuse infiltrates, subepidermal blisters, and spongiosis. Rarely, the epidermis has shown focal

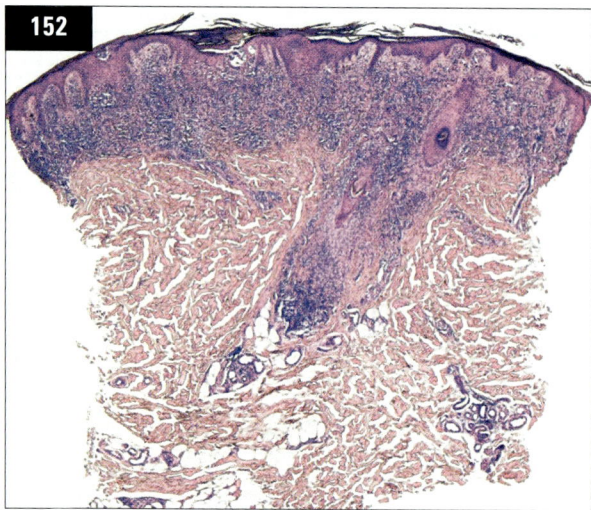

152 Low power view of lichenoid photodermatitis demonstrating features similar to those seen in lichen planus: hyperkeratosis, mild acanthosis, hypergranulosis, saw-toothing of the rete ridges, pigment incontinence, and a lichenoid infiltrate composed mostly of lymphocytes.

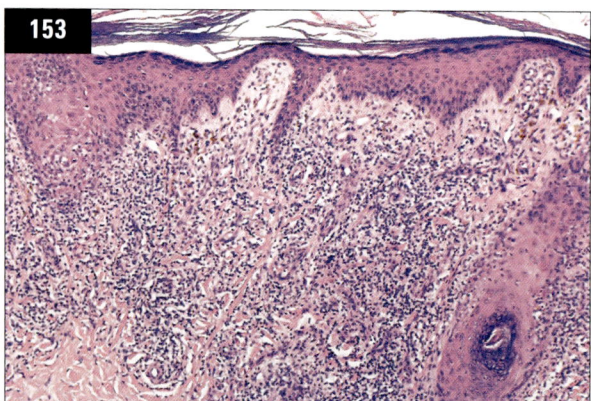

153 Higher power view shows the lichenoid infiltrate and incontinence of pigment in the upper dermis.

atrophy centrally and laterally surrounding the dermal infiltrate, imparting a 'ball and claw' morphology similar to that seen in lichen nitidus.[15] In specimens from depigmented areas, there is absence of melanocytes in the epidermis along the dermoepidermal junction and marked decreased of S100-positive cells in the basement membrane zone.[15] The presence of mild papillary dermal edema should also be noted as this is characteristic of photo-induced lichenoid eruptions, while not a typical feature of classic lichenoid lesions.

DIAGNOSIS

All patients with this type of eruption should be questioned carefully about exposure to medications that may serve as allergens or photosensitizing agents.[3] It is essential to evaluate the timing and nature of the onset of the eruption and to inquire thoroughly about all medications patients may have been taken including over-the-counter agents, especially NSAIDs.[15]

MANAGEMENT

There is an unfortunate lack of large randomized trials evaluating the efficacy of various drugs and treatment regimes for lichenoid eruptions. Most patients show at least some improvement with complete avoidance of potentially photosensitizing medications and the use of sunscreens and sun-protective measures. However, as with CAD, disease activity often persists despite following this regimen.[15] In some patients, acitretin has shown benefit,[17] and is now considered a first-line treatment. As with all systemic retinoids, these drugs should be avoided by women who plan to become pregnant. Other treatments such as topical cyclosporine and extracorporeal photochemotherapy may also be effective, but have yet to be evaluated in large clinical trials.[17] Additionally, antihistamines such as fexofenadine can be used for associated symptoms such as pruritis.[16]

PHOTODISTRIBUTED HYPERPIGMENTATION

DEFINITION/OVERVIEW

Photodistributed hyperpigmentation, a condition of abnormally amplified melanogenesis of sun-exposed areas, has been observed in HIV-infected patients who have had no exposure to photosensitizing stimuli. It is a relatively rare cutaneous manifestation of HIV infection and, as with lichenoid photo-dermatitis, is seen with marked predominance in African-American patients with advanced AIDS. While it is always photodistributed, it may be due either to photosensitivity or phototoxicity.

PATHOGENESIS/PATHOPHYSIOLOGY

It is thought that in HIV patients affected by this condition, solar radiation induces strikingly increased melanogenesis and melanin deposition similar to sunlight-induced tanning. However, it is not clear why this process occurs abnormally in HIV-infected patients and why there is such a marked predominance in African-American patients with advanced AIDS, specifically with absolute CD4+ T cell counts below $200 \times 10^6/l$.

Melanin is composed of conjugated pi-systems and nitrogen atoms, indole rings, and quinones, which are building blocks of the antioxidants and free radical scavenger molecules that protect the body against oxidative damage. In HIV-infected patients who are subject to intensified oxidative stress and a waning capacity to manage it, the melanin synthesis pathway may be up-regulated as a means of protection. The resources of the body may be shunted toward melanin production to increase the presence of a reducing agent in an attempt to deal with, and compensate for, the oxidative imbalances that cannot otherwise be adequately controlled. In HIV-infected patients this pathway may be utilized more than in normal physiology, simply because other antioxidant and free radical scavenging pathways have been reduced to substandard levels of functioning. Perhaps this abnormality is more pronounced in those of darker skin types due to the greater capacity for efficient melanin production in the skin of these patients. Thus darker skin would be more readily equipped to protect itself from oxidative stress using the melanin pathway and more likely to show a more apparent reaction when faced with one of the major causes of oxidative stress found in nature, sunlight.

Since hyperpigmentation often follows inflammation and injury to the skin, a significant component of this condition could represent postinflammatory hyperpigmentation from subclinical UV light-induced inflammation. As viral load is lower and CD4+ cell counts are somewhat recovered in hyperpigmentation reactions *vs.* eczematous and lichenoid reactions,[1] these lesions may sometimes represent relic of past dermatoses, where postinflammatory markings of eczema or a burned out dermatitis of lichenoid origin are manifested as hyperpigmentation.

CLINICAL FEATURES

Photodistributed hyperpigmentation manifests primarily in individuals with skin type V or VI, and most commonly in patients of African-American descent. Virtually all patients have absolute CD4+ T cell counts below $200 \times 10^6/l$. Clinically, there is marked hyperpigmentation in a photodistributed pattern involving the face, neck, V-pattern on the upper chest and back, and the dorsa of the hands. As previously noted, while all cases are induced by light, there are both photosensitive and nonphotosensitive forms. The photosensitive form is distinguished by its additional feature of painful irritation.

HISTOPATHOLOGY

Tissue specimens from hyperpigmented areas demonstrate increased melanin within keratinocytes and along the dermoepidermal junction, as well as numerous melanophages in the upper reticular dermis. No heavy metal deposits or evidence of pigment related to drugs have been noted.[3]

DIAGNOSIS

The diagnosis of HIV-related photodistributed hyperpigmentation is primarily one of exclusion. The differential diagnosis includes drug-induced post-inflammatory hyperpigmentation from prior inflammatory skin diseases and endocrine causes of hyperpigmentation. These must be excluded based on clinical history of past skin reactions and medications the patient has taken, as well as by laboratory studies screening for imbalances in blood chemistry, thyroid function, and other hormone abnormalities, and nutritional deficiencies. In those with HIV-related photodistributed hyperpigmentation, laboratory studies are normal with respect to blood chemistries, thyroid function studies, and levels of corticotropin, cortisol, and α-melanocyte-stimulating hormone. A deficiency in niacin can cause pellagra that may appear similar and this and should also be excluded.

Medications causing photosensitivity and commonly associated with hyperpigmentation include some of the tetracyclines, antimalarials, certain hormones, chemotherapeutic agents, phenothiazines, and NSAIDs.[3] The catalyzing effect or possibly eclipsing contribution to hyperpigmentation that can be made by these drugs must be ruled out. Many HIV-seropositive patients are administered regimens that included zidovudine; however, the patients originally studied for photodistributed hyperpigmentation had not displayed any of the pigmentary changes of nails, palms, or mucosal surfaces that are associated with this drug, so it is unlikely to be related.[3] Furthermore, a number of these patients had hyperpigmentation before the diagnosis of HIV had been established.

MANAGEMENT

Treatment of hyperpigmentation disorders is notoriously difficult in immunocompetent individuals and is even more challenging in the HIV-infected population. It entails the balance of efficacy in reducing excess pigment in affected areas while avoiding hypopigmentation or irritation in the normal surrounding skin. This is especially complicated in darker skinned patients who are most commonly affected.

First-line therapy involves use of broad-spectrum sunscreens that absorb both UVA and UVB radiation. These are used in combination with phenolic agents such as hydroquinone and N-acetyl-4-cystaminylphenol (NCAP), or nonphenolic agents such as tretinoin, adapalene, topical corticosteroids, azelaic acid, arbutin, kojic acid, and licorice extract.

A common mechanism of many of these therapies is inhibition of tyrosinase, the enzyme that converts DOPA to melanin, thereby reducing the production of melanin. Corticosteroids exert their effect by decreasing the endoplasmic reticulum secretory function of melanocytes. Tretinoin, salicylic acid, and glycolic acid act by removing melanin from the epidermis via exfoliation.

Hydroquinone, a hydroxyphenol, is considered the most effective of all and is generally used in concentrations ranging from 2–10%. While more potent and more rapidly acting, compounds with 5–10% hydroquinone are often unstable and are more irritating. Side-effects of these treatments include postinflammatory hyperpigmentation, cutaneous ochronosis, allergic contact dermatitis, nail discoloration, and hypopigmentation of surrounding skin. As these effects may be as disfiguring as the condition itself, it is essential that treatment be carefully monitored and tailored for each patient. Antioxidants such as vitamin C, retinoids, and alphahydroxy acids used with hydroquinone may enhance efficacy so that lower concentrations may be used. Furthermore, the free radical scavenger properties of these agents may impart a protective effect in reducing oxidative damage and sensitivity and serve to lessen the likelihood of developing this complication.

PORPHYRIA CUTANEA TARDA

DEFINITION/OVERVIEW

Porphyrias are a group inherited or spontaneous disorders characterized by decreased activity of enzymes that synthesize heme groups from their precursor molecules, porphyrins. Among the porphyrias, PCT is the most common, the term 'tarda' referring to the relatively late onset of the condition that usually first presents in the late thirties.[18] It arises from insufficiency of the enzyme uroporphyrinogen decarboxylase and has been associated with a number of factors including genetic, environmental, neoplastic, and infectious among others. Hepatitis C virus (HCV) in particular is a well documented contributing factor in the development of PCT. In the last two decades, increasing reports of HIV-associated cases of PCT and the observation that porphyrin metabolism is often abnormal in those with HIV disease have brought to light the existence of a relationship, the possible role of HIV in the development of PCT, and the possibility that PCT could be marker of underlying HIV disease.

PATHOGENESIS/PATHOPHYSIOLOGY

Porphyrins are the building blocks of a group of heme-containing photoactive molecules that perform essential oxidation–reduction reactions of the body. Notable members of this family include hemoglobin, myoglobin, cytochromes, and catalase, the detoxification enzyme that protects the body from toxins such as alcohol, formaldehyde, and hydrogen peroxide. Porphyrins and their metabolites are normally cleared from the body via secretion into bile and via urinary excretion. If present in excess, these compounds are deposited in tissue including the skin where they result in cutaneous photosensitivity, pruritus, increased fragility, bullae, hypertrichosis, dyspigmentation, sclerodermoid features, and scarring.

PCT is the disorder that arises from decreased activity of the enzyme uroporphyrinogen decarboxylase which converts uroporphyrin to coprophyrin in the fifth step of the heme biosynthesis pathway. Its deficiency can arise either in inherited fashion, in which the enzyme deficiency is found in both erythrocytes and hepatocytes, or as an acquired disorder in which only hepatocytes are affected. The acquired form is thought to represent approximately 80% of cases, though this is difficult to verify as many affected individuals may be asymptomatic. This enzyme abnormality leads to enhanced oxidation of uroporphyrogen to uroporphyrin which is a photoactive compound.[19,20]

Acquired PCT is associated with many factors including exogenous substances such as estrogens, ethanol, iron, and hepatotoxic aromatic hydrocarbons, infectious agents such as HCV and HIV, and hepatic neoplasms. Some forms of acquired PCT have genetic abnormalities such as mutant uroporphyrinogen decarboxylase or hemochromatosis genes. A common thread of these etiologies is liver damage. Development of PCT is associated with liver dysfunction, with 82% of patients manifesting elevated transaminase levels.[18] Liver damage results in the impairment of uroporphyrin decarboxylase,[21] and in fibrosis, which may impede biliary clearance of porphyrin precursors and breakdown products that accumulate due to this enzyme deficiency. Obstruction of bile flow as a result of fibrosis may cause toxic substances meant for biliary excretion to accumulate in the blood stream and cause systemic effects such as pruritus that is characteristically seen with primary biliary cirrhosis and primary sclerosing cholangitis. Furthermore, since the liver synthesizes free radical scavenger molecules such as glutathione (GSH) that alleviate porphyrin-induced pathology,[22,23] progressive liver damage both contributes to the pathogenesis of PCT and depletes the body's natural safeguards against it. While the mechanism of cutaneous sensitization by porphyrins remains unclear, it is considered a photodynamic process that involves radiant energy, molecular oxygen, and an oxidizable substrate.[24,25]

HIV may contribute to the development of PCT in multiple ways, largely via generating hepatic inflammation and accelerated fibrosis. Through up-regulation of proinflammatory cytokines including TNF-α, IL-1, and IL-6, HIV generates and maintains a state of inflammation, manifest as a low-grade hepatitis. This inflammatory state, in addition to byproducts of the oxidative damage such as lipid peroxides, contributes to apoptosis and necrosis of hepatic parenchyma and stimulates the collagen-producing stellate cells. The stellate cells begin proliferating and over-actively making collagen, and the end result is accelerated fibrosis eventually contributing to cirrhosis and liver failure.

The majority of HIV-infected patients with PCT are coinfected with viral hepatitis, particularly with hepatitis B (HBV) and HCV.[26–31] These diseases are associated with cirrhosis, end-stage liver disease, and liver cancer. While increased vulnerability of HIV patients to other infections or yet unexplained links between HIV and HCV may help account for this, the coexistence of these two diseases likely results from their acquisition via the same high-risk behaviors, e.g. IV drug use and having multiple sexual partners. Infection with HIV and often HCV usually predates the presentation of PCT and the hepatic changes observed in HIV-associated PCT patients are accelerated in those with both diseases.

While hepatic inflammation and injury alone may cause diminished function of uroporphyrinogen decarboxylase, there is evidence that viral diseases such HIV and HCV can alter porphyrin metabolism directly, precipitating the clinical manifestation of PCT in susceptible patients.[32] In coinfected patients, HIV is the primary driving factor as PCT and porphyrin abnormalities have been found in HIV-infected patients in the absence of HCV, although the reverse is only rarely demonstrated.[33] In fact, among patients with HCV who have abnormal porphyrin metabolism, all have some type of AIDS-defining illness and more pronounced immune suppression, having mean CD4+ cell counts of 34×10^6/l, than those without porphyrin abnormalities who have mean CD4+ cell counts of 145×10^6/l.[34] Furthermore, PCT is not found in immunocompromised patients who do not have HIV infection,[35] a finding that supports the theory that it is the combination of HIV and HCV infection that leads to the development of PCT. A marked rise in HCV ribonucleic acid (RNA) levels in patients coinfected with HCV and HIV has been observed, which suggests that HIV infection exacerbates the course of HCV infection, worsening liver damage and thereby causing PCT to become clinically apparent.[34]

Factors other than viral coinfection can also predispose HIV patients to liver disorders including PCT. Patients with PCT have increased iron levels in the body, much of which localizes to the liver.

Increased alcohol intake or exogenous iron from other sources can increase the demand for the heme group products of the porphyrin pathway, and overload the enzymes such as uroporphyrinogen decarboxylase required to make them. Furthermore, genetic factors, such as mutations in the HFE gene which codes for a protein that regulates iron absorption from the body and can result in iron overload disorders such as hemochromatosis, also increases the demand on these pathways. The combination of increased demand and reduced activity of uroporphyrinogen decarboxylase disrupts heme production and allows byproducts of these pathways to accumulate in the body, specifically the skin, triggering the signs and symptoms of PCT.

Besides coinfection with HCV, other factors have may be associated with PCT in these patients. These include hepatotoxic drugs such as those in highly active antiretroviral therapy (HAART) regimens, antibiotics, other antiretroviral agents, certain antifungal and antituberculous drugs, alcohol use, coexisting hepatic neoplasms, hepatitis A and B coinfection, and relative estrogen excess. Bacterial, mycobacterial,[36] and fungal infections may also affect the liver, worsening the process.[37]

In several studies, a number of patients with abnormal porphyrin metabolism were taking zidovudine. Onset of PCT has coincided with deteriorating immune function and initiation of zidovudine therapy. Since AZT is usually only initiated when CD4+ cells fall to levels of 500×10^6/l or less, and as such, the possibility of it inducing PCT has not been evaluated independent of immune suppression.[34]

Independent of other contributing factors, abnormal porphyrin metabolism in HIV-infected patients[34] can be significant enough to cause subclinical PCT. Porphyrin excretion in HIV-infected patients is similar to that found in PCT even when there is no clinical evidence of the disease.[38] These elevated porphyrin levels may play a role in photosensitivity in general; thus it is recommended that HIV-positive patients with idiopathic photosensitivity eruptions have their porphyrin levels evaluated. Likewise, any patient who presents with nonfamilial PCT should be screened for underlying viral infection of both HCV and HIV.

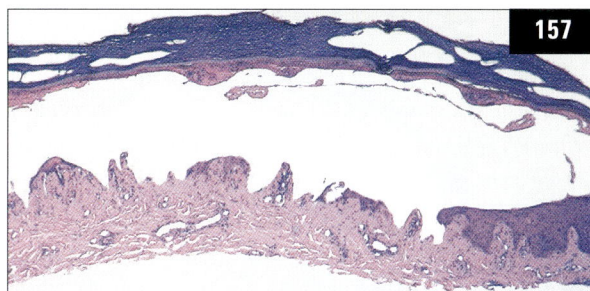

154 Porphyria cutanea tarda. Tense bullae and scarring on the dorsal hands.

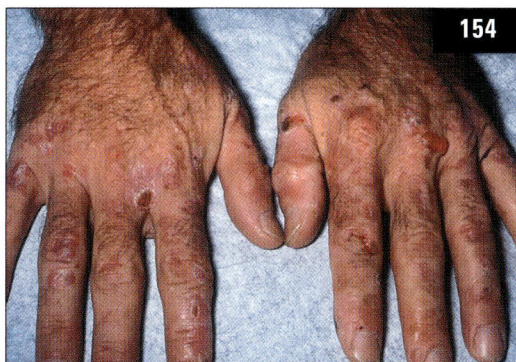

155 Large, tense bulla on the left thumb and extensive scarring of the dorsal hand.

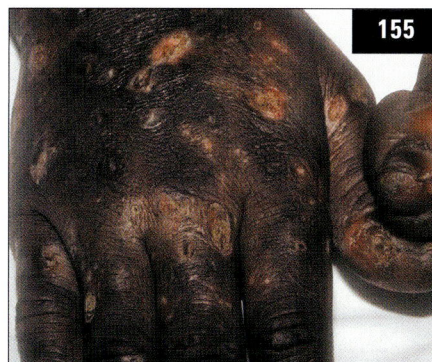

156 Hyperpigmentation, lichenification, and several areas of erosions on the face in the same patient.

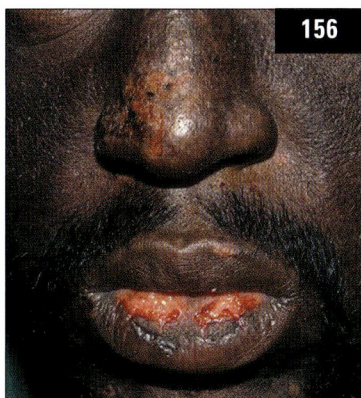

157 Cell-poor subepidermal blister on acral skin in porphyria cutanea tarda, with characteristic caterpillar bodies and festooning (preservation of dermal papillae at the base of the blister).

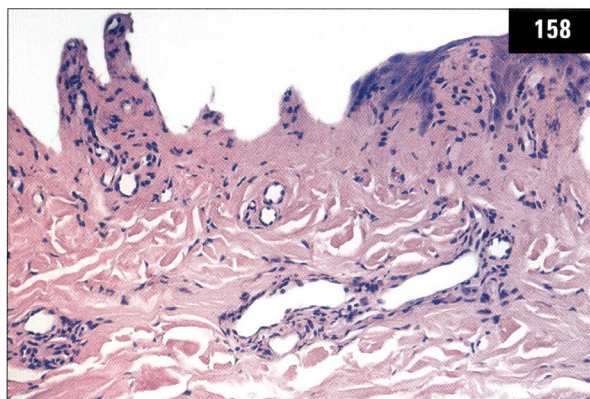

158 Higher power view of the blister cavity demonstrating thickening of the superficial dermal blood vessel walls.

CLINICAL FEATURES

The skin abnormalities of PCT are characteristically distributed on sun-exposed areas, especially the dorsal surface of the hands and arms (**154, 155**) but also the face (**156**). The initial clinical manifestations are vesicles that soon become bullae associated with skin fragility. The blisters are usually painless and often demonstrate a positive Nikolsky sign, expanding and sloughing off on pressure, in spite of their being formed beneath the epidermis, which is a consequence of the cutaneous fragility. Later, there is scarring with milia formation, hypertrichosis, especially of the face, and hyperpigmentation. Scleroderma-like change especially of the V-area of the chest is another late manifestation of PCT though less commonly observed.

The acquired form of PCT is far more common than the familial form and accounts for about 80% of all cases. Men are affected more commonly than women and the mean age of onset is 36.6 years.[18]

HISTOPATHOLOGY

Classically, there is a cell-poor subepidermal blister with minimal inflammation and marked thickening of the walls of superficial dermal vessels. There is often preservation of the dermal papillae at the base of the blister, so-called 'festooning'. Individually necrotic keratinocytes are present in the epidermis and these may be present in number and coalesce into what have been termed 'caterpillar' bodies (**157, 158**). While the underlying pathogenesis of these changes remains unclear, immunoglobulins including IgG, A, M, and/or complement are commonly found as diffuse thick deposits in the walls of blood vessels in the dermis, at the dermoepidermal junction, and around sweat glands when specimens are evaluated using direct immunofluorescence. The combination of these immune complexes and porphyrins in the skin may lead to increased skin fragility following UV light exposure, so that minor trauma results in blistering. There is not yet an established explanation for the development of facial hypertrichosis.

DIAGNOSIS

Laboratory analysis of PCT patients shows increased urinary uroporphyrins at levels two to five times above coproporphyrins, reflecting diminished activity of the uroporphyrin decarboxylase enzyme. Iron levels and liver function tests are generally elevated, likely related to conditions with which PCT is associated. While red blood cell counts and hematocrit are classically elevated, patients with HIV-associated PCT may be anemic.

One disorder that must be excluded in the diagnosis of PCT is pseudoporphyria or pseudo-PCT. While distinct from PCT in its underlying pathophysiology, pseudo-PCT can be virtually identical clinically. Blood and urine analyses are normal in pseudo-PCT and there is usually no evidence of coinfection with HBV or HCV, although IgG antibodies to hepatitis A virus have been found in some cases. Onset of pseudo-PCT has also been reported following exposure to certain drugs, hemodialysis, and UVA radiation in tanning salons.[3]

MANAGEMENT

Since strategies for inducing remission of this condition may involve treatments that are not appropriate for other porphyrias or pseudo-porphyrias, accurate diagnosis is essential. The principle of management is to treat the disease by eliminating its causes, such as circulating toxins or excessive iron levels. Serial phlebotomy, in which patients are bled until hemoglobin and hematocrit levels fall to the point of slight anemia in order to purge the body of the heme byproducts contributing to skin disease, is the classic first-line treatment.

Phlebotomy can be combined with drugs such as, deferoxamine, a chelating agent that sequesters excess iron from the blood, and erythropoietin, which stimulates bone marrow production of red blood cells and subsequently the demand for heme groups.[39]

As noted above, many HIV-infected patients with PCT are anemic, so phlebotomy is not an option. Antimalarial agents such as chloroquine and hydroxycholoroquine, enteric absorbents, and metabolic alkalinization of the blood may also be useful as they enhance excretion of porphyrins. For those with coexisting HCV, therapeutic regimens should include interferon (IFN)-α and other appropriate treatments to control the viral hepatitis. Other treatments that have shown promise include vitamin E and C supplementation, plasmapheresis and plasma exchange, high-flux hemodialysis, and cimetidine; some of these may act to slow and/or inhibit steps of porphyrin synthesis pathways in the liver. Additionally, avoidance of sunlight, alcohol, and potentially hepatotoxic drugs is also important.[39]

Finally, it is important to note that universal precautions must be taken in providing skin care for PCT lesions as HIV has been isolated from the blister fluid of patients with PCT.[40] Thus, fluid contained in skin lesions is one of the body fluids that contains virus in addition to semen, tears, cerebrospinal fluid, breast milk, alveolar fluid, and vaginal secretions. Furthermore, clinicians must practice an extreme degree of caution when performing phlebotomy on these patients.

PHOTOSENSITIVE GRANULOMA ANNULARE

DEFINITION/OVERVIEW

Granuloma annulare (GA) is a chronic inflammatory condition characterized by dermal papules, plaques, or nodules that assume an annular configuration. First described as a 'ringed eruption of the fingers', it is a benign and often self-limited condition that is usually confined to an extremity, though it may persist for years. GA has traditionally been associated with diabetes mellitus, and less commonly with autoimmune thyroiditis and various neoplastic conditions. In more recent years, an association with HIV infection has been established. HIV-related cases tend to present in an unusual fashion, such as in generalized and photodistributed distributions.

PATHOGENESIS/PATHOPHYSIOLOGY

The cause of GA, both in unaffected and HIV-infected individuals, remains unknown. Lesions have been observed to follow certain traumatic events such as excessive sun exposure, insect bites, tuberculin tests, and blunt trauma, as well as other stimuli such as following intake of allopurinol. A number of infections other than HIV have been associated with GA including those induced by Epstein–Barr virus, herpes simplex and varicella zoster viruses, HCV, *Borrelia* spp., and several mycobacteria and fungi. However, GA most commonly develops in healthy individuals without an identified cause.

GA has been theorized as a reaction pattern to traumatic insult or aberrant immune response in the skin. Though purpura are rarely seen, there may be inflammation within dermal blood vessels, consistent with a mild vasculitis, especially in the center of palisaded granulomas of early lesions. This may result from deposition of circulating immune complexes which have been found in the serum of patients with GA. A cell-mediated immune response via the secretion of cytotoxic mediators has also been proposed. Possible inciting antigens could be viruses, infectious agents from arthropods, or altered collagen or elastic fibers causing immune complex-mediated vasculitis and/or a delayed type hypersensitivity (DTH) reaction. There is support histologically for a type IV reaction (DTH), though an initiating antigen

remains to be identified. Some delayed type hypersensitivity reactions such as reactions to intradermally injected bovine collagen, display histology similar to that of GA. Furthermore treatment with medications such cyclosporine, a drug whose primary action is to block production of lymphokines such as IL-2 by activated helper T cells, as well as the photosensitizing compounds in 5-aminolevulinic acid that preferentially accumulate and cause apoptosis in activated T cells, have both proven effective causing resolution of lesions in some patients.[41,42] It is theorized that Th-1 cells, a subset of helper T cells known to interact with macrophages to yield DTH reactions, are necessary to form lesions of GA, just as an individual must have a sufficiently capable cell-mediated immunity to produce a positive skin reaction to the tuberculin test (also a form of DTH). If this is the case, then immunocompromised individuals such as HIV patients should theoretically only be able to form GA lesions in the early stages of their disease while they still retain enough viable Th-1 cells. However, GA lesions have been seen in some patients with AIDS.

Another theory is that granuloma formation may be independent of T cells,[43] and may rather reflect a poorly regulated cell-mediated axis with abnormal release and activity of related cytokines. Abnormal activity of tissue monocytes causes cutaneous granulomas via the secretion of IL-1 and TNF-α in athymic mice,[44] and similar alterations could contribute to the development of GA in humans. Furthermore, IFN-γ from Th-1 lymphocytes activates macrophages to secrete TNF-α and metalloproteinases that cause matrix degradation.[45] Cyclosporine may exert its action by inhibiting the production of these cytokines.[41] Resident tissue macrophages may also contribute to granuloma formation via secretion of lysozomal enzymes that cause collagen degeneration, and by the release of cytokines that activate fibroblasts to increase production of type III procollagen and fribronectin routinely found in GA lesions.

Thus, the concept of GA arising secondary to immune dysregulation is more consistent with the observation that GA lesions occur with greater frequency in patients in advanced stages of AIDS

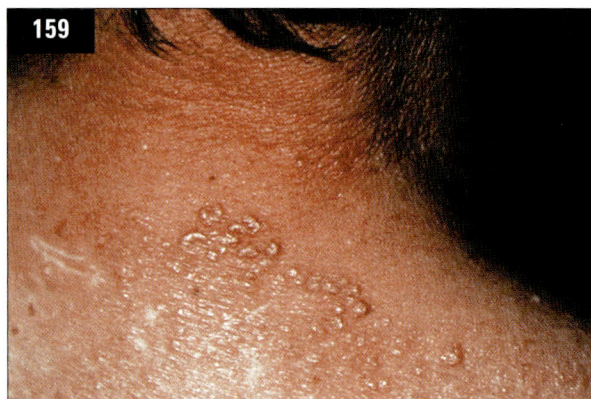

159 Granuloma annulare.

immunocompetent individuals. However, as noted above, the distribution may be more widespread (**159**). While lesions are typically painless and confined to the extremities, they are sometimes painful in HIV-infected individuals and may appear in unusual locations such as the face, neck, and, in a few cases, even in the mouth. As the face is a sun-exposed site, it is likely that facial lesions are photoinduced.

Most cases of GA are seen in children and young adults under the age of 30, and it is twice as common in females as in males. However, this demographic differs in the HIV-infected population as the mean age of onset is approximately 40 years of age and males are more commonly affected. Thus, in contrast to CAD where HIV-related disease occurs at an abnormally low age of onset, GA develops later in life in HIV-infected patients.

as well as in those with autoimmune diseases. The photodistributed nature of GA lesions in HIV patients, who exhibit heightened sensitivity to UVB light upon phototesting, may be a form of hypersensitivity due to some self-antigen altered by UV light and/or cell-mediated immune dysregulation.

GA has been observed in identical twins, siblings, and across generations in the same family, suggesting a genetic component. Generalized GA is found more frequently in individuals with HLA phenotypes BW35 and A29.

CLINICAL FEATURES

The classical picture of GA is that of a child or young adult with skin-colored, erythematous, or violaceous plaques or dome-shaped papules arranged into either a complete ring or half-circle on the extensor surface of an extremity, such as the dorsal surface of the hand or foot. Other forms include generalized, perforating, macular-atrophic, and subcutaneous types. Healthy individuals with GA typically have a localized form with over 50% having only one lesion. In cases with multiple lesions, the distribution may be either generalized or localized or, in rare cases, in a photodistributed pattern. It is typically asymptomatic and the epidermal surface is intact except in the perforating forms where there is often focal crusting.

The morphology of individual GA lesions in HIV-infected patients is often the same as those in

HISTOPATHOLOGY

Aside from certain HIV-associated findings, such as the coexistence of KS in occasional biopsy specimens, the histology of GA lesions in HIV patients is virtually identical to that seen in immunocompetent patients.[46] Microscopic examination of biopsy specimens typically shows a normal epidermis with a diffuse infiltrate of histiocytes in the dermis, with deposition of mucin and focal degeneration of collagen demonstrating the palisaded granulomatous pattern. There is also usually an infiltrate of lymphocytes around superficial blood vessels. Another pattern consists of a diffuse infiltrate of histiocytes between and among collagen with poorly formed palisaded granulomas, the interstitial pattern. Dermal mucin deposition can be observed as a grayish-blue substance with hematoxylin and eosin stain and can be highlighted with the Alcian blue stain. Multinucleated histiocytes may be prominent in some lesions and in some cases, there may be scattered eosinophils and plasma cells.[46]

Some cases may demonstrate subcutaneous involvement, the so-called 'pseudorheumatoid' nodule. This form is most commonly seen near tendons in children. Rarely, lesions may show features of vasculopathy or abundant extravascular neutrophils and such patients are more likely to have underlying systemic disease.

When evaluating biopsy specimens of GA lesions from sun-exposed areas in particular, it is important to search for other features of HIV-associated photodermatoses including necrotic keratinocytes, spongiosis, exocytosis, and vacuolar or lichenoid interface changes as there may be overlap among these conditions.[47]

DIAGNOSIS

In all forms of GA, the diagnosis hinges on clinical features coupled with histologic evaluation. As the clinical picture of HIV-related dermatoses including GA tends to be unusual, and because HIV-infected patients may suffer from various bacterial, viral, and fungal infections that can present clinically and histologically similar to GA, biopsy is often necessary to ensure accurate diagnosis and to exclude infectious causes.

GA may be mistaken for cutaneous manifestations of rheumatoid arthritis (RA), especially when nodules appear around the joints. RA may be excluded by the lack of detection of rheumatoid factor in the serum, and the lack of clinical features of arthritis. Rheumatoid nodules tend to be larger and more deeply situated in the skin than lesions of subcutaneous GA, although this is not always the case.

The differential diagnosis of HIV-associated GA includes many different conditions including a number of infections, granulomatous lymphoproliferative disorders, granulomatous drug reactions, lichenoid and granulomatous dermatitis of AIDS (LGDA), and KS.[46] Distinguishing GA from KS microscopically is important and in some cases may be challenging as they may be present simultaneously, and may appear similar as both demonstrate an increased number of ovoid and spindle cells between collagen bundles in the reticular dermis. They can be differentiated on the basis of architectural and cytologic components; in KS, the increase in spindle cells is pronounced around adnexal structures and pre-existing blood vessels. There are also slit-like vascular spaces around vascular structures and between and among reticular collagen bundles. Additionally plasma cells are commonly seen in the perivascular infiltrate while none of these features are present in GA lesions.[46]

As many infectious pathogens may elicit granulomatous responses and cause infections in HIV-infected individuals, it is important to differentiate HIV-induced GA from infectious conditions which are usually distinct, demonstrating features such as tubercles of epithelioid histiocytes, foamy histiocytes, plasma cells, caseating necrosis, or neutrophilic abscesses.[46] The absence of spirochetes, mycobacteria, spores, and hyphae with special stains such as the Warthin–Starry silver, Fite, and Gomori methenamine silver (GMS) helps to confirm the diagnosis.[46] While postviral granulomatous reactions may resemble HIV-associated GA, they are distinct in that those due to herpes simplex and varicella zoster are generally confined to areas of past viral infection and contain viral DNA, while those of chronic EBV infections are marked by neutrophils and lack the mucin and collagen changes seen with GA.[46]

Granulomatous reactions may also develop in several different lymphoproliferative disorders and these should also be excluded. These include granulomatous mycosis fungoides, granulomatous slack skin syndrome, and angiocentric lymphomas such as lymphomatoid granulomatosis, natural killer/T cell lymphoma, and angiocentric T cell lymphoma. HIV-associated GA lacks the architectural and cytologic features seen in these conditions. In mycosis fungoides, there is a band-like infiltrate of lymphoid cells and histiocytes with cytologic atypia, epidermotropism, and fibrosis of the papillary dermis. In granulomatous slack skin syndrome, there are large histiocytes with multiple nuclei, many of which may have engulfed atypical lymphocytes. Angiocentric lymphomas demonstrate atypical lymphocytes within the walls of affected blood vessels.[48]

A few other conditions may also simulate GA such as interstitial granulomatous drug reactions (IGDRs) and LGDA. Both may demonstrate an interstitial infiltrate of histiocytes, and LGDA may have a distribution quite similar to that of disseminated GA. IGDR differs from GA as it is manifest as violaceous plaques mostly in intertriginous zones and the medial portions of thighs and arms. Histologically, it may demonstrate interface change as well as the interstitial granulomatous infiltrate.[49] LGDA papules are more lichenoid and superficial in nature and biopsy specimens show a lichenoid lymphohistiocytic infiltrate without mucin deposition.[50,51]

MANAGEMENT

GA is difficult to treat in all patients and even more so in HIV-infected patients who often manifest generalized and atypical forms. First-line treatment is typically administration of topical and intralesional steroids which may result in either minimal improvement or complete resolution. Skin atrophy is a common side-effect.[42] Rarely, postinflammatory hyperpigmentation may supervene. In some patients addition of zidovudine to steroid regimens may augment resolution by improvement of the immune status. Addition of dapsone may also be beneficial and it has the added benefit of prophylaxis for *Pneumocystis carinii* pneumonia.

In severe, refractory cases, treatment with cyclosporin as monotherapy is also effective and has led to complete resolution in some patients.[41] While the drug should not be given to patients with renal failure or hypertension, it is generally well tolerated. Blood pressure and serum creatinine levels should be monitored throughout the course of treatment, which on average is approximately 3 months. Cyclosporine acts to suppress cell-mediated immunity by inhibiting the production of IL-2 from activated T cells as well as IL-1 and TNF-α.[41] It may seem counterintuitive and of concern to use an immunosuppressant medication in patients with HIV infection; however, cyclosporin is effective and has been associated with few side-effects. Nevertheless, it should be used with extreme caution in HIV-infected patients.

The treatment regimen of cyclosporin begins with a dose of 3 mg/kg body weight per day for the first month during which time most lesions gradually flatten and disappear. It is then tapered over the course of 2 additional months and then discontinued.[41] Lower dosages may be required if the microemulsion form of the drug is used, likely due to increased bioavailability.[41]

Photodynamic therapy (PTD) for the treatment of GA has also been used in some cases. Treatments are administered with a light emitting diode of 630 ± 5 nm at an intensity of 100 mW/cm^2 and a dose of 120 J/cm^2, with 5-aminolevulinic acid administered as a 20% topical ointment applied 5 hours prior to irradiation weekly. Lesions flatten and decrease in size with each treatment over 4 weeks with a cumulative dose 480 J/cm^2. A slight burning sensation during treatment is the only side-effect that has been reported, and this subsides shortly afterward. This treatment causes accumulation of the active photosensitizing agent protoporphyrin IX in lymphocytes which, when activated by light of the appropriate wavelength, generates free radicals such as singlet oxygen, thereby blocking T cell proliferation.[52–55] Although it has been used mainly in the treatment of nonmelanoma skin cancer, it is being used more frequently in inflammatory and proliferative skin conditions such as psoriasis and GA.[42]

Topical application of 5% imiquimod cream has also been used in the treatment of GA. It acts by binding to Toll-like receptors on monocytes, macrophages, and dendritic cells, inducing secretion of proinflammatory cytokines. It exerts an apoptotic effect on tumor cells in addition to exerting antiviral activity. While its role in the treatment of GA has not been well established, it may dampen the delayed type hypersensitivity reaction which is thought to lead to GA lesions.[45]

Other approaches to treatment have included isotretinoin (40 mg daily for 4 months),[56] PUVA, intralesional IFN-γ therapy,[57] topical tacrolimus,[58] TNF-α inhibitors such as infliximab,[59] dapsone, alkylating agents, and antimalarial drugs such as hydroxychloroquine. It remains to be seen, however, whether the efficacy of these treatments will be supported in large-scale studies. Cryotherapy with liquid nitrogen may clear lesions in some cases; however, it induces hypopigmentation.

CHAPTER 12
CUTANEOUS NEOPLASTIC MANIFESTATIONS OF HIV DISEASE

Cindy Berthelot and Clay J. Cockerell

KAPOSI'S SARCOMA

DEFINITION/OVERVIEW

Kaposi's sarcoma (KS) is the most frequent neoplastic disorder encountered in human immun-odeficiency virus (HIV)-infected patients, and was first described by Moritz Kaposi in 1872 as 'idio-pathic, multiple, pigment sarcoma'.[1] KS was considered to be a relatively rare, slow-growing malignancy, most commonly seen in middle-aged and elderly men. However, this changed in 1981, with Alvin Friedman-Kein's report of what eventually proved to be HIV-associated (epidemic) KS.[1,2] This report described more than 50 previously healthy, young homosexual men with KS involving the lymph nodes, viscera, mucosa, and skin.[2] Concurrent life-threatening opportunistic infections were associated with profound immunosuppression, a syndrome now recognized as acquired immunodeficiency syndrome (AIDS). While the different KS subtypes run different clinical courses, what remains constant are the phenotypic features of the proliferating vascular elements (*Table 10*).

KS is a hallmark of AIDS and in the setting of HIV infection is considered an AIDS-defining condition in the US Center of Disease Control Guidelines. The incidence of patients with AIDS presenting with KS fell dramatically from 40% of cases in 1981 to less than 20% in 1992, and its overall incidence in all AIDS patients has also fallen dramatically.[3]

Table 10 Kaposi's sarcoma variants

VARIANT	GROUPS AT RISK	MEDIAN SURVIVAL
Classic	Elderly men of eastern European or Mediterranean origin	Years to decades
Endemic	African children and adults	Months to years
Immunosuppression	Organ transplant recipients	Months to years
Epidemic	AIDS-associated, especially homosexual or bisexual men	Weeks to months

This trend has been attributed to the introduction of highly active antiretroviral therapy (HAART), safer sexual practices in the homosexual community, and changes in sexual behavior (use of condoms and avoidance of certain high-risk sexual activities).[4] KS is rare in women, intravenous drug users, hemophiliacs, recipients of blood transfusion, and children born to HIV-positive mothers. In contrast, in some regions of Africa, the incidence of KS in women is much greater, and is responsible for up to 40% of the total number of HIV-related KS.[5] In addition to homosexual men, KS has also been reported in a group of homosexual men without AIDS, and these patients tend to have a more indolent course of disease.[6]

PATHOGENESIS/PATHOPHYSIOLOGY

The discovery of human herpesvirus-8 (HHV-8) in all KS variants and the increased frequency of KS in men who have intercourse with men suggested an infectious etiology of KS. After identification of HHV-8, various cytokines and molecular mechanisms have been identified as to how this agent initiates and sustains KS growth and proliferation. As such, it is no longer considered a true neoplasm by most experts and is thought to represent a diffuse vascular proliferation.

The search for an infectious agent was initiated by Giraldo and coworkers who observed herpes-like particles in cell cultures from classic and endemic KS.[7] They also found a serologic association between cytomegalovirus (CMV) and classic endemic KS. During the outbreak of the AIDS epidemic and the increase in KS patients, isolated reports appeared that suggested *Mycoplasma penetrans*, hepatitis B virus, and human papilloma virus (HPV) as possible causal agents of KS.[8] In 1994, Chang *et al.* identified deoxyribonucleic acid (DNA) sequences in AIDS-KS coding for amino acids that shared striking homology (30–50%) with two oncogenic gamma-herpesviruses: herpesvirus saimiri and Epstein–Barr virus (EBV).[9] These findings suggested that a new herpesvirus, designated as human herpesvirus type 8 (HHV-8) or KS-associated herpesvirus (KSHV) could possibly be the causative agent of KS. In addition, it is the only virus of the genus Rhadinovirus known to infect human beings.

Infections with HHV-8 is ubiquitous, occurring in infancy or childhood, with 70–90% of patients with KS having positive serologic studies.[10,11] In most patients with KS and AIDS, seroconversion from negative to positive antibodies against KSHV-related nuclear antigens occurs before the clinical appearance of KS.[11] There are three general modes of transmission of HHV-8: vertical, casual, and sexual. In KS patients, HHV-8 is frequently detectable in saliva and nasal secretions, and only rarely in semen and cervicovaginal fluid.[12] In HIV-positive homosexual men, viral shedding of HHV-8 occurs mostly in the oral mucosa. HHV-8 may replicate in the oropharynx and salivary contact could contribute to KSHV transmission, whether from sexual exposure or nonsexual contact (close contacts among families, siblings, mother and child).[12]

The 165 kb HHV-8 genome was sequenced within 2 years after its discovery, providing clues about the way the virus may induce uncontrolled cellular proliferation.[13] HHV-8 encodes proteins that are homologous to human oncoproteins, including a cyclin that controls the G1 to S-phase of cell growth.[14] In addition, other regulatory proteins include a G-protein coupled receptor, an inhibitor of apoptosis mediated by Fas-associated death domain-like interleukin-1β-converting enzyme (FLICE) pathway, a constitutively activated immunoreceptor, and an inhibitor of the IFN signaling pathway.[15–17] HHV-8 also encodes interleukin-6 (IL-6) and chemokines that affect the replication and migration of uninfected cells. The viral cytokine IL-6 induces B cell proliferation, whereas the chemokines may activate angiogenesis and inhibit immune type 1 helper T cell responses.[18]

HHV-8 has been identified in peripheral blood mononuclear cells in more than 50% of AIDS patients.[19,20] Moreover, the detection of HHV-8 may precede the onset of KS lesions by months, therefore strengthening the hypothesis that it represents the causative agent of KS. Currently, four HHV-8 subtypes, designated A–D, have been identified, and each has a close association with the geographic and ethnic background of the infected individual.[21] Molecular studies have localized HHV-8 in cells surrounding slit-like vessels and in greater than 90% of spindle cells, but not in normal vascular endothelium. Immunomorphologic studies that used monoclonal antibodies against the major viral latency-associated nuclear antigen (LANA-1) have corroborated these findings, showing expression of LANA-1 in almost all HHV-8 infected cells.[22] During the evolution of KS lesions from patch to nodular stage, there is progressive increase in spindle cells that contain LANA-1.

Several factors required for growth and stimulation of KS cell proliferation have been recognized. All patients with KS, independent of their HIV status, are infected with HHV-8, and the virus is present in all subtypes of KS.[23] Persistence of HHV-8 antibodies indicates that continuous antigen stimulation is occurring, suggesting the virus may be present in a latent form of replication.[24] One report showed the time from seroconversion in HIV-positive individuals to overt KS may be as long as 15 years (median 63.5 months), with a higher incidence of KS when HIV was acquired before HHV-8.[25] There is also evidence supporting the association of KS with promiscuous sexual behavior.[4] Epidemiologic data show a higher rate of HHV-8 seropositivity in patients who acquired HIV via sexual contacts than compared to people who acquired HIV through blood products.[26]

Several studies indicate HIV gene products and chronic immune stimulation caused by the release of inflammatory cytokines may contribute to the pathogenesis of KS. KS cells express receptors for several proinflammatory cytokines including intercellular adhesion molecule (ICAM-1), platelet activating factor, monocyte chemotactic protein, IL-6, and IL-8. Inflammatory cells attracted to the affected area stimulate growth through the secretion of oncostatin-M, IL-1, tumor necrosis factor (TNF)-α, IFN-γ, and granulocyte macrophage colony-stimulating factor. Receptors for endothelial cell mitogens such as platelet-derived growth factor (PDGF)-β and IL-1 are also expressed on KS cells.[27] HHV-8 encodes several factors also shown to promote KS cell growth, including viral IL-6, viral interferon regulatory factor (vIRF), and v-cyclin.[28] Other factors inhibit KS cell apoptosis, for example, vFLIP, LANA, vBcl-2, K15/LAMP, and vIRF.

Studies have also suggested that HIV-gene products may contribute to the pathogenesis of KS. This was first demonstrated when male, HIV-tat transgenic mice developed KS-like skin lesions.[29] As the tat-expression in these mice was confined mostly to the epidermis, it is possible that spread to the dermis may provide appropriate mitogenic stimulation required for the progression of KS lesions.[30]

In summary, data suggest that HHV-8 is exogenously acquired and subsequently enters a latent phase of infection. The virus is activated as a consequence of immunosuppression or other mechanisms, and provides activation and transcription of HHV-8 genes. Infection with HHV-8 causes cytokine production, proteins that stimulate inflammation and cell proliferation, and other proteins that inhibit apoptosis production. Inflammatory cells attracted by HHV-8 gene products provide additional support for the proliferation of KS cells, increasing the release of tumor-promoting mediators.

CLINICAL FEATURES

HIV-associated KS displays a variety of distinct clinical features which often differ from other forms of KS (160–163). Early lesions appear as violaceous or sometimes even yellowish-green ecchymotic macules and patches that may simulate trauma, insect bite reactions, or dermatofibromas.[31] In time, these enlarge or become confluent forming papules, plaques, nodules and tumors that are violaceous, red, pink, tan, and eventually, brown-purple. Lesions may initially occur at sites of trauma such as venipuncture sites, contusions, or cutaneous abscesses.[32] Lesions are usually unilateral at the onset of disease and usually progress to become bilateral over time. A disseminated multifocal centripetal pattern may develop as the disease progresses. Initial lesions of KS frequently develop on the face, especially the tip of the nose, periorbital areas, scalp, and ears.[33] Lesions on the trunk also appear early and are usually widespread, typically arranged parallel to skin tension lines. Patients with KS may have lesions on the legs and feet, and as these lesions age, they may

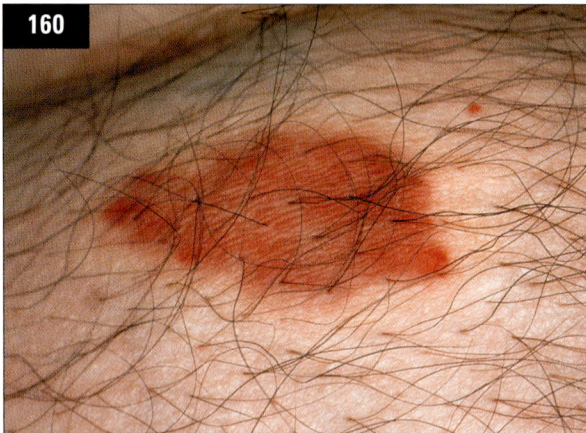

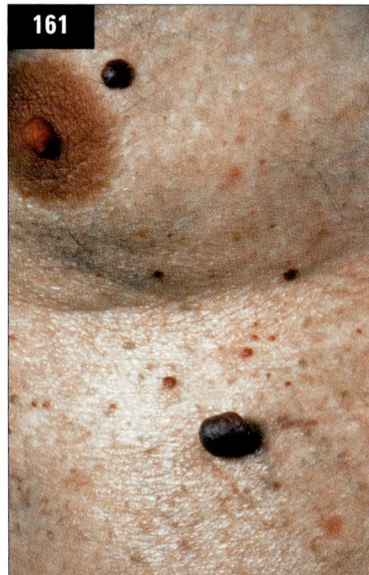

160 Kaposi's sarcoma. Early lesion presenting as a yellow-red plaque on the trunk.

161 Kaposi's sarcoma. Violaceous papules and nodules resembling angiomas.

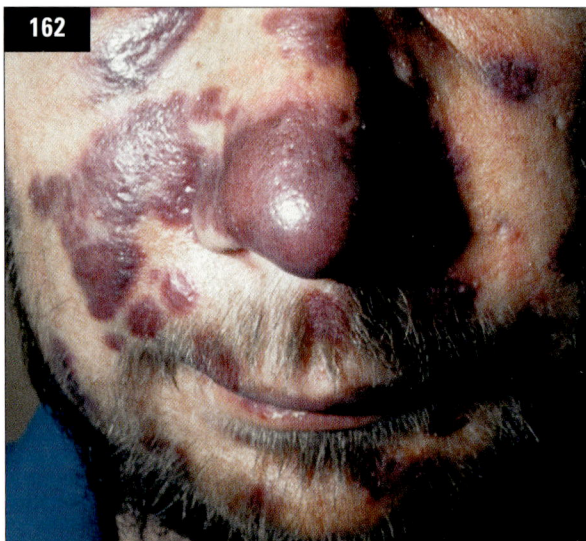

162 Extensive violaceous nodules and papules coalescing into plaques on the face in an AIDS patient with KS.

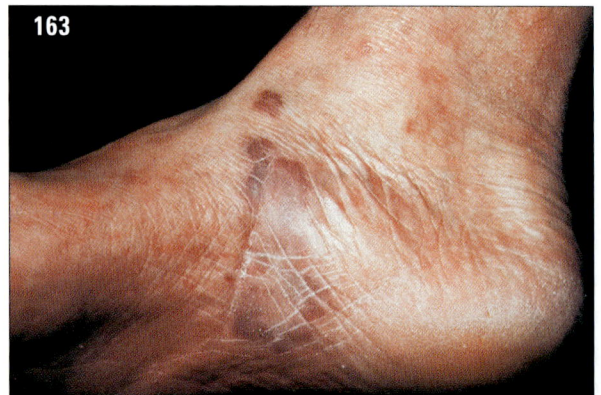

163 Kaposi's sarcoma. Violaceous plaque on the medial foot.

erode, ulcerate, or display a verrucous or hyper-keratotic surface. While early lesions may be somewhat soft or rubbery to the touch, older lesions are firm and may display a greenish hemosiderin halo. KS may also demonstrate crusting and spongiotic features in the epidermis, especially if edema and stasis changes are present. Lymphedema of the involved areas may be present and is secondary to confluent lesions involving lymphatics and lymph nodes.[34] Edema may be pronounced on the lower extremities and can involve the entire lower leg, genitalia, and face.[35] Initially the edema is pitting, although it often evolves to a brawny, firm nonpitting edema over time. Internal organ involvement is common and, as a general rule, one internal lesion develops for every five skin lesions.[36]

In addition to cutaneous lesions, KS may develop on mucous membranes, especially the oral cavity. Oral involvement with KS is often a marker for CD4+ T cell counts of <200 × 10⁶/l.[37] Intraoral lesions are most frequently located on the hard palate (50% of patients), appearing first as a violaceous stain, which evolves into papules and nodules with a cobblestone appearance. KS can also arise on the soft palate, uvula, pharynx, gingiva, and tongue. These lesions may cause considerable discomfort, respiratory distress, and may interfere with eating and speech.

Extracutaneous KS is also frequently encountered in the lymph nodes, gastrointestinal tract, and lungs. Gastrointestinal involvement is found in up to 80% of AIDS patients, especially those with extensive cutaneous involvement.[38] Although rare, gastro-intestinal KS can occur in the absence of cutaneous disease.[38] Lesions are most commonly located in the stomach and duodenum which can cause nausea, ulceration and perforation, bleeding, protein-losing enteropathy, and ileus. Pulmonary KS, reported in 20–50% of patients, may clinically cause symptoms such as bronchospasm, coughing, and respiratory insufficiency and is often mistaken for an oppor-tunistic infection. Radiologic findings include nodular, interstitial, or alveolar infiltrates. Isolated pulmonary nodules, pleural effusions, as well as hilar or mediastinal lymphadenopathy are often found. Bronchoscopy with bronchoalveolar lavage is the most appropriate tool to diagnose pulmonary KS.

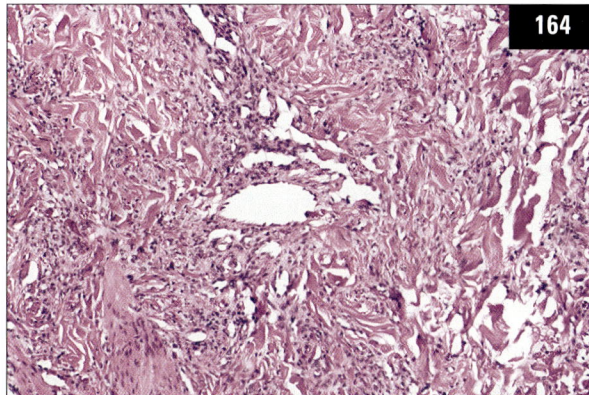

164 Histology of plaque stage Kaposi's sarcoma. Multiple irregular, slit-like vascular spaces and a spindle cell proliferation extending diffusely between dermal collagen bundles.

HISTOPATHOLOGY

The histopathologic findings in KS vary with the stage of the lesion in question. Early patch lesions are manifested as proliferations of spindle-shaped endo-thelial cells surrounding normal pre-existing blood vessels, forming small jagged vascular slits that may be subtle and difficult to recognize. Scattered sidero-phages, extravasated red blood cells, and a few plasma cells may be noted. Plaque stage lesions are characterized by a more diffuse interstitial pro-liferation with spindle cells expanding throughout dermal collagen bundles (**164**). There is a pro-liferation of jagged, irregular, slit-like spaces forming irregular, cleft-like, angulated vascular channels containing red blood cells, hemosiderin deposition in the dermis, and an infiltrate of plasma cells. Small, pink, hyaline globules representing breakdown products of erythrocytes are characteristically seen. Nodules and tumors appear as diffuse sheets and fascicles of spindle-shaped cells with mild-to-moderate cytologic atypia, single cell necrosis, and mitoses. Small vascular slits and extravasated erythrocytes may be observed. Resolved KS appears as a diffuse infiltrate of siderophages with few residual vascular slits. Immunoperoxidase studies are often positive for vascular-associated antigens such as Factor VIII and *Ulex europaeus*; however, staining with these markers is often variable.[39] CD31, Factor XIIIa, and vimentin are also variably positive.[40] HHV-8 staining is positive.

DIAGNOSIS

Diagnosis is generally based on the finding of violaceous skin lesions in the appropriate clinical setting in conjunction with histologic findings. A skin biopsy is usually used for confirmation of KS. In children and women, the diagnosis of HIV-related KS should be considered carefully as the neoplasm occurs only rarely in these patients.

A number of different cutaneous disorders, both inflammatory and neoplastic, may be easily be mistaken for KS. Purpura, hematomas, hemangiomata, angiomas, dermatofibroma, lichen planus, pityriasis rosea, mycosis fungoides, nevi, malignant melanoma, cutaneous lymphoma, secondary syphilis, and bacillary angiomatosis have all been reported as clinical simulators of KS.[41] Histologically, simulators include microvenular hemangioma, targetoid hemosiderotic hemangioma, proliferative angiomata, severe stasis dermatitis, granuloma annulare, and dermatofibroma. Clinical correlation and/or stains are often required to render an unequivocal diagnosis.

MANAGEMENT

Recent advances in the elucidation of the pathogenesis of KS continue to uncover potential targets for therapies (*Table 11*). Such targets include HHV-8 as well as the processes of angiogenesis and cellular differentiation. Although a number of advances in the treatment of KS have been achieved over the past few years, a gold standard therapy for KS has not yet been defined and treatment must be tailored to individual needs.[42] Since the availability of HAART, there has been both a decreased proportion of new AIDS-defining KS cases and a regression in the size and number of existing KS lesions, making HAART an essential treatment for KS. However, in patients

---

Table 11 Treatment options for Kaposi's sarcoma

Local treatment	Liquid nitrogen
	Radiation
	Electron beam
	Photodynamic therapy
	Intralesional vinca alkaloids
	Intralesional interferon
	Topical 9-cis retinoic acid (alitretinoin)
Systemic treatment	Antiviral therapy
	Liposomal doxyrubicin/daunorubicin
	Paclitaxel
	Vinca alkaloids
	Bleomycin
	Interferon-alpha
	Thalidomide
	Systemic retinoids
	Human chorionic gonadotropin

with more severe cases of KS, including those with visceral involvement and life-threatening KS, chemotherapy, radiotherapy, and immunotherapy should be considered. Newer cytotoxic agents including liposomal anthracyclines and paclitaxel are highly effective, and have been approved by the US Food and Drug Administration (FDA) as first- and second-line agents for advanced KS.[43,44] Furthermore, a greater understanding of the pathogenesis of KS has led to the development of experimental agents.

Local treatment

There are several options for local approaches, indicated for cosmetically troublesome lesions that are small and thin. Local modalities for treating KS include local radiation therapy, cryosurgery, laser surgery, excisional surgery, and electrocauterization. Radiotherapy has become the most important therapy in the local treatment of KS.[45] Fractioned focal X-ray therapy in doses up to 40 Gy produces higher response rate and control of cutaneous KS than a single treatment of 8 Gy.[45] Intralesional injections of vinblastine, vincristine, and interferon-alpha (INF-α) have been reported to be effective local treatments.[46,47] Other local treatment options include electron beam photodynamic therapy, topical 9-cis retinoic acid gel (alitretinoin), and liquid nitrogen.

Systemic chemotherapy

Chemotherapy, although not curative, can result in rapid tumor regression and palliation of symptoms. It is typically reserved for the treatment of pulmonary KS, symptomatic visceral disease, KS-related symptoms, and rapidly progressive cutaneous lesions. The most active cytotoxic agents include vinblastine, vincristine, bleomycin, etoposide, liposomal and nonliposomal anthracyclines (doxorubicin and daunorubicin), and paclitaxel.[48–50]

Single agent chemotherapy has been largely used in the past decade with good overall clinical response. However, toxicity often limited therapy and relapses occurred shortly after treatment ended. Combination therapy with low-dose bleomycin (10 mg/m^2), vincristine (1.4 mg/m^2), plus doxorubicin (20 mg/m^2) given every 2–3 weeks, was previously considered the standard treatment for advanced KS.[51] This regimen produced a complete and partial tumor remission rate of 88% with manageable toxicity and a clear superiority over doxorubicin monotherapy. Subsequent trials of the same regimen failed to reproduce these results and this combination has largely been replaced by newer drugs.[52]

In aggressive KS, liposomal daunorubicin and liposomal doxorubicin, two liposome-encapsulated anthracyclines, are first-line chemotherapeutics. The most common toxicities associated with liposomal anthracyclines are bone marrow suppression and hand–foot syndrome, whereas alopecia and cardiac toxicity appeared to be limited.[53] Paclitaxel, recently recognized as an active agent for the treatment of relapsed AIDS-related KS, has a response rate of 59–71%. It exerts its effects by formation of stable bundles of microtubules, thereby interfering with the normal function of cellular microtubules.[54–56]

Biological response modifiers

INF-α has been shown to produce a response in 20–40% of AIDS-KS patients.[57] INF-α is especially beneficial in those with disease limited to the skin and with lymphocyte count >400 × 10^6/l. IFN-α-induced tumor regression has also been associated with suppression of HIV, as measured by serum p24 antigen concentrations and peripheral blood virus cultures.[57] Recent clinical trials have reported a synergistic effect between IFN and zidovudine (AZT) with respect to anti-KS activity.[57–59] Major dose-limiting toxicities were AZT-related neutropenia and IFN-related hepatotoxicity.

Pathogenesis-based treatments

The critical role of angiogenesis and viral and host cytokines in the pathogenesis of KS have led to the identification of a variety of potential targets for KS therapy. Studies have demonstrated that a metabolite of thalidomide has an antiangiogenic activity by inhibition of basic fibroblastic growth factor (b-FGF)-induced vascular proliferation, TNF-α production, intercellular adhesion, basement membrane formation, and vascular maturation.[60] A study of oral thalidomide in 20 AIDS-KS patients showed partial response in 8 of 17 (47%) patients, with a median duration of 7 months.[61] The angiogenesis inhibitor TNP-470 is a semisynthetic fumagillin analog that inhibits *in vitro* b-FGF-induced spindle cell proliferation. In a study of 38 patients with diffuse mucocutaneous KS lesions treated with weekly intravenous dose of TNP-470, the drug was well tolerated and it induced partial remissions in 18% of patients.[62] However, the duration of response (median 11 weeks) and unpredictable adverse effects (neutropenia, hemorrhage, and urticaria) has limited its use in KS treatment.

Tecogalan is a sulfated polysaccharide isolated from the cell membrane of a bacterium, *Arthrobacter* species AT-25. It has been shown to inhibit the growth of KS-derived spindle cells *in vitro* and KS cell-induced capillary permeability in the murine model.[63,64] Several studies were conducted in patients with AIDS-KS using various dosing schedules, showing clinical improvement and a reduction of tumor-associated edema. However, no objective responses were observed.[64–66] IM-862 is a dipeptide of L-glutamiyl-L-tryptophan, initially isolated from the thymus. In animal studies, it has shown antiangiogenic effects by inhibiting production of vascular endothelial growth factor and by activation of natural killer cell function.[67] A randomized phase II study has been conducted in 44 AIDS patients with advanced mucocutaneous KS; a significant response was achieved in 36% of patients, lasting a median of 33 weeks.[67] Stable disease was documented in 48% of patients, for a median of 31 weeks. All but five patients during the study were concomitantly treated with protease inhibitors. Despite promising phase I and phase II studies, a phase III trial of IM-862 was not superior to placebo and may accelerate time to progression.[68]

Retinoids

Retinoids are derived from vitamin A, which has been shown to be depleted in some HIV-infected patients. They act by binding to specific nuclear retinoic acid receptors (α, β, γ) and retinoic X receptors (RXRs). The first of the systemic retinoids to be used to treat KS is all-trans-retinoic acid (ATRA; tretinoin). Other retinoids used *in vitro* and in human clinical studies include 13-cis-retinoic acid (isotretinoin) and 9-cis-retinoic acid (alitretinoin). ATRA induces objective responses in patients with

AIDS-KS and may block angiogenesis and proliferation of KS cell lines *in vitro*.[69] In a study of 27 patients with mucocutaneous, nonvisceral AIDS-KS receiving ATRA, partial response was observed in 17% of patients after a median time of 22 weeks.[70] Adverse effects consisted of transient mild to moderate headaches, mild to moderate xerosis, cheilitis, and nausea and vomiting. Hematologic toxicities included hypertriglyceridemia, anemia, and neutropenia. In a second study of 20 HIV-positive patients with low-risk KS treated with ATRA, partial response was observed in eight patients with a median response time of 56 days.[71] The duration of the response was 332 days. The main toxicities observed included cheilitis, headaches, and xerosis.

Nine-cis-retinoic acid, or alitretinoin, has been evaluated both systemically and topically. In one study. A significant response was observed in 37% of patients treated with oral 9-cis-retinoic acid.[72] Tumor response was associated with improved quality-of-life measures. The most common side-effects included headache, fatigue, alopecia, xerosis, and hypertriglyceridemia. Topical 0.1% alitretinoin gel was approved by the FDA in 1999 for the local treatment of KS.[73] It is a valuable option for the treatment of KS both in those with limited cutaneous disease as well as in widespread KS with lesions that persist after chemotherapy.

Matrix metalloproteinase inhibitors

The matrix metalloproteinase (MMP) inhibitors are a family of enzymes localized at the cell surface, and have been shown to play a prominent role in tumor angiogenesis. MMP expression is increased in KS lesions, suggesting its inhibition would be beneficial in treatment of KS.[74,75] One study of MMP inhibitors administered to patients with AIDS-related KS had antitumor activity noted in 44% patients.[76] It was well tolerated, with the most common adverse effect being dose-related photosensitivity.

Hormonal agents

Human chorionic gonadotropin (hCG) is suggested as having a protective effect against intrauterine transmission of KS. Cases of spontaneous regression of KS during pregnancy have been reported and hCG has shown anti-KS activity in several clinical trials. One study showed that hCG given intralesionally induced dose-dependent tumor regression and apoptotic cell death in up to 83% of KS lesions.[77] A subsequent phase I study was conducted using subcutaneous injections of hCG with antitumor response in 33% of cases, lasting from 200 to over 500 days.[78] A third study demonstrated that the urinary hCG beta-subunit, hCG beta-core, and to a lesser extent recombinant hCG, directly inhibit MMPs.[79]

Highly active antiretroviral therapy

Beginning in 1997, several anecdotal reports described regression of KS after the administration of HAART.[80] One retrospective study reported 78 patients who received prior anti-KS treatment such as local chemo/radiotherapy (87% of cases) or systemic chemotherapy (17% of cases) and subsequently received HAART.[81] It was shown to have an additive effect on anti-KS treatment, significantly prolonging the time to treatment failure. In a study of 10 patients with stable or progressive KS, antiviral therapy alone resulted in an 80% clinical regression.[82] The time to achieve complete response ranged between 2 and 14 months. Therapy was associated with both decreased levels of HIV ribonucleic acid (RNA) plasma levels and HHV-8 viremia in the peripheral blood mononuclear cells (PBMCs). HAART-induced clinical response of KS lesions has been confirmed by several additional studies. These findings suggest that the immune restoration induced by HAART is able to control KS effectively. However, another possible mechanism of KS regression induced by HAART is a direct antiviral effect as HIV-tat protein has been shown to promote the growth of KS-derived spindle cells, angiogenesis, and the induction of a cytokines such as IL-6. As such, an effective antiretroviral regimen should be initiated in most, if not all, patients with AIDS-related KS. Treatment of life-threatening, aggressive visceral KS often requires a more complex regimen including chemotherapy, radiotherapy, and immunotherapy, in addition to HAART.[83]

Anti-HHV-8 therapy

The use of antiviral agents with activity against HHV-8 has also been considered a therapeutic option. Data from 935 homosexual men with AIDS show a reduction in the relative risk for the development of KS in 46% and 60% of patients treated with ganciclovir and foscarnet, respectively.[84] These results have been confirmed by a second study which showed a reduction of 61% in the occurrence of KS in patients treated with ganciclovir or foscarnet.[85]

PRIMARY CUTANEOUS NEOPLASMS

DEFINITION/OVERVIEW

The development of epithelial neoplasms in patients infected with HIV is markedly increased, especially in oral and anogenital sites. Neoplasms grow more rapidly and are often more aggressive in patients with HIV than in other groups of patients. Oncogenic factors, including sunlight exposure and HPV-infection, have been associated with the development of skin cancer in these patients, and their growth is compounded in the setting of decreased cellular immunity. Epithelial neoplasms, including basal cell carcinoma (BCC), squamous cell carcinoma (SCC), Bowen's disease, and malignant melanoma in the setting of HIV infection will be discussed.

PATHOGENESIS/PATHOPHYSIOLOGY

In the setting of HIV infection, patients have a 3–5-fold increase risk of developing nonmelanoma skin cancer. In 1984, Slazinski and associates described a patient with AIDS in whom a BCC had developed.[86] Risk factors for BCC and SCC are similar to those for HIV-negative patients: sun exposure, blond hair, blue eyes, fair skin, and family history of skin cancer.[87,88] In one study spanning 36 months, the second most common cancer in 724 HIV-positive patients was BCC (1.8%).[89] In a retrospective review of 166 HIV-positive patients with nonmelanoma skin cancers, 87% of cases were BCC, mostly superficial (67%) and located on the trunk (62%).[88] The pathogenesis of BCC is due to damage to cellular DNA, most often caused by ultraviolet (UV) irradiation. BCC is more frequent in patients who have experienced considerable exposure to sunlight and have a low CD4/CD8 ratio than in those who have had less sunlight exposure and high CD4/CD8 ratios.

Most cases of Bowen's disease (SCC *in situ*) in HIV-positive patients tend to arise in the anogenital area. Bowenoid papulosis refers to SCC *in situ* that develops as a consequence of infections with HPV types 16 and 18, occurring mainly in the genital area.

SCC in HIV-infected patients may occur in the anogenital areas, skin, cervix, oral cavity, and conjunctiva. SCC of the anus is increasing in incidence among homosexual men and is similar in frequency to HPV-associated cervical lesions found in HIV-seropositive women. The increased risk is due to infection with oncogenic strains of HPV in the setting of immunosuppression.[90] Anal intercourse predisposes to condyloma, and the risk increases with the frequency of intercourse. In one study of 116 patients infected with HIV in whom nonmelanoma skin cancers developed, 13% had low-grade SCC, most commonly on the head and neck region.[88] The clinical course of cutaneous SCC in HIV-infected patients is typically progressive, with a higher propensity to metastasize. In another study, five out of 10 patients died of metastatic SCC within 7 years of their initial diagnosis despite treatment.[91] HIV stage and the degree of immunosuppression were not associated with increased morbidity and mortality. Aggressive SCCs in HIV-infected patients present at a younger age and prognosis is poor in these patients, with a 50% mortality rate (between 6 and 84 months). HIV-positive women with persistent HPV cervical infection have an increased risk of SCC of the cervix and have significantly more advanced disease than those not infected with HIV.[92] In oral SCC, HPV may collaborate with other carcinogenic factors, such as tobacco and alcohol.

Epidermodysplasia verruciformis, a premalignant condition associated with HPV infection, has also been observed in some HIV-infected patients. UV light is a major risk factor for the development of carcinoma in patients with this condition.

Melanoma involving HIV-infected patients has also been sporadically observed, with more than 20 reports of melanoma in HIV-infected patients.[93,94] Although no definitive data exist about the relationship between melanoma and HIV, multiple primary and early nodular lesions have been noted. It is unclear whether this finding is the result of increased surveillance, detection, and reporting, or an actual increase of melanoma in these patients. It has been demonstrated that HIV-positive patients with melanoma have a significantly decreased disease-free survival, with no association between

165 Basal cell carcinoma. Erythematous, pearly papule with telangiectasias and central ulceration on the nasal ala.

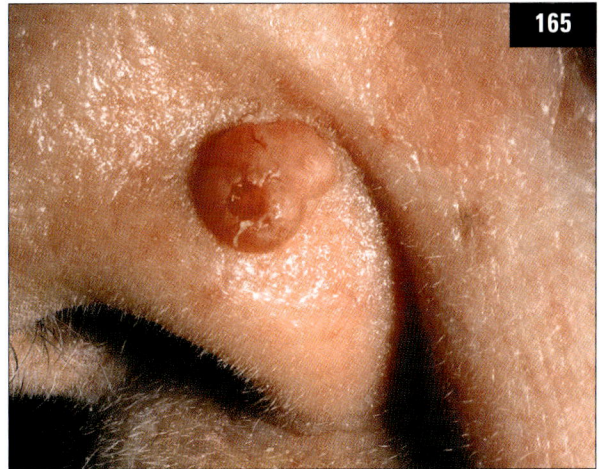

166 Squamous cell carcinoma. Crusted, hyperkeratotic papule on the tip of the nose in a patient with severely sun-damaged skin.

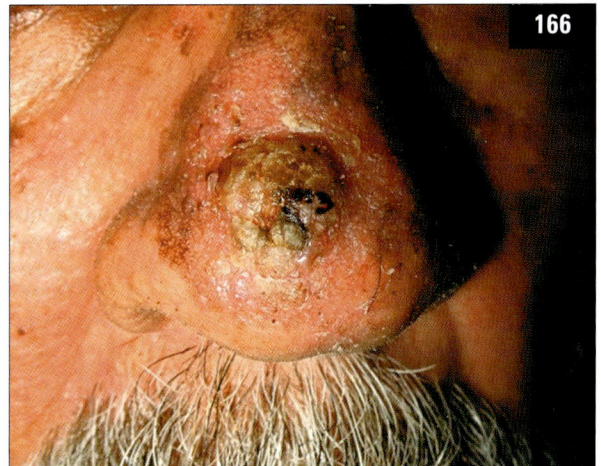

the depth of the melanoma and CD4+ count.[95] However, lower CD4 counts are predictive of a poorer prognosis. The poor prognosis may be attributed to altered host immune responses to the tumor, factors such as systemic illnesses or coexisting skin lesions, which can delay the diagnosis of melanoma in these patients. These patients also have a more aggressive course and are more likely to present with metastasis. One study described seven AIDS patients with no previous history of dsyplastic nevi or family history of melanoma, who noted the sudden appearance of multiple new nevi on the trunk and upper extremities at the same time their AIDS became symptomatic.[96]

CLINICAL FEATURES
BCC and SCC in HIV-positive patients usually have similar clinical appearances to those in immuno-competent hosts although they may develop on nonsun-exposed sites. Clinically, BCCs are typically small, pearly papules or nodules with rolled borders and telangiectatic vessels. They slowly enlarge and may undergo central ulceration (**165**).[97] In rare cases, metastasis of BCC may occur, most likely as a consequence of immunosuppression. Most metastases are to draining lymph nodes and the lungs. SCC lesions may present as erythematous, ulcerated, hyperkeratotic papules or plaques (**166**), or areas of persistent ulceration.

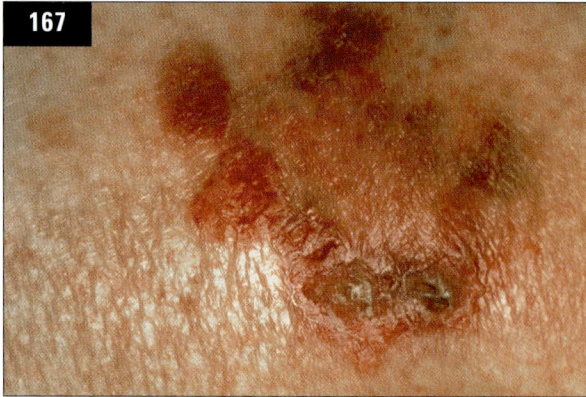

167 Squamous cell carcinoma *in situ* (Bowen's disease). This is a pigmented lesion of Bowen's disease presenting on sun-damaged skin as a hyperpigmented plaque with areas of erythema and crusting.

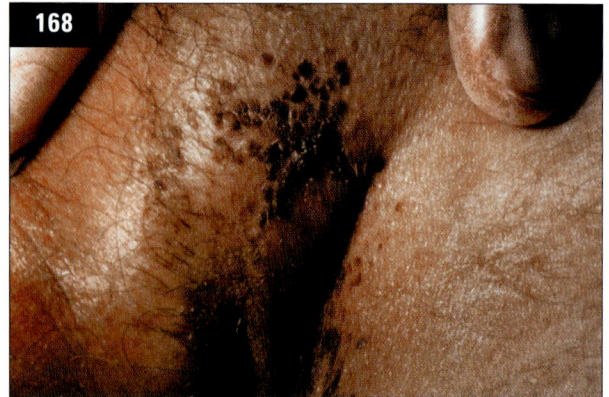

168 Bowenoid papulosis. Hyperpigmented, flat-topped papules on the penile shaft and lateral thigh.

Lesions of Bowen's disease (SCC *in situ*) present as erythematous, sometimes brown, papules or plaques with or without scaling and crusting (**167**). HPV-induced SCC *in situ* (bowenoid papulosis) presents on the labia or penile skin as brown flat-topped papules or plaques (**168**). Epidermodysplasia verruciformis has a clinical appearance of widespread warty pink to erythematous papules. These may simulate widespread warts, erythroderma, or widespread erythematous scaly dermatoses. Melanoma usually presents as an irregularly pigmented macule or papule (**169**), although many of the melanomas described in association with HIV have atypical manifestations, being multiple or metastatic.

HISTOPATHOLOGY

BCC appears histologically as islands of basophilic cells extending from the epidermis into the dermis (**170**) The histopathologic findings of SCC range from subtle atypical intraepithelial proliferations to full thickness involvement of the epithelium. Epithelial rete ridges are expanded and may be replaced by atypical cells, many of which are pleomorphic and in mitosis. As lesions progress, aggregations of neoplastic cells extend into the underlying dermis (**171**). Involvement of deeper soft tissue, nerves, and blood vessels may occur. Lesions are often digitated,

verrucous, and associated with ulceration or necrosis.

Bowen's disease has similar histopathologic features to those seen in HIV-negative patients, namely full thickness keratinocytic atypia with overlying parakeratosis. Bowenoid papulosis similarly exhibits full thickness keratinocytic atypia (**172**) and may have a histologic architecture similar to that of condyloma acuminatum, showing evidence of HPV viral changes. Epidermodysplasia verruciformis is characterized by the presence of koilocytes or a diffuse infiltrate of pale-appearing cells with slate-gray cytoplasm in the epidermis. There is dyskeratosis and there may be characteristic 'corps rond-like' structures in the stratum corneum.

DIAGNOSIS

The diagnosis of all the cutaneous neoplasms is established primarily on the basis of clinical appearance and skin biopsy.

MANAGEMENT

Any neoplasm that develops should be destroyed or excised. Primary prevention with sun avoidance and the use of sunscreen, as well as diligent skin examinations are of great importance in these individuals. After treatment, patients should have regular follow-up visits with careful examination

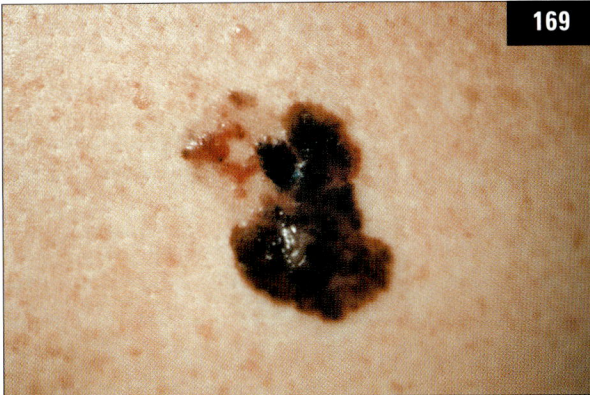

169 Malignant melanoma. Hyperpigmented plaque with irregular border, color variation from light brown to black, and an area of hypopigmentation indicative of regression.

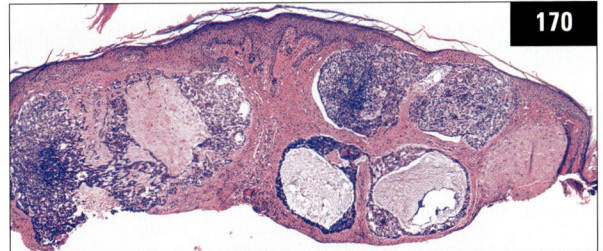

170 Histology of basal cell carcinoma. Multiple islands of basophilic cells extend from the epidermis into the dermis, which shows extensive solar elastosis. There is retraction of the tumor lobules from the surrounding stroma and abundant mucin deposition. x40.

171 Histology of squamous cell carcinoma. Proliferation of atypical keratinocytes with extension into the dermis. Islands of keratinization, pleomorphic cells, and multiple mitotic figures are seen. x200.

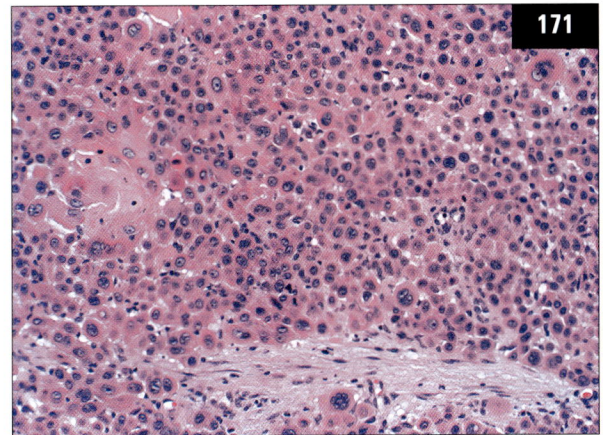

172 Histology of bowenoid papulosis. There is parakeratosis and full thickness keratinocytic atypia with multiple mitotic figures.

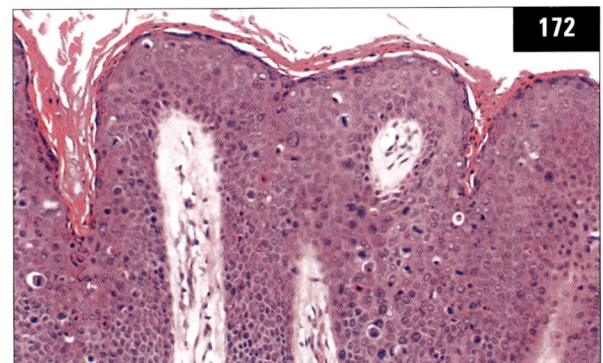

for local reoccurrence and nodal metastasis. Early biopsy of suspicious lesions is imperative. Morbidity and mortality from aggressive SCC in HIV-infected patients is dependent on the initial control of local or metastatic disease.[91] Patients with SCC should undergo resection with control of the margins, and those with high-risk tumors or with an extensive tumor burden should be considered for local or regional adjunctive radiation, chemotherapy, or both. Regardless of CD4+ count, sentinel node biopsies should also be considered. Bowen's disease, although often treated with cryotherapy, or topical 5-fluorouracil or imiquimod in immunocompetent hosts, should be treated surgically with histologic confirmation of removal. Those at risk for the development of anal SCC should be screened for anal dysplasia by Pap smears of the lower rectum, squamocolumnar junction, and anal canal. Persons with abnormal Pap smears should be examined with high-resolution anoscopy and biopsy of visible lesions. Women should also undergo regular cervical Pap smears.

Although there is no evidence that BCCs in HIV-infected patients require more aggressive therapy, there is a higher potential for metastasis. After standard treatment (elecrodesiccation and curettage, surgical resection), the recurrence rate of BCC was 5.4% at 12 months.[95]

There are no standard guidelines of the treatment of primary cutaneous melanoma in HIV-infected individuals. Full skin examinations are recommended yearly for all high-risk patients, namely those with a personal or family history of melanoma, a history of blistering sunburn, and patients with dysplastic nevi. At the time of diagnosis, a search for metastatic disease should be undertaken as melanoma has a more aggressive course in HIV-infected patients. In addition to excision of the melanoma, sentinel node biopsy should be considered, even on thinner melanomas.[98,99] Yearly chest X-rays, routine laboratory tests, including a evaluation of serum lactate dehydrogenase (LDH) levels, and collaboration with an oncologist should be considered. The safety of INF-α-2b has not been studied in this population.

LYMPHORETICULAR MALIGNANCIES

DEFINITION/OVERVIEW

Lymphoma refers to a malignancy of lymphoid cells presenting in the lymph nodes, skin, viscera, or bone marrow. Although likely a manifestation of altered immunity, HIV itself may be a direct cause of AIDS-related lymphoma. HIV induces the expression of a variety of cytokines that are associated with the proliferation, stimulation, and activation of lymphocytes. Most cases of lymphoma in HIV-infected patients involve visceral sites, although it may first appear in the skin. If the lymphoma first appears on the skin, it is in the form of primary cutaneous lymphomas originating from cutaneous lymphocytes. Skin homing markers, such as the chemokine receptor CCR4 and cutaneous lymphocyte antigen, are displayed on cutaneous lymphocytes which guide them to the skin. This section will focus on cutaneous lymphomas associated with HIV infection.

PATHOLOGY/PATHOGENESIS/CLINICAL FEATURES

Cutaneous T cell lymphomas (CTCLs), characterized by clinical phenotype and surface markers, are speculated to arise from clonal expansion of skin homing lymphocytes. Mycosis fungoides (MF), the most common variant, may require persistent antigen or superantigen stimulation. HIV-associated CTCL is a rare complication of HIV, and presents similarly to that seen in HIV-negative individuals. MF affects the skin variably by flat patches, thin plaques, or tumors (**173**).[100] Several studies have isolated CD8+ cytotoxic T lymphocyte lines from the skin of patients and demonstrated specific cytotoxic activity against HIV-1 gag-, pol-, or env-expressing cells.[101] While CTCL is well documented in HIV-infected patients, there is a condition that may simulate CTCL, referred to as pseudo-CTCL, pseudo-Sézary, CTCL-simulant, and atypical cutaneous lymphoproliferative disorder.[102] This condition may reflect reactive cutaneous infiltration by HIV-specific cytotoxic T cells. Pseudo-CTCL presents in a manner similar to CTCL, with persistent, generalized erythematous pruritic patches, plaques, or tumors. Pigment changes, including hyperpigmentation and hypopigmentation are common.[102] Pseudo-CTCL can be distinguished from classic CTCL by the predominance of CD8+ T cells versus CD4+ T cells. Pseudo-CTCL may also mimic other diseases, such as drug or photodistributed eruptions and deep ulcers of the skin.

CD30+ large-cell lymphoma may occur as a visceral disease or present with only skin involvement. In contrast to CTCL, these lymphomas are predominately of B cell origin. This lymphoma has been sporadically described in HIV-positive patients, and typically presents with a single or clustered rapidly growing deep skin nodule(s).[103]

HISTOPATHOLOGY

When the skin is involved by lymphoma, histologically there is a diffuse infiltrate of atypical lymphoid cells that are monomorphous in appearance. Many of the cells are large and pleomorphic in appearance and may be in mitosis. The infiltrate can be deeply situated, involving the lower dermis and subcutaneous fat. There is often extensive necrosis and obliteration of adjacent adnexal structures.

CTCL is typically manifested histologically by psoriasiform hyperplasia of the epidermis, as well as a band-like infiltrate of atypical lymphocytes with convoluted nuclei with a cerebriform appearance. Atypical cells are also present in the epidermis, a phenomenon referred to as epidermotropism (**174**). In pseudo-CTCL, lesional biopsies are characterized by a superficial and deep polymorphous infiltrate with atypical lymphocytes with a CD8+ predominance, negative Ki-1, and occasionally CD7 antigen depletion. However, distinguishing CTCL from pseudo-CTCL by the predominance of CD8+ T cells is not absolute, as a minority of CTCLs have a CD8+ phenotype. T cell receptor gene rearrangement studies must be performed to determine clonality, as most cases of CTCL are clonal, whereas in pseudo-CTCL the proliferation is polyclonal.[104]

The histology of CD30+ large-cell lymphomas resembles that seen on sections obtained from non-HIV-infected individuals. There are dermal aggregates of cells with pale eosinophilic cytoplasm. Also seen are large, pleomorphic vesicular nuclei containing large, eosinophilic nucleoli. Mitotic figures, which occasionally are atypical, are often present. The epidermis may be uninvolved, hyperplastic, or ulcerated.

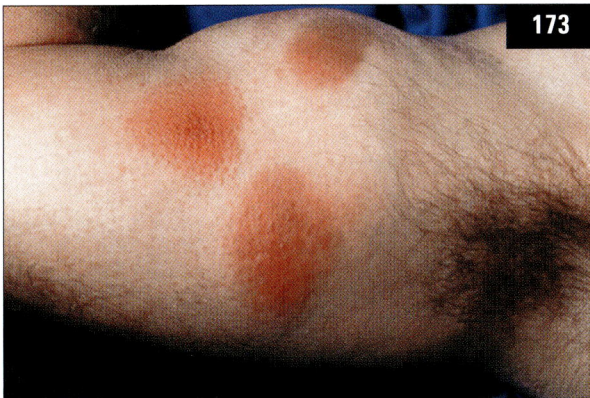

173 Mycosis fungoides. Erythematous patches and plaques on the arm.

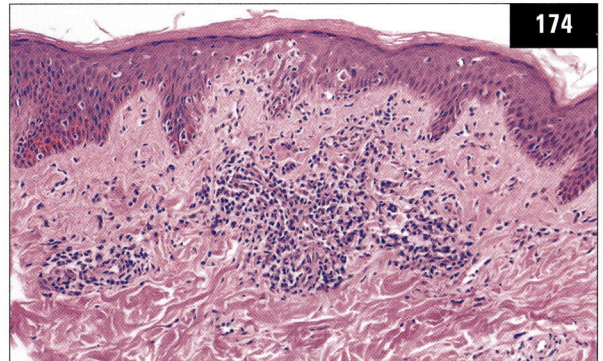

174 Histology of mycosis fungoides. There is mild acanthosis and focal spongiosis with a perivascular infiltrate of atypical lymphocytes, many of which are lined up at the dermoepidermal junction or are migrating up into the epidermis.

DIAGNOSIS

The diagnosis of these lymphomas is based on clinical appearance and histologic features. Further studies such as gene rearrangement studies, flow cytometry, and the use of DNA probes are often necessary. Immunophenotyping of CTCL in HIV patients is usually characterized by an infiltrate of CD4+ lymphocytes but, in some cases, may be comprised of monoclonal CD8+ cells.

In CD30+ large-cell lymphoma, immunohistochemical findings include a CD3+ phenotype, CD30 positivity, and staining with EBV latent membrane protein antiserum.[104] These studies are especially helpful in the cases of pyogenic cutaneous lymphoma, in which the neoplastic cells are not easily seen secondary to the extensive infiltration of neutrophils.

MANAGEMENT

In HIV-infected patients, clinical examination should begin with examination of lymph nodes, biopsy of an enlarged node if present, imaging studies, and bone marrow biopsy. Treating AIDS patients with lymphoma is of concern because even standard doses of chemotherapy can further compromise immune function. Treatment consists of myelosuppressive chemotherapy regimens containing anthracyclines, cyclophosphamide, vinca alkaloids, methotrexate, and corticosteroids. As with KS, selecting optimal therapy must take into account the patient's prognosis, quality of life, and general clinical condition. Palliative therapy may be more appropriate in patients with advanced disease.

CTCL may respond to psoralen and UV light therapy, total body electron beam therapy, and/or application of nitrogen mustard. These lymphomas tend to be more aggressive in HIV-infected patients, and survival ranges between 5 and 10 months after diagnosis. Pseudo-CTCL responds to conservative treatment with topical steroids or psoralen with ultraviolet A (PUVA). One report describes a patient with pseudo-CTCL successfully treated with HAART therapy alone.[105]

Patients with CD30+ large-cell lymphoma should also undergo evaluation for concurrent systemic involvement. Isolated lesions are treated with surgical excision, radiation, or both. Multiple lesions or clinically aggressive lesions may require multiagent chemotherapy. Most patients with CD30+ large-cell lymphoma do well. There are no studies regarding the prognosis of CD30+ large-cell lymphoma in the setting of HAART.

CHAPTER 13

CUTANEOUS MANIFESTATIONS OF SEXUALLY TRANSMITTED DISEASE IN THE HIV-POSITIVE PATIENT

Bryan Gammon, Antoanella Calame, and Clay J. Cockerell

INTRODUCTION

Sexually transmitted diseases (STDs) have been a medical and public health concern for generations. With the advent of the human immunodeficiency virus (HIV) pandemic, these have assumed an even greater significance as they may be more aggressive and may elude diagnosis. HIV has been shown to be synergistic with some STDs accelerating their progression and severity. It can likewise alter the clinical presentation of disease resulting in unusual phenotypes. On the other hand, STDs have also been shown to influence transmission of HIV. Early detection and treatment of STDs is therefore critical to preventing HIV spread. Dermatologists are particularly suited to this task due to the prominent cutaneous manifestations of many STDs. This chapter reviews common STDs and pays particular attention to the ways in which the disease interacts with HIV.

GENITAL ULCERATIVE DISEASE

The genital ulcerative diseases (GUD) herpes simplex virus (HSV), syphilis, and chancroid have all been associated with an increased risk of acquiring and transmitting HIV. Cross-sectional studies performed in Kenya have consistently shown higher HIV seropositivity in patients with current symptoms or a history of GUD,[1-4] while a prospective study showed an increased risk for HIV-seroconversion in patients with GUD.[5] There is clearly an association between GUD and HIV and a Tanzanian study supports the assertion that prevention of GUD should diminish transmission of HIV. In that study, improved recognition and treatment of STDs led to decreased incidence of HIV.[6]

GUD is thought to facilitate transmission of HIV by disrupting the genital mucosa which can serve as a portal of entry for HIV. It is also associated with an inflammatory infiltrate of CD4+ T cells and macrophages which may provide cellular targets for HIV infection.[7-10]

HERPES SIMPLEX VIRUS

Genital herpes is the most common cause of genital ulceration worldwide (**157**).[11] It is classically caused by herpes simplex virus type 2 (HSV-2) although an increasing number of cases are caused by HSV-1.[12] The association between HSV and HIV was noted as early as 1981.[13] Refer to Chapter 2 (Viral Infections in HIV Disease), for a complete review of HSV in the HIV patient.

SYPHILIS

DEFINITION/OVERVIEW

Syphilis has been a recognized public health problem since the late fifteenth century when an Italian physician, Nicolaus Leonicenus, first described the disease. The disease was presumably brought to Europe by Columbus' sailors upon return from the New World, but the true origin of the disease is debatable. In 1530 an Italian poet, Hiero Fracastor, wrote a poem with an infected shepherd, Syphillus, as the protagonist. It is from Syphillus that the disease draws its name. The disease quickly became endemic in Europe earning the moniker the Great Pox. It was not until 1837 that Philippe Ricord, a French venereologist, distinguished syphilis from gonorrhea through a series of experiments with inoculations of syphilitic chancres. Ricord also was among the first to differentiate among the syphilitic phases: primary, secondary, and tertiary.

While the devastating consequences of the disease were easily observed, treatment of the disease eluded the medical community until the discovery of salvasaran by Paul Ehrlich in 1910. Salvasaran was an improvement over the antecedent treatment modalities, i.e. mercury, and vapor baths. The disease, however, remained so prevalent that in 1937 the US Surgeon General Thomas Parran postulated that 10% of Americans would be infected in their lifetime.[14] In 1943 penicillin was recognized to be an effective treatment for syphilis and rates of primary and secondary syphilis steadily declined, reaching their nadir in 2000.

Syphilis is caused by the spirochete *Treponema pallidum*, a thin helical bacterium approximately 0.15 μm × 6–50 μm. It is thought to be microaerophilic and humans are its only known reservoir.

Since 2000, incidence of syphilis among women and infants has continued to decline but overall rates have risen. The total number of reported cases in the US rose from 6103 to 6862 from 2001 to 2002.[15] The observed increase was seen only among men, particularly among men who have sex with men (MSM).[16] The observed outbreaks could further be demographically characterized as occurring among MSM populations with high rates of HIV coinfection, as well as high-risk sexual behavior.[17,18] These trends continued through 2004 when the male:female infection rate was observed to have increased from 1.5 in 2000 to 5.9 in 2004.[19] Further, the incidence of primary and secondary syphilis was observed to rise in the south of the US, and among African-Americans, particularly males, for the first time since 1993.[19] Perhaps even more troubling and indicative of the resurgence of the problem is the observed stabilization in the rate of primary and secondary syphilis among women; 2004 was the first year in more than ten that the rate did not decline among women.

Syphilis has long been implicated in increasing the likelihood of transmission of HIV,[20] likely from ulcers that serve as portals of entry. From an epidemiologic standpoint, it is at least certain that there is a higher prevalence of syphilis among HIV-positive populations. That relationship is particularly prominent in the country with the world's highest number of HIV afflicted, South Africa, where the rate of seropositivity for *T. pallidum* among women in the general population ranged from 4.5–18.7%.[21]

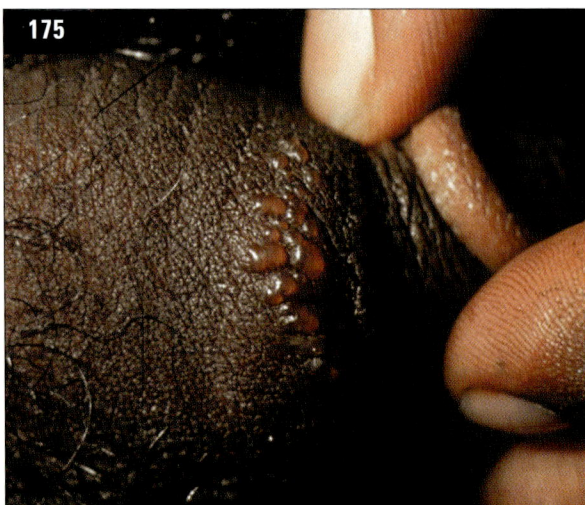

175 Genital herpes simplex virus infection. Grouped, clear-fluid-filled vesicles on the penile shaft.

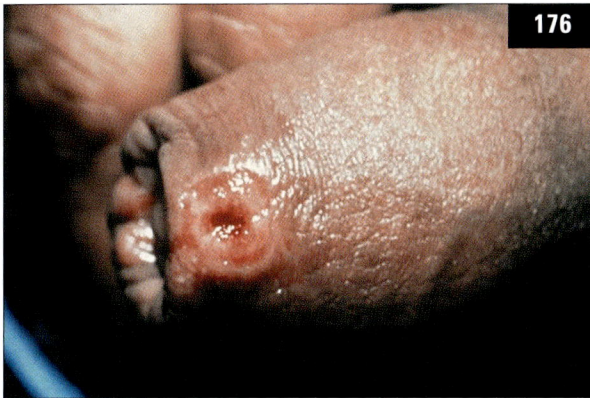

176 Primary syphilis. Nonpurulent ulceration with raised edges (chancre) on the penile shaft.

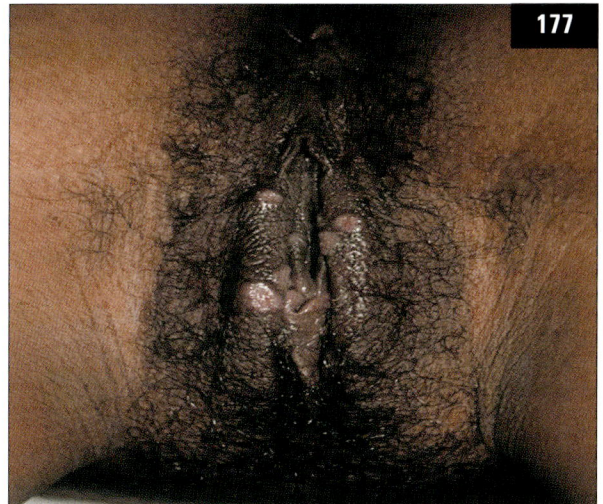

177 Multiple chancres on the labia in a female patient.

PATHOGENESIS/PATHOPHYSIOLOGY/CLINICAL FEATURES

Humans are the only known reservoir for *T. pallidum*. The organism enters the host through normal mucosal tissue or breaches in glabrous skin (**175**).[22] Syphilis is generally transmitted via sexual contact, with a transmission rate between persons with primary or secondary syphilis of 50–75%.[23] However, it can also be transmitted via transfusion of blood from infected persons.[24] Organisms can also cross the placenta and infect the fetus. If the disease is acquired in a woman 4 years preceding pregnancy, the fetus is infected greater than 70% of the time. The risk of transmission is much higher in early stages of the disease. Maternal–fetal transmission may cause premature birth, fetal demise, or congenital syphilis. The stigmata of congenital syphilis, which may develop before or after birth, include corneal opacities, saddle nose, yellowish-brown skin, radiating fissures at the angle of the mouth, around the nares and anus (rhagades), pegged lateral and notched central incisors (Hutchinson's teeth), and molar teeth with rounded rudimentary enamel cusps on the crown surface (mulberry molars). Further, the newborn may have a mucopurulent nasal discharge (snuffles), alopecia, nail dystrophy, condyloma lata, or a palmar plantar bullous eruption.[25,26]

Sexually acquired exposures are characterized by the development of chancres. Typically 3 weeks after exposure, the infected person develops a nontender, indurated, clean-based, nonpurulent ulcer (chancre) at the site of inoculation (**176, 177**). The chancre, the hallmark of primary syphilis, usually has scant serous exudates and raised edges with distinct cartilaginous consistency. The formation of the chancre is typically accompanied by regional lymphadenopathy. The chancre induces a delayed type hypersensitivity (DTH) immune response in the host that is important in clearing the initial infection.[27,28] Humoral immunity clearly plays a role, though, as circulating antibodies are detectable in the serum at the time of the presence of the chancre. Both spirochete-specific antibodies, such as *T. pallidum* particle agglutination (TPPA) and fluorescent treponemal antibodies (FTA-abs), as well as antigens cross-reactive with host particles such as the rapid plasma reagin (RPR) and Venereal Disease Research Laboratory (VDRL) tests are detectable.

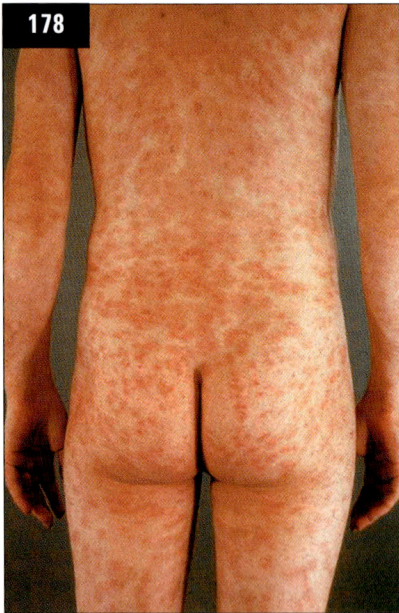

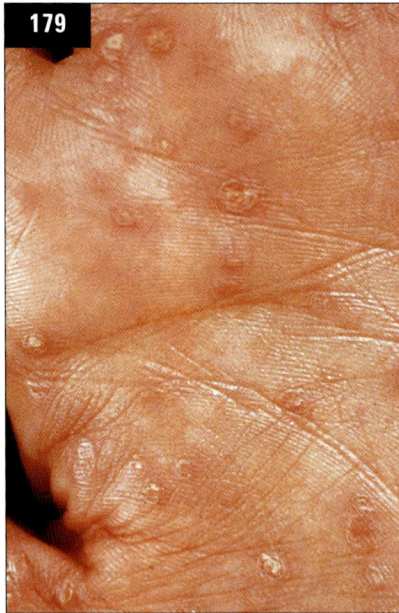

178 Secondary syphilis. Widespread erythematous, scaly papules.

179 Erythematous scaly papules of secondary syphilis on the palms.

180 Widespread scaly papules and plaques of secondary syphilis, resembling pityriasis rosea.

181 Confluent verrucous papules and nodules with ostraceous scale in secondary syphilis.

After 3–6 weeks the chancre clears often leaving an atrophic scar although lymphadenopathy persists longer. Usually 4–10 weeks after the chancre formation, the signs and symptoms of secondary syphilis develop. A cutaneous eruption is found more than 90% of the time.[29] The eruption is commonly composed of symmetric and generalized distribution of numerous erythematous macules and papules, particularly on the face, trunk, palms, soles, and genital region (178–181). Later, the lesions can involve the mucous membranes and smooth, round, coppery, scaly papules on the palms and soles can be seen. During this period the DTH response is down-regulated. The sharp increase in the number of previously controlled spirochetes spurs a rise in circulating antibody levels. Escape from host immunity appears to be secondary to down-regulation of Th-1 type helper T cells.[30] Host humoral responses are insufficient to clear the spirochetes, conceivably because the outer membrane of *T. pallidum* lacks the usual antigens present on gram-negative bacteria.[31]

Additional features which may be seen include condyloma lata, moist verrucous papules seen in the anogenital and orolabial regions. Pharyngeal erythema and a typical hair loss pattern with loss of the lateral eyebrows and 'moth-eaten' patchy alopecia are common findings in secondary syphilis. Signs and symptoms of secondary syphilis usually

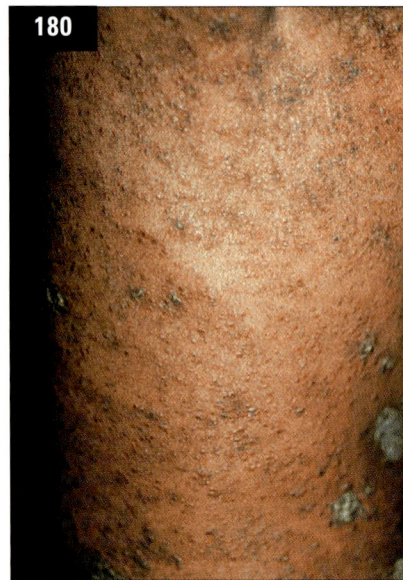

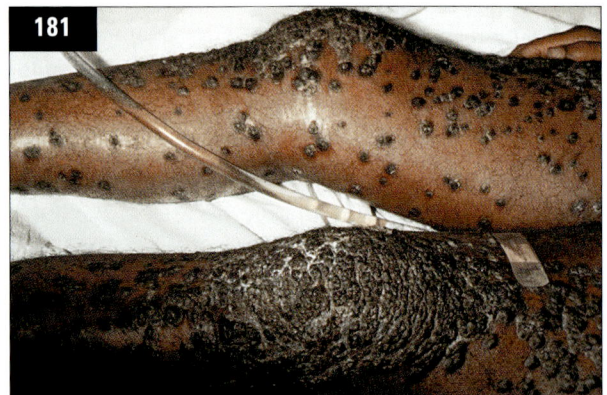

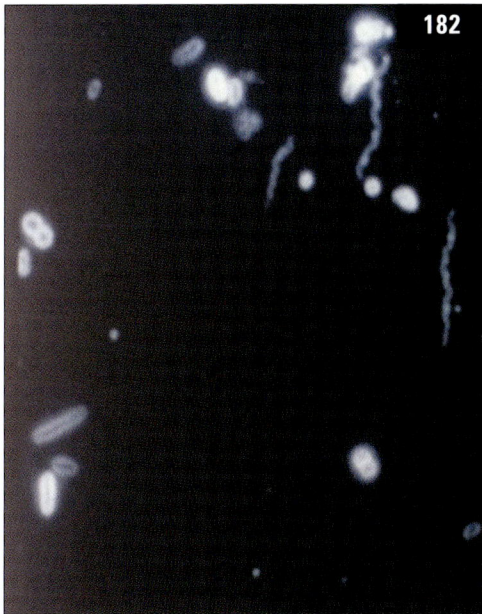

182 Darkfield slide preparation showing three *Treponema pallidum* spirochetes.

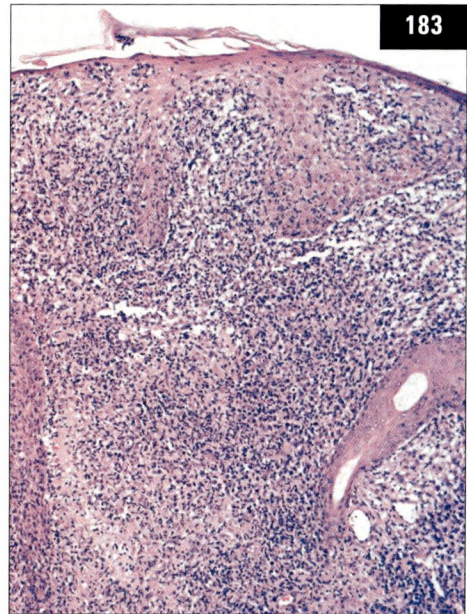

183 Histology of secondary syphilis. Dense mixed infiltrate with numerous plasma cells (×100).

resolve spontaneously, although 25% of untreated secondary syphilis patients relapse. Relapse occurs most commonly in the first year following infection.

Latent syphilis is the asymptomatic period following the resolution of secondary syphilis. This stage can last indefinitely but one-third of untreated patients develop tertiary symptoms 3–15 years after initial infection. There are three forms of late syphilitic disease: benign, cardiovascular, and neurosyphilis. All three are secondary to a DTH response to the persistent low levels of treponemes in the tissue. Late benign disease may affect nearly any tissue in the body except the cardiovascular system and the central nervous system (CNS) by definition. Skin manifestations are the most common and include cutaneous granulomas, psoriasiform papules and plaques, as well as painless indurated dusky-red nodules with serpiginous borders known as gummas. Gummas ulcerate and are destructive to host tissue. Early neurosyphilis, which is often aymptomatic, can cause meningitis or cranial neuritis. The classic findings of neurosyphilis include tabes dorsalis and loss of pupillary light reflex with preserved accommodation, the so-called Argyll–Robertson pupil. General paresis is also observed in a small

minority of patients. Cardiovascular manifestations of tertiary syphilis are varied and include aortitis with destruction of the intima and aneurysm development, endocarditis, myocarditis, and ostial stenosis with secondary myocardial infarction.

DIAGNOSIS/MANAGEMENT

T. pallidum cannot be cultured but it can be demonstrated by darkfield microscopy (**182**) and via light microscopy of specially stained histologic sections (**183**). Visualization using darkfield micros-copy is most often successful in examination of the chancre of primary syphilis or the moist, verrucous lesions of secondary syphilis. Darkfield examination or direct fluorescent antibody tests of lesion exudates or tissue provides the definitive diagnosis,[32] but sensitivity is poor and can be worsened by topical application by the patient of toxic compounds to the lesions. Examination of exudates from tissue has largely been supplanted by serologic diagnosis and routine histologic evaluation.

For serologic diagnosis, suspected patients are first tested using one of the nonspecific antibody tests, RPR or VDRL. These tests have a sensitivity of approximately 80% in primary syphilis, nearly

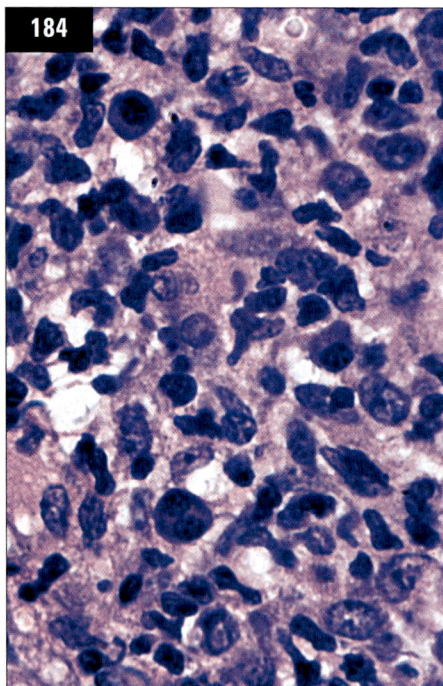

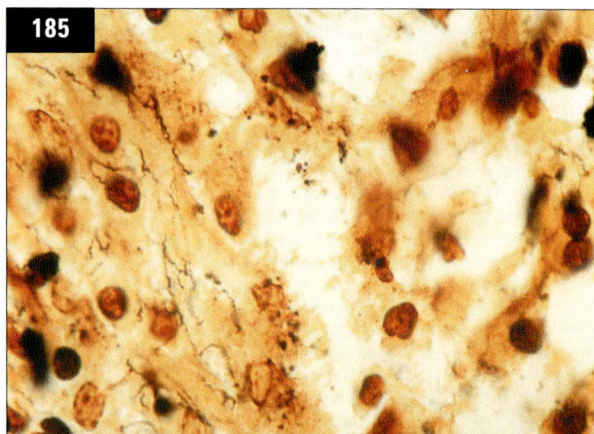

184, 185 Histology of secondary syphilis. Higher power of the dense mixed infiltrate with numerous plasma cells seen in **183** (**184**, ×200). Warthin–Starry stain showing numerous spirochetes (**185**, ×400).

100% in secondary syphilis, and 95% in latent syphilis. False-positive results are not infrequent, however, and are due to many different causes including collagen–vascular disease, intravenous drug use, pregnancy, HIV infection, vaccinations, malaria, and bacterial endocarditis.[29] Therefore, a positive result prompts a confirmatory treponema-specific test such as TPPA or FTA-abs.[33]

Histologically, syphilis has different manifestations depending on when the biopsy is performed. Chancres characteristically reveal an ulcer with a dense infiltrate of lymphocytes, plasma cells, and prominent blood vessels. The findings are relatively nonspecific and special stains are required to demonstrate spirochetes. Silver stains such as the Gomori–methenamine and Bosma–Steiner demonstrate the characteristic thin coiled organisms in the subepithelial tissue and within and around blood vessels in variable numbers. However, the stain is noted for its difficulty in being interpreted, as other argyrophilic structures in the skin such as dendritic melanocytes and melanophages may inhibit visualization of organisms. Recently, a monoclonal anti-body directed to *T. pallidum* has become commercially available and is more sensitive and easier to interpret.

Secondary syphilis may demonstrate a number of different histologic patterns and in HIV-seropositive immunocompromised patients, unusual patterns may be observed. The classic finding is that of a superficial and deep psoriasiform lichenoid dermatitis with parakeratosis containing neutrophils and abundant plasma cells in the dermis, especially in the depth of the infiltrate (**183–185**). Other patterns include a sparse superficial perivascular dermatitis with scattered plasma cells and scattered dyskeratotic keratinocytes, a diffuse granulomatous infiltrate, and leukocytoclastic vasculitis. The number of spirochetes is variable ranging from only a few to thousands.

Tertiary syphilis classically demonstrates a diffuse dermatitis and often panniculitis with extensive granulomatous inflammation, caseation degeneration, and usually ulceration. Spirochetes can usually be found but their number is generally less than that in secondary or primary lesions.

Patients with HIV infection, especially when

immunocompromised, may demonstrate unusual histologic patterns and have shown features of primary, secondary, and even tertiary lesions within the same patient all at the same time and often early in the course of the disease.

The treatment for syphilis is parenteral penicillin G. It is highly effective in healing the mucosal lesions, preventing transmission of the disease and preventing late sequelae. Dosage and length of treatment are stage dependent. There is limited evidence for the efficacy of alternative therapies for penicillin-allergic patients, especially in HIV-positive patients, although doxycycline and tetracycline have established treatment guidelines and can be considered. Alternative therapies should be avoided in the pregnant or neurosyphilitic patient as they are unproven in these cases. If a penicillin allergy is reported, these patients should undergo allergy testing to verify allergy and then should be desensitized prior to penicillin administration to prevent an anaphylactic reaction.

Nontreponemal antibody tests can be then used to monitor therapeutic response. A fourfold change in titer is the threshold for a clinically significant response to treatment. Generally, nontreponemal tests become nonreactive after appropriate treatment while the treponemal tests stay reactive for the lifetime of the patient. Failure to demonstrate a four-fold decrease in nontreponemal titers in 6 months or the persistence of signs and symptoms of primary or secondary syphilis is indicative of either treatment failure or reinfection. Patients in whom either treatment failure or reinfection is suspected should be retested, retreated, and tested for HIV infection. As treatment failure could stem from undiagnosed neurosyphilis, a cerebrospinal fluid (CSF) examination should be performed.

IMPLICATIONS OF HIV COINFECTION

The interactions of syphilis with HIV were recognized as early as 1987, when a case series described HIV-infected patients with syphilis that was either rapidly progressive or refractory to appropriate therapy.[34] Since then, multiple investigators have observed an accelerated progression of the disease which may be related to the level of

immunosuppression. One study described HIV-infected patients presenting with undiagnosed secondary syphilis when their CD4 counts were <500 × 10⁶/l.[35] Others reported an association between accelerated ulcerating syphilis or accelerating progression to neurosyphilis and advancing HIV disease.[36] The topic is somewhat controversial, however, as Dowell et al. found no association between HIV stage and syphilis progression or recalcitrance to therapy.[37]

The clinical presentation of syphilis is usually similar in HIV-infected patients and non-HIV-infected individuals. However, unusual features may be seen in immunocompromised hosts. These include multiple extensive chancres (159),[38] lues maligna (syphilis with vasculitis), ostraceous lues (163) as well as rapid progression to neurosyphilis despite appropriate therapy.[34] Syphilis is protean in its presentation in immunocompetent hosts so it comes as no surprise that unusual manifestations have been documented in immunocompromised patients.[39,40]

The standard diagnostic tests for syphilis can generally be interpreted in the HIV-infected person as they would be in an otherwise healthy patient,[32] although atypical serologic responses have been noted on occasion. Most atypical serologic results are false-positive nontreponemal antibody tests (VDRL or RPR), the so-called biologic false-positive.[41,42] On the other hand, seronegative syphilis, accelerated loss of antibody reactivity after treatment, and titers becoming nonreactive with progression of immuno-suppression have also been described.[43–46] Delayed antibody titer response to treatment has also been observed.[47,48] These observations are controversial, however, as other studies have documented normal responses to treatment in HIV-infected patients.[49] Thus, if serologic test results conflict with clinical suspicion, a definitive diagnosis should be obtained via biopsy and search for spirochetes.

The aforementioned reports of accelerated progression to neurosyphilis in HIV-positive patients has prompted some individuals to suggest CSF examination be performed prior to treatment of HIV-positive patients with primary or secondary syphilis. The prognostic utility of this has not been determined, however, as there are CSF abnormalities seen in association with HIV infection in the absence of syphilis, including elevated protein and mononuclear pleocytosis. Current recommendations include CSF examination in the HIV-positive patient with late latent syphilis and syphilis of unknown duration.

In general, the treatment of primary or secondary syphilis in HIV-positive patients is similar to that in HIV-negative patients, i.e. 2.4 million units of penicillin G delivered in an intramuscular injection.[32] HIV-positive patients should be followed closely for clinical or serologic evidence of treatment failure at 3, 6, 9, 12, and 24 months after therapy. HIV-positive patients meeting the criteria for treatment failure should be treated identically to their HIV-negative counterparts, with CSF examination and retreatment. Strong consideration should be given to CSF examination if the titers are slow to fall in the properly treated patient.

Treatment of late latent syphilis or syphilis of unknown duration is 2.4 million units of intramuscular penicillin G each week for 3 weeks. Follow-up should include clinical and serologic examinations at 6, 12, 18, and 24 months after therapy. Those with clinical signs or symptoms of neurosyphilis should receive 3–4 million units of aqueous crystalline penicillin G intravenously every 4 hours for 10–14 days. Recommended follow-up includes CSF examinations every 6 months for up to 24 months until CSF abnormalities normalize.

The efficacy of alternative treatment regimens for use in the penicillin-allergic patient has not been studied. Those HIV-seropositive patients with primary or secondary syphilis should be treated following the guidelines for HIV-negative patients, e.g. doxycycline, ceftriaxone, or azithromycin with close follow-up. Latent or tertiary syphilis should be treated with penicillin after desensitization.

CHANCROID

DEFINITION/OVERVIEW

A gram-negative intracellular facultatively anaerobic pleomorphic bacillus named *Haemophilus ducreyi* is the causative pathogenic organism of chancroid. Chancroid is a sexually transmitted infection characterized by painful ulcers, bubo formation, and inguinal lymphadenopathy.

Chancroid is rare and decreasing in incidence in the US, with the number of reported cases falling from 4986 cases in 1987 to 30 in 2004,[50,51] although it is believed to be an underreported disease secondary to the difficulty in establishing the diagnosis.[52] Over half of reported cases in the US in 2004 occurred in New York City, Texas, South Carolina or Louisiana.[51] While chancroid is uncommon in the US, it remains the leading cause of genital ulceration in Africa,[53] and has been estimated by some to exceed syphilis is worldwide incidence.[54] Men are more commonly affected than women.

PATHOGENESIS/PATHOPHYSIOLOGY/CLINICAL FEATURES

H. ducreyi enters the skin through a defect in the epithelial barrier usually from minor sexually-induced trauma. Invasion of the organism induces the production of proinflammatory cytokines which induce neutrophils and macrophages to form intradermal pustules. The organism secretes a cyto-lethal distending toxin (HdCDT) that causes apoptosis and necrosis of myeloid cells, epithelial cells, keratinocytes, and primary fibroblasts. This toxin inhibits cell proliferation and induces cell death causing the characteristic ulceration seen in chancroid.

Typically 2 days to 3 weeks after exposure, an erythematous papule develops at the site of inoculation. The initial lesion sloughs leaving an ulcer which may be solitary or multiple and is accompanied by usually unilateral inguinal lymphadenitis in 40–70% of cases.[55] The ulcer is typically painful, deep and nonindurated, having soft, ragged edges and a foul-smelling purulent exudate (**186**).[56] As the disease progresses, autoinoculation may occur forming the classic 'kissing' lesions in sites of skin apposition such as the labia. The inguinal lymphadenitis often evolves into a bubo that can rupture spontaneously if not aspirated.

DIAGNOSIS/MANAGEMENT

Diagnosis based solely upon morphologic features yields an accuracy of 30–50%.[57–59] Histologic appearance of a gram stain of exudate from a lesion typically reveals pleomorphic coccobacilli in parallel chains and clusters, the so-called 'school of fish'. While such a finding is highly suggestive of chancroid, it is insufficient for diagnosis especially given the high incidence of polymicrobial contamination of the ulcer. Definitive diagnosis therefore requires culture of the organism which is a somewhat difficult process requiring special media and has a sensitivity of <80%.[32] Polymerase chain reaction (PCR) may aid in diagnosis,[60] but there is no FDA-approved PCR test for *H. ducreyi* available in the US. The US Centers for Disease Control (CDC) suggests that a probable diagnosis may be made if the patient presents with clinical features typical of chancroid and a subsequent laboratory evaluation rules out *T. pallidum* and HSV.[32]

There are four effective antibiotic therapies available for the treatment of chancroid. These therapeutic options include a single 1 g dose of oral azithromycin; a single 250 mg dose of intramuscular ceftriaxone; 500 mg of ciprofloxacin orally twice a day for 3 days; or 500 mg of erythromycin orally three times a day for 7 days. Azithromycin and ceftriaxone offer the obvious benefit of single dose therapy; isolates with intermediate resistance to ciprofloxacin and erythromycin have been reported so that these agents will likely be used more frequently.[32]

IMPLICATIONS OF HIV COINFECTION

The presentation of those infected with both HIV and chancroid does not different markedly from that of non-HIV-infected chancroid patients. Ulcer size is not different,[61–64] and histologic examination of punch biopsy specimens of lesions in HIV-negative and HIV-positive patients demonstrate no significant differences.[64,65] Some of the most significant differences include longer ulcer duration,[63,64] and increased numbers of ulcers at initial presentation.[63] Atypical presentations have been reported, however, as exemplified by an HIV-seropositive patient with chancroid that presented as a chronic penile ulcer with multiple ulcers on the legs and digits.[66]

Chancroid recalcitrance to therapy also occurs at a higher rate in the HIV-positive population.[61–64,66] Several clinical trials have investigated the efficacy of antibiotic therapy with respect to the HIV serologic status.[62–64,67–69] Studies of quinolone-based therapy showed differences in response rates,[62,67,68] and studies of single-dose azithromycin and single-dose ceftriaxone therapy demonstrated statistically significant increases in failure rates among HIV-positive chancroid patients when compared to HIV-negative patients.[69] Erythromycin is significantly less effective at curing chancroid in HIV-positive patients at weeks 1 and 2 after initiation of therapy,[63,64] but the differences between the two populations disappear at week 3.[64] The CDC notes that because treatment failure can occur on any regimen and occurs with higher frequency in the HIV-positive population, these patients should receive the same treatment as their HIV-negative counterparts but, in addition, should receive close follow-up as they may need an extended course of medication.[32]

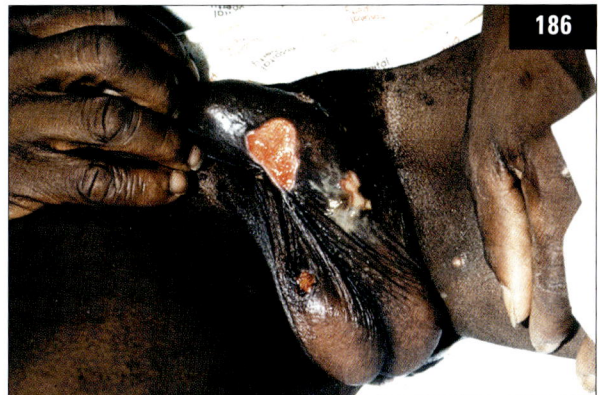

186 Chanchroid.

GRANULOMA INGUINALE

DEFINITION/OVERVIEW

Granuloma inguinale, also known as donovanosis, is a rare cause of chronic genital ulceration worldwide. The pathogenic organism is *Calymmatobacterium granulomatis*, a gram-negative, encapsulated, facultatively aerobic, obligate intracellular pleomorphic bacillus. The disease is sexually transmitted and is therefore most prevalent in more sexually active age groups. More than 70% of cases occur between the ages of 20 and 40 years,[70] with the highest rate of incidence in the third decade.[71] Cases occur in 'hotspots' worldwide, most notably Papua New Guinea, South Africa, India, Brazil, and among the Aboriginal population of Australia,[72] but are extremely rare in North America.[73] While recent accurate epidemiologic data on the prevalence of donovanosis is limited, the disease appears on the decline. In a study conducted at five health centers in Papua New Guinea in 1989–90, donovanosis was the second most common cause of genital ulcerative disease behind only genital herpes.[74] A more recent World Health Organization (WHO) consensus report, however, states that donovanosis has become very rare in Papua New Guinea.[75] Similarly in Australia, subsequent to the induction of a proactive public health program, the incidence dropped from 121 in 1994 to 13 in 2005 and 2 in 2006.[76] The incidence in the US has been consistently very low and only 8 cases were reported in 1997.[77]

PATHOGENESIS/PATHOPHYSIOLOGY/CLINICAL FEATURES

Transmission of donovanosis is usually via sexual contact, but transmission also occurs during vaginal delivery and careful cleaning of neonates born to infected mothers is therefore recommended.[78] The disease is only mildly contagious and repeated exposure is thought to be necessary for development of the disease. The infectivity rate among sexual partners is variable but low ranging from 0.4% to 52%.[70,79,80]

After a variable incubation period most likely in the neighborhood of 50 days,[72] a single or multiple firm papules or subcutaneous nodules develop at the site of inoculation. In the most common type of donovanosis, the ulcerogranulomatous form, the primary lesions grow and ultimately ulcerate to form the classic painless 'beefy red' ulcers with clean, friable bases and distinctive raised, rolled edges (**187**).[56] Without treatment, ulcers can enlarge, become confluent, and cause extensive local destruction. Autoinoculation is common leading to the classic 'kissing' lesions at sites of skin apposition.[56] Less common alternative presentations include hypertrophic or verrucous ulcers, deep necrotic foul-smelling ulcers, or sclerotic lesions. Granuloma inguinale is usually limited to a localized infection and infected persons, therefore, do not often have constitutional symptoms.[81] These local lesions occur in the genitalia in approximately 90% of cases, with the remainder of cases occurring in the inguinal area. Ulcers more commonly occur in uncircumcised men and are linked to poor hygiene. Extragenital cases comprise a small minority of cases but have been reported in the literature at anatomic sites largely contained within the oro- or nasopharynx.[82] Disseminated donovanosis may rarely occur and is thought to be associated with pregnancy and cervical infection.

Genital ulcers are rarely accompanied by true regional adenopathy; the development of adenopathy is an indication of bacterial superinfection of the open wound. However, subcutaneous granulomas, or pseudobuboes, may arise in the inguinal lymph node region. These pseudobuboes may enlarge and ulcerate through skin or underlying organs including the bladder, bone, or bowel causing significant local destruction.[83,84] Development of systemic symptoms in the presence of ulcerative buboes would suggest hematogenous spread of disease and a probable increase in mortality.

DIAGNOSIS/MANAGEMENT

The ulcers of donovanosis may be difficult to distinguish clinically from the chancre of primary syphilis, the ulcer of chancroid, or large HIV-associated herpetic ulcers. Cervical or extensively necrotic penile lesions may be confused with carcinoma.[85] The organism is extremely difficult to culture so that diagnosis is usually made by direct visualization of bipolar-staining intracytoplasmic inclusion bodies within histiocytes.[86] These so-called Donovan bodies are pin-shaped and easily visualized microscopically when examining tissue crush preparations, smears, or skin biopsy specimens stained by the Giemsa or Wright method.[72] Visualization of Donovan bodies is diagnostic in all cases and they are also seen in lesions in HIV-infected patients.[32] However, in some cases they may be difficult to see which may make establishment of the diagnosis somewhat difficult. Recent advances in culture technique have made isolation of the causative organism easier.[87,88]

Optimal management of donovanosis is dependent upon early diagnosis and treatment. Effective treatment is readily available and the disease is relatively benign if caught early, but as noted earlier, disease progression may lead to extensive local tissue destruction, significant morbidity, and increased likelihood of hematogenous dissemination and possible mortality. Treatment halts the progression of existing lesions, although extended courses of appropriate therapy may be required for complete re-epithelialization. Relapse up to 18 months after appropriate therapy is also possible. Current first-line CDC-recommended treatments are either doxycycline 100 mg orally twice a day or trimethoprim–sulfamethoxazole (800 mg/160 mg) orally twice a day.[32] Ciprofloxacin 750 mg orally twice a day, erythromycin base 500 mg orally four times a day, or azithromycin 1 g orally per week are alternative treatment regimens which are quite successful.[32] All therapies should be continued for a minimum of 3 weeks or until lesions have completely healed. If no clinical improvement is noted within the first few days of treatment, parenteral aminoglycosides may need to be added.[32]

IMPLICATIONS OF HIV COINFECTION

Scant data exist on the effects of HIV infection on donovanosis, although HIV-positive patients often present with more persistent ulcers that require more intensive antibiotic therapy.[89] A prospective case-control study of 50 patients performed in India found that while ulcer size and clinical presentation were comparable in the HIV-positive and HIV-negative patient, the HIV-positive patient presented

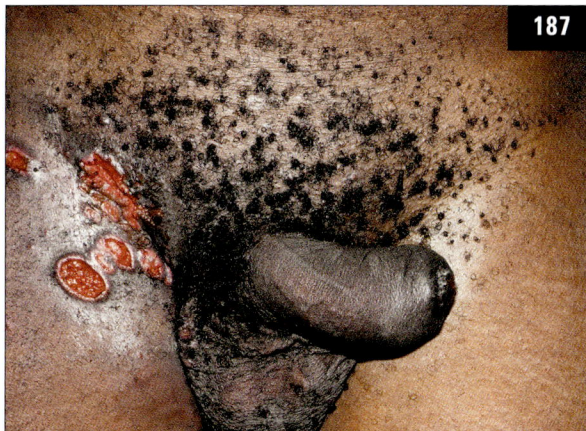

187 Granuloma inguinale. Multiple ulcers with clean bases and rolled edges.

with ulcers that were slow to respond to treatment and caused more extensive local tissue destruction.[90] A retrospective study of pregnant women with donovanosis demonstrated no effect on pregnancy outcome with respect to HIV serologic status.[91] Further, while disseminated donovanosis has been reported in association with HIV infection,[92] it is less common than recalcitrance to treatment.

Despite the literature documenting resistance to treatment in the HIV-positive patient, the CDC currently recommends the same treatment for granuloma inguinale in HIV-positive and HIV-negative patients, although consideration should be given to the use of parenteral amioglycosides (e.g. gentamicin 1 mg/kg IV every 8 hours) in HIV-positive patients.[32]

LYMPHOGRANULOMA VENEREUM

DEFINITION/OVERVIEW

Lymphogranuloma venereum (LGV) is a STD that primarily infects the lymphatics and has the development of inguinal buboes as its prime clinical manifestation. LGV is caused by the L1, L2, and L3 serotypes of *Chlamydia trachomatis*. The remaining chylamidial serovars, A–K, are known to cause trachoma and superficial genital tract infections by infecting the squamocolumnar cells of the genitourinary tract. The L1–3 serotypes, on the other hand, infect macrophages and produce systemic disease as evidenced by the presence of fever and leukocytosis.[93,94]

LGV is a rare disease in the industrialized world and is endemic mainly in the developing world. Regional zones with significant incidence include Africa, Asia, parts of the Caribbean, and South America. In 1997, only 113 cases were reported in the US,[77] although this figure may be artificially low due to underreporting.[56] Reliable epidemiologic data are scant, as the disease is difficult to distinguish clinically from other genital ulcerative diseases with lymphadenopathy including chancroid and donovanosis. Recent investigations in South Africa have reported that LGV accounts for 11% of patients presenting with genital ulceration.[95] Similarly, in a study performed in Nassau, Bahamas of 47 patients presenting with GUD, 17 had LGV confirmed by PCR or immunofluorescence.[96] Like other STDs, LGV shows highest incidence among ages of peak sexual activity, from age 15–40 years.[60] The disease is more common in men.

While still uncommon, since 2003 LGV has been reported with increased frequency in the industrialized world in certain populations such as MSM, particularly those practicing receptive anal intercourse.[97–102] Retrospective studies on anal swabs taken from STD clinic visitors in San Francisco and Amsterdam revealed that the current epidemic is caused by the L2b strain of *C. trachomatis*.[103,104] Presence of the L2b has been documented since 1981 in the US and since 2000 in Europe, leading some in the field to declare this a 'slow epidemic'.[105] The undetected spread of LGV among the MSM population is attributed to testing procedures employed prior to 2003, when positive anal swabs were recorded simply as *Chlamydia* proctitis without the performance of further serotyping. This was due to the presumed paucity of cases of LGV outside of endemic countries.[105] Recently developed real-time polymerase chain reaction (RT-PCR) test designed specifically for LGV serotypes can lessen diagnostic difficulties as the test is rapid, highly specific, and can be performed under routine microbiological laboratory conditions.[106]

PATHOGENESIS/PATHOPHYSIOLOGY/CLINICAL FEATURES

C. trachomatis gains entry to the body via skin breaks or microabrasions, although it can pass through epithelial cells of mucous membranes. It travels through the lymphatics and multiplies in the mononuclear phagocytic cells of the regional lymph nodes where it causes a characteristic disease pattern. LGV has been described as having three distinct stages. After an uncertain incubation period thought to be 1–2 weeks, a small painless papule or pustule appears at the site of inoculation, usually the glans or prepuce in men and the vulva or vaginal wall in women. The lesion usually erodes forming a small, asymptomatic shallow ulcer. If it develops, the ulcer heals without scarring within a week. Largely due to the location of the lesions in the genital area and the absence of symptoms, the initial lesion is often not noticed. In one study of 27 patients with advanced disease, only five patients recalled the presence of a primary lesion in the weeks preceding onset of systemic disease.[107] Mucopurulent discharge from the urethra in males or the cervix in females should cause the clinician to suspect the diagnosis.

Within 6 weeks after the onset of the initial lesion, the second, or inguinal, phase begins. The hallmark of this stage of disease is intense lymphadenitis. Infected macrophages migrate from the site of inoculation to draining regional nodes causing painful enlargement. The overlying skin reddens and becomes edematous and thick and develops a violaceous hue.[108] Commonly affected nodes include the inguinal and femoral nodes, although deep pelvic nodes may be involved in female patients.[109] The lymph nodes may become fluctuant, forming buboes with a tendency to rupture (**188**). Following rupture, infected lymph nodes drain via fistula formation in approximately one-third of patients.[93] In other cases, buboes form hard, nonsuppurative masses.[110] Bubo formation with enlargement of both the inguinal nodes above and femoral nodes below Poupart's ligament is known as the 'groove sign', a classic but nonspecific manifestation observed in a minority of patients.[111] The majority of buboes heal without complications, but the second stage of disease is marked by the onset of systemic complaints including arthralgias, myalgias, low-grade fevers, chills, and general malaise.[112]

Anorectal involvement in early LGV is a well known phenomenon and largely occurs in women and homosexual men who present with acute hemorrhagic proctitis and systemic complaints. Granular or ulcerative proctitis confined to the distal 10 cm of the anorectal canal is visible on proctoscopy.[113,114] The clinical presentation is similar to that of ulcerative colitis.

In contrast to early anorectal involvement mentioned above, the third stage is also manifest as anorectal and genital damage and is known as the genitoanorectal syndrome. This is characterized by healing and fibrosis of ulcers with destruction of anal and rectal tissue.[115] It is most commonly seen in women and men who practice receptive anal intercourse.[13,60] Typical presentation is that of proctocolitis followed by perirectal abscesses, fistulae, and finally the development of stenoses and rectal strictures.[116,117] Persistent bacteria in the anorectal tissue cause a chronic inflammatory response and hyperplasia of the perirectal and intestinal lymphatics.[118] Lymphatic obstruction can result in elephantiasis of the genitalia in either sex. Tenesmus, fever, and rectal pain are also common.

DIAGNOSIS/MANAGEMENT

Until recently, the diagnosis of LGV has been difficult, and complicated by the numerous serotypes of the pathogenic organism.[118] Culture, isolation, and serotyping of the organism have been the traditional methods of diagnosis. An aspirate of an inflamed lymph node is the preferred sample, although a swab of infected tissue may yield good results.[56] Cultures are expensive, not widely available, and technically difficult as evidenced by the low 30% recovery rate in most laboratories.[119] Serologic testing may be a useful adjunct given the difficulty of isolating the causative organism via culture. Complement fixation takes advantage of the vigorous immune response to LGV and can be used as an adjunctive means of diagnosis.[120] A complement fixation titer of 1:64 or greater in the presence of clinical signs or symptoms is diagnostic.[56,60] Titers to typical chlamydial cervicitis, conjunctivitis, or urethritis caused by serovars D–K, in contrast, rarely exceed 1:16.[121] Complement fixation is usually positive within 2 weeks of contracting the disease and a fourfold rise in titer further supports the diagnosis.[56] PCR and immunofluorescence testing with monoclonal antibodies are largely research techniques today, although will likely be used more routinely in the future.[122,123] Of particular interest is the previously mentioned rapid and LGV-specific RT-PCR test which should ease the difficulty associated with diagnosis.[106]

The treatment regimen recommended by the CDC for LGV is 100 mg of oral doxycycline twice daily for 21 days or, alternatively, erythromycin 500 mg orally four times a day for 21 days.[32] These recommendations are the same for HIV-positive patients although the CDC notes that slow resolution

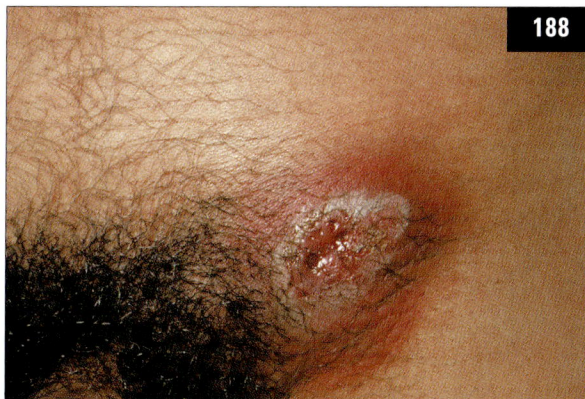

188 Lymphogranuloma venereum. Enlarged lymph node with extensive overlying erythema, central necrosis, and ulceration.

of symptoms necessitating prolonged therapy may occur in these individuals.[32] Others recommend 1 g azithromycin weekly for 3 weeks although there is no formal clinical data to support the efficacy of this regimen.[32] Aspiration or incision and drainage of fluctuant lymph nodes prevents ulceration and relieves pain and should be undertaken when possible.[32,56] Surgical correction of strictures and other late complications of LGV may also be required.[124]

IMPLICATIONS OF HIV COINFECTION

There is relatively minimal published material about the clinical manifestations of LGV in HIV-infected patients, although since the current outbreak in western Europe there have been several recent studies. A retrospective review of 6 patients coinfected with HIV and LGV demonstrated no significant differences in clinical presentation between those with and without HIV infection.[107] A case report in 2003 noted LGV presenting as a perianal ulcer mimicking HSV with inguinal adenopathy in a bisexual HIV-positive male,[125] and a report of two cases of LGV in HIV-positive patients from Dresden described one with classic genital ulceration and inguinal adenopathy and a second with ulcerative proctitis.[126] Thus, although the clinical presentation of LGV in HIV-positive patients is not significantly different from that in HIV-negative patients, HIV-positive MSM present more commonly with anorectal complaints. This is due to the site of inoculation being the rectum during receptive anal intercourse. Primary infection of the penis, anterior urethra, vulva, and anus is associated with formation of inguinal buboes, while infection of the posterior urethra, vagina, cervix, or rectum leads to involvement of the nonpalpable perirectal or deep inguinal nodes.[99]

As noted above, western Europe is in the midst of an epidemic of LGV caused by the newly identified *C. trachomatis* serovar L2b variant. It affects MSM primarily and the majority are HIV-positive.[98] As of March 2005, there were 144 confirmed cases in Amsterdam, 142 cases in France, and 34 cases in the United Kingdom.[98] Four confirmed cases were recently reported in New York City, all of whom

were HIV-positive MSM.[99] The majority of the above cases presented with severe anorectal infections and behavioral risk factors including unprotected receptive anal intercourse and having had sex with multiple anonymous partners.[98] A recent retrospective case-control study performed at Municipal Health Services in Amsterdam found that HIV seropositivity was the strongest predictor of LGV infection, with an odds ratio of 9.3 versus control patients. Clinical predictors of LGV infection include proctoscopic findings of inflamed, edematous mucosa or mucopurulent discharge, and an elevated white blood cell (WBC) count on anorectal smear. Concurrent ulcerative sexually transmitted infection (STI), previously diagnosed STI, and unprotected anal intercourse were other independent risk factors. When an individual was found to have HIV infection and clinical findings of elevated WBC count with proctitis, there was a positive predictive value of 89% sensitivity and 50% specificity for LGV infection.[127]

Recent reports of clusters of acute hepatitis C virus (HCV) infections among LGV patients raise further public health concerns. Sexual transmission of HCV has been long reported to occur at a low rate, with prevalence among spouses of chronic HCV patients averaging 1.5%.[128,129] Furthermore, prevalence of HCV among MSM who deny other risk factors has been reported to be no higher than that of heterosexuals.[130,131] Recently, however, a study involving a group of 17 MSM, 15 of whom had a new diagnosis of LGV, found that seven of the subjects had recently seroconverted positive for HCV. Of the seven, six had concomitant LGV proctitis and HIV infection. Of note, unprotected anal fisting was reported in all of the HCV seroconverters and only two of the non-HCV-infected patients.[132]

HUMAN PAPILLOMAVIRUS

DEFINITION/OVERVIEW

Human papillomavirus (HPV) is the etiologic agent of anogenital warts, also known as condylomata acuminata. HPV is a nonenveloped double-stranded deoxyribonucleic acid (DNA) virus of which there are over 120 identified genotypes.[133,134] Forty-five genotypes are known to affect the genital epithelium,[135] and 13 to 18 of those are identified as probable or definite high oncogenic risk HPV (HR-HPV). The most commonly encountered types of HR-HPV are types 16, 18, 31, 33. It is now widely known that HPV infection is a necessary component for the development of nearly all cases of cervical cancer worldwide, as well as a great number of anogenital neoplasms and oral squamous cell carcinoma (SCC). However, infection with low-risk HPV types such as 6 or 11 may also result in significant morbidity from the formation of multiple large condylomata.

HPV is the most commonly diagnosed STD.[136] It affects 30–50% of sexually active adults.[137] Highest rates of infection are found in women aged 19–22 years and men aged 22–26 years.[138–140] While the prevalence of HPV among sexually active persons is high, the majority of infections are subclinical or asymptomatic as clinically apparent anogenital warts are found in only 1–2% of sexually active persons.[141–143] Risk factors for the acquisition of condylomata in women include number of sexual partners, frequency of intercourse, and presence of warts on the sexual partner.[144–146] Men are primarily at risk if they fail to use a condom during sexual intercourse.[147] Smoking is a controversial risk factor, with some studies reporting increased incidence among smokers,[142,147] while other studies did not.[148]

PATHOGENESIS/PATHOPHYSIOLOGY/CLINICAL FEATURES

Factors associated with transmission and infectivity of HPV remain somewhat unclear,[149] but it is thought that transmission is facilitated by the presence of anogenital warts.[150] Transmission via sexual contact is well established, although the role of fomites is not clear. Although HPV DNA has been recovered from surgical gloves and under-garments,[151] the risk of transmission during exposure to this DNA is unknown.[152] Infection of the fetus during delivery occurs rarely, although reports of infants developing laryngeal papillomas[153–155] and anogenital warts[156,157] in the months subsequent to delivery indicate that vertical transmission is possible.

Infectivity between sexual partners is estimated to be 60%.[155] Commonly affected sites include the fourchette in women and the subpreputial region in men. These sites are particularly vulnerable to infection because of the epithelial damage incurred there during intercourse.[158] HPV virions travel from the epithelial cells of the infected partner to the basal cell layer of the recipient through these sites of damage.[151] Once in the basal layer, the virions may remain latent causing a subclinical infection[159] or they may replicate resulting in a condyloma. Only surface epithelial cells are infected and viremia does not occur.[160]

Cell-mediated immunity has been found to be essential in clearing HPV infection. Regressing lesions display an abundance of CD4+ and CD8+ T cells as well as mRNA transcripts.[161,162] Patients with deficient cell-mediated immune systems, such as those with acquired immunodeficiency syndrome (AIDS) and immunosuppressed transplant patients, frequently experience more severe sequelae from HPV-induced disease such as refractory condylomata or anogenital malignancies.[163–166]

HPV avoids clearance by the immune system in a variety of ways, one of which is to induce a Th-2 immune response, downregulating key inflammatory cytokines and minimizing local inflammation. Failure of the virus to be detected by the host's immune system is a key event in the development of malignancy. Another important factor is the overproduction of viral proteins E6 and E7 in infected cells. These proteins interfere with cell cycle regulators, induce genetic instability, and drive the selection of oncogenic intracellular alterations.[167] It is therefore not surprising that these proteins are highly expressed on HR-HPV subtypes 16 and 18.[168]

The clinical manifestations of HPV infection that are expressed depend to some degree on the infectious subtype. HPV types 6 and 11 are most commonly associated with anogenital warts, along with types 16, 18, 31, 33, 35, 39, 41–45, 51, 56, and 59.[139] The majority of condylomata are secondary to infection with HPV-6 and -11, however. In one study of 52 condylomata tested for HPV DNA, 83% were found to contain HPV-6 and/or -11 while only 6% were positive for HPV type 16.[169] These types are only rarely associated with cervical or genital cancer.[170] An exception to this rule is the uncommon giant condyloma acuminata of Buschke and Lowenstein. This lesion is a form of verrucous carcinoma that is locally aggressive but rarely metastatic and is associated with HPV types 6 and 11.

HR-HPV subtypes, on the other hand, rarely produce condyloma,[148] and commonly present as a subclinical infection.[170] HPV types 16 and 18 are the HPV types most commonly associated with genital malignancy[135,171] and are commonly implicated in bowenoid papulosis (BP). HPV types 31, 33, 35, 39, 45, 51, 52, 54, 56, and 58 also show either intermediate or high risk for the development of genital malignancy, especially cervical carcinoma.[172] Notably, nearly 100% of cervical neoplasms and 90% of other anogenital malignancies are related to infection with HR-HPV.

Condylomata are most often located at sites with increased friction for reasons discussed above (**189**).[173] These sites in men are the glans, prepuce, coronal sulcus, shaft and scrotum. Commonly affected sites in women are the labia, vaginal introitus, and perineum. Intravaginal or cervical condylomata can occur, but these sites more often harbor subclinical infection.[173] One-third of women with extravaginal lesions had concomitant intravaginal warts,[174] highlighting the need for a gynecologic examination. Perianal warts or warts in the anal canal are particularly common among MSM and heterosexual females practicing receptive anal intercourse.

Condyloma can present with a variety of different morphologies: small verrucous papules, sessile smooth papules, or large exophytic fungating masses. Individual lesions are rarely larger than a few centimeters unless they coalesce. Their color ranges from skin-colored to pink to reddish-brown. Lesions are most often asymptomatic although patients may complain of pruritus or burning.

Bowenoid papulosis (BP) is much rarer than condyloma acuminata and usually presents as sharply demarcated 2–3 mm papules grouped on the external genitalia or perianal region. Papules are typically reddish brown or darkly hyperpigmented. In some cases, it may appear as a flat brown plaque. As mentioned previously, BP is most often caused by HR-HPV type 16 and although it histologically demonstrates features of SCC arising as a condyloma, it usually demonstrates a benign behavior, rarely extending beneath the epidermis.[175,176] Histologically, BP may be indistinguishable from the more aggressive Bowen disease and erythroplasia of Queyrat, although clinical features usually allow the conditions to be distinguished from one another. While BP is commonly found in young patients, Bowen disease and erythroplasia of Queyrat are infrequently encountered in individuals younger than 50 years.[177] BP is usually manifest as multiple papules with a reddish-brown hue in contrast to Bowen disease which is a solitary verrucous or crusted plaque, or erythroplasia of Queyrat which is an erosive red patch or plaque.

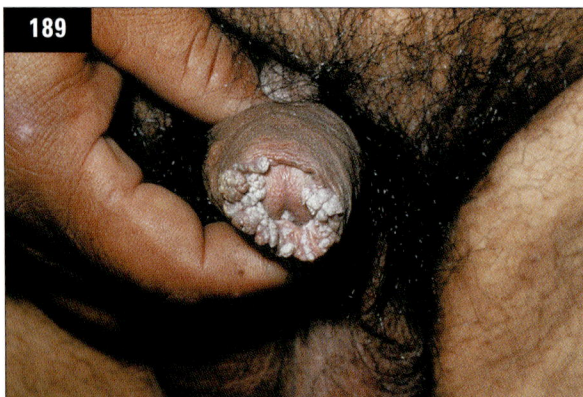

189 Condyloma acuminata. Confluent verrucous papules on the foreskin and glans.

A number of anogenital malignancies, most of which are SCC, are also caused by HPV infection. HPV is found in 70–100% of anal cancers,[178–180] in 60% of vaginal carcinomas,[181] and in 30–42% of penile carcinomas.[182,183] Pruritus is a common symptom of all of these malignancies. Vulvar, anal and penile lesions are usually characterized as sharply demarcated, slightly raised plaques with irregular borders. Pigmentation is variable from white to red to brown. Vaginal SCC appear as white, sharply demarcated multifocal plaques and are often clinically described as leukoplakia. The above-mentioned giant condyloma acuminata of Buschke and Lowenstein, attributable to HPV-6 and -11, present as large, locally destructive, exophytic tumors several centimeters in diameter.

Cervical carcinoma is the most common HPV-associated malignancy and is the second most common malignancy in women worldwide. While the vast majority of cases occur in the developing world,[184] it also remains a problem in developed countries. In the US, the incidence is 8.7 cases per 100,000 women with a mortality rate of 2.5 per 100,000.[185] HPV DNA is found in greater than 94% of all cases.[186–189] Preclinical and early lesions are usually discovered by exfoliative cytology, known commonly as the Pap smear. When Pap smears demonstrate frank atypia, colposcopy with biopsy is performed to establish a tissue diagnosis and determine if invasive carcinoma has developed.

Without treatment, the natural history of HPV infection is variable. Condyloma may regress, enlarge, or remain unchanged. Approximately 10–30% of lesions regress spontaneously within 3 months,[149,190] and the 1-year regression rate of low-grade squamous intraepithelial lesions (LSILs) is over 60%.[191] Regression of HPV infection is dependent on an intact cell-mediated immune system, however, and in those with impaired immunity, the incidence of spontaneous regression is lower.

DIAGNOSIS/MANAGEMENT

Diagnosis of condylomata acuminata is usually readily made by clinical findings alone. Entities in the differential diagnosis include seborrheic keratoses, nevi, molluscum contagiosum (MC), syphilitic condyloma lata, and pearly penile papules. Aceto-whitening is a technique that can be uses to confirm the diagnosis of condyloma acuminate and is performed by application of 5% acetic acid for 5 minutes which produces whitening of HPV-infected epithelium. False-positive results as high as 25% have been reported with this procedure,[192] however, and for this reason, it is not universally recommended. If the diagnosis remains in question, confirmatory histopathologic examination of a tissue biopsy specimen can be performed. Histopathologic findings include papillomatosis, acanthosis, elongation and branching of rete ridges, and hyperkeratosis. Diffusely disseminated large vacuolated keratinocytes with clumped keratohyalin granules known as koilocytes are also often apparent. Some cases demonstrate more subtle findings, however, with only gentle, dome-shaped papules with slight acanthosis. In cases that are difficult to diagnose, studies to search for the presence of HPV may be performed, although *in situ* hybridization studies commonly demonstrate false-negative results.

Although condylomata may be treated, eradication of HPV infection is not possible because of the surrounding subclinical infection.[193] The goal of treatment is removal of clinical lesions which may reduce transmissibility of the virus although this is controversial. Following treatment, most patients experience wart-free periods, but complete removal of anogenital warts remains difficult. All treatment modalities have a high rate of recurrence and patients usually need multiple treatments. The four main treatment options for condyloma include antiproliferative agents, destructive therapies, antiviral agents, and immunomodulators.

Podophyllotoxin is the prototype of the antiproliferative therapies. It is derived from podophyllin. Podophyllin itself is not used as frequently today as in the past, as it contains two significant mutagens and must be applied by the treating physician.[194] Podophyllotoxin, in contrast, does not contain these mutagens but has the same degree of efficacy. Its mechanism of action is by arresting cell division in mitosis by binding to microtubules.[195] It is available in a solution and a cream and can be applied by the patient at home.

Destructive modalities include cryotherapy, topical trichloroacetic acid, electrocautery, CO_2 laser treatment, and surgical excision. Regardless of modality, recurrence rates within the first 3 months after treatment are greater than 25%,[190] which is thought to be secondary to surrounding subclinical infection.[196]

Cidofovir and interferons are antiviral agents that have been used to treat condyloma acuminata, although their use in clinical practice is limited. Topical cidofovir has been used experimentally with moderate success,[197] although its use is limited by cost and difficulty in preparation. Interferons, while somewhat effective, have proven disappointing either as adjuvant or primary therapy largely because of cost and the fact that they must be administered by injection.

Imiquimod is a relatively new immunomodulatory agent that is a preferred agent for condyloma therapy. Imiquimod activates toll-like receptors on antigen presenting cells in the skin and up-regulates the cell-mediated immune response integral to HPV clearance. Recent studies have shown a significantly lower recurrence rate after therapy with imiquimod compared to other comparable therapies.[198,199] While effective in approximately 60% of cases, irritation is a potentially limiting toxicity.

Destructive modalities are preferred in pregnant patients for a number of reasons but especially due to the uncertain safety of other modalities. In nonpregnant patients, the choice of therapy is dictated by location, size, and number of lesions, patient preference, physician experience, and cost. There is a high risk for concomitant infection with HR-HPV and for that reason, patients and their partners should be given thorough genital and anal examinations including anoscopy where appropriate.

Successful treatment of anogenital neoplasia is dependent on early recognition and intervention. For low-grade squamous intraepithelial lesions (LGSILs) of the cervix, conservative therapy is appropriate while high-grade lesions are treated with excision of the transformation zone. Therapy for noncervical high-grade squamous intraepithelial lesions is site dependent. Vulvar lesions are often excised although imiquimod is being used more frequently. Vaginal lesions are also usually excised for fear of compli-cations associated with topical therapy.[200] On the other hand, surgical modalities should be avoided when possible for anal lesions as postoperative stenosis and other complications may supervene.[200] Imiqimod can be used as either primary or adjuvant therapy for ablative treatment.[201,202]

The FDA recently approved a prophylactic HPV vaccine effective against HPV types 6, 11, 16, and 18 and shortly thereafter, the Advisory Committee on Immunization Practice added the vaccine to its list of recommended vaccines.[203] The vaccine is also available in Europe, although the UK is the only country that has implemented a national vaccination program. Recent data from Europe show that widespread vaccination is currently being deployed by the countries with the lower cervical cancer rates, while those with higher rates have yet to implement vaccination.[204] In the US, the vaccine is approved for use in females aged 9–26 years. Early vaccination is imperative as the vaccine is only effective prior to development of persistent HPV infection. Given the high rate of infection with HPV in the first few years of sexual activity, vaccination of older women is of uncertain benefit, although clinical trials are underway to evaluate this. It is certain, however, that the availability of the vaccine will dramatically reduce cervical cancer among those women not already infected with HR-HPV. In fact, it is estimated that the vaccine will prevent 70% of cervical cancers in that population.[205]

IMPLICATIONS OF HIV COINFECTION

When compared with age-matched controls, HPV infections occur more often in HIV-infected patients.[206–210] These individuals are also more likely to have widespread, diffuse infections, more HPV-associated neoplasia, as well as more extensive subclinical infections compared to HIV-negative patients.[211] HIV-positive patients also tend to be infected with more HPV subtypes than HIV-negative controls.[208,212,213] The extent of HPV disease and viral shedding increases as CD4 cell count falls and there are data to suggest that HIV infection potentiates HPV replication and disease progression[166,212] as HIV influences gene transcription of HPV.[215,216]

Given the higher prevalence of subclinical, neoplastic, and diffuse infections in the HIV-positive population, it is not surprising that this same population has a higher incidence of cervical, anal, and other genital cancers. Anal cancer is the fourth highest reportable cancer in HIV-positive males[217] and cervical cancer is an AIDS-defining illness in HIV-infected individuals.[218] Patients who have a history of anal condyloma or who practice receptive anal intercourse and women with a history of abnormal Pap smear results are particularly at risk.

The morbidity and mortality associated with HPV-associated malignancies is of increasing importance since the advent of highly active antiretroviral therapy (HAART). Although gamma-herpesvirus-associated malignancies are on the decline in the era of HAART, no such decline in incidence or regression of precursor lesions has been observed for HPV-associated malignancies.[219] For this reason, aggressive screening for anal and cervical malignancies in HIV-positive patients is indicated. Full genital examinations are imperative and the CDC recommends a pelvic examination and two Pap smears in the first year after initial diagnosis of HIV infection.[32] There is no established screening routine for anal malignancies although external inspection, aceto-whitening, and anoscopy should be considered.

The number and extent of condylomata are also potentiated by the presence of HIV. HIV-positive patients may present with larger or more numerous warts and may experience more frequent recurrences following treatment.[220,221] Despite these findings, the CDC does not recommend different treatment regimens for condylomas in this patient population.[32] Given their propensity for malignant transformation, condylomatous anogenital lesions should be biopsied before therapy so that neoplastic changes can be accurately diagnosed.

MOLLUSCUM CONTAGIOSUM

DEFINITION/OVERVIEW

Molluscum contagiosum virus (MCV) is a highly infectious virus of the Molluscipox genus that is trophic for the skin and mucous membranes. MCV replicates in the stratum spinosum and induces abnormal proliferation of epithelial cells.[222–224] It occurs worldwide, although it is more prevalent in tropical climates and it afflicts children, sexually active adults, and the immunocompromised most commonly. Since the 1960s, the incidence has been rising in the US, principally as a sexually transmitted disease,[225] although its prevalence is increasing worldwide.[226,227] The majority of cases occur in patients between the ages 15 and 29 years.[225] There are four subtypes of MCV based upon DNA analysis: type I, Ia, II, and III, with the latter being extremely rare.[228–231] MCV-I is more prevalent except in HIV-positive patient populations[232] and is the etiologic agent in most childhood infections. The incidence among children exposed to swimming pools has been found to be twice that of those who do not swim in public pools.[233] Further, atopic dermatitis may predispose children to severe, disseminated infections.[234] MCV-II, on the other hand, is more often sexually transmitted and tends to infect older patients. In one study of 90 patients, MCV-II was not found in patients less than 15 years of age.[228] Infection with either subtype, however, can result in genital or extragenital lesions.

PATHOGENESIS/PATHOPHYSIOLOGY/CLINICAL FEATURES

Skin-to-skin contact is the mechanism of transmission in most cases, although autoinoculation and fomites also facilitate spread.[235] After an incubation period from 1 week to several months,[236] clinical evidence of infection first appears. Efforts to grow the organism reproducibly in cell cultures have been unsuccessful to this point, hindering study of the mechanism by which it causes disease and escapes immune detection. Clinical lesions are caused by infected keratinocytes enlarging and increasing in number and, as viral particles are extruded from cells, they coalesce producing a central aggregate of viral structures known as Henderson–Patterson

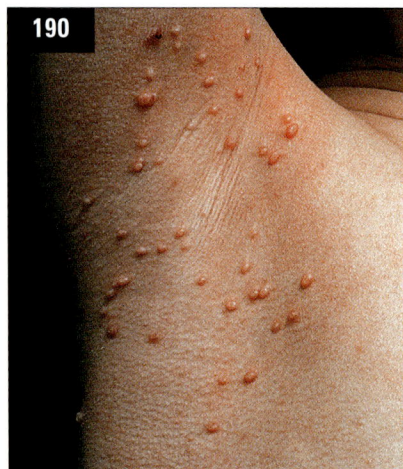

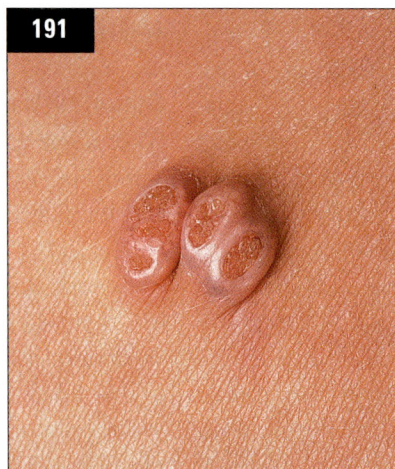

190, 191 Molluscum contagiosum. (Courtesy of St John's Institute of Dermatology [King's College], Guy's Hospital, London.)

bodies.[235] Escape from immunologic recognition is thought to be secondary to sequestration of large numbers of virions in the molluscum bodies which are sealed intracellularly by a collagenized sac-like structure.[237] Several proteins produced by MCV further impair immune function by blocking pro-inflammatory cytokines and chemotaxis of immune effector cells.[222,223] When lesions rupture, the protective barrier induced by the lesion is lost and an intense immune response develops.

The typical lesion is a small, firm, white or flesh-colored dome-shaped papule with central umbilication. They range in size from 1 mm to greater than 1 cm in diameter. In smaller lesions, the umbilication may be difficult to observe and lesions may be confused with an acneiform process. There are typically between 10 and 20 lesions which are present for months before they spontaneously resolve in most cases (**190, 191**). Individual lesions last for 2 months or more.[238] The lesions are usually limited to the skin although they are rarely noted on mucosal surfaces of the mouth[239] and conjunctivae.[240] Intertriginous regions are commonly affected sites including the groin, axillae, antecubital, and popliteal fossae. As mentioned previously, the lesions in adults are most often sexually transmitted and are caused by MCV-II. While the individual lesions of MCV-II are indistinguishable from those caused by MCV-I, they are usually located in the groin, on genital skin, on the thighs, or abdomen owing to their mode of transmission. Childhood MCV-I lesions may occur in the genital as well as extragenital regions.

An inflammatory reaction with abundant crusting around a molluscum papule is seen in approximately 30% of patients[241] which is indicative of a host immune response to the viral antigen.[242,243] In most cases, molluscum papules resolve after development of this reaction. Unusual clinical lesions may also develop when hair follicles are involved,[244] and secondary abscesses may develop following manipulation.[245] Unilateral chronic conjunctivitis has also been described with involvement of the eyelid.[246] Giant molluscum, which clinically mimics condyloma acuminata or verruca vulgaris, is a clinical variant that can be found on any part of the body.[247,248] Rarely, an id reaction has been described in association with MCV, possibly precipitated when more than 20 lesions are treated in one session.[241]

DIAGNOSIS/MANAGEMENT

The diagnosis of molluscum contagiosum (MC) is usually made on the basis of clinical examination alone, but in certain patients the diagnosis can be challenging. Use of a magnifying lens may aid visualization of central umbilication in smaller lesions. If the diagnosis remains in doubt, a smear of a scraping of a lesion examined microscopically followed application of potassium hydroxide (KOH) or by Wright or Giemsa staining (known as Tzanck preparation) is a useful bedside procedure. The molluscum bodies can be visualized by light microscopy as football-shaped oval structures with the KOH preparation or as fuschia-colored structures on Tzanck preparation. Analysis of lesions by biopsy where pathognomic molluscum bodies are readily seen can yield a definitive diagnosis. In most cases, there are tightly circumscribed groups of infected keratinocytes with numerous discrete ovoid intracytoplasmic inclusion bodies. On hematoxylin and eosin staining, the inclusion bodies are eosinophilic but basophilic at the surface. A polyclonal antibody has been developed that recognizes MCV in fixed tissue via immunohisto-chemical techniques,[249] and *in situ* hybridization for MCV DNA has also been used,[250]although these are rarely necessary.

MC is a benign, usually self-limited disease although most clinicians treat lesions to reduce the risk of spread, especially via sexual transmission, and autoinoculation. Furthermore, many patients experience pain and discomfort which is another indication for treatment. Immunocompromised individuals are also at risk for superinfection.

MC lesions can be treated identically to warts caused by HPV. Smaller lesions are commonly physically ablated by curettage, electrocautery, or cryoablation. These procedures are associated with pain and inflammation but usually leave only minimal scar. The success rate of ablative treatments has not been rigorously studied and placebo-controlled studies are lacking, although general clinical experience suggests a success rate of about 85%.[251,252] More recently, successful treatment of molluscum lesions with laser therapy has been reported.[253,254] Chemical ablation with trichloroacetic acid has also been employed and although the depth of penetrance of the agent is difficult to control and it can be associated with scarring, inflammation, and pain, good results have been reported.[255] Podophyllin has also been used although many physicians no longer recommend its use because of its limited efficacy and associated toxicity.[256,257] Retinoic acid, while not as effective as other modalities mentioned above, is a chemo-ablative agent that has the advantage in that it can be applied directly by the patient.[258] The imidazo-quinolones, of which the best characterized is imiquimod, exert antiviral activity by up-regulating Th-1 type proinflammatory cytokines, notably interferon-alpha (INF-α) and tumor necrosis factor-alpha (TNF-α).[259,260] Imiquimod is approved as a 5% cream for the treatment of perianal and genital condyloma, although there are a number of reports citing efficacy against molluscum.[261–264]

IMPLICATIONS OF HIV COINFECTION

The association between MCV and HIV was first reported in 1983 in an autopsy study of 10 patients with AIDS.[265] Since then, reports of recalcitrant, severe, and atypical presentations have been published. The incidence of MCV among AIDS patients ranges from 5–18%,[266–269] and is manifest most prominently at severely depressed levels of immune function. The appearance of multiple mollusca has been used as a clinical sign of pro-gression of HIV disease in numerous studies.[270-274] The incidence rises dramatically when CD4+ cell counts fall to <200×10^6/l.[275]

It is unclear at this point whether the appearance of mollusca in an AIDS patient is evidence of reactivation of a latent infection or represents a new infection in a vulnerable host. In an Australian study evaluating both HIV-positive and HIV-negative subjects, the incidence of antimolluscum antibodies was 23% and rose progressively with age.[276] These findings support the assertion that infection with MCV in AIDS patients represents reactivation of latent disease.[277] However, previously mentioned work showing that MCV-I is the etiologic agent of childhood infections and MCV-II afflicts only adult populations casts some doubt on this theory,[228,232] and an earlier study found that HIV-positive patients were much more likely than controls to be infected with MCV-II.[278] These findings suggest that HIV-positive patients are likely presenting with an infection acquired as an adult rather than a reactivation of a childhood infection.

There are differences in the clinical presentation of HIV-positive and HIV-negative patients. Young, healthy adults tend to develop lesions on the lower abdomen, groin, and thighs whereas HIV-positive patients tend to develop mollusca on the face and neck.[279] Ophthalmic manifestations are commonly reported including numerous and giant eyelid mollusca.[280–283] Like their HIV-negative counterparts, HIV-positive patients with MC are prone to autoinoculation. In males, shaving the beard area has resulted in severe infection.[155,284]

HIV-positive patients may also present with atypical lesion morphology. Clinical similarity with basal cell carcinoma, keratoacanthoma, abscess, furuncle, comedone, ecthyma, nevus sebaceous of Jadassohn, cutaneous horn, and syringoma has been reported.[245,285–289] While some lesions may be atypical in appearance, the classic waxy papules must be differentiated from disseminated fungal infections that afflict AIDS patients. *Cryptococcus neoformans*, *Penicillium marneffei*, and *Histoplasma capsulatum* have all been reported to mimic MCV clinically.[290–292] One case of disseminated *Pneumocystis carinii* infection was also reported to simulate MC.

The higher prevalence of atypical mollusca and the fact that lesions may be simulated by serious infections often necessitate diagnosis by biopsy in HIV-positive patients. Microscopic and ultrastructural features of MC are identical in HIV-negative and HIV-positive patients,[277,293] although viral particles in skin adjacent to the molluscum lesions have been observed in HIV-positive patients and have only rarely been observed in immunocompetent hosts.[294,295]

Unlike HIV-negative hosts, molluscum shows minimal or no tendency to regress in HIV-positive patients without treatment. Furthermore, lesions are notoriously recalcitrant to treatment.[296] Curettage[297] is commonly used, and daily application of topical tretinoin is a useful adjunct.[280] Trichloroacetic acid peels and interferon, both lesional and systemic, have both been used with moderate results.[255,298,299] There are also several reports of resolution of lesions following application of topical imiquimod 5% cream.[262,300] Laser therapy has also been used successfully and is another treatment option for recalcitrant lesions in this population.[254,301,302] Cidofovir is an antiviral agent commonly used to treat CMV retinitis and when applied topically, it has been shown to be effective in clearing mollusca in HIV-positive patients.[303,304] Mucosal erosions are a common side-effect.[305] Most lesions develop in patients with low CD4+ counts; institution of HAART, which is associated with diminution of HIV viral load and increase in CD4+ cell number, has been shown to decrease the number of lesions.[283,306,307] However, at least one study showed that this effect was minimal as the prevalence of molluscum among HIV-positive patients receiving HAART was 5.78% *vs.* 2.63% for patients not receiving antiretroviral therapy (p<0.03).[308] Thus, while HAART may result in resolution of molluscum lesions in some patients, in others it may have only minimal effect.

HUMAN HERPESVIRUS-8

Human herpesvirus-8 (HHV-8), originally known as Kaposi's sarcoma-associated herpesvirus owing to its original discovery in Kaposi's sarcoma (KS) of AIDS patients,[309] is associated with KS but also other malignancies including primary effusion lymphoma[310] and the plasma cell variant of Castleman's disease.[311,312] Although the biology of HHV-8 is incompletely understood, transmission of the disease appears to be sexual in the US and western Europe. A complete review of HHV-8 is found in Chapter 12 Cutaneous Neoplastic Manifestations of HIV Disease.

SCABIES AND PEDICULOSIS

Scabies, a common parasitic infestation worldwide, is caused by the mite *Sarcoptes scabiei*. Worldwide prevalence is estimated to be 300 million,[313] and it is seen in all socioeconomic groups. It is particularly problematic in the developing world where most affected patients are under the age of 15 years.[314] Studies in the 1970s indicated that most cases were family household infections brought to the home by children or adolescents,[315,316] although since then, a great number of cases have been reported in elderly care facilities. Transmission is via skin-to-skin contact, making sexual transmission common (**192**). A complete review of scabies in the HIV patient is found in Chapter 5 Cutaneous Manifestations of Parasitic Infections in HIV/AIDS.

Phthirus pubis louse infestation of the pubic hair, is another common parasitic infestation of sexually active individuals.

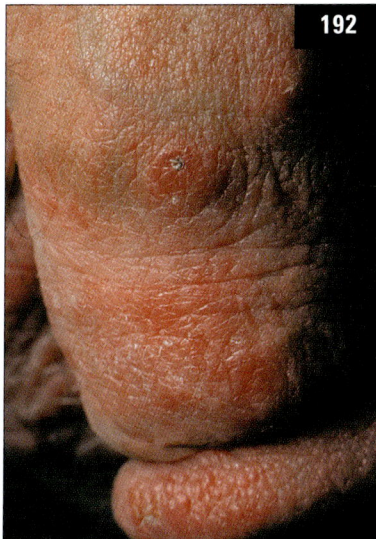

192 Scabies infestation. Erythematous papules and nodules on the penile shaft.

HEPATITIS C VIRUS

DEFINITION/OVERVIEW

Hepatitis C virus (HCV) is a RNA virus with at least six major genotypes and more than 90 subtypes[317] that was discovered in 1989.[318] Over 70% of infected persons in the US are infected with genotype 1. The virus is endemic worldwide and has a prevalence estimated by the WHO to be 2% or 123 million people as of 2004.[319] A recent study of the prevalence in the US from 1999–2002 estimated it to be similar at 1.6% or 4.1 million people. The peak prevalence in this study occurred in ages 40–49 years, and 48.4% of seropositive individuals reported a history of intravenous drug use (IVDU). While IVDU was the strongest identified risk factor for HCV infection, 20 or more lifetime partners was also a risk factor underscoring the potential for sexual transmission of the virus.[320] While sexual transmission does occur, it should be noted that it is much less efficient than other sexually transmitted viruses. Recent studies indicate in particular, that transmission among long-term monogamous couples is extremely rare.[321,322]

Parenteral injections with reuseable glass syringes is a major source of infection in resource-poor countries with an estimated 2–5 million cases of HCV being attributed to unsafe injections.[323,324] The use of disposable syringes has eliminated this problem in the western world and the reported risk of transmission from needlestick is likewise low at 1–3%.[325,326]

PATHOGENESIS/PATHOPHYSIOLOGY/CLINICAL FEATURES

After a mean incubation period of 6–8 weeks,[327,328] a minority of acutely infected patients, 25–40%, will manifest symptoms.[329] Of note, the average time from exposure to seroconversion is 8–9 weeks leading to the possibility of onset of symptoms prior to seroconversion.[330] The symptom complex of acute infection is similar to that of infection with hepatitis A or B, i.e. malaise, fatigue, anorexia, abdominal pain, jaundice, myalgias, and a morbilliform eruption. The course of acute HCV infection is characterized by elevated serum hepatocellular enzyme levels. Of acutely infected individuals, 75–85% will be unsuccessful at clearing the infection and will progress to chronic disease.[331–333] Fulminant hepatic failure, however, is rare.[334,335]

Chronic infection causes chronic mild inflammation of the liver evidenced by persistent or fluctuating alanine transferase (ALT) levels observed in 60–70% of chronically infected individuals.[327,328,336] The course is often insidious progressing without signs or symptoms for the first two or three decades after infection. Eventually, the cyclic inflammation, necrosis, and apoptosis lead to fibrosis and nodular regeneration known as cirrhosis of the liver. Progression to cirrhosis is slow although factors increasing the rate of progression are male gender, longer duration of infection, immune suppression such as that caused by HIV, concomitant HBV infection, ethanol abuse, and obesity.[337–342] After 20–30 years of infection, the risk of cirrhosis is 2–20%; once cirrhosis develops, the risk of hepatocellular carcinoma is 1–4% per year.[342,343] Evidence of late disease includes spider angiomata, palmar erythema, jaundice, splenomegaly, esophageal varices, ascites, and hepatic encephalopathy.

While hepatocytes are the primary site of infection, there is a growing body of evidence suggesting that HCV can efficiently replicate in extrahepatic tissue leading to a variety of extrahepatic clinical manifestations.[344] Extrahepatic disease in HCV is actually quite common and in one large prospective study, 74% of patients reported at least one extrahepatic clinical manifestation.[345] HCV is associated with number of dermatologic diseases including lichen planus (LP), porphyria cutanea tarda (PCT), mixed cryoglobulinemia, and the more recently described necrolytic acral erythema.

The association between HCV and LP is controversial with a reported prevalence of LP among HCV patients varying from 0.1% to 35%.[346–351] Data are similarly conflicting concerning the prevalence of anti-HCV antibodies among patients with LP. Two French studies failed to find any link between the two diseases,[352,353] while studies conducted in Japan,[354] the US,[355] and Germany[356] reported a significantly higher rate of HCV in LP patients versus control. It has been postulated that HCV may not be the actual cause of LP, rather acting as a triggering factor.[357]

Sporadic PCT shows a much stronger association with HCV. Evidence of HCV is present in 62–100% of patients presenting with PCT,[358–363] whereas the rate of HCV positivity in controls was less than 5%. It is therefore recommended that all patients presenting with sporadic PCT be tested for HCV.[364] It has been hypothesized that liver disease caused by HCV triggers PCT in susceptible individuals.[364]

The association between mixed cryoglobulinemia and HCV is well established. It is reported to occur in 35–45% of patients with chronic HCV infection.[365] Only a minority of those affected, however, develop clinical evidence of systemic vasculitis including palpable purpura, neuropathy, urticaria, or Raynaud's phenomenon.[365] Cryoprecipants in symptomatic patients are found to be composed of HCV RNA, anti-HCV antibodies, and HCV particles at 20–1000 times greater than levels measured in the serum.[366–368] The mechanism by which HCV induces these cryoprecipitants remains to be elucidated. Intermittent purpura of the lower extremities is the most common presentation and is the result of immune complex deposition in the dermal capillaries. The severity of the purpura correlates with the level of HCV viremia but not the level of serum cryoglobulins. Skin biopsy confirms the presence of leukocytoclastic vasculitis. Cutaneous vasculitis responds well to antiviral therapy with pegylated interferon and ribavirin.[369,370]

Necrolytic migratory erythema is a relatively newly described cutaneous manifestation of HCV infection and presents as crusted, hyperpigmented plaques present primarily on the acral surfaces of the arms and legs. Clinically there are similarities with pellagra and other deficiency syndromes, although histologically there is an interface dermatitis that demonstrates similar features to erythema multiforme or graft-versus-host disease. It resolves when the underlying HCV is treated with interferon.

DIAGNOSIS/MANAGEMENT

The initial laboratory test for diagnosis of HCV is enzyme immunoassay (EIA) for anti-HCV antibodies which detects anti-HCV in at least 97% of infected patients.[330] EIA carries a low positive predictive value due to the overall low prevalence of the disease,[371,372] so that supplemental testing with a more specific assay is used on samples with positive EIA results to eliminate false-positive results.[373]

Diagnosis of HCV can also be made based upon nucleic acid amplification techniques such as RT-PCR. HCV RNA can be detected in the serum as soon as 1–2 weeks after exposure, before elevation of liver enzymes is observed. Most RT-PCR assays have a lower limit of detection of 100–1000 copies of RNA and with optimization of the assay, approximately 75–85% of anti-HCV positive patients and greater than 95% of patients with chronic liver disease will test positive for HCV RNA.

HCV-positive patients should be evaluated for the presence and severity of chronic liver disease.[374] Given the fluctuating nature of ALT levels in chronic disease, evaluation for the presence of liver disease should include multiple serial measurements of liver enzymes. Most, if not all, patients are treated with antiviral regimens although it is especially important if the patient is deemed to be at risk for the development of cirrhosis.[374] Those at risk include patients with persistently elevated ALT levels, detectable HCV RNA, and a biopsy showing at least moderate inflammation and fibrosis.

Therapy for chronic HCV is a combination of IFN-α and ribavirin. Response rates for combination therapy are 40–50%, significantly higher than with interferon alone which are 15–25%.[375,376] However, response rates for infection with genotype 1, the most prevalent genotype in the US, remains poor at less than 30%.[330]

IMPLICATIONS OF HIV COINFECTION

The epidemiologic association between HIV and HCV is well established. Of the estimated one million Americans living with HIV, it is estimated that 300,000 have concomitant HCV. This parallels the 30% prevalence of HCV in HIV-infected persons. Ironically, with the introduction of HAART, the prognosis for HIV patients has improved dramatically and consequently, the liver disease caused by chronic HCV has become an important source of long-term morbidity and mortality.[377]

Infection with HIV is thought to facilitate the heterosexual transmission of HCV, an otherwise rare event as described above. It is postulated that the increased HCV viral load in HIV-positive patients may enhance sexual transmission,[130,378,379] particularly when other STDs are present. Furthermore, the recent report of a cluster of acute HCV cases in patients with LGV and HIV seems to lend support to the increased homosexual transmission rate of HCV among HIV-positive patients. In one study, HIV-infected patients who seroconverted to HCV-positive, practiced unprotected receptive anal intercourse and anal fisting.[132]

There is a growing consensus that HCV has a negative effect on the progression of HIV. One study found HCV to be associated with faster progression of HIV, greater numbers of opportunistic infections, and increased mortality when compared with those infected with HIV alone.[380] Further studies demonstrate faster progression to AIDS and death in HCV-infected than non-HVC-infected HIV patients when both groups were treated with similar HAART regimens.[380–383] Conversely, HIV is thought to worsen the course of HCV as HIV/HCV-coinfected patients demonstrate fibrotic liver changes that progress to cirrhosis more frequently as well as progression at a faster rate.[384–386]

Owing to the mutually deleterious effect on prognosis for HCV and HIV, most experts argue that all coinfected individuals should receive HCV treatment.[387] Coinfected individuals are treated with the standard therapy for HCV which is pegylated interferon and ribavirin. Studies from monotherapy with interferon showed that response to treatment was similar as long as the CD4 count was relatively well preserved.[388,389]

HEPATITIS B VIRUS

DEFINITION/OVERVIEW

Hepatitis B virus (HBV) is a member of the Hepdnaviridae family, a family of viruses showing a strong preference for infecting liver cells. HBV virions are double-shelled particles 40–42 nm in diameter.[390] The outer lipoprotein shell contains three glycoproteins or surface antigens,[391] while within the envelope is the core containing the viral genome, a 3.2kb duplex strand of DNA, and a viral polymerase. The HBV genome has four reading frames from which a number of proteins are generated, most importantly, a surface antigen (HBsAg), a core antigen (HBcAg), and HBeAg. HBeAg has an immunomodulatory role, the mechanism of which remains largely unknown.

HBV infects over one million people worldwide and is particularly prevalent in Asia, Africa, southern Europe, and South America where vertical or horizontal transmission are the most common. Infection in childhood or infancy correlates with a greater likelihood for development of chronic disease.[392] Childhood and vertical transmission have been virtually eliminated in the US by a comprehensive vaccination program instituted in 1991.[393] Prior to institution of the program, approximately 30–40% of chronic infections were believed to result from perinatal or childhood transmission, even though less than 10% of reported cases of hepatitis B occurred in children less than 10 years old.[394] Over the years 1990–2004, coincident with vaccination, the incidence of acute hepatitis B declined 75% and the incidence among children and adolescents declined 94%.[395]

While a dramatic decline in vertical and childhood transmission in North America and western Europe was observed, transmission of the disease sexually and through IVDU remains problematic.[392] Notably, among the reported cases of HBV in the US from 1990–2002, the number of heterosexuals reporting multiple sexual partners increased from 14% to 29% and the number of self-identified MSM rose from 7% to 18%. Coincident with this, the total incidence of HBV was 8064 in 2002.[396] Further support for the importance of sexual transmission comes from a study of heterosexual women without other risk factors which found that seroprevalence of HBV among women with fewer than five sexual partners in the preceding 4 months was 5% while there was a 31% prevalence in women with more than five partners.[397] In additional studies, acquisition of HBV has been associated with male homosexual activity, prostitution, and having sex under the influence of drugs.[397–400] Thus, it is increasingly apparent that HBV is a disease of unvaccinated adults with high-risk behaviors.

PATHOGENESIS/PATHOPHYSIOLOGY/CLINICAL FEATURES

HBV preferentially infects hepatocytes although it is not directly cytotoxic. There are many asymptomatic HBV carriers with minimal liver injury yet who demonstrate extensive intrahepatic viral replication.[401] Rather than the virus itself causing damage, the host immune response to viral antigens determines the extent of hepatocellular injury. Consistent with this notion is the observation that immunodeficient individuals show minimal liver injury but high rates of viral carriage.[402] The type of immune response appears to correlate with the natural history of infection. Acute self-limited hepatitis correlates with strong viral-specific T cell responses in peripheral blood,[403] whereas chronic infection is associated with an attenuated T cell response. Vigorous antibody production occurs in either case and the presence of persistent circulating immune complexes in chronic infections is a contributing factor in the pathogenesis of extrahepatic manifestations.[404] In self-limited infections, mice studies have shown that both liver injury and viral clearance are not directly mediated by the cytotoxic T cells but are due to by-products of the immune response including TNF, free radicals, proteases,[405] as well as natural killer T cells.[406]

Primary HBV infection can be either symptomatic or asymptomatic. A serum sickness-like prodrome develops in 20–30% of infected patients,[404,407] and is manifest by arthropathy, proteinuria, hematuria, and angioedema. Characteristic skin findings include urticaria and necrotizing vasculitis which result from deposition of immune complexes composed of HBsAg, C3, IgM, or IgG antibodies.[408,409] Urticaria, if present, may be associated with a transient hypocomplementemia.[410]

Polyarteritis nodosa (PAN) is also associated with

HBV infection,[411,412] and tends to occur weeks to months after the acute episode[413] in approximately 2 out of 500 cases.[414] It has been suggested that half of all cases of PAN are associated with HBV.[404] It is a systemic disease that affects the small and medium sized vessels of many different organs most notably the kidneys and CNS. Common presenting complaints include arthralgias, fever, malaise, mononeuritis, and renal disease. Skin lesions only develop in 10–15% of cases[410] and include nodules, livedo, urticaria, ulcerations, or acral gangrene.[404]

Like hepatitis C, chronic HBV infections predispose patients to mixed cryoglobulinemia. Presenting signs and symptoms include weakness, purpura, arthropathy, and renal disease.[415,416] Histologic examination of skin biopsy specimens reveals necrotizing vasculitis.[404] Cryoprecipitates are composed of IgM, IgG, HBsAg, and HBsAb.[415,417]

Several other skin conditions have been reported to be associated with HBV infection including erythema nodosum,[418] LP,[419,420] leukocytoclastic vasculitis,[421] pyoderma gangrenosum,[422] and a dermatomyositis-like syndrome.[423] In pediatric patients with HBV, papular acrodermatitis of childhood has also been described.[417,424]

In most cases, HBV infection is generally self-limiting with viral clearance and immunity from reinfection.[425,426] Approximately 5% of infections in healthy adults result in persistent infection with continual viremia and intrahepatic replication of the virus. Those with abnormal histologic liver features on biopsy and elevated liver enzymes in the presence of viremia have chronic HBV infection, while those without histologic or laboratory abnormalities are carriers. Nodular cirrhosis develops in 20% of patients.

Serologic evidence of hepatitis B infection, in the form of HBsAg antigenemia, is detectable after a 4–10 week incubation period. Presence of anti-HBc, or core antibodies, follows shortly after the appearance of HBsAg. Antibodies are of IgM type in acute infection.[425] HBeAg becomes detectable in most cases and animal models indicate that presence of this antigen is associated with infection of 75–100% of hepatocytes.[427] The observed high rate of infectivity during acute infections[428] is not surprising given the extent of infection. Liver injury in acute infection occurs after the establishment of viremia, indicative of the time needed to mount an immune response to viral antigens. Once the host mounts a T cell-mediated immune response, viral titers begin to fall. Clearance is associated with a fall in HBsAg, HBeAg, and appearance of anti-HBs.

In persistent infection, HBsAg titers do not fall and viral replication continues. Typically, levels of viremia are much lower than in the primary infection although persistent HBeAg is associated with high viral load and high infectiousness.[429] HBsAg usually persists for life although levels decline. HBeAg may disappear from the blood along with appearance of anti-HBe, and seroconversion to anti-HBe correlates with a reduction in viremia as large as five orders of magnitude.[430] Ongoing immune attack in persistent infection is successful at controlling levels of infection but incapable of eradicating it.

Chronically infected patients have a risk of developing hepatocellular carcinoma that is 100 times that of noncarriers.[431] The risk is even higher in the HBeAg positive subset of chronic carriers.[432] The cellular and molecular mechanisms by which HBV causes hepatocellular carcinoma are incompletely understood.[433–435]

DIAGNOSIS/MANAGEMENT

Diagnosis of acute or chronic HBV infection requires serologic testing. HBsAg is present in both acute and chronic infections. The presence of IgM antibody to hepatitis core antigen (IgM anti-HBc) is diagnostic of acute or recently acquired infection, while antibody to HBsAg is indicative of either a cleared infection or immunization. Presence of HBsAg with positive total anti-HBc and negative IgM anti-HBc is diagnostic of chronic infection.[32]

There is no specific therapy for acute HBV infection and treatment is supportive. For chronic HBV infection, the CDC recommends referral to a specialist experienced in the management of chronic liver disease.[32] Goals of therapy are reduction of viremia and restoration of hepatic function although treatment is not indicated for all HBV carriers. The increased risk of hepatocellular carcinoma in HBeAg-positive carriers is a clear indication for treatment. By contrast HBeAg-negative chronic carriers without elevation of liver enzymes enjoy a good prognosis and are rarely offered treatment. Regardless, true cure of chronic infection occurs infrequently with treatment. Markers of treatment success include loss of HBeAg, seroconversion to anti-HBe-positive, and reduction of viral load.[405] The treatment markers for HBeAg-negative chronic hepatitis have not yet been agreed upon.

Administration of 5–10 million units of IFN-α subcutaneously three times per week for at least 3 months has long been the standard of care. Response rate with this therapy is approximately 30%.[436] Treatment is contraindicated in advanced liver disease as a flare in liver injury is often seen with therapy and clearance of the virus may precipitate overt liver failure.

Lamivudine is one of a class of drugs that directly inhibits viral replication by targeting viral reverse transcriptase. It was first developed for the management of HIV infection but a fall in HBV viremia was observed in both HIV-positive and HIV-negative patients.[437,438] Treatment is associated with rapid fall of HBV DNA, loss of HBeAg, seroconversion to anti-HBe-positive, and normalizing of liver enzymes within the first 3 months. Lamivudine is not immuno-modulatory and is not contraindicated in advanced liver disease.[439] Induction of viral resistance is the main limitation of lamivudine monotherapy. Adefovir and tenofovir are approved by the FDA and both show efficacy even against lamivudine-resistant HBV.[440–443]

IMPLICATIONS OF HIV COINFECTION

Of the estimated 40 million people infected worldwide with HIV, approximately 2–4 million are estimated to be chronically infected with HBV.[444] This estimate is based largely upon high prevalence of chronic HBV infection in sub-Saharan Africa which accounts for 65% of HIV cases worldwide. Prevalence of chronic HBV infection in this region is high because of the high rates of perinatal and childhood transmission which are associated with high rates of chronic carriage as described above. Since sexual exposure accounts for most cases of HBV infection in developed countries, rates of chronic carriage are much lower. However, rates of chronic HBV infection among HIV-positive individuals may be tenfold higher than background prevalence.[444] Among HIV-positive individuals in the US and western Europe, rates of chronic HBV carriage range from 6–14% .[445–447]

There are different explanations offered for the increased prevalence of HBV in HIV-positive indivuals. Individuals that are HIV-positive at the time of HBV exposure are at higher risk for becoming chronic carriers.[448–453] On the other hand, individuals previously exposed to HBV who then become immunosuppressed secondary to HIV infection may experience reactivation of previous HBV infections that are anti-HBs-positive.[452,454,455] There is also evidence that HIV-infected individuals who are exposed to HBV are more likely to have a high viral replication rate and remain HBeAg-positive for a longer period of time, thereby increasing HBV transmissibility.[448,453]

HIV immunosuppression may reduce liver damage as a result of attenuating the immune response to HBV;[448,453] however, HIV infection may exacerbate liver disease. Recent studies suggest that HIV–HBV coinfected individuals are at increased risk of dying from liver failure and that the risk increases with induction of HAART.[446] There have been further reports of hepatotoxicity[456] and reactivation[457] of HBV infection when using HAART.

Occult HBV infection, defined by the presence of HBV DNA in the absence of HBsAg, is being increasingly detected in HIV-positive individuals worldwide.[458–460] This finding has obvious implications for diagnosis and screening for HBV.

As in HIV-negative patients, lamivudine is the drug of choice in HIV-positive patients as HIV-seropositive patients do not respond well to IFN.[448,453] Further, lamivudine displays activity against both HBV and HIV and should be considered for inclusion in the HAART regimen of any coinfected individual.[453]

CHAPTER 14

ORAL AND OCULAR MANIFESTATIONS OF HIV INFECTION

Robert H. Cook-Norris, Antoanella Calame, and Clay J. Cockerell

ORAL LESIONS

INTRODUCTION

There is a number of oral manifestations of human immunodeficiency virus (HIV) infection, many of which may be the first clinical indicators of infection and some may predict progression of HIV disease to acquired immunodeficiency syndrome (AIDS). Therefore, knowledge and proper identification of these lesions are critical as they may be determinants of opportunistic infection, they may be used in staging and classification systems, and they may be used to monitor disease progression as well as response to therapy. Oral lesions that have been strongly associated with HIV infection include oral candidiasis, linear gingival erythema, necrotizing ulcerative gingivitis, necrotizing ulcerative periodontitis, oral hairy leukoplakia, Kaposi's sarcoma (KS), and non-Hodgkin's lymphoma (NHL).[1] These lesions have been documented in up to 50% of HIV-positive individuals and up to 80% of individuals with AIDS[1] and their frequency tends to be correlated with decreasing CD4 count and increasing viral load.[2] When presenting in individuals of unknown HIV status, they are strong indicators of HIV infection[3] and are often used as entry or end-points in determining prophylaxis and therapy.[2,4]

The advent and now frequent use of highly active antiretroviral therapy (HAART) in HIV-infected individuals has decreased the prevalence of oral candidiasis, oral hairy leukoplakia, and HIV-associated periodontal disease in adults.[5–7] The same trend has not been documented in children receiving HAART, however.[8,9] Interestingly, increased preva-lence of benign human papillomavirus (HPV)-associated oral lesions and HIV-associated salivary gland disease have been observed[5,6,10] and the prevalence of KS has remained unchanged.[5,11]

OPPORTUNISTIC INFECTIONS: FUNGAL INFECTIONS

ORAL CANDIDIASIS

Oral candidiasis is an opportunistic, superficial fungal infection that is a feature of primary HIV infection[12] and is commonly found in late-stage disease of patients progressing to AIDS.[13–16] The species most commonly isolated in HIV-infected individuals with low CD4 counts is *Candida albicans* although other species have been documented, albeit less frequently.[17] Since *C. albicans* is part of normal flora, infection is an indicator of immunosuppression. As would be expected, declining CD4 counts are correlated with an increased prevalence of oral candidiasis.[1,18,19] Epidemiologic studies have documented that 43–93% of individuals with AIDS have oral candidiasis.[20] Oral candidiasis presenting in HIV-infected individuals receiving HAART is a clinical marker of immune failure and, although it is strongly associated with HIV infection, it is also seen in xerostomia, diabetes, antibiotic and steroid use, with other medications, as well as in other immunosuppressive conditions.[21]

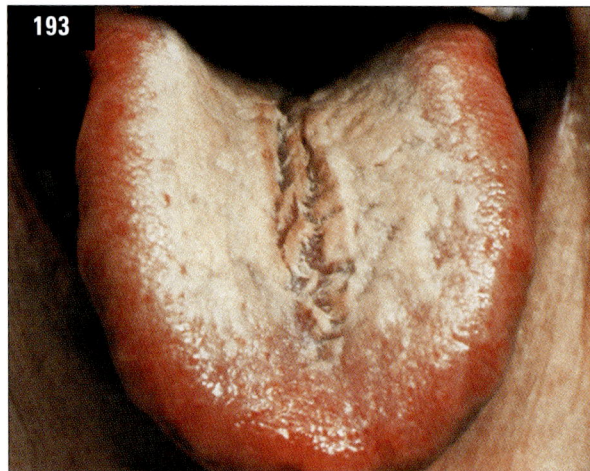

193 Pseudomembranous candidiasis of the tongue.

Four major types of oral candidiasis have been described in HIV-infected individuals: pseudomembranous candidiasis, erythematous (atrophic) candidiasis, hyperplastic candidiasis, and angular cheilitis. Pseudomembranous candidiasis, commonly called thrush, presents on the oral mucosa as white to yellow removable curdlike plaques (**193**). Upon wiping, an erythematous often bloody base is revealed. Symptoms include oral discomfort and dysphagia.[22] The presence of this lesion in HIV-infected individuals indicates progression to AIDS.[23,24]

Erythematous candidiasis, as the name implies, appears clinically as red macules that are most commonly located on the surface of the palate and dorsal tongue.[25] Lesions on the tongue may have associated depapillated areas. This form is often asymptomatic and not readily apparent on gross examination, but close examination typically reveals the subtle findings. Despite the subtle clinical appearance, detection is crucial because when present in an HIV-infected individual, it is predictive of progression to AIDS.[24]

The hyperplastic type of oral candidiasis is characterized by thick white plaques of the buccal mucosa that, unlike pseudomembranous candidiasis, are not removed with scraping. Compared to immunocompetent individuals who commonly have this form of candidiasis on the oral commissures, HIV-infected individuals rarely have lesions in this location.[20]

Angular cheilitis is seen regularly in the elderly but when seen in a young individual, it may indicate HIV infection. In angular cheilitis, prominent cracks, fissures, and/or ulcers are noted on the oral commissures. On close inspection small white plaques may be seen. This form of candidiasis can occur alone or in conjunction with the other types.

The diagnosis is usually easily made based on the characteristic clinical appearance, especially in the pseudomembranous type and angular cheilitis. If the lesion is not characteristic, as is often the case in the erythematous and hyperplastic forms, diagnosis is aided by simple tests such as a smear from the lesion. Smears examined histologically after being treated with potassium hydroxide (KOH) or stained with periodic acid-Schiff (PAS) usually reveal fungal hyphae. Although culture is helpful in determining the species involved, it is usually not necessary. Biopsy with histologic examination is occasionally performed for the hyperplastic form, due its similarity to other diseases.[25]

The associated pain, burning, and dysphagia are often relieved by the use of topical or systemic antifungal agents.[26] Topical medications include clotrimazole oral troches (10 mg, 1 tablet five times a day) and nystatin oral pastille (200,000 units, 1–2 pastilles five times/day). Topical antifungal creams (miconazole cream, clotrimazole cream, keto-conazole cream) are useful in the treatment of angular cheilitis. Systemic therapy has the advantage of once daily dosing but has the potential to interfere with other systemic medications. Some of these include fluconazole (100 mg, 1 tablet taken for 7–14 days)[27] and ketoconazole (200 mg, 1–2 tablets taken with food for 7–14 days) as well as itra-conazole and amphotericin B.[25] Fluconazole, although more expensive, does not require gastric acidity and therefore avoids the ineffectiveness occasionally seen with ketoconazole due to poor absorption in individuals with hypochlorhydria or other gastrointestinal problems.[22] When possible, topical therapy is preferred due to the emergence of systemic antifungal-resistant organisms.[28]

OTHER OPPORTUNISTIC FUNGAL INFECTIONS

Several other less common opportunistic oral fungal infections have been reported in HIV patients includ-ing histoplasmosis,[29–32] cryptococcosis,[33,34] and aspergillosis.[35] When presenting in a HIV-infected individual these conditions indicate severe immuno-suppression and disseminated disease. Oral involve-ment typically presents clinically as nonspecific mucosal ulceration, so that diagnosis is established by biopsy and histologic examination utilizing special stains to identify fungal micro-organisms as well as by cultures. Treatment consists of systemic antifungal agents that have shown to have activity against the organism identified (see Chapter 4).

VIRAL INFECTIONS

ORAL HAIRY LEUKOPLAKIA

Oral hairy leukoplakia (OHL) represents a manifes-tation of Epstein–Barr virus (EBV) infection that was first described in HIV-infected individuals. It has since been reported to occur in non-HIV-infected individuals, especially immunosup-pressed transplant recipients, albeit rarely.[36–38] Its appearance in an HIV-infected individual indicates progression to AIDS.[1,39,40] Greenspan and Greenspan documented that of 155 HIV-seropositive patients with OHL, 30% progressed to AIDS in 36 months, 47% did so by 2 years, and 67% by 4 years.[41]

OHL (**27, 28**) presents almost exclusively on the lateral tongue as white irregular plaques with a corrugated to 'hairy' surface that does not rub off in contrast to pseudomembranous candidiasis. Often, only one lesion is present. In known HIV-infected individuals, the clinical appearance is usually diagnostic.[39,42] If the patient's HIV status is unknown and/or if the diagnosis is not clear on examination, a biopsy is useful to distinguish it from other white oral lesions including lichen planus, frictional keratosis, idiopathic leukoplakia, geographic tongue, hyperplastic candidiasis, and white sponge nevus.[43]

Histologic examination (**29**) reveals a corrugated, hyperkeratotic, acanthotic epidermis with prominent clumps of enlarged prickle cells that resemble koilocytes and only a sparse superficial infiltrate.[21, 22] *In situ* hybridization demonstrates EBV deoxyri-bonucleic acid (DNA) within epithelial cells and confirms the diagnosis. Infected cells demonstrate a perinuclear clear halo and a nucleus with peripheral chromatin clumping. These characteristic changes are not only seen on routine hematoxylin and eosin stained permanent specimens but also on a mucosal smear of scraped lesion tissue stained with hema-toxylin and eosin or Papanicolau stain.[25]

Treatment is generally not necessary; however, the patient may desire therapy for cosmesis and/or discomfort. Oral acyclovir therapy typically results in lesion regression but it usually recurs once therapy is discontinued.[44] Other therapies that have been used with variable success include topical application of podophyllin resin,[45] topical application of desciclovir[46] and oral zidovudine.[47] However, some authors have reported lesion clearance followed by recurrence with zidovudine therapy.[48] Topical tretinoin, applied daily for 1–2 weeks has also been proposed as an effective treatment.[49]

HERPES SIMPLEX

Oral mucosal ulceration due to herpes simplex virus (HSV) is common in HIV-infected individuals.[50,51] HSV has been found in up to 9% of individuals with AIDS and in 29% of those with the AIDS-related complex.[52] Immunosuppressed individuals, in contrast to those with an intact immune system, tend to develop extensive, persistent, painful, superficial ulcers that are most commonly located on the palate (**194**) but have been reported to occur anywhere in the oral cavity.[24,53–55] In HIV-infected individuals, spontaneous resolution is uncommon. Furthermore, HSV-associated ulcers that are refractory to treatment suggest immunodeficiency, and persistence over 1 month in a known HIV-infected individual is considered an AIDS-defining opportunistic disease.[56]

The diagnosis can be made from viral culture of early lesions, from examination of smears of lesions that reveal multinucleated epithelial giant cells, and/or response to antiviral treatment.[24,57] If need be, more accurate confirmation can be obtained by a culture, by positive monoclonal antibody test, by histologic examination of a biopsy, or by immuno-fluorescence techniques.[21]

Standard treatment consists of oral administration of acyclovir 200 mg, five times a day. If no response is seen after 3–5 days, a higher dose is indicated, i.e. 800 mg, five times a day. Topical acyclovir is ineffective in treating intraoral HSV infection[58] and acyclovir-resistant lesions are becoming increasingly common.[59,60] Lesions that fail to respond to acyclovir should be cultured to confirm the etiology and once verified as acyclovir-resistant HSV, intravenous foscarnet at a dose of 40 mg/kg, three times a day or 60 mg/kg, twice daily should be initiated as soon as possible. If therapy with foscarnet fails, intravenous cidofovir or vidarabine may be effective. Lesions reoccurring at the same site should be treated with high-dose oral acyclovir or intravenous foscarnet, while recurrence of disease at a different site should be initially treated with standard-dose oral acyclovir 200 mg, five times a day.[61]

HUMAN PAPILLOMAVIRUS

Human papillomaviruses (HPVs), with over 100 genotypes, are well-known causes of viral-induced oral lesions in immunosuppressed individuals (**195**). Oral HPV lesions in HIV-infected individuals are

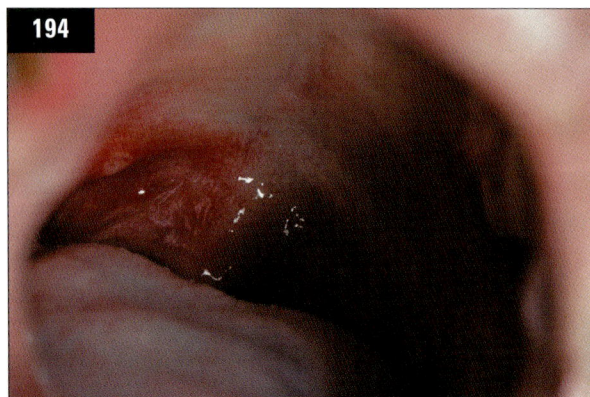

194 Herpes simplex virus infection with ulceration of the palate.

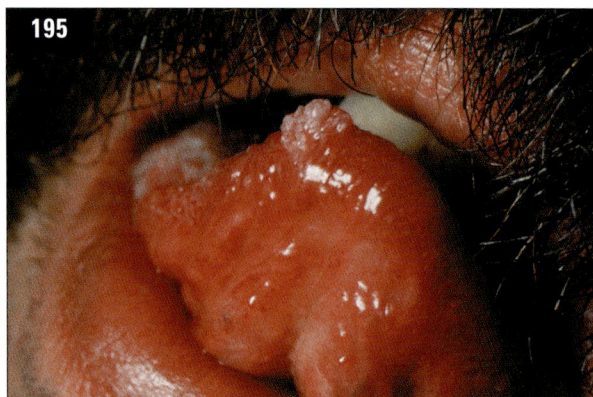

195 Mucosal verruca on the tip of the tongue.

often multiple and may appear exophytic, papillary, or flat.[25] Papillomatous lesions are commonly due to HPV-7, a subtype commonly found in the warts of butchers.[62] Oral flat warts, also called focal epithelial hyperplasia, are associated with HPV-13 and -32.[63,64]

The clinical appearance of multiple papillary lesions is often diagnostic. Histologic examination reveals a characteristic pattern of acanthosis, an increased granular cell layer, and epithelial koilocytosis. Further confirmation is achieved by identification of HPV-infected epithelial cells using immunofluorescence or immunoperoxidase stains.

Treatment options include excision, cryosurgery, electrosurgery, application of podophyllin resin and imiquimod for lesions that are primarily cutaneous.[25] In HIV-infected individuals, HPV lesions tend to recur no matter which treatment is used.

OTHER VIRAL INFECTIONS

HIV-infected individuals may experience other viral infections such as herpes zoster (HZ) and cytomegalovirus (CMV). Oral HZ is the result of latent varicella virus reactivation resulting in a painful prodrome followed by grouped vesicles distributed in a dermatomal distribution. Many HIV-seropositive individuals with HZ develop AIDS within a relatively short time, i.e. 23% within 2 years and 46% within 4 years.[65,66] Treatment, consisting of high-dose acyclovir 4 g/day as tablets, or intravenous at 10 mg/kg every 8 hr, is essential to prevent ocular lesions. Ocular lesions due to HZ are termed herpes zoster opthalmicus and are discussed in further detail in the ocular section in this chapter.[22]

CMV-induced oral ulceration is a rare cause of ulceration that may occur anywhere in the mouth including the gingiva.[67–70] The ulcers are often clinically similar to those caused by HSV so that biopsy or viral culture is required to make a definitive diagnosis. The presence of CMV-induced oral ulceration represents disease progression to AIDS.[22] Treatment with ganciclovir or foscarnet is indicated.

BACTERIAL INFECTIONS

NECROTIZING ULCERATIVE PERIODONTAL DISEASE

Necrotizing ulcerative periodontal disease (NUPD) represents an aggressive form of periodontal disease that is distinctly different from periodontal disease seen in immunocompetent individuals. NUPD is characterized by painful gingival ulceration and rapid loss of the bone supporting the teeth.[71] This represents a bacterial infection from gingival flora and while the causal bacteria may be identical to those causing periodontal disease in immunocompetent individuals,[72] a recent study found a difference in the cause of periodontal disease in these two groups.[73] Proper management includes early intervention with local debridement and administration of systemic antibiotics such as metronidazole, penicillin, and tetracycline.

BACILLARY ANGIOMATOSIS

Bacillary epithelioid angiomatosis (BA) is a manifestation of *Bartonella henselae* or *B. quintana* infection that presents as violaceous papulonodular lesions most commonly on the skin and occasionally the oral cavity.[74] Oral BA is characterized by blue to purple macules or papules most commonly of the palate and gingiva. Overlying exudate and ulceration have been described in a few cases.[74] Constitutional symptoms such as fever, chills, headache, and malaise are often present and are clinically helpful in establishing the diagnosis. Distinction from KS can be very difficult and a biopsy is often needed. Histologic examination reveals lobular vascular proliferations and a moderate neutrophilic infiltrate containing argyrophilic microorganisms that can be visualized with a silver stain such as the Warthin–Starry stain (**40–42**). Polymerase chain reaction (PCR) can also be performed which allows precise identification of the organism. Erythromycin at a dose of 250–500 mg four times/day is considered first-line treatment although ceftazidime, ciprofloxacin, doxycycline, and azithromycin have also been reported to be effective.[74]

NECROTIZING STOMATITIS

Necrotizing stomatitis is characterized as chronic ulceration of the periodontal mucosa that results in destruction of the soft tissues as well as the bone (196). Several authors have proposed a bacterial cause of the process and, recently, symbiotic overgrowth with fusiform bacteria and *Borrelia* spirochetes has been implicated.[75] Interestingly, a histopathologic study of 18 cases in HIV-positive individuals revealed a prominent infiltrate of histiocytes[76] suggesting that much of the destruction seen in ulcerative stomatitis represents an immune response to pathogens. Local debridement in conjunction with antibiotics and topical corticosteroid therapy have both been reported as effective therapies.

OTHER BACTERIAL INFECTIONS

Several other, less common, bacterial infections with oral manifestations have been reported in HIV-infected individuals.[25] These include infection with *Mycobacterium avium intracellulare*, *Myocobacterium tuberculosis*, *Klebsiella pneumoniae*, *Enterobacter cloacae*, *Actinomyces israelii*, and *Escherichia coli*. Diagnosis typically requires biopsy and tissue culture. Treatment with antibiotics should be targeted to the specific micro-organism identified by culture.

NEOPLASMS

KAPOSI'S SARCOMA

As previously discussed in Chapter 12 (Cutaneous Neoplastic Manifestations of HIV Disease), KS represents a vascular neoplasm resulting from KS-associated herpesvirus or human herpesvirus-8 infection in the presence of immunosuppression and cytokine-induced growth. In HIV-infected individuals, the oral mucosa is frequently the initial site of involvement, occurring as the initial site in 22% of cases in one series.[77] The palate and gingiva are the two most common oral locations.[25] KS lesions are typically reddish to purple macules or papules that range from a few millimeters up to several centimeters in size (197, 198). Occasionally, KS behaves quite aggressively, growing rapidly and interfering with swallowing and/or breathing. The diagnosis is made by clinical inspection and histologic examination which reveals a proliferation of spindle-shaped cells and prominent slit-like vascular spaces with extra-vasated red blood cells and hemosiderin deposits.

KS may be treated successfully with radiation, systemic chemotherapy, intralesional chemotherapy, and injection with sclerosing agents.[25] In a recent study examining the efficacy of intralesional vinblastine or 3% sodium tetradecyl sulfate for the treatment of oral KS, no difference in efficacy was identified.[78] Surgical excision can also be a useful adjunct to therapy. Good

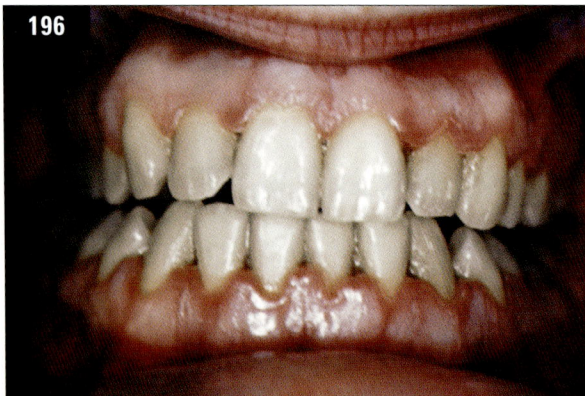

196 Necrotizing stomatitis. (Courtesy CDC/ Minnesota Department of Health, R.N. Barr Library; Librarians Melissa Rethlefsen and Marie Jones.)

oral hygiene consisting of professional teeth cleaning and oral rinsing with chlorhexidine, is necessary to prevent secondary infection which may mimic HIV-associated periodontitis.[21,25]

NON-HODGKIN'S LYMPHOMA

Of the lymphomas associated with HIV-infection, NHL is the most common and the only type having documented oral manifestations.[20] Intraoral NHL may be the presenting sign of this malignancy and it does not necessarily indicate disseminated disease. Plasmablastic lymphoma, a type of NHL, has recently been documented in up to 3% of HIV-infected individuals.[79] Oral lesions of NHL are quite variable and no consistent clinical pattern has been identified[25,80,81] although they often appear as necrotic or ulcerated tumors or plaques or as non-ulcerated areas of firm painless swelling with overlying normal-appearing mucosa.[20] Diagnosis is made on the basis of biopsy with histologic examination. Treatment consists of systemic chemotherapy in conjunction with HAART.[25]

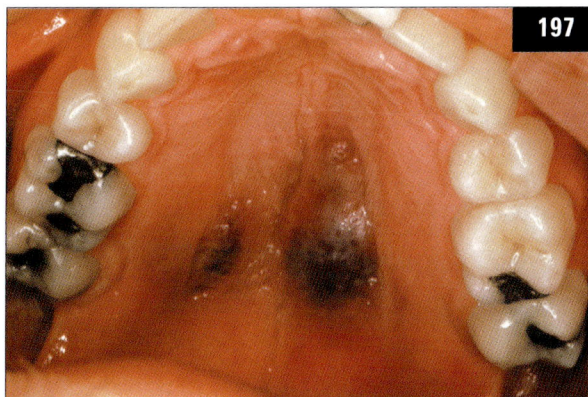

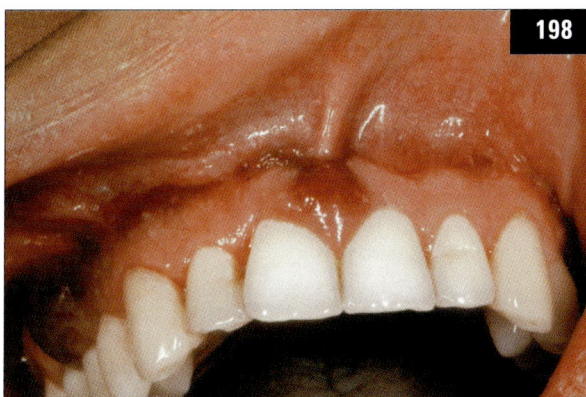

197, **198** Oral Kaposi's sarcoma. Violaceous nodules on the palate (**197**) and gingiva (**198**).

OTHER ORAL LESIONS

APHTHOUS ULCERS

Three distinct forms of aphthous ulceration have been documented in HIV-infected individuals: minor, major (**199**), and herpetiform. The most common type is minor aphthous ulcers, also known as canker sores, which occur on nonkeratinized oral mucosa.[25] Minor aphthous ulcers are painful, ill-defined, round, yellowish to white ulcers that are generally less than 1 cm in diameter. The cause of these ulcerations is unknown and to date, no causative organisms have been identified. It is generally accepted that these lesions are the result of cell-mediated immunity-induced mucosal destruction.[25] Although commonly seen in immunocompetent individuals, minor aphthous ulcers in HIV-infected individuals tend to be more severe and more frequently recurrent. The diagnosis is made based on the characteristic clinical appearance with or without biopsy to exclude other entities that may simulate them. Treatment consists of application of topical corticosteroid preparations, especially gels, coupled with supportive care such as the use of gargles and topical anesthetic agents.

Major aphthous ulcers, also known as Sutton's disease and periadenitis mucosa necrotica recurrens, are by definition larger than 1 cm in diameter and are often deeper and tend to last longer than minor aphthous ulcers.[25] They are commonly located in the posterior oropharynx. The clinical appearance may resemble other oral lesions so that a biopsy is often required to establish the diagnosis as well as to exclude other conditions. Standard therapy consists of application of topical corticosteroid agents and occasionally administration of systemic prednisone for recalcitrant lesions. Second-line treatment includes oral administration of thalidomide as well as other immunomodulators.[82,83]

Herpetiform aphthous ulcers appear as small 1–2 mm ulcers which resemble those seen in primary HSV infection.[25] However, unlike primary HSV infection there are no associated systemic symptoms, cervical lymphadenopathy, or painful gingivitis. Corticosteroid oral rinse solution and tetracycline suspension have both been reported as effective in the management of this form of aphthous ulceration.[25]

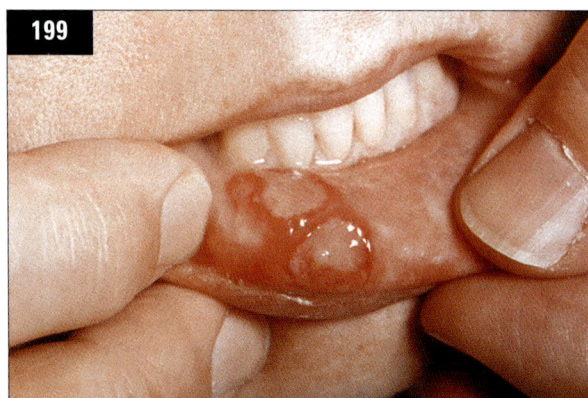

199 Major aphthous ulcer. (Courtesy CDC/ Robert E. Sumpter.)

LINEAR GINGIVAL ERYTHEMA

Linear gingival erythema is characterized by a well defined erythematous band along the gingival margin.[42,84] Its cause remains unknown although it is distinctly different from typical gingivitis, in that the erythema does not regress after removal of local irritants such as dental plaque. This lesion has been associated with oral candidiasis although it does not respond to antifungal therapy.[25] Clinical surveillance is warranted as it may progress to the more severe rapidly destructive conditions NUPD and necrotizing stomatitis.[84]

MUCOSAL MELANIN PIGMENTATION

HIV-infected patients may present with one to multiple melanotic macules of the oral mucosa. The cause remains unclear but some cases are the result of zidovudine therapy.[85] Treatment is not necessary.

ORAL MANIFESTATIONS OF HIV INFECTION IN CHILDREN

As in HIV-infected adults, children infected with HIV are also prone to developing opportunistic infections. Orofacial lesions commonly seen in HIV-infected children include oral candidiasis, HSV infection, linear gingival erythema, parotid enlargement, recurrent oral ulceration, and, less commonly, HZ and OHL.[1,86–88] Oral candidiasis is the most common of these, occurring in 67% of HIV-positive children.[1] Oropharyngeal candidiasis in children is strongly associated with failure to thrive, low CD4 counts, and the subsequent development of AIDS.[89] Parotid enlargement, on the other hand, is a predictor of positive prognosis and long-term survival in HIV-infected children.[1] HIV-infected children receiving HAART, compared to untreated controls, have a lower prevalence of oral lesions and, as would be expected, the prevalence increases as the CD4 cell count drops.[90]

OCULAR LESIONS

With the advent of HAART, ocular manifestations of HIV infection have become less common. Prior to HAART, 70–80% of HIV-infected individuals experienced HIV-associated eye disorders at some point during their illness.[91] Ocular complications still affect approximately 25% of untreated HIV-positive patients,[92] so that it is important to be aware of these manifestations as they may be the presenting sign of HIV infection.

HERPES ZOSTER OPHTHALMICUS

HZ involving the ophthalmic distribution of the trigeminal nerve is termed herpes zoster ophthalmicus (HZO) and is suspected when there is a painful eruption of tense, grouped, vesiculobullous lesions on the tip of the nose (Hutchinson's sign). HZO affects approximately 5–15% of untreated HIV-infected patients.[92] It is observed in immunocompetent elderly individuals commonly and in this setting it does not generally warrant further work-up; however, HZO presenting in individuals under 50 years of age is uncommon and suggests immunosuppression. In HIV-infected individuals, HZO occurs more frequently when the CD4 count drops below $200 \times 10^6/l$.[92] Ocular complications associated with HZO include acute retinal necrosis,[93] keratitis, scleritis, uveitis, retinitis, and optic neuritis.[92]

Treatment for HIV-infected individuals includes a 1-week course of intravenous acyclovir at a dose of 10 gm/kg every 8 hours followed by oral acyclovir at a dose of 800 mg five times a day for maintenance therapy.[92] Famciclovir, another antiviral approved for the treatment of HZO, offers the advantage of decreased dosing as it is administered in a dose of 500 mg three times a day and is equally effective.[94] Valacyclovir has also been reported as equally effective;[95] however, reports of valacyclovir-associated thrombocytopenic purpura and hemolytic uremic syndrome in HIV-positive individuals warrant caution when using this medication in these patients.[96]

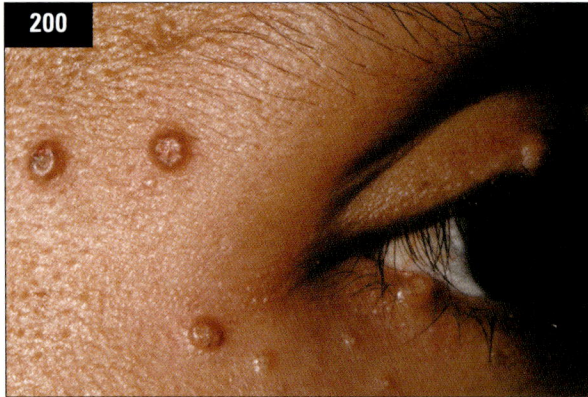

200 Molluscum contagiosum on the eyelids in a patient with advanced HIV disease and trichomegaly of eyelashes.

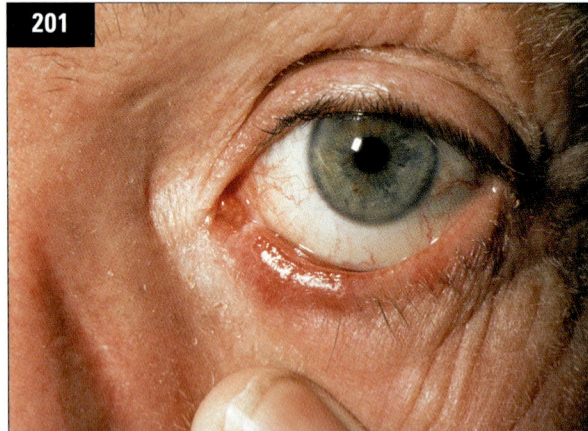

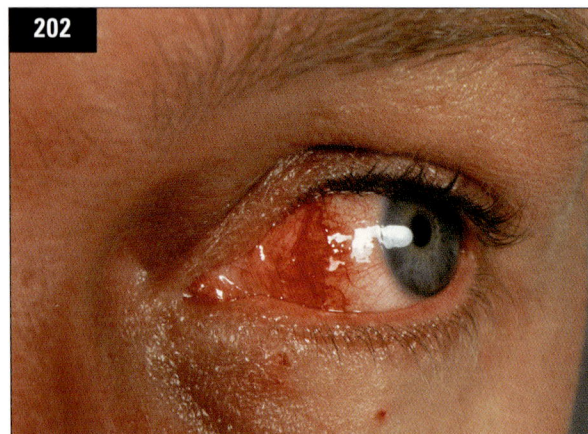

201, 202 Ocular Kaposi's sarcoma. Erythematous to violaceous plaque on the lower eyelid (**201**). Erythematous conjunctival plaque and conjunctival injection mimicking subcorneal hemorrhage (**202**).

MOLLUSCUM CONTAGIOSUM

Molluscum contagiosum (MC), a contagious manifestation of poxvirus infection, presents with multiple well defined umbilicated papules on the skin and mucous membranes. In HIV-infected individuals, MC is more common and tends to be more severe, presenting as multiple, large, rapidly growing umbilicated papules. An inverse relationship between CD4 count and the number of MC lesions has been observed.[97] MC involves the eyelids in up to 5% of HIV-infected patients (**200**), and MC of the conjunctiva has also been reported, albeit rarely.[92] MC can be treated with cryotherapy,[98] excision and curettage, or incision of the papular dome.[92] In one study, photodynamic therapy in conjunction with 5-aminolevulinic acid resulted in a substantial reduction in lesion count and severity in six patients.[99]

KAPOSI'S SARCOMA

As discussed previously, KS is a vascular proliferative condition that affects up to 25% of HIV-seropositive patients.[92] Of those individuals with KS, approximately 20% have eyelid or conjunctival involvement[100] (**201, 202**). At times, these lesions may be difficult to identify. KS on the eyelid may mimic a chalazion. Lesions involving the conjunctiva can be mistaken for subconjunctival hemorrhage. As with KS of the skin, BA may also simulate KS and should be suspected if there is a history of prior systemic *Bartonella* infection or cat-scratch disease.[92]

As stated by Brun and Jakobiec,[100] the appropriate therapeutic modality should be selected based on the overall clinical scenario, including the individual's general health, extent of disease, degree of morbidity and discomfort, and the size of the lesions to be treated. Treatment options include local radiation therapy, local cryotherapy, intralesional chemotherapy with vinblastine, and surgical excision. Radiation therapy is effective at treating both focal eyelid and conjunctival lesions. Surgical excision is often reserved for conjunctival lesions due to the prominent bleeding associated with excision of lesions on the eyelid. Small lesions of the eyelid may also respond to cryotherapy, intralesional vinblastine, or intralesional interferon-alpha.[92] Ocular lesions associated with systemic KS are best treated with systemic chemotherapy.

RARE OCULAR NEOPLASMS

HIV-infected individuals appear to be at increased risk for the development of squamous cell carcinoma (SCC) of the eyelid and conjunctiva. In one study, the relative risk for conjunctival SCC associated with HIV infection was documented to be 13:1.[101] There is good evidence suggesting that these lesions are associated with HPV infection[102] although a recent study failed to detect HPV DNA in lesions.[103] It is likely that multiple cofactors are involved, including HPV coinfection and ultraviolet light. The recommended treatment of ocular SCC is surgical excision.[92]

NHL of the eyelid is a rare manifestation of AIDS.[104] NHL, as previously discussed, is more common and tends to be more aggressive in HIV-infected individuals, but ocular lesions appear to be extremely uncommon. NHL is treated with radiation.

INFECTIOUS KERATITIS

Corneal infections occur in less than 5% of HIV-infected individuals but may result in permanent vision loss.[105] Keratitis may be due to viral, bacterial, fungal, or protozoal infections. The two most common viral causes of infectious keratitis (IK) are the varicella-zoster virus (VZV) and HSV.[106] Keratitis due to VZV occurs in up to 50% of HIV-positive patients in association with HZO, and may also occur in the absence of the cutaneous vesicular eruption (herpes zoster sine herpete).[107,108] Keratitis due to these two viral agents tends to be both more severe and more resistant to treatment in HIV-infected individuals. Treatment of VZV-associated keratitis consists of oral acyclovir at the dose used to treat HZO. HSV-associated keratitis responds to lower doses of oral acyclovir (400 mg five times a day) or famiciclovir (125–500 mg three times a day).[106] Often, long-term therapy is needed for complete clearing.

TRICHOMEGALY OF THE EYELASHES

Trichomegaly, or hyperthrichosis, of the eyelashes is relatively uncommon and, when present, tends to occur in the late stages of HIV infection[92] (200). The cause is unknown but has been postulated to be the result of elevated viral titers, drug toxicity, or poor nutrition. A recent study found no correlation between eyelash length in HIV-positive patients and CD4 cell count, viral load, and AIDS case criteria.[109] If the long lashes become bothersome they can be trimmed.

PRESEPTAL CELLULITIS

Preseptal cellulitis caused by *Staphylococcus aureus* is relatively common in HIV-seropositive patients and is not unexpected given that HIV-infected individuals carry *S. aureus* in their nares twice as often as normal individuals.[92] The infection results in periorbital swelling and must be differentiated from orbital cellulitis which carries a worse prognosis.[110] Preseptal cellulitis typically clears with a 10-day course of oral penicillinase-resistant penicillin such as methicillin, although more cases are caused by methicillin-resistant strains which require treatment with other agents such as vancomycin.[92] Failure to respond to therapy warrants hospitalization, evaluation for sinus infection, and possibly administration of intravenous antibiotics.

ORBITAL MANIFESTATIONS

Orbital manifestations affect less than 1% of HIV-infected patients and when present are associated with serious complications.[92] Patients with orbital involvement may complain of orbital pain, blurred vision, and/or diplopia. Physical signs include ptosis, proptosis, erythema, decreased extraocular movement, decreased vision, and an afferent papillary defect. Orbital cellulitis and NHL are the two most commonly encountered orbital complications of AIDS.[92] *Aspergillus* is the most common organism to be identified among HIV-infected individuals with orbital cellulitis, although several other microorganisms have also been reported.[92,106] Standard therapy for orbital cellulitis consists of systemic antibiotics and surgical debridement as indicated. As previously discussed, NHL is treated with radiation and KS is treated with chemotherapy.

OCULAR MANIFESTATIONS IN CHILDREN

Compared to adults, children are less likely to have ocular manifestations of HIV infection. The overall rate of ophthalmic involvement in HIV-infected children is approximately 35%. CMV retinitis is one of the most common findings, as are nonpurulent conjunctivitis and MC.[111] Children with ocular manifestations are at increased risk for developing central nervous system manifestations including HIV-associated neurodevelopmental delay[112] and AIDS-associated embryopathy. Fetal AIDS-associated embryopathy is a rare condition that is characterized by downward slanting eyes, prominent palpebral fissures, hypertelorism, and blue sclera.[113] HIV-infected children with or without visual symptoms or signs should be seen by an ophthalmologist for an ophthalmic screening examination.[92]

CHAPTER 15

HAIR AND NAIL MANIFESTATIONS OF HIV INFECTION

Gabriela M. Blanco, Frankie G. Rholdon, and Clay J. Cockerell

Infection with human immunodeficiency virus (HIV) may result in a variety of hair and nail changes, some of which may be the initial manifestation of the disease. Having detailed knowledge of the spectrum of hair and nail alterations is important as it may provide a clue in the diagnosis of HIV infection and prompt earlier treatment.

HAIR ABNORMALITIES

°Diffuse hair loss is the most common hair disorder in HIV-1 infected patients, occurring in almost 7%.[1] Many different forms of alopecia may be seen in these patients including telogen effluvium,[2] drug-induced alopecia,[3] alopecia areata,[4] diffuse 'involutional' alopecia,[5,6] alopecia with hair straightening,[2] and loose anagen hair syndrome.[7] Many of these and other HIV-related hair disorders are associated with advanced disease states and thus may serve as valuable markers of disease progression.

TELOGEN EFFLUVIUM

DEFINITION/OVERVIEW

Telogen effluvium, which presents as an acute to subacute diffuse noninflammatory alopecia, is the most common type of HIV-related hair loss.[8,9] The affected hairs have their anagen phase terminated abruptly and move into telogen phase prematurely, which is manifest clinically as shedding of hair. Telogen effluvium has been commonly described in advanced stages of HIV infection so that it is a potential marker of HIV progression.[2,7] However, it may also be the initial clinical feature of HIV infection and in several patients, telogen effluvium has led to early diagnosis.[8]

PATHOGENESIS/PATHOPHYSIOLOGY

The causes of telogen effluvium are multiple and frequently involve HIV infection itself, other acute and chronic infections, or medication. Other factors that may cause or potentiate telogen effluvium include protein and caloric malnutrition, deficiencies in copper, zinc, and selenium, other immunologic disturbances, and endocrine dysregulation.[2] It is assumed that apoptosis may play a role in the pathogenesis of telogen effluvium due to the characteristic histopathologic findings of apoptotic keratinocytes seen on biopsy. Barcaui *et al.* proposed the HIV-1 protein Vpr as causing stem cell apoptosis.[9] The etiology of telogen effluvium is likely to be multifactorial in HIV-positive patients making it challenging to manage effectively.

Antiretroviral agents deserve special mention as they have become increasingly common triggers of alopecia. Indinavir has traditionally been the most common culprit,[10–13] although treatment with lopinavir plus ritonavir[14] and the multidrug regimen of stavudine, lamivudine, and efavirenz[15] has also

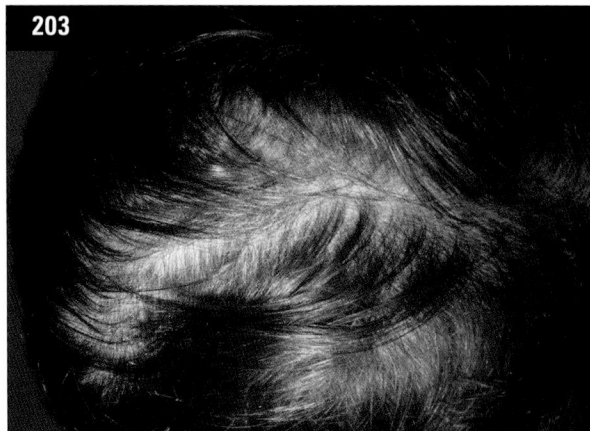

203 Diffuse hair loss consistent with telogen effluvium.

been reported to cause diffuse hair loss. Indinavir is presumed to induce alopecia via retinoid-like effects due to homologies between the amino acid sequences of the retinoic acid-binding protein and the catalytic site of HIV-1 protease, the target site of indinavir.[16] The similarity of the side-effects of indinavir and retinoids, which include hair loss, cheilitis, xerosis, and paronychia, further suggest an association. Antiretrovirals other than indinavir are thought to induce alopecia through a process similar to immune reconstitution syndrome.

Clinical features

Telogen effluvium is characterized by diffuse alopecia with a relatively even distribution of hair loss over the entire scalp (203). It usually does not become clinically evident until 25–50% of total hair loss has occurred. Associated hair findings have been noted, including finer and straighter hair as well as an increased tendency for broken hairs.[2] These changes are more common in black patients. Constitutional symptoms such as fever and weight loss from under-lying conditions are frequently observed, as most forms of telogen effluvium have been described following serious infections.[17] Hair shedding is typically seen 6 weeks to 3 months after the precipi-tating event and the hair usually regrows after the triggering insult is removed.[18] However, the hair loss may become progressive in the setting of recurrent bouts of opportunistic infections.[7] Telogen effluvium

may be the initial clinical feature of HIV infection although it generally occurs in advanced stages of the disease with CD4 counts $<200 \times 10^6/l$.[2,7,8] In a prospective study of 1161 HIV-positive patients, there was a higher prevalence of alopecia in women.[5]

Telogen effluvium is most commonly seen during the course of such diseases as syphilis, lymphoma, seborrheic dermatitis, nodular prurigo, and psoriasis.[8]

Histopathology

A scalp biopsy shows an increased number of follicles in the telogen phase with minimal inflammation. Having more than 15–25% of follicles in telogen phase is considered abnormal as this represents a significant shift from anagen to telogen. The most characteristic findings in HIV-induced alopecia are the presence of apoptotic keratinoyctes in the outer sheath at bulge level,[2] but these findings may not always be seen.[8] Some cases may demonstrate a sparse inflammatory infiltrate but this is secondary or coincidental as the process is not primarily inflam-matory in nature.

Diagnosis

Telogen effluvium is diagnosed through the combination of a detailed medical and drug history, scalp inspection, hair pull tests, direct examination of the hair shaft, and microscopic analysis of the hair. Common triggers that may serve as clues to the diagnosis include recent diagnosis of HIV or other chronic infection and a history of administration of one or more new medications, particularly anti-retroviral drugs. HIV-induced alopecia is usually accompanied by systemic symptoms such as fever, whereas drug-induced alopecia presents with hair loss and no accompanying symptoms.[12,17] A scalp examination helps determine if the hair loss is diffuse and nonscarring. Sometimes hair loss is not evident on clinical examination alone and the hair pull test is more important. The hair pull test is performed by grasping 25–30 hairs between thumb and forefinger and gently pulling, repeating the process on different areas of the scalp six to eight times. If more than five to six club hairs per clump are removed, active telogen effluvium is recognized. Club hairs are the morphologically distinct telogen phase hairs which to the naked eye show a rounded-up, bulbous, white end and on microscopic analysis look like a club.[19] This constellation of findings is usually conclusive enough to provide a diagnosis of telogen effluvium. If scalp biopsies are taken, they reveal an increased telogen phase count with minimal inflammation.

MANAGEMENT

Telogen effluvium usually resolves on its own when the precipitating event is removed. However, hair regrowth may take anywhere from 6 to 12 months. In the case of HIV, recurrent infections secondary to the immunosuppressive state as well as the HIV infection itself may create a chronic form that is difficult to treat.[7] The hair loss may improve with antiretroviral treatment.[8] If it is drug-induced, discontinuation of the drug and replacement with another in its class or switching to another equipotent agent may resolve the hair loss.[12,14] Topical agents such as minoxidil may be beneficial in enhancing hair regrowth. Providing psychologic support is critical due to the negative impact hair loss can have on self-esteem and quality of life for the patient. Patients should be counseled that telogen effluvium is potentially reversible and does not lead to total scalp hair loss[20] but that patience is required to achieve a full cosmetic effect.

ALOPECIA AREATA

DEFINITION/OVERVIEW

Alopecia areata (AA) is a focal, nonscarring alopecia of the scalp and/or body (204–206). It can be seen with the loss of eyebrow, eyelash, axillary, or pubic hair.[21] More severe forms include total loss of scalp hair (alopecia totalis) and total loss of scalp and body hair (alopecia universalis). There have been several cases published describing the occurrence of alopecia areata with HIV infection.[4,6,7,21–24] However, while AA is associated with advanced immunodeficiency,[25] there is no direct correlation between AA and decreased CD4 counts.[6]

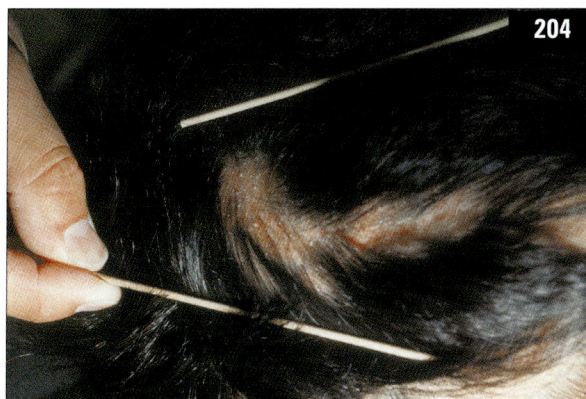

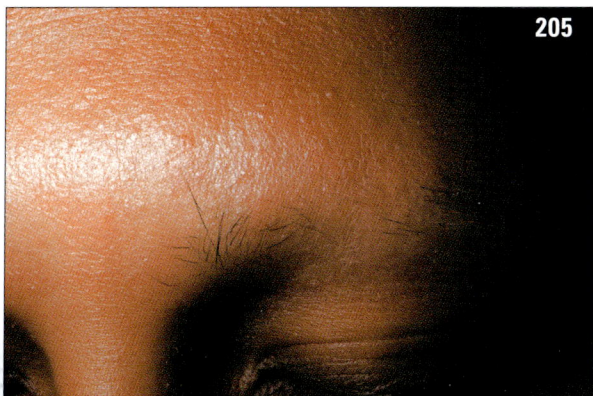

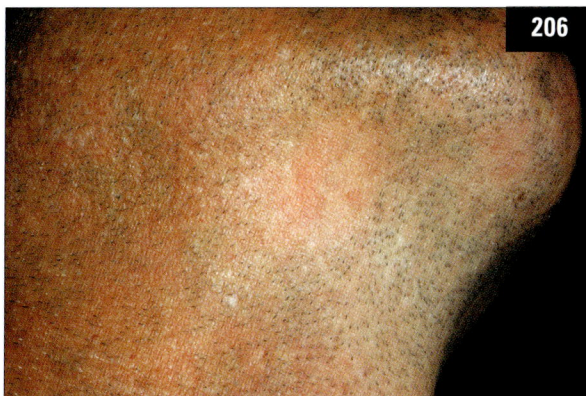

204–206 Alopecia areata. Patchy hair loss on the scalp (204), eyebrows (205), and beard (206).

PATHOGENESIS/PATHOPHYSIOLOGY

The etiology of AA is unknown although it is presumed be a form of autoimmune disease.[26–28] Several theories have been developed in efforts to explain its cause. Most authors consider AA to be a cell-mediated immune dysfunction as immune system alterations that have been reported in association include a decreased total number of helper T cells and a decreased ratio of helper T cells to suppressor T cells. It is thought that in affected patients, HIV infection itself may induce this change in the balance of helper to suppressor T cells, resulting in an influx of CD4+ lymphocytes into the areas around the anagen hair follicles.[21,29] The inflammation terminates the anagen stage shifting the hair follicles into the catagen and telogen stage prematurely. In contrast to the theory of systemic immune dysfunction causing AA, an organ-specific hypothesis has been offered. This proposes that the HIV attacks the hair follicle bulbs directly and secondarily causes an immune-mediated response that leads to alopecia.[24] Hair loss is therefore the result of an 'appropriate' immune action to HIV-infected follicles. Finally, there is a hypothesis that suggests that changes in the humoral arm of the immune system are responsible for the association between HIV infection and AA. This proposes that the virus causes generalized polyclonal B cell activation and that these activated B cells react with self-antigens located in the anagen stage hair follicles.[24] While the ultimate cause of AA is unknown, many suspect that genetic predisposition also plays an important role.[30]

Although drug-related alopecia is usually associated with telogen effluvium, a few cases of AA have been clearly associated with the institution of highly active antiretroviral therapy (HAART). Zidovudine (azidothymidine, AZT), lamivudine, and indinavir have also been reported to induce AA in HIV patients.[10,31,32] Whether the drugs themselves or immune reconstitution explains this remains to be determined.

CLINICAL FEATURES

AA is characterized by the sudden onset of focal, nonscarring hair loss, with spontaneous remissions and exacerbations. Various patterns of AA are identifiable: patchy, diffuse, totalis, universalis, and ophiasis. Patchy hair loss is the most common presentation, appearing as well demarcated 1–4 cm oval and round patches most commonly on the scalp.[33,34] Body hair such as eyebrows, eyelashes, beard, axillary, and pubic hair may also be affected. Diffuse AA refers to a decrease in the density of hair over the entire scalp. Alopecia totalis is 100% loss of scalp hair. Alopecia universalis is 100% loss of scalp and body hair. Ophiasis refers to a band-like pattern of hair loss in the parietal and temporal scalp area. This pattern of hair loss is rarely reported in HIV-seropositive patients. Alopecia lesions may be isolated or numerous and the scalp is normal in color and morphology. Typically the hair loss in AA is abrupt and asymptomatic but some patients report intense burning, itching, tenderness, and pain.[35] The periphery of the patch of alopecia has a distinctive border and may have the pathognomonic 'exclamation point' hairs. These short, broken hairs have a broad distal end and a tapered proximal end. Hair pull tests may be positive, that is six or more hair shafts removed with slight pulling, at the border of the patch indicating active disease. Nail dystrophy, especially nail pitting, is commonly associated with AA in non-HIV-infected patients.[34,36,37] However, nail changes are not commonly seen in association with AA in patients with HIV infection, perhaps since many of these patients tend to have other nail disorders as manifestations of HIV infection.

HISTOPATHOLOGY

The most characteristic histologic feature of AA is a peribulbar and intrabulbar inflammatory infiltrate of lymphocytes around the anagen follicles. The infiltrate consists predominantly of T lymphocytes and has been likened to a swarm of bees. There are also eosinophils and mast cells in the infiltrate, although less commonly.[21,27,30] As a result of the inflammation, a decreased number of anagen follicles and an increased number of catagen and telogen follicles are seen. In acute lesions, there is 'synchroniziation' of the follicular cycles of multiple follicles with many follicles being shifted into catagen simultaneously. Noninflammatory changes have also been reported, including miniaturization of hair follicles, reduced numbers of follicles, matrix degeneration, and increased numbers of follicular stelae.[21,30] Horizontal sections provide follicular counts that can help make the diagnosis of AA when a biopsy is taken between acute episodes and the characteristic inflammatory infiltrate is absent.[30,38]

DIAGNOSIS

AA is usually readily diagnosed clinically although a confirmatory scalp biopsy is sometimes necessary when the clinical presentation is ambiguous. For example, when the hair loss in AA is in a diffuse pattern, it may mimic telogen effluvium or so-called 'involutional' alopecia. The differential diagnosis of AA includes telogen effluvium, anagen effluvium, trichotillomania, and 'moth-eaten' alopecia of syphilis.

MANAGEMENT

While therapy is usually effective, some patients elect to receive no treatment as some cases resolve spontaneously, whereas others are refractory and it may require multiple injections or other long-term therapy which may be problematic for these individuals.[39] If medical treatment is attempted, it is directed at reducing the inflammation at the base of the hair follicle and involves the use of corticosteroids and immunomodulators. A wide variety of regimens is available and they are tailored to the age of the patient and the severity of hair loss (*Table 12*).

Table 12 Treatment options for alopecia areata

AGE AND SEVERITY	TREATMENT OPTIONS
Children <10 years old	Topical corticosteroid +/– minoxidil Anthralin Cosmetic aids
Children >10 years old and adults Patchy, focal AA (<50% involvement)	*Intralesional corticosteroid Topical corticosteroid with occlusion Minoxidil Short contact anthralin Minoxidil + anthralin
Extensive AA (>50% involvement)	*Topical immunotherapy (DPCP/SADBE/DNCB) Topical corticosteroid with occlusion Minoxidil Short contact anthralin Minoxidil + anthralin ±PUVA, thalidomide, anti-interferon-gamma antibodies, methotrexate, alefacept, efalizumab

*First-line therapy
±New treatments for severe, refractory alopecia areata
AA = alopecia areata; DPCP = diphenylcyclopropenone; SADBE = squaric acid dibutyl ester;
DNCB = dinitrochlorobenzene

The most popular treatment options include intralesional, topical, and systemic corticosteroids; topical immunomodulators; minoxidil; and anthralin.[35] Other treatment options that have been successful at treating more severe forms of AA are psoralen with ultraviolet A light (PUVA),[40] thalidomide,[41] anti-interferon (IFN)-gamma antibodies,[42] alefacept,[43] methotrexate,[44] efalizumab,[45] dapsone,[46] and sulfasalazine.[46] Cosmetic aids such as wigs and caps are useful alternatives, especially in patients with rapidly advancing disease. It is important to address the patient's psychologic well being and offer support and supplemental information, such as that provided by the National Alopecia Areata Foundation (www.alopeciaareata.org).

ACQUIRED TRICHOMEGALY OF THE EYELASHES

DEFINITION/OVERVIEW

Trichomegaly refers to abnormal lengthening of the eyelashes (**207**). It is usually seen in congenital diseases such as Oliver–McFarlane syndrome but it may also occur acquired from drugs, malnutrition, and chronic liver disease among others. In 1987, Casanova *et al.*[47] and Janier *et al.*[48] first independently reported elongation of eyelashes in patients with HIV infection. Long eyelashes have also been seen in several children with acquired immunodeficiency syndrome (AIDS).[49,50] Of importance is the notion that it may be a marker of late-stage disease in HIV infection.[7,51–54]

PATHOGENESIS/PATHOPHYSIOLOGY

The etiology of acquired trichomegaly remains unknown. Since most cases of acquired trichomegaly have been in patients with end stage HIV-1 disease, high viral load is presumed to play an important role in the pathogenesis. It is thought that a viral protein or immune mediator released as result of the HIV infection directly stimulates the pilosebaceous structures.[51] An argument for immune dysregulation is supported by the finding of trichomegaly in patients receiving chemotherapy with cyclosporine or IFN. However, Almagro *et al.* reported findings that suggest there is no correlation with CD4 count or viral load.[55] Thus, it remains to be determined whether eyelash tricho-

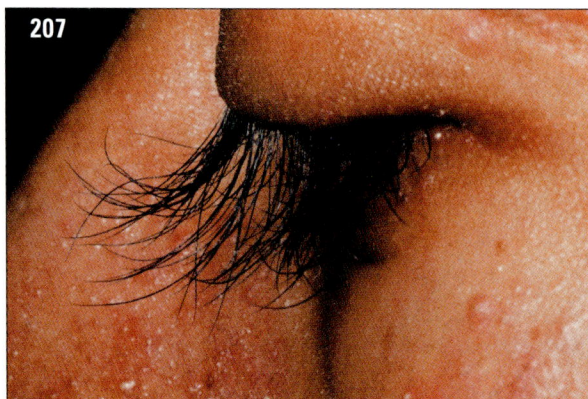

207 Trichomegaly of eyelashes in a patient with AIDS.

megaly is really a marker for more advanced stages of HIV disease. Other authors have correlated excessive eyelash growth with increased levels of zinc or endogenous IFN-α, but these relationships have not been consistently reported.[50]

CLINICAL FEATURES

HIV-positive patients with acquired trichomegaly have documented eyelash lengths from 12 mm to greater than 2 cm. It is sometimes associated with excessive growth of the eyebrows.[56] The excessive growth appears to be correlated with advanced HIV disease as most studies report the appearance of eyelash lengthening when helper T cell depletion is severe, with a range of $0–250 \times 10^6/l$.[51,53,56]

Some HIV patients with trichomegaly have demonstrated intolerance to AZT.[7] In these patients, when AZT was discontinued and another anti-retroviral agent was initiated, trichomegaly was noted to diminish.[7,51]

HISTOPATHOLOGY

Electron microscopy shows no abnormalities within the eyelashes, indicating that HIV-1 does not damage the structure of the hair shaft.[51] Histopathologic examination of affected eyelash follicles has not been undertaken to date.

DIAGNOSIS

It is generally accepted that a diagnosis of eyelash trichomegaly may be made when eyelashes measure 12 mm or greater in length.[55] As noted above, other causes of acquired trichomegaly should be excluded such as that induced by drugs (steroids, cyclosporine, IFN, AZT, and latanoprost), liver disease, malignant neoplasia, and malnutrition.

MANAGEMENT

There is no specific treatment other than controlling HIV infection and supporting the patients' nutritional status. Trimming of the eyelashes may be required as needed for comfort. The presence of trichomegaly with systemic symptoms in a patient without a known immune deficiency disorder should prompt an evaluation for such, as these may be physical signs of HIV infection.

OTHER HAIR ABNORMALITIES

Hair straightening is a characteristic sign of HIV infection, especially in black patients.[7,57–59] The hair is described as lighter, thinner, and softer,[57] and the alteration occurs predominantly in advanced HIV disease. Unfortunately, improvement of immune function with antiretroviral therapy has not been shown to reverse the changes.[7] Various explanations have been suggested for this phenomenon including HIV-induced regression of hair to its fetal stage, deficiencies in zinc, selenium, and copper, and endocrine changes. Smith *et al.* suggest that hormonal changes occurring in HIV infection such as decreased androgen levels and increased levels of estradiol, cortisol, and thyroid hormone may play a role.[2]

Premature graying of the hair (canities) has also been described in HIV-infected patients.[7,60] It is noted to occur with other signs of aging such as premature skin aging and diffuse hair loss.[61] The mechanism of action is unknown but it has been compared to a vitiligo-like process.[62] Brittle hair,[2] fine hair,[54] hypertrichosis of the eyebrows,[63] and increased hair and nail growth[64] have also been observed occasionally in patients with AIDS.

NAIL ABNORMALITIES

Nail changes are a common manifestation of HIV infection and AIDS, with a prevalence of 32–67%.[65,66] Some nail abnormalities are associated with low CD4 counts; however, there has been no correlation between nail changes and HIV viral load.[66]

ONYCHOMYCOSIS

DEFINITION/OVERVIEW

Onychomycosis is often a sign of HIV disease progression in an otherwise asymptomatic individual.[67] Onychomycosis refers to an infection of the nail that is caused by dermatophyte fungi, nondermatophyte fungi, or yeast.[68] Tinea unguium is onychomycosis that is limited to the nail plate. Infection of the nail unit of the toe is often preceded or accompanied by tinea pedis.[69]

The prevalence of onychomycosis ranges from 23%[69] to 38%,[66,70,71] which is more than twice the rate of the non-HIV-infected population. Infection is related to the degree of immune suppression. Because of this, onychomycosis is an important indicator of disease progression in HIV-positive patients as it typically develops at a CD4 count $<450 \times 10^6/l$.[72,73] Of interest, there appears to be no association between onychomycosis and HIV viral load.[66,69] Risk factors for contracting onychomycosis include a low CD4 count ($<450 \times 10^6/l$), a positive family history, a personal history of onychomycosis, and walking barefoot around swimming pools.[69]

There are four distinct patterns of nail infection that may occur either alone or simultaneously within the same nail. These include distal subungual onychomycosis (DSO), proximal subungual onychomycosis (PSO), white superficial onychomycosis (WSO), and candidal onychomycosis. DSO is the most common type of infection in both HIV-infected and non-HIV-infected individuals.[67,69] However, PSO which is most commonly due to *Trichophyton rubrum*, and candidal onychomycosis are more specific markers for HIV infection.[74,75]

PATHOGENESIS/PATHOPHYSIOLOGY

Onychomycosis is most commonly caused by *T. rubrum* in both HIV-infected and non-infected individuals. However, coinfection with mold fungi or *Candida* is much more common with HIV infection. Other dermatophytes that invade the nail unit include *T. mentagrophytes*, *T. tonsurans*, and *Epidermophyton floccosum*. The nondermatophyte molds include *Acremonium*, *Aspergillus*, *Fusarium*, *Onychocola canadensis*, *Scopulariopsis brevicaulis*, and *Scytalidium dimidiatum*.

In DSO, the organism begins invading the nail bed distally and then spreads proximally. Hyperproliferation of the nail bed epithelium in response to the infection causes hyperkeratotic, subungual debris and onycholysis. The debris can then serve as a nidus for secondary superinfection by bacteria, other molds, and yeast.

The most common organism causing WSO is *T. rubrum* in HIV-infected patients and *T. mentagrophytes* in non-HIV-infected individuals. The fungi invade the surface of the nail plate and remain confined there; therefore, they do not cause onycholysis or accumulation of hyperkeratotic debris below the nail.

In PSO organisms enter at the posterior nail fold and invade the nail plate from below. This pattern of infection accounts for only about 5% of cases of onychomycosis in HIV-infected patients.[69] Because it rarely causes onychomycosis in immunocompetent individuals (0.3%), the presence of PSO should immediately prompt evaluation of the patient's immune status.[67,69]

Candidal onychomycosis is most commonly caused by *C. albicans* and is associated with chronic mucocutaneous candidiasis. *Candida* species invade the hyponychial epithelium and spread across the entire nail plate.

CLINICAL FEATURES

The clinical presentation is divided into four patterns of infection, as previously mentioned. DSO begins as a whitish to yellow-brown discoloration of the distal or lateral edges of the nail. As the infection progresses,

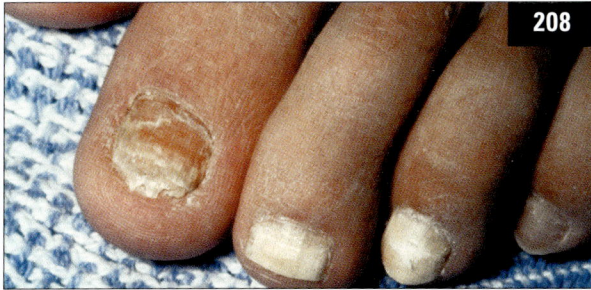

208 Onychomycosis of the toenails in a patient with HIV. The toenails are dystrophic, brittle, and discolored.

209 Histology of onychomycosis. Periodic acid-Schiff (PAS) staining of nail plate showing numerous hyphal elements.

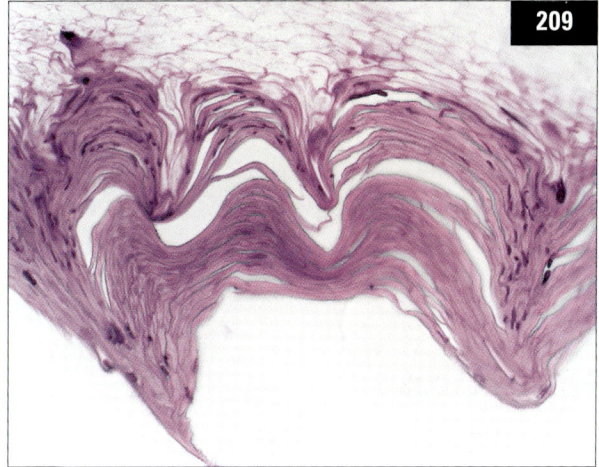

subungual hyperkeratosis causes onycholysis. The fungus grows within the substance of the nail plate causing thick, discolored brittle nails (**208**). WSO presents as white to yellow sharply demarcated patches on the surface of the nail. These areas are rough and friable. Normally WSO is confined to the toenails[67] but it may also occur on the fingernails of immunocompromised individuals. PSO begins as a whitish opacification of the proximal nail and then spreads distally to affect the entire nail eventually.

Candidal onychomycosis commonly involves all of the fingernails. It is associated with yellow-brown discoloration, onycholysis, and nail plate thickening without subungual debris accumulation. Lateral onycholysis is a major finding in candidal onychomycosis which is also present in psoriasis.[67] In contrast to the other types of onychomycosis, paronychial inflammation is often present. In HIV-infected patients, the infection is often more severe and correlates with the CD4 count.

HISTOPATHOLOGY

In DSO and PSO, hyphae can be seen between the laminae parallel to the nail's surface. The epithelium may respond to the infection with spongiosis, focal parakeratosis, and dermal inflammatory infiltrates that may be minimal or relatively intense. There is often verrucous epithelial hyperplasia with hemorrhage in the cornified layer that may simulate a wart. There may also be features similar to those seen in

psoriasis. In WSO, the organisms are seen on the dorsal nail surface. In candidal onychomycosis, pseudohyphae are present throughout the entire nail plate.

DIAGNOSIS

Onychomycosis is usually readily diagnosable clinically although it may be simulated by a number of different conditions. The prevalence of onychomycosis in HIV-positive patients with abnormal appearing nails is 50%.[69] Definitive diagnosis requires laboratory confirmation via direct microscopic examination, periodic acid-Schiff (PAS) staining of nail plate specimens (**209**), or culture. Diagnostic yield is increased when both microscopy and culture is performed as false negatives are common in each of these. Most false negatives are due to sampling error so that it is important to obtain and submit adequate amounts of nail clippings and subungual debris and when necessary, to perform repeated tests. In order to achieve adequate softening for microscopic observation, it may be necessary to soak the fragments with potassium hydroxide (KOH) in a closed container for 24 hours. When performing a culture, both the nail plate and cornified cells of the nail bed should be sampled as organisms residing in the nail plate may not be viable. Collected clippings and debris are inoculated on Sabouraud's or Dermatophyte Test medium.

MANAGEMENT

The antimicrobial susceptibility of organisms causing onychomycosis in HIV-infected patients appears to be the same as that in non-HIV-infected patients; therefore, treatment does not change based on HIV status. Nevertheless, treatment in HIV-infected patients is often more difficult due to advanced severity of the disease and the increased incidence of coinfection.

Topical agents are typically used only for WSO as they have poor penetration into the nail plate.[72] The most commonly used topical antifungal is ciclopirox. If this is used to treat onychomycosis, it is recommended as a daily application for 48 weeks.[68]

The use of systemic antifungals is far more effective than topical treatment as they have increased efficacy and can be administered for relatively short treatment regimens. A particular antifungal agent should be chosen based on the causative organism and the adverse effects of the medication. *Table 13* presents information on specific therapeutic agents employed. Of note, griseofulvin is no longer considered standard treatment for onychomycosis.[68] Refractory cases may require nail avulsion in combination with drug therapy.

HERPETIC WHITLOW

DEFINITION/OVERVIEW

Herpetic whitlow refers to a herpes simplex virus (HSV) infection of the finger. These infections are caused by either of the two different virus types, HSV-1 or HSV-2, both of which produce identical patterns of infection. HSV-1 is most commonly associated with oral labial infections while HSV-2 is associated with genital infections although either type can occur at any location. While the rate of HSV-1 infection does not vary between HIV-seropositive individuals and those who are HIV seronegative, HSV-2 is significantly more common in patients with HIV infection.[76]

Herpetic whitlow in a patient with AIDS is often more severe and may be difficult to diagnose. Most cases are associated with extreme immunodeficiency and CD4 counts below $1 \times 10^5/l$.[77] Severe herpetic whitlow may be the first sign of HIV infection.[78,79]

Table 13 Oral therapeutic agents for onychomycosis

THERAPEUTIC AGENT	INDICATION	TREATMENT REGIMEN	LENGTH OF TREATMENT	ADVERSE EFFECTS
Terbinafine	First-line therapy for dermatophytes Also treats *Aspergillus* and *Scopulariopsis*	250 mg daily	Fingernails: 6 weeks Toenails: 12 weeks	GI upset, elevated liver enzymes
Itraconazole	Alternative first-line therapy for dermatophytes Preferred use for nondermatophytes and *Candida*	200 mg daily or 400 mg daily 1 week per month	Fingernails: 6 weeks Toenails: 12 weeks	Elevated liver enzymes
Fluconazole	First-line therapy for *Candida*, but also active against dermatophytes, and some nondermatophytes	150–300 mg weekly Refractory cases: 450 mg weekly	3–12 months	GI upset, elevated liver enzymes

PATHOGENESIS/PATHOPHYSIOLOGY

Herpetic whitlow is a recognized occupational hazard of dental and medical personnel. HSV is contracted via direct inoculation from respiratory droplets, direct contact with an active lesion, or direct contact with virus-containing bodily fluids. It replicates at the site of infection causing the clinical manifestations of the disease. The virus is then transported to the dorsal root ganglia via retrograde axonal flow along the sensory neurons innervating the site of infection. It remains latent in the ganglion without clinical signs of disease. Upon reactivation of the virus secondary to skin trauma or systemic changes, the virus migrates down the peripheral nerves to the original site of infection and causes clinical disease once again.[33] HIV causes an immunocompromised state that allows for the herpes virus to replicate and destroy tissues without defense from T cells, which is necessary for adequate viral immunity.

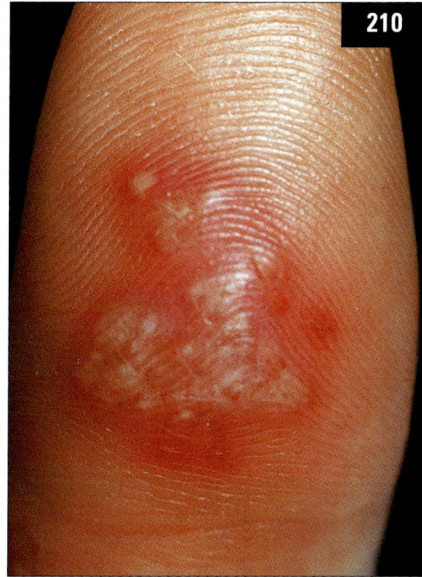

210 Herpetic whitlow. (Courtesy of St John's Institute of Dermatology (King's College), Guy's Hospital, London.)

CLINICAL FEATURES

Herpetic whitlow is characterized by erythema and edema of the periungual tissues of the finger.[76] HSV lesions typically present as grouped vesicles or pustules of uniform size on an erythematous base (**210**). The vesicles later burst to form a crust. Lesions are usually located in the paronychial, eponychial, and subungual space of the distal phalanx and are typically quite painful.[77] Fever and local lymphadenopathy are common with primary infection.[37] The disease, which is usually caused by HSV-2 infections, recurs in 20% of patients.[77]

Herpetic whitlow in immunocompromised individuals usually presents as a much more severe disease and can be difficult to recognize. In advanced stages of HIV, with CD4 counts lower than 100×10^6/l, the lesions often ulcerate and become deeply invasive. They are often slower to heal and, if left untreated, can become chronic with extensive areas of necrosis.[77,80–82] Secondary bacterial infections can distort the clinical presentation, making diagnosis even more difficult.

HISTOPATHOLOGY

Histopathology is not usually performed for periungual herpes simplex as diagnostic Tzanck smears are easily performed and give rapid results. However, tissue diagnosis should be considered in AIDS patients as there is an increased risk of multiple infections in this population. Tzanck smears reveal the characteristic multinucleated epithelial giant cells with steel blue and homogeneous nuclei classic for HSV.[74] Biopsy specimens demonstrate ballooning degeneration of epidermal cells with homogeneous eosinophilic cytoplasm.[80] Inclusion bodies are frequently seen in the nuclei of these multinucleated cells. Acantholysis is also usually present.[81] In immunocompromised patients there may be extensive infection, with numerous degenerating cells in some cases forming a syncytium.

DIAGNOSIS

Herpetic whitlow is often difficult to diagnose on clinical features alone in an immunocompromised patient due to the unusual presentations and extensive variety of diseases that affect AIDS patients. The differential diagnosis can be extensive including staphylococcal infection, streptococcal infection, *Candida* paronychia, milker's nodule, pyoderma gangrenosum, and deep fungal infection.[77] Diagnostic tests include Tzanck smear, viral culture, immunoperoxidase stains using monoclonal antibodies or viral probes, PCR, as well as routine histopathologic evaluation of biopsy specimens. Smears are taken from intact vesicles when present and can be stained with Wright or Giemsa stains or evaluated using direct immunofluorescence. Characteristic multinucleated giant cells with viral inclusions are typically seen.[74] However, Tzanck smear cannot distinguish between HSV-1 and HSV-2. A viral culture from vesicular fluid is more sensitive and specific but may take several days for results to be available. Monoclonal antibodies and PCR are more rapid and precise diagnostic tools[83] but are also more expensive.

MANAGEMENT

Treatment options include acyclovir, valacyclovir, and famciclovir. They are given orally for uncomplicated cases and often must be administered intravenously when significant systemic symptoms are present. Acyclovir is used for herpetic whitlow as well as for prophylaxis[77,80] which may help in reducing resistance to acyclovir.[82] Although there is scant data regarding the treatment of herpetic whitlow in AIDS patients, most authorities would recommend a longer course of therapy than that traditionally used in other herpetic infections.[77] Dosages of 200–800 mg every 4 hours orally administered for 5–7 days is usually successful in treating herpetic whitlow.[77,83,84] Cases resistant to acyclovir may respond to intravenous foscarnet or cidofovir.[76]

YELLOW NAILS

DEFINITION/OVERVIEW

Yellow nails are a frequent finding in HIV patients,[23,60,85,86] and are considered a marker of progression towards AIDS.[87] The presence of yellow nails in association with HIV infection is widely accepted but the existence of true yellow nail syndrome in these individuals is controversial.[74,88–91] Yellow nail syndrome was first described by Samman and White in 1964[92] and is associated with other characteristic features such as loss of the cuticle, over-curvature and thickening of the nails, shedding, onycholysis, and slowing of nail growth. Many of these features are not found in HIV-positive patients with yellow nails. Nevertheless, the presence of the nail discoloration on its own can serve as an important diagnostic clue to the presence of HIV infection and may be an indicator of the disease severity.

PATHOGENESIS/PATHOPHYSIOLOGY

The etiology of yellow nails in HIV infection is unknown although it is thought to be associated with dermatophyte infection due to the high frequency of tinea pedis in this population.[23] In many cases, however, bacterial cultures and mycologic studies have failed to reveal definitive causal microorganisms.[74,85]

CLINICAL FEATURES

The yellow discoloration is typically seen in the distal half of the nail plate although the entire nail plate may be involved. Various shades of yellow may be seen and the change to a yellow color is generally gradual (**211**). The nail involvement is progressive and asymmetric. Toe nails, particularly of the great toe, are usually affected whereas finger nails are rarely involved. Opacification, loss of lunulae, onycholysis, and transverse and longitudinal ridging may be present.[85]

HISTOPATHOLOGY

No unique pathologic findings have been reported. The yellow pigment is distributed through the entire plate thickness, not just the surface, as is seen in dermatophyte infections.[85] No infectious organisms have been detected when nail plates are specially stained.

DIAGNOSIS

The diagnosis is based on clinical features. Various degrees of yellow color may be observed but the discoloration is usually limited to the distal half of the nail plate. Several other causes of yellow nails exist and should be ruled out, including discoloration from nail polishes, chemical exposure, drugs, diabetes mellitus, or onychomycosis.

MANAGEMENT

Since the clinical appearance is similar to that of onychomycosis, it is essential to exclude it via appropriate methods such as direct microscopic examination, culture, and PAS staining.[67] There is no US Food and Drug Administration (FDA) approved medication for the treatment of yellow nails although oral vitamin E (400–1200 IU daily) has been shown to be beneficial in the classic yellow nail syndrome.[93]

ZIDOVUDINE-INDUCED NAIL DYSCHROMIA

DEFINITION/OVERVIEW

AZT, a nucleoside reverse transcriptase inhibitor (NRTI), is widely used in the treatment of HIV infection. Nail hyperpigmentation with AZT use is well documented, and appears to be more prevalent in the black population.[94–102]

PATHOGENESIS/PATHOPHYSIOLOGY

The mechanism of hyperpigmentation is unknown. Matrix melanocyte stimulation is the cause of chemotherapy-induced nail hyperpigmentation and a similar mechanism may explain the nail changes seen with AZT therapy. The nail matrix contains melanocytes that are normally quiescent. Injury to, or stimulation of, these melanocytes may cause them to become active and synthesize melanin which is transferred to the surrounding keratinocytes.[75] Cutaneous hyperpigmentation is also associated with AZT treatment and is proven to be secondary to melanin deposition in the epidermis and dermis.[99] This melanocyte stimulation hypothesis could explain the higher incidence of AZT-induced pigmentary changes seen in patients with deeper pigmentation.

CLINICAL FEATURES

Nail hyperpigmentation usually develops after 4–8 weeks of 600–1200 mg of AZT daily.[102] The nail changes are usually in the form of longitudinal bands also known as pigmented streaks (212).

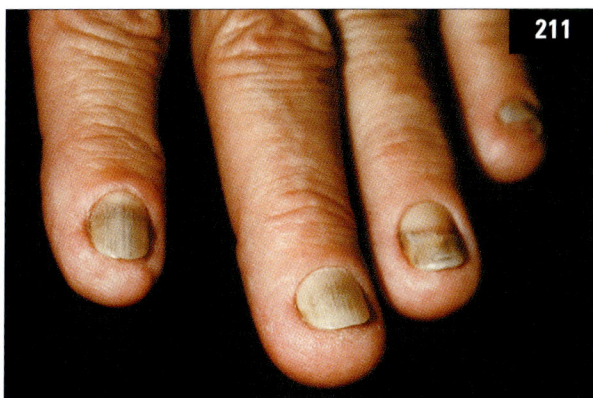

211 Yellow nails in a patient with AIDS.

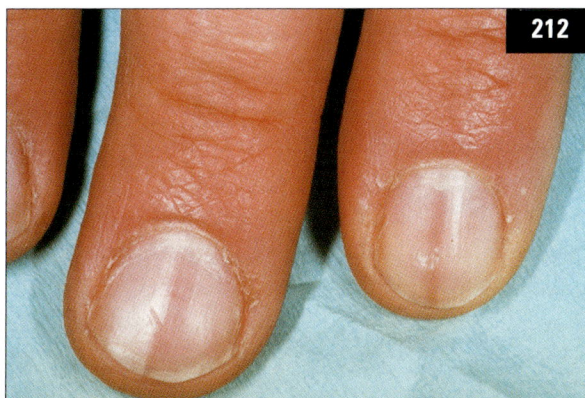

212 Longitudinal nail hyperpigmentation secondary to ingestion of AZT.

Transverse bands and complete and partial discoloration of the nail are other observed patterns. Nail discoloration varies from hues of blue to yellow-brown to black. The pigment starts at, and moves distally from, the nail base and either some or all the nails may be affected. In the majority of the patients, the thumbnail is the first nail involved and toenails develop discoloration after fingernail dyschromia.[23] Cutaneous[94,99] and mucosal[97,99] hyperpigmentation have also been documented with AZT use.

The hyperpigmentation appears to be progressive and dependent on the intrinsic skin color of the patient.[99,103] Don et al. (1990)[98] observed that black patients had more than twice the incidence of nail pigmentation abnormalities than nonblack patients.

HISTOPATHOLOGY

Fontana–Masson staining of nail clippings demonstrates deposits of melanin granules within the nail plate.[23,99] Histopathologic findings consist of increased melanocytes in the basal layers and increased melanin within melanophages of the dermis.[99,102] Transmission electron microscopy shows numerous macrophages with normal melanosomes.[99,100]

DIAGNOSIS

As HIV patients are on multiple drugs and have a chronic systemic infection, it may be difficult to delineate AZT as the agent causing nail hyperpigmentation. AZT-induced nail dyschromias should be clinically correlated with the timing of introduction of the drug. The nail changes are typically evident after 1 month of therapy but have been reported to occur up to 1 year later.[102] A diverse number of situations produce diffuse discoloration and pigmented streaks in nails. Brown, longitudinal streaks are especially common in black patients.[98,104,105] HIV itself is associated with a bluish discoloration of nails as well as longitudinal nail pigmentation.[60,106–108] Chemotherapeutic agents, especially cyclophosphamide, doxorubicin, and adriamycin, may also cause transverse, longitudinal, and diffuse discoloration. Other causes of longitudinal pigmented nail bands are nail biting, pregnancy, systemic irradiation, postinflammatory hyper-

pigmentation, Laugier–Hunziker syndrome, antimalarials, and other cytotoxic drugs.[104] Neoplastic lesions such as Bowen's disease, subungual verruca, malignant melanoma, glomus tumor, and rarely basal cell carcinoma may also produce pigmented nail changes.

MANAGEMENT

It is important to evaluate the nails of all patients before the introduction of AZT therapy in order to rule out pre-existing conditions. Nail changes during therapy should also be documented. The patient should be warned that they may develop nail hyperpigmentation while on AZT which may prevent fear of other more worrisome diagnoses such as melanoma. The effects of AZT disappear or gradually fade when the drug is discontinued.[99,102] The nail changes are a cosmetic adverse effect so that discontinuation of AZT for this reason must be balanced against the benefits of the drug in treating the HIV infection. Replacing AZT with another antiretroviral agent may be feasible.

INDINAVIR-ASSOCIATED PARONYCHIA

DEFINITION/OVERVIEW

Paronychia refers to a soft tissue infection or inflammation of the epidermis around the nail plate. In the non-HIV-infected population chronic paronychia is usually caused by contact irritants or repeated exposure to water. In HIV-infected patients, the protease inhibitor indinavir is thought to be the most common cause of chronic paronychia,[109] followed by onychomycosis and candidal infections. Although a direct cause–effect relationship has yet to be established between indinavir and paronychia, when it has been discontinued, it has been noted that the paronychia has either resolved or diminished in intensity, findings which are strongly suggestive of such a relationship.[110–112] Garcia-Silva *et al.* reported paronychia in 4–9% of HIV patients receiving indinavir,[109] and in a retrospective study by Colson *et al.*, indinavir treatment was significantly associated with a 4.7-fold increased risk of great toe paronychia.[113] Similar nail changes have also been reported in HIV-infected patients taking lamivudine[114] and AZT,[115] albeit less frequently.

PATHOLOGY/PATHOGENESIS

About 30% of patients taking indinavir develop one of many retinoid-like effects such as alopecia, xerosis, ingrown nails, and paronychia.[109] Bouscarat *et al.* suggested that protease inhibitors have a retinoid-like effect due to homologies between the amino acid sequences of retinoic acid-binding protein 1 (CRABP1) and the catalytic site of HIV-1 protease, the target site of protease inhibitors.[110] It is hypothesized that indinavir may interfere with retinoid metabolism by either enhancing the retinoid signaling pathway, increasing the synthesis of retinoic acid, or decreasing the P450-mediated oxidative metabolism of retinoic acid.

CLINICAL FEATURES

Patients typically present with intense pain, erythema, and edema along the lateral nail folds. Pyogenic granuloma-like lesions may also be evident along these folds. The nail changes appear within 1–9 months of the start of treatment with indinavir and may be associated with ingrown nails. The great toe nail is primarily affected although other toe and finger nails may be involved subsequently. Superinfection by bacteria and fungi can confuse the clinical picture. Recurrences are common while patients are receiving indinavir, occurring in up to 50% of cases.[113] Most affected usually have CD4 cell counts >200 × 10^6/l.[110,116,117] The clinical manifestations appear to be dose-dependent and are responsive to discontinuation of therapy.

HISTOPATHOLOGY

Histopathology demonstrates granulation, consisting of loose connective tissue with edema, numerous blood vessels, and a dense perivascular lymphocytic infiltrate.[114,116]

DIAGNOSIS

Paronychia is diagnosed based on the clinical findings of swollen and tender posterior or lateral nail folds. In HIV-seropositive patients, it may not be possible to determine if the paronychia is due to antiretroviral drugs, onychomycosis, or *Candida*. However, if it is thought to be due to drug therapy, the most commonly associated agent is indinavir. Tests to exclude infections such as Gram stains, KOH tests, and cultures should be performed and may reveal bacterial and/or fungal superinfection. The physician should query for a history of previous episodes of paronychia, psoriasis, local trauma, ingrown nails, or other known risk factors of paronychia. The differential diagnosis includes onychomycosis, candidal infection, herpetic whitlow, psoriasis, lupus erythematosus, dermatomyositis, and local trauma.

MANAGEMENT

Unlike infectious causes of periungual inflammation, surgical management of indinavir-induced paronychia is not recommended due to its high rate of recurrence. For minimally symptomatic patients, local measures and warm compresses may be sufficient.[118] More aggressive treatment options include changing the antiretroviral therapy to a regimen not containing indinavir, while continuing to administer other protease inhibitors such as lamivudine.[119] If it is not feasible to change therapy, topical application of a strong antimicrobial and anti-inflammatory agent may significantly improve the symptoms.[111] Treatment of secondary bacterial and fungal infections may be necessary. The physician should carefully examine the hands and feet of the patient prior to initiating therapy with indinavir and document any changes that occur during treatment. Knowledge that indinavir can cause paronychia may help avoid unnecessary and invasive procedures, such as lateral matrixectomy.

OTHER NAIL ABNORMALITIES

Squamous cell carcinoma (SCC) of the digits in HIV-infected patients is a relatively rare finding.[5] Human papillomavirus (HPV) has been detected in many of these and is regarded as the main oncogenic stimulus.[73,75,120] HPV serotypes 16[121] and 26[122] are of particular importance. Although HPV 26 is not classically considered a high risk serotype, the immunosuppression that develops in HIV-infected patients is thought to predispose to malignant transformation. Thus, any persistent periungual verrucous lesion in an HIV-infected patient should alert the physician to the possibility of SCC and a biopsy should be performed. Mohs surgery is considered the treatment of choice as lesions may be poorly circumscribed and may extend into the subungual epithelium.[120]

Clubbing (**213**) is considered by some to be part of the clinical spectrum of HIV-associated nail abnormalities, especially in the pediatric population, many of whom have underlying chronic lung disease.[66,123,124] Two studies suggest that clubbing may be related to the degree of immunosuppression.[66,124] While more common in children, it can also occur in adults,[124,125] and in one case it was the initial manifestation of HIV infection.[126]

Longitudinal melanonychia is a common finding in HIV patients taking AZT as discussed above; however, it has also been found in HIV patients not receiving any antiretroviral medications.[60,127,128] Several nails are usually involved and it is often associated with mucosal and cutaneous hyperpigmentation.[75] It is thought to be due to increased levels of α-melanocyte-stimulating hormone which is associated with the adrenal abnormalities these patients often suffer from.[129]

Blue nails, manifest as diffuse bluish-gray discoloration of multiple nail plates, may also be a sign of HIV infection. Nail dyschromia was initially described in patients taking AZT,[103] although Chandrasekar subsequently reported blue nails in two black HIV-infected patients who were not receiving medication.[130] Others have reported similar findings,[107,131] and in one study of 75 HIV-positive patients, Leppard described the discoloration as

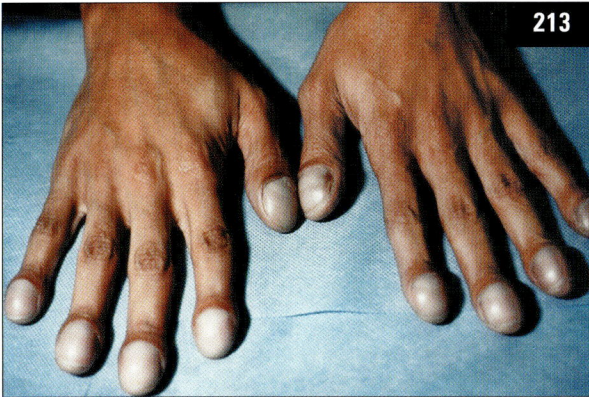

213 Clubbing of the nails in a patient infected with HIV.

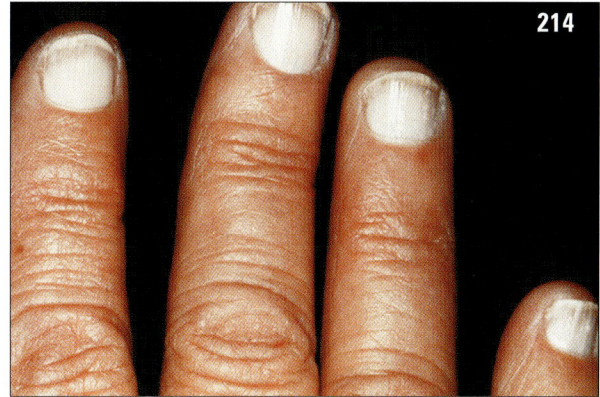

214 Leukonychia.

beginning in the lunulae with gradual, distal spread.[131] The changes were permanent and were not correlated with the immune status of the patient.[131]

Leukonychia, or 'white nails' (**214**), were found in more than 10% of a group of 155 HIV-positive patients, all of whom had low CD4 cell counts.[66] In another study, white nails were associated with severe illness and emotional stress in two children with HIV infection.[132] Terry's nails[66] and Muehrcke's nails have also been reported.[17]

Beau's lines have also been described in AIDS patients. These are manifest as transverse depressions across the nail plate and are typically seen 2–3 months after an episode of serious infection.[17] In some cases, Beau's lines may be a marker of zinc depletion in HIV-infected patients.[23]

Periungual erythema of the fingers and toes in HIV-seropositive patients was first documented in 1996.[133] Since then several case reports have correlated the presence of 'red fingers' and periungual telangiectasis with HIV infection,[66,134] although a direct relationship has not been established. Ruiz-Avila

et al. speculated that the telangiectasias are due to the production of angiogenic factors such as in HIV-associated Kaposi's sarcoma and bacillary angiomatosis.[135] Other authors suggest that the changes are due to immunologic changes secondary to HIV, hepatitis B virus, or hepatitis C virus infection.[133] Capillaroscopy is normal and histology shows dilated capillaries.[133] At present, there is no definitive treatment for this condition. Periungual changes may also be seen with other infections, psoriasis, or paronychia.

Psoriatic nail changes are a frequent manifestation of HIV infection and may be associated with widespread skin psoriasis or as a sole manifestation of the disease.[73] Key features include nail pitting, subungual keratosis, and onycholysis.[67] Paronychia may also occur. A psoriasis–Reiter's syndrome overlap process may also be seen in HIV-positive patients and the nail findings may be identical to those seen in psoriasis.

Other nail changes associated with HIV include diminished nail plate thickness, onychoschizia, opaqueness, and transverse or longitudinal ridging.[17,60,66]

REFERENCES

CHAPTER 1

1 CDC (1981). Kaposi's sarcoma and *Pneumocystis* pneumonia among homosexual men: New York City and California. *MMWR* 30(25):305–8.

2 Gottlieb GJ, Ragaz A, Vogel JV, *et al.* (1981). A preliminary communication on extensively disseminated Kaposi's sarcoma in young homosexual men. *Am J Dermatopathol* 3(2):111–14.

3 Hymes KB, Cheung T, Greene JB, *et al.* (1981). Kaposi's sarcoma in homosexual men: a report of eight cases. *Lancet* 2(8247):598–600.

4 Thomsen HK, Jacobsen M, Malchow-Møller A (1981). Kaposi sarcoma among homosexual men in Europe. *Lancet* 2(8248):688.

5 Friedman-Kien AE (1981). Disseminated Kaposi's sarcoma syndrome in young homosexual men. *J Am Acad Dermatol* 5(4):468–71.

6 Borkovic SP, Schwartz RA (1981). Kaposi's sarcoma presenting in the homosexual man: a new and striking phenomenon! *Ariz Med* 38(12):902–4.

7 Gottlieb MS, Schroff R, Schanker HM, *et al.* (1981). *Pneumocystis carinii* pneumonia and mucosal candidiasis in previously healthy homosexual men: evidence of a new acquired cellular immunodeficiency. *N Engl J Med* 305(24):1425–31.

8 Siegal FP, Lopez C, Hammer GS, *et al.* (1981). Severe acquired immunodeficiency in male homosexuals, manifested by chronic perianal ulcerative herpes simplex lesions. *N Engl J Med* 305(24):1439–44.

9 Durack DT (1981). Opportunistic infections and Kaposi's sarcoma in homosexual men. *N Engl J Med* 305(24):1465–7.

10 Masur H, Michelis MA, Greene JB, *et al.* (1981). An outbreak of community-acquired *Pneumocystis carinii* pneumonia: initial manifestation of cellular immune dysfunction. *N Engl J Med* 305(24):1431–8.

11 Brennan RO, Durack DT (1981). Gay compromise syndrome. *Lancet* 2(8259):1338–9.

12 (No authors listed) (1981). Immunocompromised homosexuals. *Lancet* 2(8259):1325–6.

CHAPTER 2

1 Kahn JO, Walker BD (1998). Acute human immunodeficiency virus type 1 infection. *NEJM* 339(1):33–9.

2 Alessi E, Cusini M (1995). The exanthem of HIV-1 seroconversion syndrome. *Int J Dermatol* 34(4):238–9.

3 Kinloch-de Loes S, de Saussure P, Saurat JH, *et al.* (1993). Symptomatic primary infection due to human immunodeficiency virus type 1: review of 31 cases. *Clin Infect Dis* 17(1):59–65.

4 Taiwo BO, Hicks CB (2002). Primary human immunodeficiency virus. *South Med J* 95(11):1312–17.

5 Vanhems P, Dassa C, Lambert J, *et al.* (1999). Comprehensive classification of symptoms and signs reported among 218 patients with acute HIV-1 infection. *J Acquir Immune Defic Syndr* 21(2):99–106.

6 Vanhems P, Beaulieu R (1997). Primary infection by type 1 human immunodeficiency virus: diagnosis and prognosis. *Postgrad Med J* 73(861):403–8.

7 Tindall B, Barker S, Donovan B, *et al.* (1988). Characterization of the acute clinical illness associated with human immunodeficiency virus infection. *Arch Internal Med* 148(4):945–9.

8 Vanhems P, Allard R, Cooper DA, *et al.* (1997). Acute human immunodeficiency virus type 1 disease as a mononucleosis-like illness: is the diagnosis too restrictive? *Clin Infect Dis* 24(5):965–70.

9 Schacker T, Collier AC, Hughes J, *et al.* (1996). Clinical and epidemiologic features of primary HIV infection. *Ann Internal Med* 125(4):257–64.

10 Mortier E, Zahar JR, Gros I, *et al.* (1994). Primary infection with human immunodeficiency virus that presented as Stevens–Johnson syndrome. *Clin Infect Dis* 19(4):798.

11 Lapins J, Lindback S, Lidbrink P, *et al.* (1996). Mucocutaneous manifestations in 22 consecutive cases of primary HIV-1 infection. *Br J Dermatol* 134(2):257–61.

12 Perlmutter BL, Glaser JB, Oyugi SO (1999). How to recognize and treat acute HIV syndrome. *Am Fam Physician* 60(2):535–42, 545–6.

13 Lindback S, Brostrom C, Karlsson A, *et al.* (1994). Does symptomatic primary HIV-1 infection accelerate progression to CDC stage IV disease, CD4 count below 200 × 10^6/l, AIDS, and death from AIDS? *BMJ* 309(6968):1535–7.

14 Keet IP, Krijnen P, Koot M, *et al.* (1993). Predictors of rapid progression to AIDS in HIV-1 seroconverters. *AIDS* 7(1):51–7.

15 Pedersen C, Lindhardt BO, Jensen BL, *et al.* (1989). Clinical course of primary HIV infection: consequences for subsequent course of infection. *BMJ* 299(6692):154–7.

16 Al-Harthi L, Siegel J, Spritzler J, *et al.* (2000). Maximum suppression of HIV replication leads to the

restoration of HIV-specific responses in early HIV disease. *AIDS* **14**(7):761–70.

17 Malhotra U, Berrey MM, Huang Y, *et al.* (2000). Effect of combination antiretroviral therapy on T-cell immunity in acute human immunodeficiency virus type 1 infection. *J Infect Dis* **181**(1):121–31.

18 Jacquez JA, Koopman JS, Simon CP, *et al.* (1994). Role of the primary infection in epidemics of HIV infection in gay cohorts. *J Acquir Immune Defic Syndr* **7**(11):1169–84.

19 Goldman GD, Milstone LM, Shapiro PE (1995). Histologic findings in acute HIV exanthem. *J Cutan Pathol* **22**(4):371–3.

20 Carcelain G, Blanc C, Leibowitch J, *et al.* (1999). T cell changes after combined nucleoside analogue therapy in HIV primary infection. *AIDS* **13**(9):1077–81.

21 Lillo FB, Ciuffreda D, Veglia F, *et al.* (1999). Viral load and burden modification following early antiretroviral therapy of primary HIV-1 infection. *AIDS* **13**(7):791–6.

22 Reichert CM, O'Leary TJ, Levens DL, *et al.* (1983). Autopsy pathology in the acquired immunodeficiency syndrome. *Am J Pathol* **112**:357–82.

23 Dann FJ, Tabibian P (1995). Cutaneous diseases in human immunodeficiency virus-infected patients referred to the UCLA Immunosuppression Skin Clinic: reasons for referral and management of selected diseases. *Cutis* **55**:85–8.

24 Tyring SK (2003). Molluscum contagiosum: the importance of early diagnosis and treatment. *Am J Obstet Gynecol* **189**(Suppl 3):S12–6.

25 Thompson CH, de Zwart-Steffe RT, Donovan B (1992). Clinical and molecular aspects of molluscum contagiosum infection in HIV-1 positive patients. *Int J STD AIDS* **3**(2):101–6.

26 Reynaud-Mendel B, Janier M, Gerbaka J, *et al.* (1996). Dermatologic findings in HIV-1 infected patients: a prospective study with emphasis on CD4+ cell count. *Dermatology* **192**:325–8.

27 Munoz-Perez MA, Rodriguez-Pichardo A, Camacho F, *et al.* (1998). Dermatological findings correlated with CD4 lymphocyte counts in a prospective 3 year study of 1161 patients with human immunodeficiency virus disease predominantly acquired though intravenous drug abuse. *Br J Dermatol* **139**:33–9.

28 Czelusta A, Yen-Moore A, Van der Straten M, *et al.* (2000). An overview of sexually transmitted diseases. Part III. Sexually transmitted diseases in HIV-infected patients. *J Am Acad Dermatol* **43**(3):409–32; quiz 433–6.

29 Bansal R, Tutrone WD, Weinberg JM (2002). Viral skin infections in the elderly: diagnosis and management. *Drugs Aging* **19**(7):503–14.

30 Konya J, Thompson CH (1999). Molluscum contagiosum virus: antibody responses in persons with clinical lesions and seroepidemiology in a representative Australian population. *J Infect Dis* **179**:701–4.

31 Matis WL, Triana A, Shapiro R, *et al.* (1987). Dermatologic findings associated with human immunodeficiency virus infection. *J Am Acad Dermatol* **17**:746–5.

32 Hira SK, Wadhawan D, Kamanga J, *et al.* (1988). Cutaneous manifestations of human immunodeficiency virus in Lusaka, Zambia. *J Am Acad Dermatol* **19**:451–7.

33 Coldiron BM, Bergstresser PR (1989). Prevalence and clinical spectrum of skin disease in patients infected with human immunodeficiency virus. *Arch Dermatol* **125**:357–61.

34 Smith KJ, Skelton H (2002). Molluscum contagiosum: recent advances in pathogenic mechanisms, and new therapies. *Am J Clin Dermatol* **3**(8):535–45.

35 Schwartz JJ, Myskowski PL (1992). Molluscum contagiosum in patients with human immunodeficiency virus infection. A review of twenty-seven patients. *J Am Acad Dermatol* **27**(4):583–8.

36 Gupta RK, Naran S, Lallu S, *et al.* (2003). Cytologic diagnosis of molluscum contagiosum in scrape samples from facial lesions. *Diagn Cytopathol* **29**(2):84.

37 Smith KJ, Skelton HG, Yeager J, *et al.* (1992). Molluscum contagiosum: ultrastructural evidence for its presence in skin adjacent to clinical lesions in patients infected with human immunodeficiency virus type I. *Arch Dermatol* **128**:223–7.

38 Ficarra G, Cortes S, Rubino I, *et al.* (1994). Facial and perioral molluscum contagiosum in patients with HIV infection: a report of eight cases. *Oral Surg Oral Med Oral Pathol* **78**:621–6.

39 Cavicchini S, Brezzi A, Alessi E (1993). Ultrastructural findings in mucocutaneous infections of patients seropositive to HIV. *Am J Dermatopathol* **15**:320–5.

40 Cronin TA, Resnik BI, Elgart G, *et al.* (1996). Recalcitrant giant molluscum contagiosum in a patient with AIDS. *J Am Acad Dermatol* **35**:266–7.

41 Diven DG (2001). An overview of poxviruses. *J Am Acad Dermatol* **44**(1):1–16.

42 Papa CM, Berger RS (1976). Venereal herpes-like molluscum contagiosum: treatment with tretinoin. *Cutis* **18**(4):537–40.

43 Silverberg NB, Sidbury R, Mancini AJ (2000). Childhood molluscum contagiosum: experience with cantharidin therapy in 300 patients. *J Am Acad Dermatol* **43**(3):503–7.

44 Garrett SJ, Robinson JK, Roenogk HH (1992). Trichloroacetic acid peel of molluscum contagiosum in immunocompromised patients. *J Dermatol Surg Oncol* **18**:855–8.

45 Nelson MR, Chard S, Barton SE (1995). Intralesional interferon for the treatment of recalcitrant molluscum contagiosum in HIV-antibody positive individuals, a preliminary report. *Int J STD AIDS* **6**:351–2.

46 Suzuki H, Wang B, Shivji GM, *et al.* (2000). Imiquimod, a topical immune response modifier, induces migration of Langerhans cells. *J Invest Dermatol* **114**(1):135–41.

47 Conant MA (2000). Immunomodulatory therapy in the management of viral infections in patients with HIV infection. *J Am Acad Dermatol* **43**(1 Pt 2):S27–30.

48 Petersen CS, Weismann K (1995). Quercetin and kaempherol: an argument against the use of podophyllin. *Genitourinary Med* **71**:92–3.

49 Safrin S, Cherrington J, Jaffe HS (1997). Clinical uses of cidofovir. *Rev Med Virol* **7**(3):145–56.

50 Hicks CB, Myers SA, Giner J (1997). Resolution of intractable molluscum contagiosum in a human immunodeficiency virus-infected patient after institution of antiretroviral therapy with ritonavir. *Clin Infect Dis* **24**(5):1023–5.

51 Akgul B, Cooke JC, Storey A (2006). HPV-associated skin disease. *J Pathol* **208**(2):165–75.

52 Berger TG, Sawchuk WS, Leonardi

C, *et al.* (1991). Epidermodysplasia verruciformis-associated papillomavirus infection complicating human immunodeficiency virus disease. *Br J Dermatol* **124**(1):79–83.

53 LeBoit PE (1992). Dermatopathologic findings in patients infected with HIV. *Dermatol Clin* **10**(1):59–71.

54 Rivera A, Tyring SK (2004). Therapy of cutaneous human papillomavirus infections. *Dermatol Ther* **17**(6):441–8.

55 Wu JJ, Huang DB, Pang KR, *et al.* (2004). Vaccines and immunotherapies for the prevention of infectious diseases having cutaneous manifestations. *J Am Acad Dermatol* **50**(4):495–528; quiz 529–32.

56 Roizman B, Carmichael LE, Deinhardt F, *et al.* (1981). Herpesviridae. Definition, provisional nomenclature, and taxonomy. *Intervirology* **16**:201–17.

57 Corey L, Spear PG (1981). Infections with herpes simplex viruses. *N Engl J Med* **314**(11): 686–91.

58 Zachariae H (1985). Herpes virus infection in man. *Scand J Infect Dis* **47**(Suppl.):44–50.

59 Whitley, RJ, Gnann, JW Jr (1992). Acyclovir: A decade later. *N Engl J Med* **327** (11):782–9.

60 Hirsch MS, Swartz MN (1980). Drug therapy: antiviral agents (second of two parts). *N Engl J Med* **302**(17):949–53.

61 Chatis PA, Crumpacker CS (1992). Minireview. Resistance of herpes viruses to antiviral drugs. *Antimicrob Agents Chemother* **36**:1589–95.

62 Levin MJ, Bacon TH, Leary JJ (2004). Resistance of herpes simplex virus infections to nucleoside analogues in HIV-infected patients. *Clin Infect Dis* **39** Suppl 5:S248–57.

63 Perry CM, Faulds D (1996). Valaciclovir. A review of its antiviral activity, pharmacokinetic properties, and therapeutic efficacy in herpesvirus infections. *Drugs* **52**(5):754–72.

64 Perry CM, Wagstaff AJ (1995). Famciclovir. A review of its pharmacological properties and therapeutic efficacy in herpes virus infections. *Drugs* **50**(2):396–415.

65 Wagstaff AJ, Bryson HM (1994). Foscarnet. A reappraisal of its antiviral activity, pharmacokinetic properties and therapeutic use in immunocompromised patients with viral infections. *Drugs* **48**(2):199–226.

66 Erlich KS, Mills J, Chatis P, *et al.* (1989). Acyclovir-resistant herpes simplex virus infections in patients with the acquired immunodeficiency syndrome. *N Engl J Med* **320**(5):293–6.

67 Trifillis AL, Cui X, Drusano GL (1993). Use of human proximal tubule cell cultures for studying foscarnet-induced nephrotoxicity *in vitro*. *Antimicrob Agents Chemother* **37**(11):2496–9.

68 Crumpacker CS (1996). Ganciclovir. *N Engl J Med* **335**(10):721–9.

69 Faulds D, Heel RC (1990). Ganciclovir. A review of its antiviral activity, pharmacokinetic properties and therapeutic efficacy in cytomegalovirus infections. *Drugs* **39**(4):597–638.

70 Markham A, Faulds D (1994). Ganciclovir. An update of its therapeutic use in cytomegalovirus infection. *Drugs* **48**(3):455–84.

71 Lea AP, Bryson HM (1996). Cidofovir. *Drugs* **52**(2):225–30.

72 Vandercam B, Moreau M, Goffin E, *et al.* (1999). Cidofovir-induced end-stage renal failure. *Clin Infect Dis* **29**(4):948–9.

73 Meier P, Dautheville-Guibal S, Ronco PM, *et al.* (2002). Cidofovir-induced end-stage renal failure. *Nephrol Dial Transplant* **17**(1):148–9.

74 Geary RS, Henry SP, Grillone LR (2002). Fomivirsen. Clinical Pharmacology and Potential Drug Interactions. *Clin Pharmacokinet* **41**(4):255–60.

75 Whitley RJ (2001). Herpes simplex viruses. In: *Field's Virology*, 4th edn. DM Knipe, PM Howley (eds.) Lippincott-Raven, Philadelphia, pp. 2461–510.

76 Corey L, Adams HG, Brown ZA, *et al.* (1983). Genital herpes simplex virus infections: clinical manifestations, courses, and complications. *Ann Internal Med* **98**:958–72.

77 Lafferty WE, Coombs RW, Benedetti J, *et al.* (1987). Recurrences after oral and genital herpes simplex virus infection. Influence of site of infection and viral type. *New Engl J Med* **316**(23):1444–9.

78 Rode OD, Lepej SZ, Begovac J (2008). Seroprevalence of herpes simplex virus type 2 in adult HIV-infected patients and blood donors in Croatia. *Coll Antropol* **32**(3):693–5.

79 McClelland RS, Lavreys L, Katingima C, *et al.* (2005). Contribution of HIV-1 infection to acquisition of sexually transmitted disease: a 10-year prospective study. *J Infect Dis* **191**(3):333–8.

80 Whitley RJ, Kimberlin DW, Roizman B (1998). Herpes simplex viruses. *Clin Infect Dis* **26**(3):541–55.

81 Foley E (2004). Treatment of genital herpes infections in HIV-infected patients. *J HIV Ther* **9**(1):14–18.

82 Severson JL, Tyring SK (1999). Relation between herpes simplex viruses and human immunodeficiency virus infections. *Arch Dermatol* **135**(11):1393–7.

83 Bagdades EK, Pillay D, Squire SB, *et al.* (1992). Relationship between herpes simplex virus ulceration and CD4+ cell counts in patients with HIV infection. *AIDS* **6**(11):1317–20.

84 Samaratunga H, Weedon D, Musgrave N, *et al.* (2001). Atypical presentation of herpes simplex (chronic hypertrophic herpes) in a patient with HIV Infection. *Pathology* **33**(4):532–5.

85 Tappero JW, Perkins BA, Wenger JD, *et al.* (1995). Cutaneous manifestations of opportunistic infections in patients infected with human immunodeficiency virus. *Clin Microbiol Rev* **8**(3):440–50.

86 Mommeja-Marin H, Lafaurie M, Scieux C, *et al.* (2003). Herpes simplex virus type 2 as a cause of severe meningitis in immunocompromised adults. *Clin Infect Dis* **37**(11):1527–33.

87 Corral I, Quereda C, Navas E, *et al.* (2005). Sacral myeloradiculitis complicating genital herpes in a HIV-infected patient. *Int J STD AIDS* **16**(2):175–7.

88 Yoritaka A, Ohta K, Kishida S (2005). Herpetic lumbosacral radiculoneuropathy in patients with human immunodeficiency virus infection. *Eur Neurol* **53**(4):179–81.

89 McSorley J, Shapiro L, Brownstein MH, *et al.* (1974). Herpes simplex and varicella-zoster: comparative histopathology of 77 cases. *Int J Dermatol* **13**:69–75.

90 Weinberg JM, Mysliwiec A, Turiansky GW, *et al.* (1997). Viral folliculitis. Atypical presentations of herpes simplex, herpes zoster, and molluscum contagiosum. *Arch Dermatol* **133**(8):983–6.

91 Vestergaard, BF (1985). Laboratory diagnosis of herpes viruses. *Scand J Infect Dis* **47**:22–32.

92 Lucotte G, Bathelier C, Lespiaux V, *et al.* (1985). Detection and genotyping of herpes simplex types 1 and 2 by polymerase chain reaction. *Mol Cell Probes* **9**(5):287–90.

93 Hardy WD (1992). Foscarnet treatment of acyclovir-resistant herpes simplex virus infection in patients with acquired immunodeficiency syndrome: preliminary results of a controlled, randomized, regimen-controlled trial. *Am J Med* **92**(2A):30s–5s.

94 Straus SE, Ostrove JM, Inchauspe G, *et al.* (1988). NIH conference. Varicella-zoster virus infections. Biology, natural history, treatment, and prevention. *Ann Internal Med* **108**(2):221–37.

95 Wharton M (1996). The epidemiology of varicella-zoster infections. *Infect Dis Clin North Am* **10**(3):571–81.

96 Kennedy PG, Grinfeld E, Gow JW (1998). Latent varicella-zoster virus is located predominantly in neurons in human trigeminal ganglia. *Proc Natl Acad Sci USA* **95**(8):4658–62.

97 Gnann JW Jr, Whitley RJ (2002). Clinical practice. Herpes zoster. *N Engl J Med* **347**(5):340–6.

98 Oxman MN (1995). Immunization to reduce the frequency and severity of herpes zoster and its complications. *Neurology* **45**(12 Suppl 8):S41–6.

99 Buchbinder SP, Katz MH, Hessol NA, *et al.* (1992). Herpes zoster and human immunodeficiency virus infection. *J Infect Dis* **166**(5):1153–6.

100 Veenstra J, Krol A, Van Praag RME, *et al.* (1995). Herpes zoster, immunological deterioration and disease progression in HIV-1 infection. *AIDS* **9**(10):1153–8.

101 Gershon AA, Mervish N, La Russa P, *et al.* (1997). Varicella-zoster virus infection in children with underlying human immunodeficiency virus infection. *J Infect Dis* **176**(6):1496–500.

102 Dworkin RH, Portenoy RK (1996). Pain and its persistence in herpes zoster. *Pain* **67**(2–3):241–51.

103 Pavan-Langston D (1995). Herpes zoster ophthalmicus. *Neurology* **45**(12 Suppl 8):S50–1.

104 Liesegang TJ (1991). Diagnosis and therapy of herpes zoster ophthalmicus. *Ophthalmology* **98**(8):1216–29.

105 Severson EA, Baratz KH, Hodge DO, *et al.* (2003). Herpes zoster ophthalmicus in olmsted county, Minnesota: have systemic antivirals made a difference? *Arch Ophthalmol* **121**(3):386–90.

106 Saint-Leger E, Caumes E, Breton G, *et al.* (2001). Clinical and virologic characterization of acyclovir-resistant varicella-zoster viruses isolated from 11 patients with acquired immunodeficiency syndrome. *Clin Infect Dis* **33**(12):2061–7.

107 Perronne C, Lazanas M, Leport C, *et al.* (1990). Varicella in patients infected with the human immunodeficiency virus. *Arch Dermatol* **126**(8):1033–6.

108 Weinberg JM, Mysliwiec A, Turiansky GW, *et al.* (1997). Viral folliculitis: atypical presentations of herpes simplex, herpes zoster, and molluscum contagiosum. *Arch Dermatol* **133**(8):983–6.

109 Requena L, Kutzner H, Escalonilla P, *et al.* (1998). Cutaneous reactions at sites of herpes zoster scars: an expanded spectrum. *Br J Dermatol* **138**(1):161–8.

110 Guill MA, Goette DK (1978). Granuloma annulare at sites of healing herpes zoster. *Arch Dermatol* **114**(9):1383–4.

111 Packer RH, Fields JP, King LE (1984). Granuloma annulare in herpes zoster scars. *Cutis* **34**(2):177–9.

112 Friedman SJ, Fox BJ, Albert H (1986). Granuloma annulare arising in herpes zoster scars. *J Am Acad Dermatol* **14**(5 Pt 1):764–70.

113 Shideler SJ, Richards M (1986). Granuloma annulare arising after herpes zoster. *J Am Acad Dermatol* **15**(5 Pt 1):1049–50.

114 Kleber R Landthaler M, Burg G (1989). Postzosterisches granuloma annulare. *Hautarzt* **40**:110–11.

115 Zanolli MD, Powell BL, McCalmont T, *et al.* (1992). Granuloma annulare and disseminated herpes zoster. *Int J Dermatol* **31**(9):55–7.

116 Hayakawa K, Mizukawa Y, Shiohara T, *et al.* (1992). Granuloma annulare arising after herpes zoster. *Int J Dermatol* **31**(10):745–6.

117 Gibney MD, Nahass GT, Leonardi CL (1996). Cutaneous reactions following herpes zoster infections: report of three cases and review of the literature. *Br J Dermatol* **134**(3):504–9.

118 Winkelmann RK, Connolly SM, Yiannias JA, *et al.* (1995). Postzoster eruptions: granuloma annulare, granulomatous vasculitis, and pseudolymphoma. *Eur J Dermatol* **5**:470–6.

119 Langenberg A, Yen TSB, LeBoit PE (1991). Granulomatous vasculitis occurring after cutaneous herpes zoster despite absence of viral genome. *J Am Acad Dermatol* **24**(3):429–33.

120 Baalbaki SA, Malak JA, Al-Khars MAA, *et al.* (1994). Granulomatous vasculitis in herpes zoster. *Int J Dermatol* **33**(4):268–9.

121 Fernández-Redondo V, Amrouni B, Varela E, *et al.* (2001). Granulomatous folliculitis at sites of herpes zoster scars: Wolf's isotopic response. *J Eur Acad Dermatol Venereol* **16**(6):628–30.

122 Toney JF (2005). Skin manifestations of herpesvirus infections. *Curr Infect Dis Rep* **7**(5):359–64.

123 Balfour HH Jr (1988). Varicella zoster virus infections in immunocompromised hosts. A review of the natural history and management. *Am J Med* **85**(2A): 68–73.

124 Antela A, Fortún J, Navas E, *et al.* (1991). Nosocomial varicella: study of an epidemic outbreak among immunosuppressed patients. *Enferm Infecc Microbiol Clin* **9**(6):357–60.

125 Cohen JI, Corey GR (1985). Cytomegalovirus infection in the normal host. *Medicine (Baltimore)* **64**(2):100–14.

126 Goldberg DE, Smithen LM, Angelilli A, *et al.* (2005). HIV-associated retinopathy in the HAART era. *Retina* **25**(5):633–49; quiz 682–3.

127 Bournérias I, Boisnic S, Patey O, *et al.* (1989). Unusual cutaneous cytomegalovirus involvement in patients with acquired immunodeficiency syndrome. *Arch Dermatol* **125**(9):1243–6.

128 Chiewchanvit S, Thamprasert K, Siriunkgul S (1993). Disseminated cutaneous cytomegalovirus inclusion disease resembling prurigo nodularis in an HIV-infected patient: case report and literature review. *J Med Assoc Thai* **76**(10):581–4.

129 Horn TD, Hood AF (1990). Cytomegalovirus is predictably present in perineal ulcers from immunosuppressed patients. *Arch Dermatol* **126**(5):642–4.

130 Penneys NS, Hicks B (1985).

Unusual cutaneous lesions associated with acquired immunodeficiency syndrome. *J Am Acad Dermatol* **13**(5 Pt 1):845–52.

131 Lee JY, Peel R (1989). Concurrent cytomegalovirus and herpes simplex virus infections in skin biopsy specimens from two AIDS patients with fatal CMV infection. *Am J Dermatopathol* **11**(2):136–43.

132 Strano AJ (1976). Light Microscopy of selected viral diseases (morphology of viral inclusion bodies). *Pathol Annu* **11**:53–75.

133 Chou S (1990). Newer methods for diagnosis of cytomegalovirus infection. *Rev Infect Dis* **12** Suppl 7:S727–36.

134 Bek B, Boeckh M, Lepenies J, *et al.* (1996). High-level sensitivity of quantitative pp65 cytomegalovirus (CMV) antigenemia assay for diagnosis of CMV disease in AIDS patients and follow-up. *J Clin Microbiol* **34**(2):457.

135 Triantos D, Porter SR, Scully C, *et al.* (1997). Oral hairy leukoplakia: Clinicopathologic features, pathogenesis, diagnosis, and clinical significance. *Clin Infect Dis* **25**(6):1392–6.

136 Epstein JB, Sherlock CH, Greenspan JS (1991). Hairy leukoplakia-like lesions following bone-marrow transplantation. *AIDS* **5**(1):101–2.

137 Macleod RI, Long LQ, Soames JV, *et al.* (1990). Oral hairy leukoplakia in an HIV-negative renal transplant patient. *Br Dent J* **169**(7):208–9.

138 Schmidt-Westhausen A, Gelderblom HR, Reichart PA (1990). Oral hairy leukoplakia in an HIV-seronegative heart transplant patient. *J Oral Pathol Med* **19**(4);192–4.

139 Eisenberg E, Krutchkoff D, Yamase H (1992). Incidental oral hairy leukoplakia in immunocompetent persons. A report of two cases. *Oral Surg Oral Med Oral Pathol* **74**(3):332–3.

140 Itin PH (1993). Oral hairy leukoplakia – 10 years on. *Dermatology* **187**(3):159–63.

141 Freedberg IM, Eisen AZ, Klaus Wolff K, *et al.* (2003). *Fitzpatrick's Dermatology in General Medicine,* 6th edn. Volume II, pp. 2067–68.

CHAPTER 3

1 Holdiness M (2002). Management of cutaneous erythrasma. *Drugs*

62(8):1131–41.

2 Granok AB, Benjamin P, Garret LS (2002). *Corynebacterium minutissimum* bacteremia in an immunocompetent host with cellulitis. *Clin Infec Dis* **35**:e40–e42.

3 Santos-Juanes J (2002). Cutaneous granuloma caused by *Corynebacterium minutissimum* in an HIV-infected man. *Eur Acad Dermatol Venereol* **16**:638–49.

4 Bandera A, Gori A, Rossi MC, *et al.* (2000). A case of costochondral abscess due to *Corynebacterium minutissimum* in an HIV-infected patient. *J Infect* **41**(1):103–5.

5 Takama H, Tamada Y, Yano K, Nitta Y, Ikeya T (1997). Pitted keratolysis: clinical manifestations in 53 cases. *Br J Dermatol* **137**:282–5.

6 Longshaw CM, Wright JD, Farrell AM, Holland KT (2002). *Kytococcus sedentarius*, the organism associated with pitted keratolysis, produces two keratin-degrading enzymes. *J Appl Microbiol* **93**(5):810–16.

7 Takama H, Tamada Y, Yokoichi K, Ikeya T (1998). Pitted keratolyisis: a discussion of two cases in nonweight-bearing areas. *Acta Derm Venereol (Stockh)* **78**(3):225–6.

8 Wohlrab J, Rohrbach D, Marsch WC (2000). Keratolysis sulcata (pitted keratolysis): clinical symptoms with different histological correlates. *Br J Dermatol* **143**(6):1348–9.

9 Tamura BM, Cuce LC, Souza RL, Levites J (2004). Plantar hyperhidrosis and pitted keratolysis treated with *Botulinum* toxin injection. *Dermatol Surg* **30**:1510–14.

10 Luelmo-Aguilar J, Santandreu MS (2004). Folliculitis. Recognition and managment. *Am J Clin Dermatol* **5**(5):301–10.

11 Rhody C (2000). Bacterial infections of the skin. *Primary Care* **27**(2):459–73.

12 Chiller K, Selkin BA, Murakawa GJ (2001). Skin microflora and bacterial infections of the skin. *J Investig Dermatol Symp Proc* **6**(3):170–4.

13 Smith KJ, Neafie R, Yeager J, Skelton HG (1999). *Micrococcus* folliculitis in HIV-1 disease. *Br J Dermatol* **141**(3):558–61.

14 Bachmeyer C, Landgraf N, Cordier F, Lematire P, Blum L (2004). *Acinetobacter baumanii* folliculitis in a patient with AIDS. *Clin Exp Dermatol* **30**(3):256–8.

15 Holmes RB, Martins C, Horn T

(2002). The histopathology of folliculitis in HIV-infected patients. *J Cut Pathol* **29**(2):93–5.

16 Ladhani S (2003). Understanding the mechanism of action of the exfoliative toxins of *Staphyloccus aureus*. *FEMS Immunol Med Microbiol* **39**(2):181–9.

17 Yamasaki O, Yamaguchi T, Sugai M, Chapuis-Cellier C, *et al.* (2005). Clinical manifestations of staphylococcal scalded-skin syndrome depend of serotypes of exfoliative toxins. *J Clin Microbiol* **43**(4):1890–3.

18 Hanakawa Y, Stanley JR (2004). Mechanisms of blister formation by staphylococcal toxins. *J Biochem* **136**(6):747–50.

19 Amagai M, Matsuyoshi N, Wang ZH, Andl C, Stanley JR (2000). Toxin in bullous impetigo and staphylococcal scalded-skin syndrome targets desmoglein 1. *Nature Med* **6**(11):1275–7.

20 Udey MC, Stanley JR (1999). Pemphigus-diseases of antidesmosomal autoimmunity. *JAMA* **282**(6): 572–6.

21 Wiley BB, Allman S, Rogolsky M, Norden CW, Glasgow LA (1974). Staphylococcal scalded skin syndrome: potentiation by immunosuppression in mice; toxin medicated exfoliation in a healthy adult. *Infect Immunol* **9**(4):636–40.

22 Patel GK, Finlay AY (2003). Staphylococcal scalded skin syndrome: diagnosis and treatment. *Am J Clin Dermatol* **4**(3):165–75.

23 Farrell AM, Ross JS, Umasankar S, Bunker CB (1996). Staphylococcal scalded skin syndrome in an HIV-1 seropositive man. *Br J Dermatol* **134**(5):962–5.

24 Rigopoulos D, Paparizos V, Katsambas A. (2004). Cutaneous markers of HIV Infection. *Clin Dermatol* **22**(6):487–98.

25 Cockerell CJ, Tierno PM, Friedman-Kien AE, Kim KS (1991). Clinical, histologic, microbiologic, and biochemical characterization of the causative agent of bacillary (epitherlioid) angiomatosis: a rickettsial illness with features of bartonellosis. *J Investig Dermatol* **97**(5):812–17.

26 Santos R, Cardoso O, Rodrigues P, *et al.* (2000). Bacillary angiomatosis by *Bartonella quintana* in an HIV-infected patient. *J Am Acad Dermatol* **42**(2):299–301.

27 Kayaselcuk F, Ceken I, Bircan S, Tuncert I (2002). Bacillary

angiomatosis of the scalp in a human immunodeficiency virus-negative patient. *Eur Acad Dermatol Venereol* **16**(6):612–614.

28 Cockerell C (1992). The causative agent of bacillary angiomatosis. *Int J Dermatol* **31**(9):615–16.

29 Wilson W, Sande M (2001). *Current Diagnosis and Treatment of Infectious Disease*, 1st edn. McGraw-Hill Medical, pp. 713–20.

30 Caplan SE, Kauffman CL (1996). Primary incoluation tuberculosis after immunotherapy for malignant melanoma with BCG vaccine. *J Am Acad Dermatol* **35**(5): 783–85.

31 Sehgal VN (1994). Cutaneous tuberculosis. *Dermatol Clin* **12**(4):645–53.

32 Barbagallo J, Tager P, Ingleton R, Hirsch RJ, Weinberg JM (2002). Cutaneous tuberculosis: diagnosis and treatment. *Am J Clin Dermatol* **3**(5):319–28.

33 Lundgren R, Norman E, Asbert I (1987). Tuberculosis infection transmitted at autopsy. *Tubercle* **68**(2):147–50.

34 Freedberg I, Eisen A, Wolff K, *et al.* (1999). Tuberculosis and other mycobacterial infections. In: *Dermatology in General Medicine*, 5th edn. EA Fitzpatrick, TB Wolff, *et al.* (eds), McGraw Hill, New York, pp. 2274–92.

35 Curco N, Pagerols X, Gomez L, Vives P (1996). *Mycobacterium kansasii* infection limited to the skin in a patient with AIDS. *Br J Dermatol* **135**(2):324–26.

36 High WA, Evans CC, Hoang MP (2004). Cutaneous miliary tuberculosis in two patients with HIV infection. *J Am Acad Dermatol* **50**(5):s110–13.

37 Tappe D, Langmann P, Zilly M, Klinker H, Schmausser B, Frosch M (2004). Osteomyelitis and skin ulcers caused by *Mycobacterium szulgai* in an AIDS patient. *Scand J Infect Dis* **36**:883–5.

38 Boyd AS, Robbins J (2005). Cutaneous *Mycobacterium avium intracellulare* infection in an HIV+ patient mimicking histoid leprosy. *Am J Dermatopathol* **27**(1):39–41.

39 Bartralot R, Pujol RM, Garcia-Patos V, Sitjas D, *et al.* (2000). Cutaneous infections due to nontuberculous mycobacteria: histopathological review of 28 cases. Comparative study between lesions observed in immunosuppressed patients and normal hosts. *J Cut Pathol* **27**(3):124–9.

CHAPTER 4

1 Ruhnke M (2004). Mucosal and systemic fungal infections in patients with AIDS: prophylaxis and treatment. *Drugs* **64**(11):1163–80.

2 Lynch, DP, Naftolin LZ (1987). Oral *Cryptococcus neoformans* infection in AIDS. *Oral Surg Oral Med Oral Pathol* **64**(4):449–53.

3 Richardson MD (2005). Changing patterns and trends in systemic fungal infections. *J Antimicrob Chemother* **56**(Suppl 1):i5–11.

4 Polis MA, Kovacs JA (1997). Fungal infections in patients with the acquired immune deficiency syndrome. In: *AIDS: Biology, Diagnosis, Treatment and Prevention*. Lippincott-Raven, Philadelphia, pp. 231–42.

5 Perfect JR, Casadevall A (2002). Cryptococcosis. *Infect Dis Clin North Am* **16**(4):837–74, v–vi.

6 Neilson JB, Fromtling RA, *et al.* (1977). *Cryptococcus neoformans*: size range of infectious particles from aerosolized soil. *Infect Immun* **17**(3):634–38.

7 Subramanian S, Mathai D (2005). Clinical manifestations and management of cryptococcal infection. *J Postgrad Med* **51**(Suppl 1):S21–6.

8 Sorrell TC (2001). *Cryptococcus neoformans* variety gattii. *Med Mycol* **39**(2):155–68.

9 Bartlett JF (2001). Causes of death in U.S. Patients dying of AIDS. In: *The Johns Hopkins Hospital 2002 Guide to Medical Care of Patients with HIV Infection*. Lipincott Williams and Wilkins, Philadelphia, p. 19.

10 Johnson RA (2000). HIV disease: mucocutaneous fungal infections in HIV disease. *Clin Dermatol* **18**(4):411–22.

11 Hakim JG, Gangaidzo IT, Heyderman RS, *et al.* (2000). Impact of HIV infection on meningitis in Harare, Zimbabwe: a prospective study of 406 predominantly adult patients. *Aids* **14**(10):1401–7.

12 Palella, FJ Jr, Delaney KM, Moorman AC, *et al.* (1998). Declining morbidity and mortality among patients with advanced human immunodeficiency virus infection. HIV Outpatient Study Investigators. *N Engl J Med* **338**(13):853–60.

13 Hajjeh RA, Conn LA, Stephens DS, *et al.* (1999). Cryptococcosis: population-based multistate active surveillance and risk factors in human immunodeficiency virus-infected persons. Cryptococcal Active Surveillance Group. *J Infect Dis* **179**(2):449–54.

14 Mehrabi M, Bagheri S, Leonard MK Jr, *et al.* (2005). Muco-cutaneous manifestation of cryptococcal infection: report of a case and review of the literature. *J Oral Maxillofac Surg* **63**(10):1543–9.

15 Levitz SM, DiBenedetto DJ (1989). Paradoxical role of capsule in murine bronchoalveolar macrophage-mediated killing of *Cryptococcus neoformans*. *J Immunol* **142**(2):659–65.

16 Huffnagle GB, Traynor TR, McDonald RA, *et al.* (2000). Leukocyte recruitment during pulmonary *Cryptococcus neoformans* infection. *Immunopharmacology* **48**(3):231–6.

17 Hill, JO (1992). CD4+ T cells cause multinucleated giant cells to form around Cryptococcus neoformans and confine the yeast within the primary site of infection in the respiratory tract. *J Exp Med* **175**(6):1685–95.

18 Feldmesser M, Tucker S, Casadevall A (2001). Intracellular parasitism of macrophages by *Cryptococcus neoformans*. *Trends Microbiol* **9**(6):273–8.

19 Crowe SM, Carlin JB, Stewart KI, *et al.* (1991). Predictive value of CD4 lymphocyte numbers for the development of opportunistic infections and malignancies in HIV-infected persons. *J Acquir Immune Defic Syndr* **4**(8):770–6.

20 Sorvillo F, Beall G, Turner PA, *et al.* (1997). Incidence and factors associated with extrapulmonary cryptococcosis among persons with HIV infection in Los Angeles County. *AIDS* **11**(5):673–9.

21 Sabetta JR, Andriole VT (1985). Cryptococcal infection of the central nervous system. *Med Clin North Am* **69**(2):333–44.

22 Hage CA, Goldman M, Wheat LJ (2002). Mucosal and invasive fungal infections in HIV/AIDS. *Eur J Med Res* **7**(5):236–41.

23 Dimino-Emme L, Gurevitch AW (1995). Cutaneous manifestations of disseminated cryptococcosis. *J Am Acad Dermatol* **32**(5 Pt 2):844–50.

24 Powderly W (1999). Fungi. In: *Textbook of AIDS Medicine*. Williams and Wilkins, Baltimore, pp. 357–71.

25 Shibuya K, Hirata A, Omuta J, *et al.* (2005). Granuloma and

cryptococcosis. *J Infect Chemother* **11**(3):115–22.

26 Zuger A, Louie E, Holzman RS, *et al.* (1986). Cryptococcal disease in patients with the acquired immunodeficiency syndrome. Diagnostic features and outcome of treatment. *Ann Internal Med* **104**(2):234–40.

27 Kovacs JA, Kovacs AA, Polis M, *et al.* (1985). Cryptococcosis in the acquired immunodeficiency syndrome. *Ann Internal Med* **103**(4):533–38.

28 Powderly WG (2000). Current approach to the acute management of cryptococcal infections. *J Infect* **41**(1):18–22.

29 van der Horst CM, Saag MS, Cloud GA, *et al.* (1997). Treatment of cryptococcal meningitis associated with the acquired immunodeficiency syndrome. National Institute of Allergy and Infectious Diseases Mycoses Study Group and AIDS Clinical Trials Group. *N Engl J Med* **337**(1):15–21.

30 Benson CA, Kaplan JE, Masur H, *et al.* (2004). Treating opportunistic infections among HIV-exposed and infected children: recommendations from CDC, the National Institutes of Health, and the Infectious Diseases Society of America. *MMWR Recomm Rep* **53**(RR-15):1–112.

31 Graybill JR, Sobel J, Saag M (2000). Diagnosis and management of increased intracranial pressure in patients with AIDS and cryptococcal meningitis. The NIAID Mycoses Study Group and AIDS Cooperative Treatment Groups. *Clin Infect Dis* **30**(1):47–54.

32 Aberg JA, Price RW, Heeren DM, *et al.* (2002). A pilot study of the discontinuation of antifungal therapy for disseminated cryptococcal disease in patients with acquired immunodeficiency syndrome, following immunologic response to antiretroviral therapy. *J Infect Dis* **185**(8):1179–82.

33 Vibhagool A, Sungkanuparph S, Mootsikapun P, *et al.* (2003). Discontinuation of secondary prophylaxis for cryptococcal meningitis in human immunodeficiency virus-infected patients treated with highly active antiretroviral therapy: a prospective, multicenter, randomized study. *Clin Infect Dis* **36**(10):1329–31.

34 Powderly WG (1996). Prophylaxis for HIV-related infections: a work in progress. *Ann Internal Med* **124**(3):342–4.

35 Lortholary O, Fontanet A, Memain N, *et al.* (2005). Incidence and risk factors of immune reconstitution inflammatory syndrome complicating HIV-associated cryptococcosis in France. *AIDS* **19**(10):1043–9.

36 Powderly WG, Landay A, Lederman MM (1998). Recovery of the immune system with antiretroviral therapy: the end of opportunism? *JAMA* **280**(1):72–7.

37 Subramanian S, Abraham OC, Rupali P, *et al.* (2005). Disseminated histoplasmosis. *J Assoc Physicians India* **53**:185–9.

38 Woods JP (2002). *Histoplasma capsulatum* molecular genetics, pathogenesis, and responsiveness to its environment. *Fungal Genet Biol* **35**(2):81–97.

39 Antinori S, Magni C, Nebuloni M, *et al.* (2006). Histoplasmosis among human immunodeficiency virus-infected people in Europe: report of 4 cases and review of the literature. *Medicine* (*Baltimore*) **85**(1):22–36.

40 Gutierrez ME, Canton A, Sosa N (2005). Disseminated histoplasmosis in patients with AIDS in Panama: a review of 104 cases. *Clin Infect Dis* **40**(8):1199–202.

41 Manfredi R, Mazzoni A, Nanetti A, Chiodo F (1994). Histoplasmosis *capsulati* and *duboisii* in Europe: the impact of the HIV pandemic, travel and immigration. *Eur J Epidemiol* **10**(6):675–81.

42 Wheat LJ, Kauffman CA (2003). Histoplasmosis. *Infect Dis Clin North Am* **17**(1):1–19, vii.

43 Goodwin RA Jr, Shapiro JL, Thurman GH (1980). Disseminated histoplasmosis: clinical and pathologic correlations. *Medicine* (*Baltimore*) **59**(1):1–33.

44 Antinori S, Ridolfo AL, Corbellino M, *et al.* (2000). Disseminated histoplasmosis in patients with AIDS. 2 case reports. *Recenti Prog Med* **91**(7–8):362–4.

45 Wheat J (1996). Histoplasmosis in the acquired immunodeficiency syndrome. *Curr Top Med Mycol* **7**(1):7–18.

46 Wheat LJ, Connolly-Stringfield PA, Baker RL, *et al.* (1990). Disseminated histoplasmosis in the acquired immune deficiency syndrome: clinical findings, diagnosis and treatment, and review of the literature. *Medicine* (*Baltimore*) **69**(6):361–74.

47 Williams B, Fojtasek M, Connolly-Stringfield PA, *et al.* (1994). Diagnosis of histoplasmosis by antigen detection during an outbreak in Indianapolis, Ind. *Arch Pathol Lab Med* **118**(12):1205–8.

48 Wheat LJ, Kohler RB, Tewari RP (1986). Diagnosis of disseminated histoplasmosis by detection of *Histoplasma capsulatum* antigen in serum and urine specimens. *N Engl J Med* **314**(2):83–8.

49 Wheat LJ, Connolly-Stringfield P, Blair R, *et al.* (1991). Histoplasmosis relapse in patients with AIDS: detection using *Histoplasma capsulatum* variety *capsulatum* antigen levels. *Ann Internal Med* **115**(12):936–41.

50 Wheat J, Sarosi G, McKinsey D, *et al.* (2000). Practice guidelines for the management of patients with histoplasmosis. Infectious Diseases Society of America. *Clin Infect Dis* **30**(4):688–95.

51 Hecht FM, Wheat J, Korzun AH, *et al.* (1997). Itraconazole maintenance treatment for histoplasmosis in AIDS: a prospective, multicenter trial. *J Acquir Immune Defic Syndr Hum Retrovirol* **16**(2):100–7.

52 Wheat LJ, Connolly P, Smedema M, *et al.* (2001). Emergence of resistance to fluconazole as a cause of failure during treatment of histoplasmosis in patients with acquired immunodeficiency disease syndrome. *Clin Infect Dis* **33**(11):1910–13.

53 Norris S, Wheat J, McKinsey D, *et al.* (1994). Prevention of relapse of histoplasmosis with fluconazole in patients with the acquired immunodeficiency syndrome. *Am J Med* **96**(6):504–8.

54 McKinsey DS, Gupta MR, Driks MR, *et al.* (1992). Histoplasmosis in patients with AIDS: efficacy of maintenance amphotericin B therapy. *Am J Med* **92**(2):225–7.

55 McKinsey DS, Wheat LJ, Cloud GA, *et al.* (1999). Itraconazole prophylaxis for fungal infections in patients with advanced human immunodeficiency virus infection: randomized, placebo-controlled, double-blind study. National Institute of Allergy and Infectious Diseases Mycoses Study Group. *Clin Infect Dis* **28**(5):1049–56.

56 Rixford E, Gilchrist T (1896). Two cases of protozoan (coccidioidal) infection of the skin and other organs. In: *Johns Hopkins Hosp*

Red pp. 209–68.

57 Ophuls W, Moffitt H (1900). A new pathogenic mould (formerly described as a protozoan *Coccidioides imminitis pyogenes*): preliminary report. *Philadelphia Med J*5:1471–2.

58 Dickson E (1937). Valley fever of the San Joaquin Valley and fungus *Coccidioides*. *Calif West Med* 47:151–5.

59 Pappagianis D (1988). Epidemiology of coccidioidomycosis. *Curr Top Med Mycol* 2:199–238.

60 Chiller TM, Galgiani JN, Stevens DA (2003). Coccidioidomycosis. *Infect Dis Clin North Am* 17(1):41–57, viii.

61 Werner SB, Pappagianis D, Heindl I, *et al.* (1972). An epidemic of coccidioidomycosis among archeology students in northern California. *N Engl J Med* 286(10):507–12.

62 Galgiani JN, Isenberg RA, Stevens DA (1978). Chemotaxigenic activity of extracts from the mycelial and spherule phases of *Coccidioides immitis* for human polymorphonuclear leukocytes. *Infect Immun* 21(3):862–5.

63 Magee DM, Cox RA (1995). Roles of gamma interferon and interleukin-4 in genetically determined resistance to *Coccidioides immitis*. *Infect Immun* 63(9):3514–19.

64 Resnick S, Pappagianis D, McKerrow JH (1987). Proteinase production by the parasitic cycle of the pathogenic fungus *Coccidioides immitis*. *Infect Immun* 55(11):2807–15.

65 Peterson CM, Schuppert K, Kelly PC, *et al.* (1993). Coccidioidomy-cosis and pregnancy. *Obstet Gynecol Surv* 48(3):149–56.

66 Gifford MA, Buss WC, Douds RJ (1936). Data on coccidioides fungus infection, Kern County, Bakersfield, CA. In: *Kern County Public Health Annual Report* 1936–1937, pp. 39–54.

67 Ampel NM, Dols CL, Galgiani JN (1993). Coccidioidomycosis during human immunodeficiency virus infection: results of a prospective study in a coccidioidal endemic area. *Am J Med* 94(3):235–40.

68 Jacobs P (1980). Cutaneous coccidioidomycosis. In: *Coccidioidomycosis*. DA Stevens (ed). Plenum Publishing, New York, pp. 213–24.

69 Banuelos AF, Williams PL, Johnson RH, *et al.* (1996). Central nervous system abscesses due to *Coccidioides* species. *Clin Infect Dis* 22(2):240–50.

70 Stockman L, Clark KA, Hunt JM, *et al.* (1993). Evaluation of commercially available acridinium ester-labeled chemiluminescent DNA probes for culture identification of *Blastomyces dermatitidis*, *Coccidioides immitis*, *Cryptococcus neoformans*, and *Histoplasma capsulatum*. *J Clin Microbiol* 31(4):845–50.

71 Galgiani JN (1993). Coccidioidomycosis. *West J Med* 159(2):153–71.

72 Beard JS, Benson PM, Skillman L (1993). Rapid diagnosis of coccidioidomycosis with a DNA probe to ribosomal RNA. *Arch Dermatol* 129(12):1589–93.

73 Fish DG, Ampel NM, Galgiani JN, *et al.* (1990). Coccidioidomycosis during human immunodeficiency virus infection. A review of 77 patients. *Medicine* (Baltimore) 69(6):384–91.

74 Kullberg BJ, Oude Lashof AM (2002). Epidemiology of opportunistic invasive mycoses. *Eur J Med Res* 7(5):183–91.

75 Denning DW (1996). Therapeutic outcome in invasive aspergillosis. *Clin Infect Dis* 23(3):608–15.

76 Holding KJ, Dworkin MS, Wan PC, *et al.* (2000). Aspergillosis among people infected with human immunodeficiency virus: incidence and survival. Adult and Adolescent Spectrum of HIV Disease Project. *Clin Infect Dis* 31(5):1253–7.

77 Woitas RP, Rockstroh JK, Theisen A, *et al.* (1998). Changing role of invasive aspergillosis in AIDS – a case control study. *J Infect* 37(2):116–22.

78 Streifel AJ, Lauer JL, Vesley D, *et al.* (1983). *Aspergillus fumigatus* and other thermotolerant fungi generated by hospital building demolition. *Appl Environ Microbiol* 46(2):375–8.

79 Mahieu LM, De Dooy JJ, Van Laer FA, *et al.* (2000). A prospective study on factors influencing *Aspergillus* spore load in the air during renovation works in a neonatal intensive care unit. *J Hosp Infect* 45(3):191–7.

80 Denning DW (1998). Invasive aspergillosis. *Clin Infect Dis* 26(4):781–803; quiz 804–785.

81 Khoo SH, Denning DW (1994). Invasive aspergillosis in patients with AIDS. *Clin Infect Dis* 19(Suppl 1):S41–8.

82 Lin SJ, Schranz J, Teutsch SM (2001). Aspergillosis case-fatality rate: systematic review of the literature. *Clin Infect Dis* 32(3):358–66.

83 Denning DW, Follansbee SE, Scolaro M, *et al.* (1991). Pulmonary aspergillosis in the acquired immunodeficiency syndrome. *N Engl J Med* 324(10):654–62.

84 van Burik JA, Colven R, Spach DH (1998). Cutaneous aspergillosis. *J Clin Microbiol* 36(11):3115–21.

85 Grossman ME, Fithian EC, Behrens C (1985). Primary cutaneous aspergillosis in six leukemic children. *J Am Acad Dermatol* 12(2 Pt 1):313–18.

86 Pursell KJ, Telzak EE, Armstrong D (1992). *Aspergillus* species colonization and invasive disease in patients with AIDS. *Clin Infect Dis* 14(1):141–8.

87 Mylonakis E, Barlam TF, Flanigan T, *et al.* (1998). Pulmonary aspergillosis and invasive disease in AIDS: review of 342 cases. *Chest* 114(1):251–62.

88 Leenders AC, Daenen S, Jansen RL, *et al.* (1998). Liposomal amphotericin B compared with amphotericin B deoxycholate in the treatment of documented and suspected neutropenia-associated invasive fungal infections. *Br J Haematol* 103(1):205–12.

89 Splendore A (1912). Zymonematosis com localizazzio ne nella cavita della bocca, osservada in Brasile. *Bull Soc Path Exot* 5:313–19.

90 Almeida OP, Jacks J Jr, Scully C (2003). Paracoccidioidomycosis of the mouth: an emerging deep mycosis. *Crit Rev Oral Biol Med* 14(5):377–83.

91 Talhari S, Garrido NR, (eds) (1997). Paracoccidioidomycoses. In: *Dermatologia Tropical*. Ed Medsi, Rio de Janeiro.

92 Restrepo A (1985). The ecology of *Paracoccidioides brasiliensis*: a puzzle still unsolved. *Sabouraudia* 23(5):323–34.

93 Benard G, Duarte AJ (2000). Paracoccidioidomycosis: a model for evaluation of the effects of human immunodeficiency virus infection on the natural history of endemic tropical diseases. *Clin Infect Dis* 31(4):1032–9.

94 Brummer E, Castaneda E, Restrepo

A (1993). Paracoccidioidomycosis: an update. *Clin Microbiol Rev* 6(2):89–117.

95 Bicalho RN, Santo MF, de Aguiar MC, *et al*. (2001). Oral paracoccidioidomycosis: a retrospective study of 62 Brazilian patients. *Oral Dis* 7(1):56–60.

96 Mendes-Giannini MJ, Moraes RA, Ricci TA (1990). Proteolytic activity of the 43,000 molecular weight antigen secreted by *Paracoccidioides brasiliensis*. *Rev Inst Med Trop Sao Paulo* 32(5):384–5.

97 Puccia R, Schenkman S, Gorin PA, *et al*. (1986). Exocellular components of *Paracoccidioides brasiliensis*: identification of a specific antigen. *Infect Immun* 53(1):199–206.

98 Flavia Popi AF, Lopes JD, Mariano M (2002). GP43 from *Paracoccidioides brasiliensis* inhibits macrophage functions. An evasion mechanism of the fungus. *Cell Immunol* 218(1-2):87–94.

99 Oliveira SJ, Mamoni RL, Musatti CC, *et al*. (2002). Cytokines and lymphocyte proliferation in juvenile and adult forms of paracoccidioidomycosis: comparison with infected and noninfected controls. *Microbes Infect* 4(2):139–44.

100 Valle ACF, Wanke B (1992). Tratamento do paracoccidioidomicose: estude retrospective de 500 casos. *Anais Brasileiros de Dermatologia* 67:251–4.

101 Castro RM, Del Negro G (1976). Clinical characteristics of paracoccidioidomycosis in children. *Rev Hosp Clin Fac Med Sao Paulo* 31(3):194–8.

102 Mendes P, Pereira PC (1992). Juvenile type of paracoccidioidomycosis: a retrospective study of 30 cases [abstract C-2/0]. *Revista Argentina de Micologia* 15(63).

103 Restrepo A, Salazar ME, Cano LE, *et al*. (1984). Estrogens inhibit mycelium-to-yeast transformation in the fungus *Paracoccidioides brasiliensis*: implications for resistance of females to paracoccidioidomycosis. *Infect Immun* 46(2):346–53.

104 Benard G, Hong MA, Del Negro GM, *et al*. (1996). Antigen-specific immunosuppression in paracoccidioidomycosis. *Am J Trop Med Hyg* 54(1):7–12.

105 McKinsey DS, Spiegel RA,

Hutwagner L, *et al*. (1997). Prospective study of histoplasmosis in patients infected with human immunodeficiency virus: incidence, risk factors, and pathophysiology. *Clin Infect Dis* 24(6):1195–203.

106 Marques SA, Conterno LO, Sgarbi LP, *et al*. (1995). Paracoccidioidomycosis associated with acquired immunodeficiency syndrome. Report of seven cases. *Rev Inst Med Trop Sao Paulo* 37(3):261–5.

107 Saraiva EC, Altemani A, Franco MF, *et al*. (1996). *Paracoccidioides brasiliensis*-gp43 used as paracoccidioidin. *J Med Vet Mycol* 34(3):155–61.

108 De Brito T, Sandhu GS, Kline BC, *et al*. (1999). *In situ* hybridization in paracoccidioidomycosis. *Med Mycol* 37(3):207–11.

109 Motoyama AB, Venancio EJ, Brandao GO, *et al*. (2000). Molecular identification of *Paracoccidioides brasiliensis* by PCR amplification of ribosomal DNA. *J Clin Microbiol* 38(8):3106–9.

110 Goldani LZ, Sugar AM (1995). Paracoccidioidomycosis and AIDS: an overview. *Clin Infect Dis* 21(5):1275–81.

111 Marques SA, Robles AM, Tortorano AM, *et al*. (2000). Mycoses associated with AIDS in the Third World. *Med Mycol* 38(Suppl 1):269–79.

112 Duong TA (1996). Infection due to *Penicillium marneffei*, an emerging pathogen: review of 155 reported cases. *Clin Infect Dis* 23(1):125–30.

113 Supparatpinyo K, Khamwan C, Baosoung V, *et al*. (1994). Disseminated *Penicillium marneffei* infection in southeast Asia. *Lancet* 344(8915):110–13.

114 Oscherwitz SL, Rinaldi MG (1992). Disseminated sporotrichosis in a patient infected with human immunodeficiency virus. *Clin Infect Dis* 15(3):568–9.

115 Carvalho MT, de Castro AP, Baby C, *et al*. (2002). Disseminated cutaneous sporotrichosis in a patient with AIDS: report of a case. *Rev Soc Bras Med Trop* 35(6):655–9.

116 (No authors listed) (1987). Revision of the CDC surveillance case definition for acquired immunodeficiency syndrome. Council of State and Territorial Epidemiologists; AIDS Program, Center for Infectious Diseases. *MMWR Morb Mortal Wkly Rep* 36(Suppl 1):1S–15S.

CHAPTER 5

1 Downs AMR, Harvey I, Kennedy CTC (1999). The epidemiology of head lice and scabies in the UK. *Epidemiol. Infect* 122:471–7.

2 Munoz-Perez MA, Rodriguez-Pichardo A, Camacho Martinez F (1998). Sexually transmitted disease in 1161 HIV-positive patients: a 38-month prospective study in southern Spain. *J Eur Acad Dermatol Venereol* 11(3):221–6.

3 Farrell AM, Ross JS, Bunker CB, Staughton RCD (1998). Crusted scabies with scalp involvement in HIV-1 infection. *Brit J Dermatol* 138:192–3.

4 Perna AB, Bell K, Rosen T (2004). Localised genital Norwegian scabies in an AIDS patient. *Sex Transmitt Infect* 80:72–3.

5 Portu JJ, Santamaria JM, Zubero Z, *et al*. (1996). Atypical scabies in HIV-positive patients. *J Am Acad Dermatol* 34(5 Pt 2): 915–17.

6 Hulbert TV, Larsen, RA (1992). Hyperkeratotic (Norwegian) scabies with gram-negative bacteremia as the initial presentation of AIDS. *Clin Infect Dis* 14:1164–5.

7 Skinner SM, DeVillez RL (1992). Sepsis associated with Norwegian scabies in patients with acquired immunodeficiency syndrome. *Cutis* 50:213–16.

8 Meinking TL, Taplin D, Herminda JL, *et al*. (1995). The treatment of scabies with ivermectin *N Engl J Med* 333:26–30.

9 Pellizer G, Betto P, Manfrin V, *et al*. (1996). Ivermectin treatment of AIDS-related crusted scabies. *Eur J Dermatol* 6:396.

10 De Almeida, HL (2005). Treatment of steroid resistant nodular scabies with topical pimecrolimus. *J Am Acad Dermatol* 53(2):357–8.

11 Holmes RB, Martins C, Horn T (2002). The histopathology of folliculitis in HIV-infected patients. *J Cutan Pathol* 29:93–5.

12 Dominey A, Rosen T, Tschen J (1989). immunodeficiency syndrome. *J Am Acad Dermatol* 20(2 Pt 1):197–201.

13 Sarro RA, Hong JJ, Elgart ML (1998). An unusual demodicidosis manifestation in a patient with AIDS. *J Am Acad Dermatol* 38(1):120–1.

14 Ashak RJ, Frost ML, Norins AL (1989). Papular pruritic eruption of *Demodex* folliculitis in patients with

acquired immunodeficiency syndrome. *J Am Acad Dermatol* **21**(2 Pt 1):306–7.

15 Redondo-Mateo J, Soto-Guzman O, Fernandez-Rubio E, Dominguez-Franjo F (1993). *Demodex*-attributed rosacea-like lesions in AIDS. *Acta Derm Venereol* **73**:437.

16 Schaller M, Sander CA, Pledwig G (2003). *Demodex* abscesses: clinical and therapeutic challenges. *J Am Acad Dermatol* **49**(5):S272–4.

17 Gonzalez MM, Gould E, Dickinson G, *et al.* (1986). Acquired immunodeficiency syndrome associated with *Acanthamoeba* infection and other opportunistic organisms. *Arch Pathol Lab Med* **110**(8):749–51.

18 Antony SJ, Lopez-Po P (1999). Genital amebiasis: historical perspective of an unusual disease presentation. *Urology* **54**:952–5.

19 Torno MS. Babapour R, Gurevitch A, Witt MD (2000). Cutaneous acanthamoebiasis in AIDS. *J Am Acad Dermatol* **42**:351–4.

20 Citronberg RJ, Semel JD (1995). Severe vaginal infection with *Entamoeba histolytica* in a woman who recently returned from Mexico: case report and review. *Clin Infect Dis* **20**:700–2.

21 Friedland LR, Raphael ES, Deutsch J, *et al.* (1992). Disseminated *Acanthamoeba* infection in a child with symptomatic human immunodeficiency virus infection. *Pediatr Infect Dis J* **11**:404–7.

22 Slater CA, Sickel GS, Visvesvara RC, *et al.* (1994). Brief report: successful treatment of disseminated *Acanthamoeba* infection in an immunocompromised patient. *N Engl J Med* **331**:85–87.

23 Helton J, Loveless M, White CR (1993). Cutaneous *Acanthamoeba* infection associated with leukocytoclastic vasculitis in an AIDS patient. *Am J Dermatopathol* **15**:146–9.

24 Levine SA, Goldstein AE, Dahdouh, M, *et al.* (2001). Cutaneous *Acanthamoeba* in a patient with AIDS: a case study with a review of new therapy. *Cutis* **67**:377–80.

25 Develoux M, Blanc L, Garba S, *et al.* (1990). Cutaneous leishmaniasis in Niger. *Am J Trop Med Hyg* **43**(1):29–30.

26 Blickstein I, Dgani R, Lifschitz-Mercer B (1993). Cutaneous leishmaniasis of the vulva. *Int J Gynaecol Obstet* **42**:46–7.

27 Rathi SK, Pandhi RK, Chopra P, Khanna N (2005). Post-kala-azar dermal leishmaniasis: a histopathological study. *Indian J Dermatol Venereol Leprol* **71**:250–3.

28 Berhe N, Wolday D, Hailu A, *et al.* (1999). HIV viral load and response to antileishmanial chemotherapy in co-infected patients. *AIDS* **13**:1921–5.

29 Gopinath R, Ostrowski M, Justement SJ, *et al.* (2000). Filarial infections increase susceptibility to human immunodeficiency virus infection in peripheral blood mononuclear cells in vitro. *J Infect Dis* **182**:1804–6.

30 Feldmeier H, Poggensee G, Krantz I, Helling-Giese G (1995). Female genital schistosomiasis. New challenge from a gender perspective. *Trop Geograph Med* **47**:2–15.

31 Helling-Giese G, Sjaastad A, Poggensee G, *et al.* (1996). Female genital schistosomiasis (FGS): relationship between gynecological and histopathological findings. *Acta Tropica* **62**:257–67.

32 Poggensee G, Feldmeier H (2001). Female genital schistosomiasis: facts and hypotheses. *Acta Trop* **79**:193–210.

33 Weinstock JV, Elliott D, Metwali A, *et al.* (1999). Immunoregulation within the granulomas of murine *Schistosoma mansoni*. *Microbes Infect* **1**:491–8.

34 Leutscher, P, Ramarokoto CE, Reimert CM, *et al.* (2000). Genital schistosomiasis in males – a community based study from Madagascar. *Lancet* **355**:117–18.

35 Karanja DM, Colley DG, Nahlen BL, *et al.* (1998). Studies on schistosomiasis in western Kenya. II. Efficacy of praziquantel for treatment of schistosomiasis in person coinfected with HIV-1. *Am J Trop Med Hyg* **59**:307–11.

36 Sentongo E, Rubaale T, Buettner DW, Brattig NW (1998). T cell responses in coinfection with *Onchocerca volvulus* and the human immunodeficiency virus type 1. *Parasite Immunol* **20**:431–39.

CHAPTER 6

1 Palella F, Delaney K, Moorman A, *et al.* (1998). Declining mortality and morbidity among patients with advanced human immunodeficiency virus infection. *N Engl J Med* **338**: 853–60.

2 Flexner C (1998). HIV-protease inhibitors. *N Engl J Med* **338**:1281–91.

3 Carr A, Samaras K, Thorisdottir A, *et al.* (1999). Diagnosis, prediction, and natural course of HIV protease-inhibitor-associated lipodystrophy, hyperlipidemia, and diabetes mellitus. *Lancet* **353**:2893–9.

4 Aftergut L, Cockerell CJ (1999). Update on the cutaneous manifestations of HIV infection. *Dermatol Clin* **17**:443–71.

5 Arner A, Myers M (1998). Nevirapine and rashes. *Lancet* **351**:1133.

6 Ward HA, Russo GG, Shrum J (2002). Cutaneous manifestations of antiretroviral therapy. *J Am Acad Dermatol* **46**:284–93.

7 Patel SM, Johnson S, Belknap SM, *et al.* (2004). Serious adverse cutaneous and hepatic toxicities associated with nevirapine use by non-HIV infected individuals. *J Acquir Immune Defic Syndr* **35**:120–5.

8 Bourezane Y, Salard V, Hoen B, *et al.* (1998). DRESS (drug rash with eosinophilia and systemic symptoms) syndrome associated with nevirapine therapy. *Clin Infect Dis* **27**:1321–2.

9 Anton P, Soriano V, Jimenez-Nacher I, *et al.* (1999). Incidence of rash and discontinuation of nevirapine using two different escalating doses. *AIDS* **12**:524–5.

10 Mills G, Morgan H, Hales G, *et al.* (1999). Acute hypersensitivity with delavirdine. *Antivir Ther* **4**:51.

11 Jover F, Cuadrado JM, Roig P, *et al.* (2004). Efavirenz-associated gynecomastia: report of five cases and review of the literature. *Breast J* **10**:244–6.

12 Domingo P, Barcelo M (2002). Efavirenz-induced leukocytoclastic vasculitis. *Arch Internal Med* **162**:355–6.

13 Bossi P, Colin D, Bricaire F, *et al.* (2000). Hypersensitivity syndrome associated with efavirenz therapy. *Clin Infect Dis* **30**:227–8.

14 Phillips EJ, Kuriakose B, Knowles SR (2002). Efavirenz-induced skin eruption and successful desensitization. *Ann Pharmacother* **36**:430–2.

15 Greenberg RG, Berger TG (1990). Nail and mucocutaneous hyperpigmentation with azidothymidine therapy. *J Am Acad Dermatol* **22**:327–30.

16 Merenich JA, Hannon RN, Gentry

RH, *et al.* (1989). Azidothymidine-induced hyperpigmentation mimicking primary adrenal insufficiency. *Am J Med* **86**:469–70.

17 Wassef M, Keiser P (1995). Hypersensitivity of zidovudine: report of a case of anaphylaxis and review of the literature. *Clin Infect Dis* **20**:1387–9.

18 Torres RA, Lin RY, Lee M, *et al.* (1992). Zidovudine-induced leukocytoclastic vasculitis. *Arch Internal Med* **152**:850–1.

19 Murri R, Antinori A, Camilli G, *et al.* (1996). Fatal toxic epidermolysis induced by zidovudine. *Clin Infect Dis* **23**:640–1.

20 Gaglioti D, Ficarra G, Adler-Storthz K, *et al.* (1991). Zidovudine-related oral lichenoid reactions. Poster presentation, *VII International Conference on AIDS* Jun 16–21;7:232.

21 Hetherington S, McGuirk S, Powell G *et al.* (2001). Hypersensitivity reactions during therapy with the nucleoside reverse transcriptase inhibitor, abacavir. *Clin Ther* **23**:1603–14.

22 Foster RH, Faulds D (1998). Abacavir. *Drugs* **55**:729–36.

23 Walensky RP, Goldberg JH, Daily JP (1999). Anaphylaxis after rechallenge with abacavir. *AIDS* **13**:999–1000.

24 Philips EJ, Sullivan JR, Knowles SR, *et al.* (2002). Utility of patch testing in patients with hypersensitivity syndromes associated with abacavir. *AIDS* **16**:2223–5.

25 Saag MS, Cahn P, Raffi F, *et al.* (2004). Efficacy and safety of emtricitabine versus stavudine in combination therapy in antiretroviral-naïve patients: a randomized trial. *JAMA* **292**:180–90.

26 Rotunda A, Hirsch RJ, Scheinfeld N, *et al.* (2003). Severe cutaneous reactions associated with the use of human immunodeficiency virus medications. *Acta Derm Venereol* **83**:1–9.

27 Herranz P, Fernandez-Diaz ML, de Lucas MR, *et al.* (1994). Cutaneous vasculitis associated with didanosine. *Lancet* **344**:680.

28 Buffet M, Schwarzinger B, Amellal K, *et al.* (2005). Mitochondrial DNA depletion in adipose tissue of HIV-infected patients with peripheral lipoatrophy. *J Clin Virol* **33**:60–4.

29 Roth VR, Kravcik S, Angel JB

(1998). Development of cervical fat pads following therapy with human immunodeficiency virus type 1 protease inhibitors. *Clin Infect Dis* **27**:65–7.

30 Chen D (2002). Lipodystrophy in human immunodeficiency virus-infected patients. *J Clin Endocrinol Metabol* **87**:4845–56.

31 Gallant JE, Staszewski S, Pozniak AL, *et al.* (2004). Efficacy and safety of tenofovir DF versus stavudine in combination therapy in antiretroviral-naïve patients: a 3-year randomized trial. *JAMA* **292**:191–201.

32 Martin A, Smith DE, Carr A, *et al.* (2004). Reversibility of lipoatrophy in HIV-infected patients 2 years after switching from a thymidine analogue to abacavir: the MITOX extension study. *AIDS* **18**:1029–36.

33 Toma E, Therrien R (1998). Gynecomastia during indinavir antiretroviral therapy in HIV infection. *AIDS* **12**:681–2.

34 Fox PA, Boang FC, Hawkins DA, *et al.* (1999). Acute porphyria following commencement of indinavir. *AIDS* **13**:622–3.

35 Fung HB, Pecini RA, Brown ST, *et al.* (1999). Indinavir-associated maculopapular eruption. *Pharmacotherapy* **19**:1328–30.

36 Teira R, Zubero Z, Munoz J, *et al.* (1998). Stevens–Johnson syndrome caused by indinavir. *Scand J Infect Dis* **340**:634–5.

37 Bouscarat F, Bouchard C (1998). Paronychia and pyogenic granuloma of the great toes in patients treated with indinavir. *N Engl J Med* **338**:1776–7.

38 Sass JO, Jakob-Solder B, Heitger A, *et al.* (2000). Paronychia with pyogenic granuloma in a child treated with indinavir: the retinoid-mediated side effect theory revisited. *Dermatology* **200**:40–2.

39 Babl FE, Regan AM, Pelton SI (2002). Xanthomas and hyperlipidemia in a human immunodeficiency virus-infected child receiving highly active antiretroviral therapy. *Pediatr Infect Dis J* **21**:259–60.

40 Darvay A, Acland K, Lynn W, *et al.* (1999). Striae formation in two HIV-positive persons receiving protease inhibitors. *J Am Acad Dermatol* **41**:467–9.

41 Dank JP, Colven R (2000). Protease inhibitor-associated angiolipomas. *J Am Acad Dermatol* **42**:129–31.

42 Pedneault L, Brothers C, Pagano G,

et al. (2000). Safety profile and tolerability of amprenavir in the treatment of adult and pediatric patients with HIV infection. *Clin Ther* **22**:1378–94.

43 Chapman TM, Plosker GL, Perry CM (2004). Fosamprenavir: a review of its use in the management of antiretroviral therapy-naïve patients with HIV infection. *Drugs* **64**:2101–24.

44 Murphy RL, Sanne I, Cahn P, *et al.* (2003). Dose-ranging, randomized, clinical trial of atazanavir with lamivudine and stavudine in antiretroviral-naïve subjects: 48-week results. *AIDS* **17**:2603–14.

45 Wilde JT, Lee CA, Collins P, *et al.* (1999). Increased bleeding associated with protease inhibitor therapy in HIV-positive patients with bleeding disorders. *Br J Haematol* **107**:556–9.

46 Kawsar M, El-Gadi S (2002). Subcutaneous granulomatous lesions related to ritonavir therapy in HIV-infected patients. *Int J STD AIDS* **13**:273–4.

47 Prins JM, Schellekens PT, Reiss P (1998). Continued therapy with HIV-1 protease inhibitors, despite previous hypersensitivity reactions through coadministration of prednisone. *Scand J Infect Dis* **30**:612–13.

48 Fortuny C, Vicente MA, Medina MM, *et al.* (2000). Rash as a side-effect of nelfinavir in children. *AIDS* **114**:335–6.

49 Smith KJ, Yeager J, Skelton H (2000). Fixed drug eruptions to human immunodeficiency virus-1 protease inhibitor. *Cutis* **66**:29–32.

50 Carr A, Cooper DA, Penny R (1991). Allergic manifestations of human immunodeficiency virus infection. *J Clin Immunol* **11**:52–64.

51 Aquilina C, Viraben R, Roueire A (1998). Acute generalized exanthematous pustulosis. *Arch Internal Med* **158**:2160–1.

52 Heald AE, Pieper CF, Schiffman SS (1998). Taste and smell complaint in HIV-infected patients. *AIDS* **12**:1667.

53 Bonfati P, Capetti A, Riva P, *et al.* (1997). Hypersensitivity reactions during antretroviral regimens with protease inhibitors. *AIDS* **11**:1301–2.

54 Garcia-Silva JA, Almagro MA, Juega JB, *et al.* (2000). Protease inhibitor-related paronychia,

ingrown toenails, desquamative cheilitis and cutaneous xerosis. *AIDS* **14**:1289.

55 Dank JP, Cloven R (2000). Protease inhibitor-associated angiolipomatosis. *J Am Acad Dermatol* **42**:129–31.

56 Cockerell CJ, Chen TM (2003). Cutaneous manifestations of HIV infection and HIV-related disorders. In: *Dermatology,* Volume 2. J Bolognia, JL Jorizzo, RP Rapini (eds). Elsevier, London, pp. 1199.

57 Demoly P, Messad D, Trylesinski A, *et al.* (1998). Nelfinavir-induced urticaria and successful desensitization. *J Allergy Clin Immunol* **102**:875–6.

58 Rey D, Partisani M, Krantz V, *et al.* (1999). Prednisolone does not prevent the occurrence of nevirapine-induced rashes. *AIDS* **13**:2307.

59 Ball RA, Kinchelow T (2003). ISR substudy group. Injection site reactions with the HIV-1 fusion inhibitor enfuvirtide. *J Am Acad Dermatol* **49**:826–31.

60 Maggi P, Ladisa N, Cinori E, *et al.* (2004). Cutaneous injection site reactions to long-term therapy with enfuvirtide. *J Antimicrob Chemother* **53**:678–81.

61 Williamson K, Rebolli AC, Manders SM (1999). Protease inhibitor-induced lipodystrophy. *J Am Acad Dermatol* **40**:635–6.

62 Madge S, Kinloch-de-Loes S, Mercey D, *et al.* (1999). Lipodystrophy in patients naïve to HIV protease inhibitors. *AIDS* **13**:735–7.

63 Carr A, Samaras K, Chisholm DJ, *et al.* (1998). Pathogenesis of HIV-1-protease inhibitor-associated peripheral lipodystrophy, hyperlipidaemia, and insulin resistance. *Lancet* **351**:1881–3.

64 Moyle GJ, Lysakova L, Brown S, *et al.* (2004). A randomized open-label study of immediate versus delayed polyactic acid injections for the cosmetic management of facial lipoatrophy in persons with HIV infection. *HIV Med* **5**:82–7.

65 Viraben R, Aquilina C (1998). Indinavir-associated lipodystrophy. *AIDS* **12**:F37–9.

66 Dolev J, Reyter I, Maurer T (2004). Treatment of recurring cutaneous drug reactions in patients with human immunodeficiency virus 1 infection: a series of three cases. *Arch Dermatol* **140**:1051–3.

CHAPTER 7

1 Newcomer VD (1997). Human immunodeficiency virus infection and acquired immunodeficiency syndrome in the elderly. *Arch Dermatol* **133**:1311–12.

2 Sadick NS, McNutt N, Scott N, Kaplan MH (1990). Papulosquamous dermatoses of AIDS. *J Am Acad Dermatol* **22**:1270–7.

3 Kaplan MH, Sadick N, McNutt N, *et al.* (1987). Dermatologic findings and manifestations of acquired immunodeficiency syndrome *AIDS* **16**:485–506.

4 Walsh AS, Shear NH (2004). Psoriasis and the new biologic agents: interrupting a T-AP dance. *Can Med Assoc J* **22**:1933–41.

5 Nickoloff BJ, Nestle FO (2004). Recent insights into the immunopathogenesis of psoriasis provide new therapeutic opportunities. *J Clin Investig* **113**:1664–75.

6 Bolognia JL, Jorizzo JL, Rapini RP, (eds) (2003). Psoriasis. In: *Dermatology.* Mosby, London, pp. 115–36.

7 Mallon E, Young D, Bunce M, *et al.* (1998). HLA-Cw*0602 and HIV-associated psoriasis. *Br J Dermatol* **139**:527–33.

8 Mallon E, Bunce M, Savoie H, *et al.* (2000). HLA-C and guttate psoriasis. *Br J Dermatol* **143**:1177–82.

9 Rogers M (2002). Childhood psoriasis. *Curr Opin Pediatr* **14**:404–9.

10 Henseler T, Christophers E (1995). Disease concomitance in psoriasis. *J Am Acad Dermatol* **32**:982–6.

11 Tyring SK (ed) (2002). In: *Mucocutaneous Manifestations of Viral Diseases.* Marcel Dekker Inc, New York, pp. 344–51.

12 Bartke U, Venten I, Kreuter A, *et al.* (2004). Human immunodeficiency virus-associated psoriasis and psoriatic arthritis treated with infliximab. *Br J Dermatol* **150**:784–6.

13 Fischer T, Schworer H, Vente C, *et al.* (1999). Clinical improvement of HIV-associated psoriasis parallels a reduction of HIV viral load induced by effective antiretroviral therapy. *AIDS* **13**:628–9.

14 Mahoney SE, Duvic M, Nickoloff B, *et al.* (1991). Human immunodeficiency virus (HIV) transcripts identified in HIV-related

psoriasis and Kaposi's sarcoma lesions. *J Clin Investig* **88**:174–85.

15 De Socio G, Vittorio L, Simonetti S, Stagni G (2005). Clinical improvement of psoriasis in an AIDS patient effectively treated with combination antiretroviral therapy. *Case Reports* 74–5.

16 Romani J, Puig L, Baselga E, De Moragas J (1996). Reiter's syndrome-like pattern in AIDS-associated psoriasiform dermatitis. *Int J Dermatol* **35**:484–8.

17 Farber EM, Nall L (1993). Psoriasis associated with human immunodeficiency virus/acquired immunodeficiency syndrome. *Cutis* **52**:29–35.

18 Rosenberg EW, Skinner RB, Noah PW (1991). AIDS and psoriasis. *Int J Dermatol* **30**:449–50.

19 Farber EM, Nall L (1993). Pustular psoriasis. *Cutis* **51**:29–32.

20 Puig L, Fernandez-Figueras MT, Ferrandiz C, *et al.* (1995). Epidermal expression of 65 and 72 kd heat shock proteins in psoriasis and AIDS-associated psoriasiform dermatitis. *J Am Acad Dermatol* **33**:985–9.

21 Chaker MB, Cockerell CJ (1993). Concomitant psoriasis, seborrheic dermatitis, and disseminated cutaneous histoplasmosis in a patient infected with human immunodeficiency virus. *J Am Acad Dermatol* **29**:311–13.

22 Smith KJ, Decker C, Yeager J, *et al.* (1997). Therapeutic efficacy of carbamazepine in a HIV-1-positive patient with psoriatic erythroderma. *J Am Acad Dermatol* **37**:851–4.

23 Smith KC (1994). Ranitidine useful in the management of psoriasis in a patient with acquired immunodeficiency syndrome. *Int J Dermatol* **33**:220–1.

24 Bowman PH, Hogan, DJ (2000). Ulcerated atrophic striae from etretinate. *Cutis* **65**:327–8.

25 Diez F, del Hoyo M, Serrano S (1990). Zidovudine treatment of psoriasis associated with acquired immunodeficiency syndrome. *J Am Acad Dermatol* **22**: 146–7.

26 Breuer-McHam J, Marshall G, Adu-Oppong A, *et al.* (1999). Alterations in HIV expression in AIDS patients with psoriasis or pruritis treated with phototherapy. *J Am Acad Dermatol* **40**:48–60.

27 Stern RS, Mills DK, Krell K, *et al.* (1998). HIV-positive patients differ from HIV-negative patients in

indications for and type of UV therapy used. *J Am Acad Dermatol* **39**:48–55.

28 Matarasso SL (1998). Epitomes important advances in dermatology psoriasis therapy update. *WJM* **169**:221–2.

29 Freedberg IM, Eisen AZ, Wolff K, *et al.* (eds) (2003). *Fitzpatrick's Dermatology in General Medicine.* McGraw-Hill, New York, pp. 450–55.

30 Smith KJ, Nelson A, Skelton H, *et al.* (1997). Pityriasis lichenoides et varioliformis acuta in HIV-1+ patients: a marker of early stage disease. *Int J Dermatol* **36**:104–9.

31 Griffiths JK (1998). Successful long-term use of cyclosporin A in HIV-induced pityriasis lichenoides chronica. *J Acquir Immune Defic Syndr* **18**:396–7.

32 Dupin N, Franck N, Calvez V, *et al.* (1997). Lack of evidence of human herpesvirus 8 DNA sequences in HIV-negative patients with various lymphoproliferative disorders of the skin. *Br J Dermatol* **136**:827–30.

33 Klein PA, Jones EC, Nelson JL, Clark RAF (2003). Infectious causes of pityriasis lichenoides: a case of fulminant infectious mononucleosis. *J Am Acad Dermatol* **49**:S151–3.

34 Haeffner AC, Smoller BR, Zepter K, Wood GS (1995). Differentiation and clonality of lesional lymphocytes in small plaque parapsoriasis. *Arch Dermatol* **131**:321–4.

35 Weinstein A, Mirzabeigi M, Withee M, Vincek V (2004). Lymphomatoid papulosis in an HIV-positive man. *AIDS Patient Care and STDs* **18**:563–7.

36 Stergiou GD, Nicolaidi A, Evangelopoulou P, *et al.* (1996). A rare case of parapsoriasis (pityriasis lichenoides) in a patient with HIV infection. *International Conference AIDS 1996 July 7–12* (abstract no. Tu.B.2272). **11**:312.

37 Mathes BM, Douglass MC (1985). Seborrheic dermatitis in patients with acquired immunodeficiency syndrome. *J Am Acad Dermatol* **13**:947–51.

38 Mahe A, Simon F, Coulibaly S, *et al.* (1996). Predictive value of seborrheic dermatitis and other common dermatoses for HIV infection in Bamako, Mali. *J Am Acad Dermatol* **34**:1084–6.

39 Vidal C, Girard PM, Dompmartin D, *et al.* (1990). Seborrheic dermatitis and HIV infection. *J Am Acad Dermatol* **6**:1106–10.

40 Groisser D, Bottone EJ, Lebwohl M (1989). Association of *Pityrosporum orbiculare* (*Malassezia furfur*) with seborrheic dermatitis in patients with acquired immunodeficiency syndrome (AIDS). *J Am Acad Dermatol* **20**(5 Pt 1):770–3.

41 Fitzpatrick TB, Johnson RA, Wolff R, Suurmond R (2002). *Color Atlas & Synopsis of Clinical Dermatology*, 5th edn. McGraw-Hill, New York, pp. 1198–204.

42 Cockerell CJ (1991). Seborrheic dermatitis-like and atopic dermatitis-like eruptions in HIV-infected patients. *Clin Dermatol* **9**:49–51.

43 Soeprono FF, Schinella RA, Cockerell CJ, Comite SL (1986). Seborrheic-like dermatitis of acquired immunodeficiency syndrome. *J Am Acad Dermatol* **14**:242–8.

44 Elder DE, Elenitsas R, Johnson BL, *et al.* (eds) (2009). *Lever's Histopathology of the Skin*, 10th edn. Lippincott, Williams, &Wilkins, Philadelphia, p. 243.

45 Gonzalez-Lopez A, Velasco E, Pozo T, Del Villar A (1999). HIV-associated pityriasis rubra pilaris responsive to triple antiretroviral therapy. *Br J Dermatol* **140**:931–4.

46 Hall CB (2002). In this issue: the human herpesviruses and pityriasis rosea: curious covert companions? *J Investig Dermatol* **119**(4):793–7.

47 Perminova NG, Timofeyev IV, Paletskaya TF (1999). The laboratory diagnostic of the human herpesvirus 6 and 7 infection. *Biotekhnologiya* **0**(2):89–95.

48 Black JB, Pellett PE (1999). Human herpesvirus 7. *Rev Med Virol* **9**(4):245–62.

49 Fetil E, Ozkan S, Gurler N, *et al.* (2004). Lichen nitidus after hepatitis B vaccine. *Int J Dermatol* **43**:956–8.

50 Goerdt S, Nolle X, Ramaker J, *et al.* (1995). Pruritic papular eruption in an HIV-infected immunocompetent patient. *Eur J Dermatol* **5**(3):243–6.

51 Stricker RB (1999). Lichen nitidus and dinitrochlorobenzene. *J Am Acad Dermatol* **40**:647–8.

52 Ceballos-Salobrena A, Aguirre-Urizar JM, Bagan-Sebastian JV (1996). Oral manifestations associated with human immunodeficiency virus infection in a Spanish population. *J Oral Pathol Med* **25**(10):523–6.

53 Campisi G, Di Fede O, Craxi A, *et al.* (2004). Oral lichen planus, hepatitis C virus, and HIV: no association in a cohort study from an area of high hepatitis C virus endemicity. *J Am Acad Dermatol* **51**(3):364–70.

54 Lodi G, Scully C, Carrozzo M, *et al.* (2005). Current controversies in oral lichen planus: report of an international consensus meeting. Part 1. Viral infections and etiopathogenesis. *Oral Surg Oral Med Oral Pathol Oral Radiol Endodontol* **100**(1):40–7.

55 Ficarra G, Flaitz CM, Gaglioti D, *et al.* (1988). White lichenoid lesions of the buccal mucosa in patients with HIV infection. *Oral Surg Oral Med Oral Pathol* **76**(4):460–6.

56 Pardo RJ, Kerdel FA (1988). Hypertrophic lichen planus and light sensitivity in an HIV-positive patient. *Int J Dermatol* **27**(9):642–4.

57 Fitzgerald E, Purcell SM, Goldman HM (1995). Photodistributed hypertrophic lichen planus in association with acquired immunodeficiency syndrome: a distinct entity. *Cutis* **55**: 109–11.

58 Bessinger GT, Conologue,TD, Krivda SJ, *et al.* (2003). Violaceous plaques in a patient with acquired immunodeficiency syndrome. *Arch Dermatol* **139**:215–20.

59 Villaverde RR, Melguizo JB, Sintes RN, *et al.* (2002). Multiple linear lichen planus in HIV patient. *Eur Acad Dermatol Venereol* **16**:412–13.

60 Fivenson DP, Mathes B (2006). Treatment of generalized lichen planus with alefacept. *Arch Dermatol* **142**:151–2.

61 Ishida CE, Ramos-e-Silva M (1998). Cryosurgery in oral lesions. *Int J Dermatol* **37**:283–5.

62 Moraes M, Russo G (2001). Thalidomide and its dermatologic uses. *Am J Med Sci* **321**:321–5.

63 Schoppelrey HP, Grummer M, Emminger C, Breit R (1996). Hyperkeratotic epidermal invaginations in chronic herpes zoster. *International Conference AIDS 1996 July 7–12* **11**:302, abstract no. Tu.B.2213.

64 Rosatelli JB, Machado AA, Roselino AMF (1997). Dermatoses among Brazilian HIV-positive patients: correlation with the evolutionary phases of AIDS. *Int J Dermatol* **36**:729–34.

CHAPTER 8

1 Kaye B (1996). Rheumatologic manifestations of HIV infections. *Clin Rev Allergy Immunol* **14**:385–416.

2 Friedman-Kien AE, Cockerell CJ (1996). Cutaneous manifestation of HIV infection: vasculitis and other vascular-related abnormalities. In: *Color Atlas of AIDS*, 2nd edn. WB Saunders, Philadelphia, pp.134–5.

3 Chetty R (2001). Vasculitides associated with HIV infection. *J Clin Pathol* **54**:275–8.

4 Grisselbrecht M, Cohen P, Lortholary O, *et al.* (1997). HIV related vasculitis: clinical presentation and clinical approach of six patients. *AIDS* **11**:121–2.

5 Friedman PC (2005). Nodular tuberculid in a patient with HIV. *J Am Acad Dermatol* **53**(2 Suppl 1):S154–6.

6 Hewitt RG (2002). Abacavir hypersensitivity reaction. *Clin Infect Dis* **34**:1137–42.

7 Koopmans PP, van der Ven AJ, Vree TB, van der Meer JW (1995). Pathogenesis of hypersensitivity reactions to drugs in patients with HIV infection: allergic or toxic? *AIDS* **9**:217–22.

8 Pantaleo G, Graziosi C, Fauci AS (1993). Immunopathogenesis of human immuno-deficiency virus infection. *N Engl J Med* **328**:327–35.

9 Coleman JW (1998). Protein haptenation by drugs. *Clin Exp Allergy* **28**(Suppl 4):79–82.

10 Chren MM, Silverman RA, Sorensen RU, Elmets CA (1993). Leukocytoclastic vasculitis in a patient infected with HIV. *J Am Acad Dermatol* **28**:919–22.

11 Hall TN, Brennan B, Leahy MF, Woodroffe AJ (1998). Henoch–Schönlein purpura associated with human immunodeficiency virus. *Nephr Dial Transplant* **13**:988–90.

12 Stein CM, Thomas JE (1991). Behçet's disease associated with HIV infection. *J Rheumatol* **18**:1427–8.

13 Gherardi R, Belec L, Mhiri C, *et al.* (1993). The spectrum of vasculitis in human immunodeficiency virus-infected patients. *Arthritis Rheum* **36**:1164–74.

14 Libman BS, Quismoro FP, Stimmler MM (1995). Polyarteritis nodosa-like vasculitis in human immunodeficiency virus infection. *J Rheumotol* **22**:351–5.

15 Johnson RM, Little JR, Storch GA (2001). Kawasaki-like syndromes associated with human immunodeficiency virus infection. *Clin Infect Dis* **32**:1628–34.

16 Mckee P, Calonje E, Granter S (2005). Vascular diseases. In: *Pathology of the Skin with Clinical Corelation*, 3rd edn. Vol 1. Elsevier, Mosby, London, pp. 709–73.

17 Ryan TJ (1999). Common mistakes in the clinical approach to vasculitis. *Clin Dermatol* **17**:555–7.

18 Cornely OA, Hauschild S, Weise C, *et al.* (1999). Seroprevalence and disease association of antineutrophilic cytoplasmic autoantibodies and antigens in HIV infection. *Infection* **27**:92–6.

19 Lebwohl M, Heymann W, Berth-Jones J, Coulson I (eds) (2002). *Treatment of Skin Disease: Comprehensive Therapeutic Strategies.* Mosby, St Louis.

20 Rostoker G, Desvaux-Belghiti D, Pilatte Y, *et al.* (1994). High-dose immunoglobulin therapy for severe IgA nephropathy and Henoch–Schönlein purpura. *Ann Internal Med* **120**:476–84.

21 Kim H (2003). Erythema elevatum diutinum in an HIV-positive patient. *J Drugs Dermatol* **2**(4):411–12.

22 Fakheri A, Gupta SM, White SM, *et al.* (2001). Erythema elevatum diutinum in a patient with human immunodeficiency virus. *Cutis* **68**(1):41–2, 55.

23 Muratori, Carrera, Gorani, Alessi (1999). Erythema elevatum diutinum and HIV infection: a report of five cases. *Br J Dermatol* **141**(2):335.

24 Martin JL, Dronda F, Chaves F (2001). Erythema elevatum diutinum, a clinical entity to be considered in patients infected with HIV-1. *Clin Exp Dermatol* **26**(8):725–6.

25 Soni BP, Wiliford PM, White WL (1998). Erythematous nodules in a patient infected with the human immunodeficiency virus. Erythema elevatum diutinum (EED). *Arch Dermtol* **134**(2):232–3,235–6.

26 Suarez M, *et al.* (1998). Nodular erythema elevatum diutinum in an HIV-1 infected woman: response to dapsone and antiretroviral therapy. *Br J Dermatol* **138**:717.

27 Requena L, Sanchez Yus Y, Martin L, *et al.* (1991). Erythema elevatum diutinum in a patient with acquired immunodeficiency syndrome. Another clinical simulator of Kaposi's sarcoma. *Arch Dermatol* **127**:1819–22.

28 Walker KD, Badame AJ (1990). Erythema elevatum diutinum in a patient with Crohn's disease. *J Am Acad Dermatol* **22**:948–52.

29 Nakajima H, Ikeda M, Yamamoto Y, *et al.* (1999). Erythema elevatum diunitum complicated by rheumatoid arthritis. *J Dermatol* **26**:452–6.

30 LeBoit PE (2002). Granuloma faciale: a diagnosis deserving of dignity. *Am J Dermatopathol* **24**(5):440–3.

31 Kanitakis J, *et al.* (1993). Ultrastructural study of chronic lesions of erythema elevatum diutinum: 'Extracellular cholesterosis' is a misnomer. *J Am Acad Dermatol* **29**:363.

32 LeBoit PE, Cockerell CJ (1993). Nodular lesions of erythema elevatum diutinum in patients with human immunodeficiency infection. *J Am Acad Dermatol* **28**:919–22.

33 Gasquet S, Maurin M, Brouqui P, *et al.* (1998). Bacillary angiomatosis in immunocompromised patients. *AIDS* **12**(4):1793–803.

34 Kempf VA, Schairer A, Neumann D, *et al.* (2005). *Bartonella henselae* inhibits apoptosis in Mono Mac 6 cells. *Cell Microbiol* **7**(1):91–104.

35 Cockerell CJ, Whitlow MA, Webster GF, Friedman–Kien AE. (1987). Epithelioid angiomatosis: a distinct vascular disorder in patients with acquired immunodeficiency syndrome or AIDS-related complex. *Lancet* **2**:654.

36 Stoler MH, Bonfiglio TA, Steigbigel MT, Pereira M, (1983). An atypical subcutaneous infection associated with acquired immune deficiency syndrome. *Am J Clin Pathol* **80**:714–18.

37 Gasquet S, *et al.* (1998). Bacillary angiomatosis in immunocompromised patients. *AIDS.* **12**(4):1793–803.

38 Welch DF, Hensel DM, Pickett DA, *et al.* (1993). Bacteremia due to *Rochalimaea henselae* in a child: practical identification of isolates in the clinical laboratory. *J Clin Microbiol* **31**:2381–6.

39 Megarbane B, Carbon C (1996). Unusual presentations of bacterial skin and soft-tissue infections and their treatment. *Curr Opin Infect Dis* **9**:58–62.

40 Mientjes GH, *et al.* (1992). Prevalence of thrombocytopenia in HIV-infected and non-HIV infected drug users and homosexual men. *Br J Haematol* **82**:615.

41 Volberding PA (2008). Hematology and oncology in AIDS. In: *Goldman: Cecil Textbook of Medicine*, 23rd edn. Goldman L, Ausiello D (eds). Saunders Elsevier, Philadelphia, pp. 2601–6.

42 Najean Y, Rain JD (1994). The mechanism of thrombocytopenia in patients with HIV infection. *J Lab Clin Med* **123**:415.

43 Li Z, Nardi MA, Karpatkin S (2005). Role of molecular mimicry to HIV-1 peptides in HIV-1 related immunologic thrombocytopenia. *Blood* **106**(2):572–6.

44 Levine AM (2009). Hematologic manifestations of AIDS. In: *Hoffman: Hematology: Basic Principles and Practice*, 5th edn. Hoffman R, Benz Jr, EJ, Shattil SJ, *et al.* (eds). Churchill Livingstone Elsevier, Philadelphia, pp. 2321–40.

45 Nicolle M, Levy S, Amrhein E, *et al.* (1998). Normal platelet numbers correlate with plasma viral load and CD4+ cell counts in HIV-1 infection. *Eur J Haematol* **61**:216.

46 Scaradavou A (2002). HIV-related thrombocytopenia. *Blood Rev* **16**:73.

47 Ramratnam B, *et al.* (1996). Short course dexamethasone for thrombocytopenia in AIDS. *Am J Med* **100**:117.

48 Majluf-Cruz A, *et al.* (1998). Usefulness of a low-dose intravenous immunoglobulin regimen for the treatment of thrombocytopenia associated with AIDS. *Am J Hematol* **59**:127.

49 Lord RV, Coleman MJ, Milliken ST (1998). Splenectomy for HIV-related immune thrombocytopenia: comparison with results of splenectomy for non-HIV immune thrombocytopenic purpura. *Arch Surg* **133**:205.

50 Fallon T Jr, *et al.* (1986). Telangiectasia of the anterior chest in homosexual men, *Ann Internal Med* **105**:679.

51 MacFarlane DF, Gregory N (1994). Telangiectases in human immunodeficiency virus-positive patients. *Cutis* **53**(2):79–80.

52 Jimenez-Acosta F, Fonseca E, Magallon M (1998). Response to tetracycline in a male hemophiliac with human immunodeficiency virus infection. *J Am Acad Dermatol* **19**(2 Pt 1):369–70.

53 Abramson SB, Odajnk CM, Grieco AJ, Weissmann G, Rosenstein E (1985). Hyperalgesic pseudothrombophlebitis. New syndrome in male homosexuals. *Am J Med* **17**(2):317–20.

54 Montfort-Gouraund M, Duyckaerts V, Boccara F, de Boissieu D, Guillou MA, Badoual J (1991). Superficial pseudophlebitis in a HIV seropositive child. *Arch Fr Pediatr* **48**(3):205–6.

CHAPTER 9

1 Fisher BK, Warner LC (1987). Cutaneous manifestations of the acquired immunodeficiency syndrome. *Int J Dermatol* **26**(10):615–30.

2 Colebunders R, Mann JM, Francis H, *et al.* (1987). Generalized papular pruritic eruptions in African patients with HIV infection. *AIDS* **1**(2):117–21.

3 Hira SK, Wadhawan D, Kamanga J, *et al.* (1988). Cutaneous manifestations of human immunodeficiency virus in Lusaka, Zambia. *J Am Acad Dermatol* **19**(3):451–7.

4 Liautaud B, Pape JW, DeHovitz JA, *et al.* (1989). Pruritic skin lesions: a common initial presentation of acquired immunodeficiency syndrome. *Arch Dermatol* **125**(5):629–32.

5 Bason MM, Berger TG, Nesbitt LT Jr (1993). Pruritic papular eruption of HIV-disease. *Int J Dermatol* **32**(11):784–9.

6 Rosatelli JB, Machado AA, Roselino AM (1997). Dermatoses among Brazilian HIV-positive patients: correlation with the evolutionary phases of AIDS. *Int J Dermatol* **36**(10):729–34.

7 Boonchai WB, Laohasrisakul R, Manonukul J, Kulthanan K (1999). Pruritic papular eruption in HIV seropositive patients: a cutaneous marker for immunosuppression. *Int J Dermatol* **38**(5):348–50.

8 Sanchez M, Fotiades J, Soter NA, *et al.* (1993). The characterization of HIV-associated papular eruptions. *International Conference on AIDS*, **9**(1):447.

9 Eisman S (2006). Pruritic papular eruption in HIV. *Dermatol Clin* **24**(4):449–57.

10 Resneck JS, Van Beek M, Furmanski L, *et al.* (2004). Etiology of pruritic papular eruption with HIV infection in Uganda. *JAMA* **292**(21):2614–21.

11 Duvic M (1987). Staphylococcal infections and the pruritis of AIDS-related complex. *Arch Dermatol* **123**(12):1599.

12 Hevia O, Jimenez-Acosta F, Celballos PI, *et al.* (1991). Pruritic papular eruptions of the acquired immunodeficiency syndrome: a clinicopathologic study. *J Am Acad Dermatol* **24**(2 Pt 1):231–5.

13 Fearfield LA, Rowe A, Francis N, *et al.* (1999). Itchy folliculitis and human immunodeficiency virus infection: clinicopathological and immunological features, pathogenesis and treatment. *Br J Dermatol* **141**(1):3–11.

14 Kinloch-de Loes S, Didierjean L, Rieckerhoff-Cantoni L, *et al.* (1991). Bullous pemphogoid autoantibodies, HIV-infection and pruritic papular eruption. *AIDS* **5**(4):451–4.

15 Gelfand JM, Rudikoff D (2001). Evaluation and treatment of itching in HIV-infected patients. *Mt Sinai J Med New York* **68**(4-5):298–308.

16 Rosatelli JB, Soares FA, Roselino AM (2000). Pruritic papular eruption of the aquired immunodeficiency syndrome: predominance of CD8 + cells. *Int J Dermatol* **39**(11):873–4.

17 Pardo RJ, Bogaert MA, Penneys NS, *et al.* (1992). UVB phototherapy of the pruritic papular eruption of the acquired immunodeficiency syndrome. *J Am Acad Dermatol* **26**(3 Pt 2):423–8.

18 Valerie K, Delers A, Bruck C, *et al.* (1988). Activation of human immunodeficiency virus type 1 by DNA damage in human cells. *Nature* **333**(6168):78–81.

19 Cavard C, Zider A, Vernet M, *et al.* (1990). *In vivo* activation of human immunodeficiency virus type 1 long terminal repeat. *J Clin Investig* **86**(4):1369–74.

20 Meola T, Soter NA, Ostreicher R, *et al.* (1993). The safety of UVB phototherapy in patients with HIV infection. *J Am Acad Dermatol* **29**(2 Pt 1):216–20.

21 Berman B, Flores F, Burke G (1998). Efficacy of pentoxifylline in the treatment of pruritic papular eruption of HIV-infected persons. *J Am Acad Dermatol* **38**(6 Pt 1):955–9.

22 Payne CM, Wilkinson JD, Mckee PH, *et al.* (1985). Nodular prurigo – a clinicopathologic study of 46 patients. *Br J Dermatol* **113**(4):431–9.

23 Payne CME (1994). Prurigo

nodularis. In: *Itch: Mechanisms and Management of Pruritis*. JD Bernard (ed). McGraw-Hill, New York, p. 103.

24 Matthews SN, Cockerell CJ (1998). Prurigo nodularis in HIV-infected individuals. *Int J Dermatol* 37(6):401–9.

25 Anzala A, Wambugu P, Bosire M, *et al*. (1990). The rate of development of HIV-1 infection related illness in women with a known duration of infection. *International Conference on AIDS*, Jun 20–23, 6:143.

26 Wambugu P, Plummer FA, Anzala AO, *et al*. (1990). Clinical manifestations of HIV-1 infection among women working as prostitutes in Nairobi. *International Conference on AIDS*, Jun 20–23, 6:260.

27 Lee MR, Shumack S (2005). Prurigo nodularis: a review. *Austr J Dermatol* 46(4):211–18.

28 Diven DG, Newton RC, Ramsey KM (1988). Heightened cutaneous reactions to mosquito bites in patients with acquired immunodeficiency syndrome receiving zidovudine. *Arch Internal Med* 148(10):2296.

29 Penney NS, Nayar JK, Bernstein H, Knight JW (1989). A chronic eruption in patients with AIDS associated with increased antibody titers to mosquito salivary gland antigens. *J Am Acad Dermatol* 21(2 Pt 2):421–5.

30 Cockerell CJ (1994). The itches of HIV and AIDS. In: *Itch: Mechanisms and Management of Puritis*. JT Bernard (ed). McGraw Hill, New York, pp. 281–98.

31 Matis WL, Lavker RM, Murphy GF (1990). Substance P induces the expression of an endothelial-leukocyte adhesion molecule by microinvasion endothelium. *J Investig Dermatol* 94(4):492–5.

32 Wakeel RA, Urbaniak SJ, Armstrong SS, *et al*. (1994). Idiopathic CD4+ lymphocytopenia associated with chronic pruritic papules. *Br J Dermatol* 131(3):371–5.

33 Belsito DV, Sanchez MR, Baer RL, Valentine F, *et al*. (1994). Reduced Langerhans cells Ia antigen and ATPase activity in patients with the acquired immunodeficiency syndrome. *N Engl J Med* 310(20):1279–82.

34 Berger TG, Hoffman C, Thieberg MD (1995). Prurigo nodularis and photosensitivity in AIDS: treatment with thalidomide. *J Am Acad Dermatol* 33(5-Pt 1):837–38.

35 Maurer T, Poncelet A, Berger T (2004). Thalidomide treatment for prurigo nodularis in human immunodeficiency virus-infected subjects. *Arch Dermatol* 140(7):845–9.

36 Elder DE, Elenitsas R, Johnson BL, *et al*. (2009). *Lever's Histopathology of the Skin*, 10th edn. Lippincott, Williams & Wilkins, Philadelphia, p. 173.

37 Doyle JA, Connolly SM, Hunziker N, Winkelmann RK (1979). Prurigo nodularis: a reappraisal of the clinical and histologic features. *J Cut Pathol* 6(5):392–403.

38 Perez GL, Peters MS, Reda AM, *et al*. (1993). Mast cells, neutrophils, and eosinophils in prurigo nodularis. *Arch Dermatol* 129(7):861–5.

39 Feuerman EJ, Sandbank M (1975). Prurigo nodularis. Histological and electron microscopical study. *Arch Dermatol* 111(11):1472–7.

40 Sandbank M (1976). Cutaneous nerve lesions in prurigo nodularis: electron microscopic study of two patients. *J Cut Pathol* 3(3):125–32.

41 Runne U, Orfanos CE (1977). Cutaneous neural proliferation in highly pruritic lesions of chronic prurigo. *Arch Dermatol* 113(6):787–91.

42 Herranz P, Pizarro A, De Lucas R, *et al*. (1998). Treatment of AIDS-associated prurigo nodularis with thalidomide. *Clin Exp Dermatol* 23(5):233–5.

43 Tupker RA, Coenraads PJ, van der Meer JB (1992). Treatment of prurigo nodularis, chronic prurigo and neurodermatitis circumscripta with topical capsaicin. *Acta Derm Venereol* 72(6):463.

44 Lindley RP, Rowland Payne CM (1989). Neural hyperplasia is not a diagnostic prerequisite in nodular prurigo. A controlled morphometric microscopic study of 26 biopsy specimens. *J Cut Pathol* 16(1):14–18.

45 Hann SK, Cho MY, Park YK (1990). UV treatment of generalized prurigo nodularis. *Int J Dermatol* 29(6):436–7.

46 Winkelmann RK, Connolly SM, Doyle JA, Padilha-Goncalves A (1984). Thalidomide treatment of prurigo nodularis. *Acta Derm Venereol* 64(5):412–17.

47 Dimopoulos MA, Eleutherakis-Papaiakovou V (2004). Adverse effects of thalidomide administration in patients with neoplastic diseases. *Am J Med* 117(7):508–15.

48 Gunzler V (1992). Thalidomide in human immunodeficiency virus (HIV) patients. A review of safety considerations. *Drug Safety* 7(2):116–34.

49 Ofuji S, Ogino A, Horio T, *et al*. (1970). Eosinophilic pustular folliculitis. *Acta Derm Venereol* 50(3):195–203.

50 Soeprono F, Schinella RA (1986). Eosinophilic pustular folliculitis in patients with acquired immunodeficiency syndrome. *J Am Acad Dermatol* 14(6):1020–2.

51 Buchness MR, Lim HW, Hatcher VA, *et al*. (1988). Eosinophilic pustular folliculitis in acquired immunodeficiency syndrome: treatment with ultraviolet B phototherapy. *N Engl J Med* 318(18):1183–6.

52 Jenkins D, Fisher B, Chalvardjian A, Adam P (1988). Eosinophilic pustular folliculitis in a patient with AIDS. *Int J Dermatol* 27(1):34–5.

53 Rosenthal D, LeBoit P, Klumpp L, Berger TG (1991). Human immunodeficiency virus-associated eosinophilic folliculitis. *Arch Dermatol* 127(2):206–9.

54 Basarab T, Jones RR (1996). HIV-associated eosinophilic folliculitis: case report and review of the literature. *Br J Dermatol* 134(3):499–503.

55 Uthayakumar S, Nandwani R, Drinkwater T, *et al*. (1997). The prevalence of skin disease in HIV infection and its relationship to the degree of immunosuppression. *Br J Dermatol* 137(4):595–8.

56 Simpson-Dent S, Fearfield LA, Staughton RC (1999). HIV-associated eosinophilic folliculitis – differential diagnosis and management. *Sex Transmitt Infect* 75(5):291–3.

57 McCalmont TH, Altemus D, Maurer T, Berger TG (1995). Eosinophilic folliculitis: the histologic spectrum. *Am J Dermatopathol* 17(5):439–46.

58 Ferrandiz C, Ribera M, Barranco JC, *et al*. (1992). Eosinophilic pustular folliculitis in patients with acquired immunodeficiency syndrome. *Int J Dermatol* 31(3):193–5.

59 Berger TG, Heon V, King C, *et al*. (1995). Itraconazole therapy for human immunodeficiency virus-associated eosinophilic folliculitis.

Arch Dermatol **131**(3):358–60.

60 Haupt HM, Stern JB, Weber CB (1990). Eosinophilic pustular folliculitis: fungal folliculitis? *J Am Acad Dermatol* **23**(5 Pt 2):1021–4.

61 Otley CC, Avram MR, Johnson RA (1995). Isotretinoin treatment of human immunodeficiency virus-associated eosinophilic folliculitis: results of an open, pilot trial. *Arch Dermatol* **131**(9):1047–50.

62 Amerio P, Verdolini R, Proietto G, *et al.* (2001). Role of Th2 cytokines, RANTES and eotaxin in AIDS-associated eosinophilic folliculitis. *Acta Derm Venereol* **81**(2):92–5.

63 Harris DWS, Ostlere L, Buckley C, *et al.* (1992). Eosinophilic pustular folliculitis in an HIV-positive man: response to cetirizine. *Br J Dermatol* **126**(4):392–4.

64 Frentz G, Niordson AM, Thomsen K (1989). Eosinophilic pustular dermatosis: an early skin marker of infection with human immunodeficiency virus? *Br J Dermatol* **121**(2):271–4.

65 Magro CM, Crowson AN (2000). Necrotizing eosinophilic folliculitis as a manifestation of the atopic diathesis. *Int J Dermatol* **39**(9):672–7.

66 Takematsu H, Nakamura K, Igarashi M, Tagami H (1985). Eosinophilic pustular folliculitis: report of two cases with a review of the Japanese literature. *Arch Dermatol* **121**(7):917–20.

67 Buchness MR, Gregory N, Lim HW, Soter NA (1989). The role of mast cells and eosinophils in eosinophilic pustular folliculitis of the acquired immunodeficiency syndrome. *J Investig Dermatol* **92**(3):408.

68 Ellis E, Scheinfeld N (2004). Eosinophilic pustular folliculitis: a comprehensive review of treatment options. *Am J Clin Dermatol* **5**(3):189–97.

69 Grange F, Schoenlaub P, Tortel MC, *et al.* (1996). AIDS-related eosinophilic folliculitis: efficacy of high-dose topical corticotherapy. *Ann Derm Venereol* **123**(8):456–9.

70 Blauvelt A, Plott RT, Spooner K, *et al.* (1995). Eosinophilic folliculitis associated with the acquired immunodeficiency syndrome responds well to permethrin. *Arch Dermatol* **131**(3):360–1.

71 Moyle M, Woolley IJ, Thevarajan I, Korman TM (2004). Eosinophilic folliculitis: an example of 'immue reconstitution folliculitits'? *AIDS* **18**(17):2350–2.

72 Rajendran PM, Dolev JC, Heaphy MR, Maurer T (2005). Eosinophilic folliculitis: before and after the introduction of antiretroviral therapy. *Arch Dermatol* **141**(10):1227–31.

CHAPTER 10

1 Neuman MG, Malkiewicz IM, Phillips EJ, *et al.* (2002). Monitoring adverse drug reactions to sulfonamide antibiotics in human immunodeficiency virus-infected individuals. *Therap Drug Monitor* **24**(6):728–36.

2 Roujeau JC, Stern RS (1994). Medical progress: severe adverse cutaneous reactions to drugs. *N Engl J Med* **331**(19):1272–85.

3 Coopman SA, Johnson RA, Platt R, *et al.* (1993). Cutaneous disease and drug reactions in HIV infection. *N Engl J Med* **328**(23):1670–4.

4 Pirmohamed M, Park BK (1994). HIV and drug allergy. *Curr Opin Allergy Clin Immunol* **1**(4):311–16.

5 Hussain H, Beall G, Sanwo M (1997). Drug reactions in HIV/AIDS. *Western J Med* **167**(5):344.

6 Mitsuyasu R, Groopman J, Volberding P (1983). Cutaneous reaction to trimethoprim–sulfamethoxazole in patients with AIDS and Kaposi's sarcoma. *N Engl Med* **308**:1535–36.

7 Gordin FM, Simon GL, Wofsy CB, *et al.* (1984). Adverse reactions to trimethoprim–sulfamethoxazole in patients with the acquired immunodeficiency syndrome. *Ann Internal Med* **100**:495–9.

8 Sattler FR, Cowan R, Nielsen DM, *et al.* (1988). Trimethoprim–sulfamethoxazole compared with pentamidine for treatment of *Pneumocystis carinii* pneumonia in the acquired immunodeficiency syndrome: a prospective, noncrossover study. *Ann Internal Med* **109**:280–7.

9 Small CB, Harris CA, Friedland GH, *et al.* (1985). The treatment of *Pneumocystis carinii* pneumonia in the acquired immunodeficiency syndrome. *Arch Internal Med* **145**:837–40.

10 Kovacs JA, Hiemenz JW, Macher AM, *et al.* (1984). *Pneumocystis carinii* pneumonia: a comparison between patients with the acquired immunodeficiency syndrome and patients with other immunodeficiencies. *Ann Internal Med* **100**:663–71.

11 Medina I, Mills J, Leoung G, *et al.* (1990). Oral therapy for *Pneumocystis carinii* pneumonia in the acquired immunodeficiency syndrome: a controlled trial of trimethoprim–sulfamethoxazole *vs.* trimethoprim–dapsone. *N Engl J Med* **323**:776–82.

12 Jick H (1982). Adverse reactions to trimethoprim–sulfamethoxazole in hospitalized patients. *Rev Infect Dis* **4**:426–8.

13 Friedman-Kien AE, Cockerell CJ (eds) (1996). Cutaneous manifestations of HIV infection: cutaneous drug eruptions. In: *Color Atlas of AIDS*, 2nd edn. WB Saunders, Philadelphia, pp. 138–41.

14 Nguyen MT, Weiss PJ, Wallace MR (1995). Two-day oral desensibilization to trimethoprim–sulfamethoxazole in HIV-infected patients. *AIDS* **9**:573–5.

15 Hennesy D, Strom BL, Berlin JA, *et al.* (1995). Predicting cutaneous hypersensitivity reactions to cotrimoxazole in HIV-infected individuals receiving primary *Pneumocystis carinii* pneumonia prophylaxis. *J Gen Internal Med* **10**:380–6.

16 Carr A, Tindall B, Penny R, *et al.* (1993). Patterns of multiple-drug hypersensitivities in HIV-infected patients. *AIDS* **7**:1532–33.

17 Kennedy CA, Pimentel JA, Lewis DE, *et al.* (1993). Crossover of human immunodeficiency virus-infected patients from aerosolized pentamidine to trimethoprim–sulfamethoxazole: lack of hematologic toxicity and relationship of side-effects to CD4$^+$ lymphocyte count. *J Infect Dis* **168**:314–17.

18 Veenstra J, Veugelers PJ, Keet IPM, *et al.* (1997). Rapid disease progression in human immunodeficiency virus type 1-infected individuals with adverse reactions to trimethoprim–sulfamethoxazole prophylaxis. *Clin Infect Dis* **24**:936–41.

19 Smith KJ, Skelton HG, Yeager J, *et al.* (1997). Increased drug reactions in HIV-1-positive patients: a possible explanation based on patterns of immune dysregulation seen in HIV-1 disease. *Clin Exp Dermatol* **22**:118–23.

20 Carr A, Swanson C, Penny R, *et al.* (1993). Clinical and laboratory markers of hypersensitivity to

trimethoprim–sulfamethoxazole in patients with *Pneumocystis carinii* pneumonia and AIDS. *J Infect Dis* **167**:180–5.

21 Carr A, Gross AS, Hoskins JM, *et al.* (1994). Acetylation phenotype and cutaneous hypersensitivity to trimethoprim–sulfamethoxazole in HIV-infected patients. *AIDS* **8**:333–7.

22 Buhl R, Jaffe HA, Holroyd KJ, *et al.* (1989). Systemic glutathione deficiency in symptom-free HIV seropositive individuals. *Lancet* **334**:1294–8.

23 Dannemann B, McCutchan JA, Israelski D, *et al.* (1992). Treatment of toxoplasmic encephalitis in patients with AIDS. *Ann Internal Med* **116**:33–43.

24 Caumes E, Roudier C, Rogeaux O, *et al.* (1994). Effects of corticosteroids on the incidence of adverse reactions to trimethoprim–sulfamethoxazole during treatment of AIDS-associated *Pneumocystis carinii* pneumonia. *Clin Infect Dis* **18**:319–23.

25 Walmsley S, Levinton C, Brunton J, *et al.* (1995). A multicenter randomized double-blind placebo controlled trial of adjunctive corticosteroids in the treatment of *Pneumocystis carinii* pneumonia complicating the acquired immune deficiency syndrome. *J Acquir Immune Defic Syndr* **8**:348–57.

26 Eliaszewicz M, Flahault A, Roujeau JC, *et al.* (2002). Prospective evaluation of risk factors of cutaneous drug reactions to sulfonamides in patients with AIDS. *J Am Acad Dermatol* **47**(1):40–6.

27 Sullivan JR, Shear NH (2001). The drug hypersensitivity syndrome: what is the pathogenesis? *Arch Dermatol* **137**:357–64.

28 Ott M, Emiliani S, Van Lint C, *et al.* (1997). Immune hyperactivation of HIV-1 infected T cells mediated by Tat and the CD28 pathway. *Science* **275**:1481–5.

29 Pantaleo G, Fauci AS (1995). New concepts in the immunopathogenesis of HIV infection. *Ann Rev Immunol* **13**:487–512.

30 Baier-Bitterlich G, Fuchs D, Wachter H (1997). Chronic immune stimulation, oxidative stress, and apoptosis in HIV infection. *Biochem Pharmacol* **53**:755–63.

31 Lee BL, Wong D, Benowitz NL, *et al.* (1993). Altered patterns of drug metabolism in patients with acquired immunodeficiency syndrome. *Clin Pharmacol Therap* **53**:529–35.

32 Reilly TP, Ju C (2002). Mechanistic perspectives of sulfonamide-induced cutaneous drug reactions. *Curr Opin Allergy Clin Immunol* **2**:307–15.

33 Heller HM (2000). Adverse cutaneous drug reactions in patients with human immunodeficiency virus-1 infection. *Clin Dermatol* **18**(4):485–9.

34 Carr A, Tindall B, Penny R, *et al.* (1993). *In vitro* cytotoxicity as a marker of hypersensitivity to sulphamethoxazole in patients with HIV. *Clin Exp Immunol* **94**:21–5.

35 Smith CL, Brown I, Torraca BM (1997). Acetylator status and tolerance of high-dose trimethoprim–sulfamethoxazole therapy among patients infected with human immunodeficiency virus. *Clin Infect Dis* **25**:1477–8.

36 Lee B, Wong D, Benowitz NL, *et al.* (1993). Altered patterns of drug metabolism in patients with acquired immunodeficiency syndrome. *Clin Pharmacol Therap* **53**:529–35.

37 Rose EW, McCloskey WW (1998). Glutathione in hypersensitivity to trimethoprim/sulfamethoxazole in patients with HIV infection. *Ann Pharmacotherap* **32**:381–3.

38 Cribb AE, Spielberg SP, Griffin GP (1995). N-4-hydroxylation of sulfamethoxazole by cytochrome P450 of the cytochrome P4502C subfamily and reduction of sulfamethoxazole hydroxylamine in human and rat hepatic microsomes. *Drug Metab Dispos* **23**:406–14.

39 van der Ven AJ, Vree TB, van Ewijk-Beneken Kolmer EW, *et al.* (1995). Urinary recovery and kinetics of sulphamethoxazole and its metabolites in HIV-seropositive patients and healthy volunteers after a single oral dose of sulphamethoxazole. *Br J Clin Pharmacol* **39**:621–5.

40 Reilly TP, Lash LH, Doll MA, *et al.* (2000). A role for bioactivation and covalent binding within epidermal keratinocytes in sulfonamide-induced cutaneous drug reactions. *J Investig Dermatol* **114**:1164–73.

41 Baron JM, Holler D, Schiffer R, *et al.* (2001). Expression of multiple cytochrome P450 enzymes and multidrug resistance-associated transport proteins in human skin keratinocytes. *J Investig Dermatol* **116**:541–8.

42 Naisbitt DJ, Hough SJ, Gill HJ, *et al.* (1999). Cellular disposition of sulphamethoxazole and its metabolites: implications for hypersensitivity. *Br J Pharmacol* **126**:1393–407.

43 Hertl M, Jugert F, Merk HF (1995). CD8(+) dermal T cells from a sulfamethoxazole-induced bullous exanthema proliferate in response to drug-modified liver microsomes. *Br J Dermatol* **132**:215–20.

44 Kauppinen K, Stubb S (1984). Drug eruptions: causative agents and clinical types: a series of in-patients during a 10-year-period. *Acta Derm Venereol* **64**:320–4.

45 Coopman SA, Stern RS (1991). Cutaneous drug reactions in human immunodeficiency virus infection. [comment]. *Arch Dermatol* **127**(5):714–17.

46 Porteous DM, Berger TG (1991). Severe cutaneous drug reactions (Stevens–Johnson syndrome and toxic epidermal necrolysis) in human immunodeficiency virus infection. *Arch Dermatol* **127**:740–1.

47 Hira SK, Wadhawan D, Kamanga J, *et al.* (1988). Cutaneous manifestations of human immunodeficiency virus in Lusaka, Zambia. *J Am Acad Dermatol* **19**:451–7.

48 Navin TR, Miller KD, Satriale RF, *et al.* (1985). Adverse reactions associated with pyrimethamine–sulfadoxine prophylaxis for *Pneumocystis carinii* infections in AIDS. *Lancet* **1**:1332.

49 Raviglione MC, Dinan WA, Pablos-Mendez A, *et al.* (1988). Fatal toxic epidermal necrolysis during prophylaxis with pyrimethamine and sulfadoxine in a human immunodeficiency virus-infected person. *Arch Internal Med* **148**:2863–5.

50 Guillaume JC, Roujeau JC, Revuz J, *et al.* (1987). The culprit drugs in 87 cases of toxic epidermal necrolysis (Lyell's syndrome). *Arch Dermatol* **123**:1166–70.

51 Prins C, Kerdel F, Padilla S, *et al.* (2003). Treatment of toxic epidermal necrolysis with high-dose intravenous immunoglobulin. *Arch Dermatol* **139**:26–32.

52 Chosidow O, Bourgault I, Roujeau JC (1994). Drug rashes: what are the targets of cell-mediated cytotoxicity? *Arch Dermatol* **130**:627–9.

53 Greenberger RG, Patterson R (1987). Management of drug allergy in patients with acquired immunodeficiency syndrome. *J Allergy Clin Immunol* **79**:484–8.

54 Raviglione MC, Dinan WA, Pablos-

Mendez A. *et al.* (1988). Fatal toxic epidermal necrolysis during prophylaxis with pyrimethamine and sulfadoxine in a human immunodeficiency virus-infected person. *Arch Internal Med* **148**:2683–5.

55 Berger TG, Tappero JW, Leoung GS, *et al.* (1989). Aerosolized pentamadine and cutaneous eruptions (letter). *Ann Internal Med* **110**:1035–6.

56 O'Brien JG, Dong BJ, Coleman RL, *et al.* (1997). A 5-year retrospective review of adverse drug reactions and their risk factors in human immunodeficiency virus-infected patients who were receiving intravenous pentamidine therapy for *Pneumocystis carinii* pneumonia. *Clin Infect Dis* **24**(5):854–9.

57 Snider DE, Graczyk J, Bek E, *et al.* (1984). Supervised six-month treatment of newly diagnosed pulmonary tuberculosis using isoniazid, rifampin, and pyrazinamide with and without streptomycin. *Am Rev Respir Dis* **130**:1091–4.

58 Eriki P, Okwera A, Aisu T, *et al.* (1991). The influence of human immunodeficiency virus infection on tuberculosis in Kampala, Uganda. *Am Rev Respir Dis* **143**:185–7.

59 Hawken M, Nunn P, Gathua D, *et al.* (1993). Increased recurrence of tuberculosis in HIV-1-infected patients in Kenya. *Lancet* **342**:332–7.

60 Jayaweera DT (1997). Minimizing the dosage-limiting toxicities of foscarnet induction therapy. *Drug Safety* **16**(4):258–66.

61 Garman M, Tyring S (2002). The cutaneous manifestations of HIV infection. *Dermatolog Clin* **20**:193–208.

62 Wald A, Mattson D, Schubert MA (1999). Photo quiz. Foscarnet-induced genital ulcers. *Clin Infect Dis* **28**(1):139.

63 Brown TJ, Vander Straten M, Tyring SK (2001). Antiviral agents. *Dermatolog Clin* **19**(1):23–34.

64 Van Der Pijl JW, Frissen PH, Reiss P, *et al.* (1990). Foscarnet and penile ulceration (letter). *Lancet* **335**:286.

65 Gross AS, Dretler RH (1993). Foscarnet-induced penile ulcer in an uncircumcised patient with AIDS. *Clin Infect Dis* **17**:1076–7.

66 Lacey HB, Ness A, Mandal BK (1992). Vulval ulceration associated with foscarnet.
Genitourinary Med **68**:182.

67 Blanshard C (1991). Generalized cutaneous rash associated with foscarnet usage in AIDS. *J Infect Dis* **23**:336–7.

68 Gill PS, Loureiro C, Bernstein-Singer M, *et al.* (1989). Clinical effects of glucocorticoids on Kaposi's sarcoma related to the acquired immunodeficiency syndrome. *Ann Internal Med* **110**:937–40.

69 Dolev J, Reyter I, Maurer T (2004). Treatment of recurring cutaneous drug reactions in patients with human immunodeficiency virus 1 infection. *Arch Dermatol* **140**:1051–3.

70 Brown P, Crane L (2001). Avascular necrosis of bone in patients with human immunodeficiency virus infection: report of 6 cases and review of the literature. *Clin Infect Dis* **32**:1221–6.

71 Vittorio CC, Muglia JJ (1995). Anticonvulsant hypersensitivity syndrome. *Arch Internal Med* **155**(21):2285–90.

72 Patterson R, DeSwarte RD, Greenberger PA, *et al.* (1995). Individual drugs or problems: summary of useful techniques. In: *Drug Allergy and Protocols for Management of Drug Allergies.* Oceanside Publications, Providence, pp. 9–18.

73 Tilles SA (2001). Practical issues in the management of hypersensitivity reactions: sulfonamides. *Southern Med J* **94**(8):817–24.

74 Sanwo M, Nwadiuko R, Beall G (1996). Use of intravenous immunoglobulin in the treatment of severe cutaneous drug reactions in patients with AIDS. *J Allergy Clin Immunol* **98**:1112–15.

75 Viard I, Wehrli P, Bullani R, *et al.* (1998). Inhibition of toxic epidermal necrolysis by blockade of CD95 with human intravenous immunoglobulin. *Science* **282**:490–3.

CHAPTER 11

1 Bilu D, Mamelak AJ, Nguyen RHN, *et al.* (2004). Clinical and epidemiologic characterization of photosensitivity in HIV-positive individuals. *Photodermatol Photoimmunol Photomed* **20**:175–83.

2 Stanley SK, Fauci A (1989). UV-induced DNA damage as an intermediate step in UV-induced
expression of human immunodeficiency virus type 1, collagenase, C-foas, and metallothionein. *Mol Cell Biol* **9**:5169.

3 Gregory N, DeLeo VA (1994). Clinical manifestations of photosensitivity in patients with human immunodeficiency virus infection. *Arch Dermatol* **130**:630–3.

4 Zmudska BZ (1992). Activation of HIV by UVB radiation and PUVA treatment *in vitro*: an evaluation of the safety of medical procedures and cosmetic applications. *Photochem Photobiol* **55**:895–905.

5 Miller SA, Beer JZ, Strickland AG, Zmudska BZ (1993). Spectral effects in activation of the HIV promoter by PUVA. *Photochem Photobiol* **57**:945.

6 Smith KJ, Skelton HG, Tuur S, *et al.* (1997). Increased cutaneous toxicity to ionizing radiation in HIV-positive patients. *Int J Dermatol* **36**:779–82.

7 Smith KJ, Skelton HG, Tuur S, *et al.* (1997). Histopathologic features seen in cutaneous photoeruptions in HIV-positive patients. *Int J Dermatol* **36**:745–53.

8 Meola T, Sanchez M, Lim HW, *et al.* (1997). Chronic actinic dermatitis associated with human immunodeficiency virus infection. *Br J Dermatol* **137**:431–6.

9 Humbert P, Drobacheff C, Vigan M, *et al.* (1991). Chronic actinic dermatitis responding to danzol. *Br J Dermatol* **124**:195–7.

10 Murphy GM, Maurice PDL, Norris PG, *et al.* (1989). Azathioprine treatment in chronic actinic dermatitis: a double-blind controlled trial with monitoring of exposure to ultraviolet radiation. *Br J Dermatol* **121**:639–46.

11 Wong SN, Khoo LSW (2003). Chronic actinic dermatitis as the presenting feature of HIV infection in three Chinese males. *Clin Exp Dermatol* **28**:265–8.

12 Pappert A, Grossman M, DeLeo V (1994). Photosensitivity as the presenting illness in four patients with human immunodeficiency viral infection. *Arch Dermatol* **130**:618–23.

13 Toback AC, Longley J, Cardullo A, *et al.* (1986). Severe chronic photosensitivity in association with acquired immunodeficiency syndrome. *J Am Acad Dermatol* **15**:1056–7.

14 Wolf P, Mullegger R, Cerroni L, *et*

al. (1996). Photoaccentuated erythroderma associated with CD4+ T lymphocytopenia: successful treatment with 5-methoxypsolaren and UVA, interferon alfa-2b, and extracorporeal photophoresis. *J Am Acad Dermatol* **35**:291–4.

15 Berger TG, Dhar A (1994). Lichenoid photoeruptions in human immunodeficiency virus infection. *Arch Dermatol* **130**:609–13.

16 Villaverde RR, Melguizo JB, Sintes RN, *et al.* (2002). Multiple linear lichen planus in an HIV patient. *JEADV* **16**:411–27.

17 Cribier B, Frances C, Chosidow O (1998). Treatment of lichen planus: an evidence-based medicine analysis of efficacy. *Arch Dermatol* **134**:1521–30.

18 Blauvelt A, Harris HR, Hogan DJ, *et al.* (1992). Porphyria cutanea tarda and human immunodeficiency virus infection. *Int J Dermatol* **31**:472–9.

19 Sampietro M, Fiorelli G, Fargion S (1999). Iron overload in porphyria cutanea tarda. *Haematologica* **84**:248–53.

20 Kushner JP, Steinmuller DP, Lee GR (1975). The role of iron in the pathogenesis of porphyria cutanea tarda, II: inhibition of uroporphyrinogen decarboxylase. *J Clin Invest* **56**:661–7.

21 Blauvelt A (1996). Hepatitis C virus and human immunodeficiency virus infection can alter porphyrin metabolism and lead to porphyria cutanea tarda. *Arch Dermatol* **132**:1503–4.

22 Shigesawa TP-L, Marumo FSC (1992). Significance of plasma glutathione determination in patients with alcoholic and nonalcoholic liver disease. *J Gastoenterol Hepatol* **7**:7–11.

23 Del Nero E, De Lorenzi E, Granata K, *et al.* (1990). Therapeutic use of glutathione. *Clin Ther* **132**:167–71.

24 Ostrowski J, Kosecki P, Martynska M, Milewski B (1984). Urinary porphyrins and liver disease. *Scand J Gastroenterol* **19**:862–6.

25 Bickers DR (1991). Photosensitization by porphyrins. In: *Physiology, Biochemistry, and Molecular Biology of the Skin*, 2nd edn. AN Goldsmith (ed). Oxford University Press, New York, pp. 957–75.

26 Fargion S, Piperno A, Cappellini MD, *et al.* (1992). Hepatitis C virus and porphyria cutanea tarda. *Hepatology* **16**:1322–6.

27 DeCastro M, Sanchez J, Herrera JF, *et al.* (1993). Hepatitis C virus antibodies and liver disease in patients with porphyria cutanea tarda. *Hepatology* **17**:551–7.

28 Herrero C, Vincent A, Bruguera M, *et al.* (1993). Is hepatitis C virus infection a trigger of porphyria cutanea tarda? *Lancet* **341**:788–9.

29 Lacour JP, Bodokh I,Castanet J, *et al.* (1993). Porphyria cutanea tarda and antibodies to hepatitis C virus. *Br J Dermatol* **128**:121–3.

30 Koester G, Feldman J, Bigler C (1994). Hepatitis C in patients with porphyria cutanea tarda. *J Am Acad Dermatol* **31**:1054.

31 Lim HW (1995). Hepatitis C virus infection in patients with porphyria cutanea tarda evaluated in New York, NY. *Arch Dermatol* **131**:849.

32 Coburn PR, Coleman JC, Cream JJ, *et al.* (1985). Porphyria cutanea tarda and porphyria variegata unmasked by viral hepatitis. *Clin Exp Dermatol* **10**:169–73.

33 O'Reilly FM, Darby C, O'Moore R, *et al.* (1995). Porphyrin metabolism in hepatitis C infection secondary to anti-D immunoglobulin and intravenous drug use. *Br J Dermatol* **132**:656.

34 O'Connor WJ, Murphy GM, Darby C, *et al.* (1996). Porphyrin abnormalities in acquired immunodeficiency syndrome. *Arch Dermatol* **132**:1443–7.

35 Reynaud P, Goodfellow K, Svec F (1990). Porphyria cutanea tarda as the initial presentation of the acquired immunodeficiency syndrome in two patients. *J Infect Dis* **161**:1032–3.

36 Larnier C, Avenel M, Rousselet MC, *et al.* (1987). Granulomatous hepatitis caused by *Mycobacterium avium* in AIDS detected by porphyria cutanea tarda [in French]. *Gastroenterol Clin Biol* **11**:264–5.

37 Cappell MS (1991). Hepatobiliary manifestations of the acquired immune deficiency syndrome. *Am J Gastroenterol* **86**:1–15.

38 Wissel PS, Sordillo P, Anderson KE, *et al.* (1987). Porphyria cutanea tarda associated with the acquired immunodeficiency syndrome. *Am J Hematol* **25**:107–33.

39 Poh-Fitzpatrick M (2002). Porphyria cutanea tarda. In: *Treatment of Skin Disease, Comprehensive and Therapeutic Strategies*. M Lebwohl (ed). Harcourt Publishers Ltd, London, pp. 493–5.

40 Supapannachart N, Breneman DL, Linnemann CC Jr (1991). Isolation of human immunodeficiency virus type 1 in cutaneous blister fluid. *Arch Dermatol* **127**:1198–200.

41 Fiallo P (1998). Cyclosporin for the treatment of granuloma annulare. *Br J Dermatol* **138**:357–73.

42 Kim YJ, Kang HY, Lee ES, Kim YC (2006). Photodynamic therapy for granuloma annulare. *J Dermatol* **33**:642–3.

43 Epstein WL, Okamoto M, Suya H, Fukuyama K (1986/1987). T cell independent transfer of organized granuloma formation. *Immunol Lett* **14**:59–63.

44 Suya H, Fujioka A, Pincelli C, *et al.* (1988). Skin granuloma formation in mice immunosuppressed by cyclosporine. *J Invest Dermatol* **90**:430–3.

45 Badavanis G, Monastirli A, Pasmatzi E, Tsambaos D (2005). Successful treatment of granuloma annulare with imiquimod cream 5%: a report of four cases. *Acta Derm Venereol* **85**:547–8.

46 Fiallo P (1998). Cyclosporine for the treatment of granuloma annulare. *Br J Dermatol* **138**(2):357–73.

47 Toro JR, Crawford R, Berger TG, LeBoit PE (1997). Photodermatitis in human immunodeficiency viral infection: a histological and immunohistochemical study. *J Cutan Pathol* **24**:89.

48 LeBoit PE, Beckstead JH, Bond, B, *et al.* (1987). Granulomatous slack skin: clonal rearrangement of the T cell receptor beta gene is evidence for the lymphoproliferative nature of cutaneous elastolytic disorder. *J Invest Dermatol* **89**:183–6.

49 Magro CM, Crowson AN, Schapiro BL (1998). The interstitial granulomatous drug reaction: a distinctive clinical and pathological entity. *J Cut Pathol* **25**:72–8.

50 Toro JR, McCalmont TH, Leonardi C, Berger TG (1995). Lichenoid and granulomatous dermatitis: a cuntaneous eruption seen in late-stage human immunodeficiency virus infection [abstract]. *J Cutan Pathol* **22**:91.

51 Viraben R, Dupre A (1998). Lichenoid granulomatous papular dermatosis associated with human immunodeficiency virus infection: an immunohistochemical study [letter]. *J Am Acad Dermatol* **18**(pt 1):1140–1.

52 Gad F, Viau G, Boushira M, *et al.*

(2001). Photodynamic therapy with 5-aminolaevulinic acid induces apoptosis and caspase activation in malignant T cells. *J Cut Med Surg* 5:8–13.

53 Wang I, Bauer B, Andersson-Engels S, *et al.* (2003). Photodynamic therapy with topical -aminolaevulinic acid for treatment of cutaneous carcinomas and cutaneous T cell lymphoma. *J Invest Dermatol* 100:602.

54 Zeitouni NC, Oseroff AR, Shieh S (2003). Photodynamic therapy for nonmelanoma skin cancers. *Mol Immunol* 39:1133–6.

55 Morton CA(2004). Photodynamic therapy for non-melanoma skin cancer – and more? *Arch Dermatol* 140:116–20.

56 Ratnavel RC, Norris PG (1995). Perforating granuloma annulare; response to treatment with isotretinoin. *J Am Acad Dermatol* 32(1):126–7.

57 Weiss JM, Muchenberger S, Schopf E, Simon JC (1998). Treatment of granuloma annulare by local injections with local-dose recombinant interferon gamma. *J Am Acad Dermatol* 39:117–19.

58 Jain S, Stephens CJM (2004). Successful treatment of disseminated granuloma annulare with topical tacrolimus. *Br J Dermatol* 150:1042–3.

59 Hertl MS, Haedle I, Schuler HG, Hertl M (2005). Rapid improvement of recalcitrant disseminated granuloma annulare upon treatment with the tumour necrosis factor-inhibitor, infliximab. *Br J Dermatol* 152:552–5.

CHAPTER 12

1 Sternbach G, Varon J (1995). Moritz Kaposi: idiopathic pigmented sarcoma of the skin. *J Emerg Med* 13(5):671–4.

2 Friedman-Kien AE (1981). Disseminated Kaposi's sarcoma syndrome in young homosexual men. *J Am Acad Dermatol* 5(4):468–71.

3 Biggar RJ, Rabkin CS (1996). The epidemiology of AIDS-related neoplasms. *Hematol Oncol Clin North Am* 10(5):997–1010.

4 Beral V, Bull D, Jaffe H, *et al.* (1991). Is risk of Kaposi's sarcoma in AIDS patients in Britain increased if sexual partners came from United States or Africa? *BMJ* 302(6777):624–5.

5 Friedman-Kien AE, Saltzman BR (1990). Clinical manifestations of classical, endemic African, and epidemic AIDS-associated Kaposi's sarcoma. *J Am Acad Dermatol* 22(6 Pt 2):1237–50.

6 Friedman-Kien AE, Saltzman BR, Cao YZ, *et al.* (1990). Kaposi's sarcoma in HIV-negative homosexual men. *Lancet* 335(8682):168–9.

7 Giraldo G, Beth E, Kyalwazi SK (1984). Role of cytomegalovirus in Kaposi's sarcoma. *IARC Sci Pub* 63:583–606.

8 Wang RY, Shih JW, Weiss SH, *et al.* (1993). Mycoplasma penetrans infection in male homosexuals with AIDS: high seroprevalence and association with Kaposi's sarcoma. *Clin Infect Dis* 17(4):724–9.

9 Chang Y, Cesarman E, Pessin MS, *et al.* (1994). Identification of herpesvirus-like DNA sequences in AIDS-associated Kaposi's sarcoma. *Science* 266(5192):1865–9.

10 Miller G, Rigsby MO, Heston L, *et al.* (1996). Antibodies to butyrate-inducible antigens of Kaposi's sarcoma-associated herpesvirus in patients with HIV-1 infection. *N Engl J Med* 334(20):1292–7.

11 Gao SJ, Kingsley L, Hoover DR, *et al.* (1996). Seroconversion to antibodies against Kaposi's sarcoma-associated herpesvirus-related latent nuclear antigens before the development of Kaposi's sarcoma. *N Engl J Med* 335(4):233–41.

12 Koelle DM, Huang ML, Chandran B, *et al.* (1997). Frequent detection of Kaposi's sarcoma-associated herpesvirus (human herpesvirus 8) DNA in saliva of human immunodeficiency virus-infected men: clinical and immunologic correlates. *J Infect Dis* 176(1):94–102.

13 Russo JJ, Bohenzky RA, Chien MC, *et al.* (1996). Nucleotide sequence of the Kaposi sarcoma-associated herpesvirus (HHV8). *Proc Natl Acad Sci USA* 93(25):14862–7.

14 Chang Y, Moore PS, Talbot SJ, *et al.* (1996). Cyclin encoded by KS herpesvirus. *Nature* 382(6590):410.

15 Thome M, Schneider P, Hofmann K, *et al.* (1997). Viral FLICE-inhibitory proteins (FLIPs) prevent apoptosis induced by death receptors. *Nature* 386(6624):517–21.

16 Lee H, Veazey R, Williams K, *et al.* (1998). Deregulation of cell growth by the K1 gene of Kaposi's sarcoma-associated herpesvirus.

Nature Med 4(4):435–40.

17 Gao SJ, Boshoff C, Jayachandra S, *et al.* (1997). KSHV ORF K9 (vIRF) is an oncogene which inhibits the interferon signaling pathway. *Oncogene* 15(16):1979–85.

18 Stine JT, Wood C, Hill M, *et al.* (2000). KSHV-encoded CC chemokine vMIP-III is a CCR4 agonist, stimulates angiogenesis, and selectively chemoattracts TH2 cells. *Blood* 95(4):1151–7.

19 Whitby D, Howard MR, Tenant-Flowers M, *et al.* (1995). Detection of Kaposi sarcoma-associated herpesvirus in peripheral blood of HIV-infected individuals and progression to Kaposi's sarcoma. *Lancet* 346(8978):799–802.

20 Parry JP, Moore PS (1997). Corrected prevalence of Kaposi's sarcoma (KS)-associated herpesvirus infection prior to onset of KS. *AIDS* 11(1):127–8.

21 Boshoff C, Weiss RA (2001). Epidemiology and pathogenesis of Kaposi's sarcoma-associated herpesvirus. *Philos Trans R Soc Lond B Biol Sci* 356(1408):517–34.

22 Dupin N, Fisher C, Kellam P, *et al.* (1999). Distribution of human herpesvirus-8 latently infected cells in Kaposi's sarcoma, multicentric Castleman's disease, and primary effusion lymphoma. *Proc Natl Acad Sci USA* 96(8):4546–51.

23 Katano H, Iwasaki T, Baba N, *et al.* (2000). Identification of antigenic proteins encoded by human herpesvirus 8 and seroprevalence in the general population and among patients with and without Kaposi's sarcoma. *J Virol* 74(8):3478–85.

24 Goudsmit J, Renwick N, Dukers NH, *et al.* (2000). Human herpesvirus 8 infections in the Amsterdam Cohort Studies (1984–1997): analysis of seroconversions to ORF65 and ORF73. *Proc Natl Acad Sci USA* 97(9):4838–43.

25 O'Brien TR, Kedes D, Ganem D, *et al.* (1999). Evidence for concurrent epidemics of human herpesvirus 8 and human immunodeficiency virus type 1 in US homosexual men: rates, risk factors, and relationship to Kaposi's sarcoma. *J Infect Dis* 180(4):1010–7.

26 Greenblatt RM, Jacobson LP, Levine AM, *et al.* (2001). Human herpesvirus 8 infection and Kaposi's sarcoma among human immunodeficiency virus-infected and -uninfected women. *J Infect Dis*

183(7):1130–4. Epub 2001 Mar 8.

27 Koster R, Blatt LM, Streubert M, *et al.* (1996). Consensus-interferon and platelet-derived growth factor adversely regulate proliferation and migration of Kaposi's sarcoma cells by control of c-myc expression. *Am J Pathol* 149(6):1871–85.

28 Zimring JC, Goodbourn S, Offermann MK(1998). Human herpesvirus 8 encodes an interferon regulatory factor (IRF) homolog that represses IRF-1-mediated transcription. *J Virol* 72(1):701–7.

29 Vogel J, Hinrichs SH, Reynolds RK, *et al.* (1988). The HIV tat gene induces dermal lesions resembling Kaposi's sarcoma in transgenic mice. *Nature* 335(6191):606–11.

30 Rappersberger K, Gartner S, Schenk P, *et al.* (1988). Langerhans' cells are an actual site of HIV-1 replication. *Intervirology* 29(4):185–94.

31 Cheuk W, Wong KO, Wong CS, *et al.* (2004). Immunostaining for human herpesvirus 8 latent nuclear antigen-1 helps distinguish Kaposi sarcoma from its mimickers. *Am J Clin Pathol* 121(3):335–42.

32 Janier M, Morel P, Civatte J (1990). The Koebner phenomenon in AIDS-related Kaposi's sarcoma. *J Am Acad Dermatol* 22(1):125–6.

33 Schwartz RA (2004). Kaposi's sarcoma: an update. *J Surg Oncol* 87(3):146–51.

34 Ruocco V, Schwartz RA, Ruocco E (2002). Lymphedema: an immunologically vulnerable site for development of neoplasms. *J Am Acad Dermatol* 47(1):124–7.

35 Nasti G, Vaccher E, Errante D, *et al.* (1997). Malignant tumors and AIDS. *Biomed Pharmacotherap* 51(6-7):243–51.

36 Aftergut K, Cockerell CJ (1997) (1999). Update on the cutaneous manifestations of HIV infection. Clinical and pathologic features. *Dermatol Clin* 17(3):445–71, vii.

37 Crowe SM, Carlin JB, Stewart KI, *et al.* (1991). Predictive value of CD4 lymphocyte numbers for the development of opportunistic infections and malignancies in HIV-infected persons. *J Acquir Immune Defic Syndr* 4(8):770–6.

38 Ioachim HL, Adsay V, Giancotti FR, *et al.* (1995). Kaposi's sarcoma of internal organs. A multiparameter study of 86 cases. *Cancer* 75(6):1376–85.

39 Gray MH, Trimble CL, Zirn J, *et al.* (1991). Relationship of factor XIIIa-positive dermal dendrocytes to

Kaposi's sarcoma. *Arch Pathol Lab Med* 115(8):791–6.

40 Way DL, Witte MH, Fiala M, *et al.* (1993). Endothelial transdifferentiated phenotype and cell-cycle kinetics of AIDS-associated Kaposi sarcoma cells. *Lymphology* 26(2):79–89.

41 Reis-Filho JS, Souto-Moura C, Lopes JM (2002). Classic Kaposi's sarcoma of the tongue: case report with emphasis on the differential diagnosis. *J Oral Maxillofac Surg* 60(8):951–4.

42 Krown SE (1998). Clinical overview: issues in Kaposi's sarcoma therapeutics. *J Natl Cancer Inst Monogr* 23:59–63.

43 Cattelan AM, Trevenzoli M, Aversa SM (2002). Recent advances in the treatment of AIDS-related Kaposi's sarcoma. *Am J Clin Dermatol* 3(7):451–62.

44 Tulpule A, Groopman J, Saville MW, *et al.* (2002). Multicenter trial of low-dose paclitaxel in patients with advanced AIDS-related Kaposi sarcoma. *Cancer* 95(1):147–54.

45 Stelzer KJ, Griffin TW (1993). A randomized prospective trial of radiation therapy for AIDS-associated Kaposi's sarcoma. *Int J Radiat Oncol Biol Phys* 27(5):1057–61.

46 McCormick SU (1996). Intralesional vinblastine injections for the treatment of oral Kaposi's sarcoma: report of 10 patients with 2-year follow-up. *J Oral Maxillofac Surg* 54(5):583–7, discussion 588–9.

47 Trattner A, Reizis Z, David M, *et al.* (1993). The therapeutic effect of intralesional interferon in classical Kaposi's sarcoma. *Br J Dermatol* 129(5):590–3.

48 Laubenstein LJ, Krigel RL, Odajnyk CM, *et al.* (1984). Treatment of epidemic Kaposi's sarcoma with etoposide or a combination of doxorubicin, bleomycin, and vinblastine. *J Clin Oncol* 2(10):1115–20.

49 Remick SC, Reddy M, Herman D, *et al.* (1994). Continuous infusion bleomycin in AIDS-related Kaposi's sarcoma. *J Clin Oncol* 12(6):1130–6.

50 Northfelt DW, Dezube BJ, Thommes JA, *et al.* (1998). Pegylated-liposomal doxorubicin versus doxorubicin, bleomycin, and vincristine in the treatment of AIDS-related Kaposi's sarcoma: results of a randomized phase III clinical trial. *J Clin Oncol* 16(7):2445–51.

51 Gill PS, Rarick M, McCutchan JA, *et al.* (1991). Systemic treatment of AIDS-related Kaposi's sarcoma: results of a randomized trial. *Am J Med* 90(4):427–33.

52 Stewart S, Jablonowski H, Goebel FD, *et al.* (1998). Randomized comparative trial of pegylated liposomal doxorubicin versus bleomycin and vincristine in the treatment of AIDS-related Kaposi's sarcoma. International Pegylated Liposomal Doxorubicin Study Group. *J Clin Oncol* 16(2):683–91.

53 Berry G, Billingham M, Alderman E, *et al.* (1998). The use of cardiac biopsy to demonstrate reduced cardiotoxicity in AIDS Kaposi's sarcoma patients treated with pegylated liposomal doxorubicin. *Ann Oncol* 9(7):711–6.

54 Horwitz SB, Cohen D, Rao S, *et al.* (1993). Taxol: mechanisms of action and resistance. *J Natl Cancer Inst Monogr* 15:55–61.

55 Klauber N, Parangi S, Flynn E, *et al.* (1997). Inhibition of angiogenesis and breast cancer in mice by the microtubule inhibitors 2-methoxyestradiol and taxol. *Cancer Res* 57(1):81–6.

56 Belotti D, Vergani V, Drudis T, *et al.* (1996). The microtubule-affecting drug paclitaxel has antiangiogenic activity. *Clin Cancer Res* 2(11):1843–9.

57 Krown SE (1991). Interferon and other biologic agents for the treatment of Kaposi's sarcoma. *Hematol Oncol Clin North Am* 5(2):311–22.

58 Fischl MA (1991). Antiretroviral therapy in combination with interferon for AIDS-related Kaposi's sarcoma. *Am J Med* 90(4A):2S–7S.

59 Krown SE, Gold JW, Niedzwiecki D, *et al.* (1990). Interferon-alpha with zidovudine: safety, tolerance, and clinical and virologic effects in patients with Kaposi sarcoma associated with the acquired immunodeficiency syndrome (AIDS). *Ann Internal Med* 112(11):812–21.

60 D'Amato RJ, Loughnan MS, Flynn E, *et al.* (1994). Thalidomide is an inhibitor of angiogenesis. *Proc Natl Acad Sci USA* 91(9):4082–5.

61 Little RF, Wyvill KM, Pluda JM, *et al.* (2000). Activity of thalidomide in AIDS-related Kaposi's sarcoma. *J Clin Oncol* 18(13):2593–602.

62 Dezube BJ, Von Roenn JH, Holden-Wiltse J, *et al.* (1998). Fumagillin analog in the treatment of Kaposi's

sarcoma: a phase I AIDS Clinical Trial Group study. AIDS Clinical Trial Group No. 215 Team. *J Clin Oncol* **16**(4):1444–9.

63 Nakamura S, Sakurada S, Salahuddin SZ, *et al.* (1992). Inhibition of development of Kaposi's sarcoma-related lesions by a bacterial cell wall complex. *Science* **255**(5050):1437–40.

64 Pluda JM, Shay LE, Foli A, *et al.* (1993). Administration of pentosan polysulfate to patients with human immunodeficiency virus-associated Kaposi's sarcoma. *J Natl Cancer Inst* **85**(19):1585–92.

65 Twardowski P, Gradishar WJ (1997). Clinical trials of antiangiogenic agents. *Curr Opin Oncol* **9**(6):584–9.

66 Eckhardt SG, Burris HA, Eckardt JR, *et al.* (1996). A phase I clinical and pharmacokinetic study of the angiogenesis inhibitor, tecogalan sodium. *Ann Oncol* **7**(5):491–6.

67 Tulpule A, Scadden DT, Espina BM, *et al.* (2000). Results of a randomized study of IM862 nasal solution in the treatment of AIDS-related Kaposi's sarcoma. *J Clin Oncol* **18**(4):716–23.

68 Noy A, Scadden DT, Lee J, *et al.* (2005). Angiogenesis inhibitor IM862 is ineffective against AIDS-Kaposi's sarcoma in a phase III trial, but demonstrates sustained, potent effect of highly active antiretroviral therapy: from the AIDS Malignancy Consortium and IM862 Study Team. *J Clin Oncol* **23**(5):990–8. Epub 2004 Dec 14.

69 Guo WX, Gill PS, Antakly T (1995). Inhibition of AIDS-Kaposi's sarcoma cell proliferation following retinoic acid receptor activation. *Cancer Res* **55**(4):823–9.

70 Gill PS, Espina BM, Moudgil T, *et al.* (1994). All-trans retinoic acid for the treatment of AIDS-related Kaposi's sarcoma: results of a pilot phase II study. *Leukemia* **8**(Suppl 3):S26–32.

71 Saiag P, Pavlovic M, Clerici T, *et al.* (1998). Treatment of early AIDS-related Kaposi's sarcoma with oral all-trans-retinoic acid: results of a sequential non-randomized phase II trial. Kaposi's Sarcoma ANRS Study Group. Agence Nationale de Recherches sur le SIDA. *AIDS* **12**(16):2169–76.

72 Miles SA, Dezube BJ, Lee JY, *et al.* (2002). Antitumor activity of oral 9-cis-retinoic acid in HIV-associated Kaposi's sarcoma.

AIDS **16**(3):421–9.

73 Duvic M, Friedman-Kien AE, Looney DJ, *et al.* (2000). Topical treatment of cutaneous lesions of acquired immunodeficiency syndrome-related Kaposi sarcoma using alitretinoin gel: results of phase 1 and 2 trials. *Arch Dermatol* **136**(12):1461–9.

74 Albini A, Fontanini G, Masiello L, *et al.* (1994). Angiogenic potential *in vivo* by Kaposi's sarcoma cell-free supernatants and HIV-1 tat product: inhibition of KS-like lesions by tissue inhibitor of metalloproteinase-2. *AIDS* **8**(9):1237–44.

75 Prakash O, Tang ZY, He YE, *et al.* (2000). Human Kaposi's sarcoma cell-mediated tumorigenesis in human immunodeficiency type 1 tat-expressing transgenic mice. *J Natl Cancer Inst* **92**(9):721–8.

76 Cianfrocca M, Cooley TP, Lee JY, *et al.* (2002). Matrix metalloproteinase inhibitor COL-3 in the treatment of AIDS-related Kaposi's sarcoma: a phase I AIDS malignancy consortium study. *J Clin Oncol* **20**(1):153–9.

77 Gill PS, Lunardi-Ishkandar Y, Louie S, *et al.* (1996). The effects of preparations of human chorionic gonadotropin on AIDS-related Kaposi's sarcoma. *N Engl J Med* **335**(17):1261–9.

78 Gill PS, McLaughlin T, Espina BM, *et al.* (1997). Phase I study of human chorionic gonadotropin given subcutaneously to patients with acquired immunodeficiency syndrome-related mucocutaneous Kaposi's sarcoma. *J Natl Cancer Inst* **89**(23):1797–802.

79 Pfeffer U, Bisacchi D, Morini M, *et al.* (2002). Human chorionic gonadotropin inhibits Kaposi's sarcoma associated angiogenesis, matrix metalloprotease activity, and tumor growth. *Endocrinology* **143**(8):3114–21.

80 Murphy M, Armstrong D, Sepkowitz KA, *et al.* (1997). Regression of AIDS-related Kaposi's sarcoma following treatment with an HIV-1 protease inhibitor. *AIDS* **11**(2):261–2.

81 Bower M, Fox P, Fife K, *et al.* (1999). Highly active antiretroviral therapy (HAART) prolongs time to treatment failure in Kaposi's sarcoma. *AIDS* **13**(15):2105–11.

82 Lebbe C, Blum L, Pellet C, *et al.* (1998). Clinical and biological impact of antiretroviral therapy with protease inhibitors on HIV-related

Kaposi's sarcoma. *AIDS* **12**(7):F45–9.

83 Krown SE (2004). Highly active antiretroviral therapy in AIDS-associated Kaposi's sarcoma: implications for the design of therapeutic trials in patients with advanced, symptomatic Kaposi's sarcoma. *J Clin Oncol* **22**(3):399–402.

84 Glesby MJ, Hoover DR, Weng S, *et al.* (1996). Use of antiherpes drugs and the risk of Kaposi's sarcoma: data from the Multicenter AIDS Cohort Study. *J Infect Dis* **173**(6):1477–80.

85 Mocroft A, Youle M, Gazzard B, *et al.* (1996). Antiherpesvirus treatment and risk of Kaposi's sarcoma in HIV infection. Royal Free/Chelsea and Westminster Hospitals Collaborative Group. *AIDS* **10**(10):1101–5.

86 Slazinski L, Stall JR, Mathews CR (1984). Basal cell carcinoma in a man with acquired immunodeficiency syndrome. *J Am Acad Dermatol* **11**(1):140–1.

87 Maurer TA, Christian KV, Kerschmann RL, *et al.* (1997). Cutaneous squamous cell carcinoma in human immunodeficiency virus-infected patients. A study of epidemiologic risk factors, human papillomavirus, and p53 expression. *Arch Dermatol* **133**(5):577–83.

88 Lobo DV, Chu P, Grekin RC, *et al.* (1992). Nonmelanoma skin cancers and infection with the human immunodeficiency virus. *Arch Dermatol* **128**(5):623–7.

89 Smith KJ, Skelton HG, Yeager J, *et al.* (1994). Cutaneous findings in HIV-1-positive patients: a 42-month prospective study. Military Medical Consortium for the Advancement of Retroviral Research (MMCARR). *J Am Acad Dermatol* **31**(5 Pt 1):746–54.

90 Palefsky JM, Gonzales J, Greenblatt RM, *et al.* (1990). Anal intraepithelial neoplasia and anal papillomavirus infection among homosexual males with group IV HIV disease. *JAMA* **263**(21):2911–6.

91 Nguyen P, Vin-Christian K, Ming ME, *et al.* (2002). Aggressive squamous cell carcinomas in persons infected with the human immunodeficiency virus. *Arch Dermatol* **138**(6):758–63.

92 Nappi L, Carriero C, Bettocchi S, *et al.* (2005). Cervical squamous intraepithelial lesions of low-grade

in HIV-infected women: recurrence, persistence, and progression, in treated and untreated women. *Eur J Obstet Gynecol Reprod Biol* 121(2):226–32. Epub 2005 Jan 18.

93 Cooley TP (2003). Non-AIDS-defining cancer in HIV-infected people. *Hematol Oncol Clin North Am* 17(3):889–99.

94 Rasokat H, Steigleder GK, Bendick C, *et al.* (1989). Malignant melanoma and HIV infection. *Z Hautkr* 64(7):581–2, 587.

95 Wilkins K, Dolev JC, Turner R, *et al.* (2005). Approach to the treatment of cutaneous malignancy in HIV-infected patients. *Dermatol Ther* 18(1):77–86.

96 Duvic M, Lowe L, Rapini RP, *et al.* (1989). Eruptive dysplastic nevi associated with human immunodeficiency virus infection. *Arch Dermatol* 125(3):397–401.

97 Rubin AI, Chen EH, Ratner D (2005). Basal-cell carcinoma. *N Engl J Med* 353(21):2262–9.

98 Rodrigues LK, Klencke BJ, Vin-Christian K, *et al.* (2002). Altered clinical course of malignant melanoma in HIV-positive patients. *Arch Dermatol* 138(6):765–70.

99 Kashani-Sabet M (2004). Melanoma genomics. *Curr Oncol Rep* 6(5):401–5.

100 Girardi M, Heald PW, Wilson LD (2004). The pathogenesis of mycosis fungoides. *N Engl J Med* 350(19):1978–88.

101 Hivnor CM, Nguyen V, Rook AH, *et al.* (2005). CD8+ lymphoma in a patient with human immunodeficiency virus. *Arch Dermatol* 141(10):1321–2.

102 Friedler S, Parisi MT, Waldo E, *et al.* (1999). Atypical cutaneous lymphoproliferative disorder in patients with HIV infection. *Int J Dermatol* 38(2):111–18.

103 Beylot-Barry M, Vergier B, Masquelier B, *et al.* (1999). The spectrum of cutaneous lymphomas in HIV infection: a study of 21 cases. *Am J Surg Pathol* 23(10):1208–16.

104 Wilkins K, Turner R, Dolev JC, *et al.* (2006). Cutaneous malignancy and human immunodeficiency virus disease. *J Am Acad Dermatol* 54(2):189–206; quiz 207–10.

105 Schartz NE, De La Blanchardiere A, Alaoui S, *et al.* (2003). Regression of CD8+ pseudolymphoma after HIV antiviral triple therapy. *J Am Acad Dermatol* 49:139–41.

CHAPTER 13

1 Kreiss JK, Koech D, Plummer FA, *et al.* (1986). AIDS virus infection in Nairobi prostitutes. Spread of the epidemic to East Africa. *N Engl J Med* 314(7):414–8.

2 Greenblatt RM, Lukehart SA, Plummer FA, *et al.* (1988). Genital ulceration as a risk factor for human immunodeficiency virus infection. *AIDS* 2(1):47–50.

3 Simonsen JN, Cameron DW, Gakinya MN, *et al.* (1988). Human immunodeficiency virus infection among men with sexually transmitted diseases. Experience from a center in Africa. *N Engl J Med* 319(5):274–8.

4 Plourde PJ, Plummer FA, Pepin J, *et al.* (1992). Human immunodeficiency virus type 1 infection in women attending a sexually transmitted diseases clinic in Kenya. *J Infect Dis* 166(1):86–92.

5 Plummer FA, Simonsen JN, Cameron DW, *et al.* (1991). Cofactors in male–female sexual transmission of human immunodeficiency virus type 1. *J Infect Dis* 163(2):233–9.

6 Grosskurth H, Mosha F, Todd J, *et al.* (1995). Impact of improved treatment of sexually transmitted diseases on HIV infection in rural Tanzania: randomised controlled trial. *Lancet* 346(8974): 530–6.

7 Cunningham AL, Turner RR, Miller AC, *et al.* (1985). Evolution of recurrent herpes simplex lesions. An immunohistologic study. *J Clin Investig* 75(1):226–33.

8 de Vincenzi I (1994). A longitudinal study of human immunodeficiency virus transmission by heterosexual partners. European Study Group on Heterosexual Transmission of HIV. *N Engl J Med* 331(6):341–6.

9 Heng MC, Heng SY, Allen SG (1994). Co-infection and synergy of human immunodeficiency virus-1 and herpes simplex virus-1. *Lancet* 343(8892):255–8.

10 Koelle DM, Abbo H, Peck A, *et al.* (1994). Direct recovery of herpes simplex virus (HSV)-specific T lymphocyte clones from recurrent genital HSV-2 lesions. *J Infect Dis* 169(5):956–61.

11 Kinghorn GR (1993). Genital herpes: natural history and treatment of acute episodes. *J Med Virol Suppl* 1:33–8.

12 Schomogyi M, Wald A, Corey L (1998). Herpes simplex virus-2 infection. An emerging disease?

Infect Dis Clin North Am 12(1):47–61.

13 Siegal FP, Lopez C, Hammer GS, *et al.* (1981). Severe acquired immunodeficiency in male homosexuals, manifested by chronic perianal ulcerative herpes simplex lesions. *N Engl J Med* 305(24):1439–44.

14 Parran T (1937). *Shadow on the Land*. Reynal & Hitchcock, New York.

15 (No authors listed) (2003). Primary and secondary syphilis – United States, 2002. *MMWR* 52(46):1117–20.

16 (No authors listed) (2002). Primary and secondary syphilis among men who have sex with men – New York City, 2001. *From the Centers for Disease Control and Prevention* 288(15):1840–2.

17 (No authors listed) (2002). Primary and secondary syphilis – United States, 2000–2001. *MMWR* 51(43):971–3.

18 Ciesielski CA, (2003). Sexually transmitted diseases in men who have sex with men: an epidemiologic review. *Curr Infect Dis Rep* 5(2):145–52.

19 (No authors listed) (2006). Primary and secondary syphilis – United States, 2003–2004. *MMWR* 55(10):269–73.

20 Fleming DT, Wasserheit JN (1999). From epidemiological synergy to public health policy and practice: the contribution of other sexually transmitted diseases to sexual transmission of HIV infection. *Sex Transmitt Infect* 75(1):3–17.

21 Johnson LF, Coetzee DJ, R. E. Dorrington RE (2005). Sentinel surveillance of sexually transmitted infections in South Africa: a review. *Sex Transmitt Infect* 81(4): 287–93.

22 Pike RM (1976). Laboratory-associated infections: summary and analysis of 3921 cases. *Health Lab Sci* 13(2):105–14.

23 Garnett GP, Aral SO, Hoyle DV, *et al.* (1997). The natural history of syphilis. Implications for the transmission dynamics and control of infection. *Sex Transmitt Dis* 24(4):185–200.

24 De Schryver A, Meheus A (1990). Syphilis and blood transfusion: a global perspective. *Transfusion* 30(9):844–7.

25 Hollier LM, Cox SM (1998). Syphilis. *Semin Perinatol* 22(4):323–31.

26 Walker DG, Walker GJ (2002).

Forgotten but not gone: the continuing scourge of congenital syphilis. *Lancet Infect Dis* 2(7):432–6.

27 Klein JR, Monjan AA (1983). Delayed-type hypersensitivity response in mice to *Treponema pallidum. Immunol Commun* 12(1):25–30.

28 Sell S, Hsu PL (1993). Delayed hypersensitivity, immune deviation, antigen processing and T cell subset selection in syphilis pathogenesis and vaccine design. *Immunology Today* 14(12):576–82.

29 Golden MR, Marra CM, Holmes KK (2003). Update on syphilis: resurgence of an old problem. *JAMA* 290(11):1510–14.

30 Fitzgerald TJ (1992). The Th1/Th2-like switch in syphilitic infection: is it detrimental? *Infect Immun* 60(9):3475–9.

31 Blanco DR, Miller JN, Lovett MA (1997). Surface antigens of the syphilis spirochete and their potential as virulence determinants. *Emerg Infect Dis* 3(1):11–20.

32 (No authors listed) (2002). Sexually transmitted diseases treatment guidelines 2002. *Centers for Disease Control and Prevention* 51(RR-6):1–78.

33 Hart G (1986). Syphilis tests in diagnostic and therapeutic decision making. *Ann Internal Med* 104(3):368–76.

34 Johns DR, Tierney M, Felsenstein D (1987). Alteration in the natural history of neurosyphilis by concurrent infection with the human immunodeficiency virus. *N Engl J Med* 316(25):1569–72.

35 Hutchinson CM, Hook EW 3rd, Shepherd M, *et al.* (1994). Altered clinical presentation of early syphilis in patients with human immunodeficiency virus infection. *Ann Internal Med* 121(2):94–100.

36 Schofer H, Imhof M, Thoma-Greber E, *et al.* (1996). Active syphilis in HIV infection: a multicentre retrospective survey. The German AIDS Study Group (GASG). *Genitourinary Med* 72(3):176–81.

37 Dowell ME, Ross PG, Musher DM, *et al.* (1992). Response of latent syphilis or neurosyphilis to ceftriaxone therapy in persons infected with human immunodeficiency virus. *Am J Med* 93(5):481–8.

38 Rolfs RT, Joesoef MR, Hendershot EF, *et al.* (1997). A randomized trial of enhanced therapy for early

syphilis in patients with and without human immunodeficiency virus infection. The Syphilis and HIV Study Group. *N Engl J Med* 337(5):307–14.

39 Morgello S, Laufer H (1989). Quaternary neurosyphilis in a Haitian man with human immunodeficiency virus infection. *Hum Pathol* 20(8):808–11.

40 Hay PE, Tam FW, Kitchen VS, *et al.* (1990). Gummatous lesions in men infected with human immunodeficiency virus and syphilis. *Genitourinary Med* 66(5):374–9.

41 Rompalo AM, Cannon RO, Quinn TC, Hook EW 3rd (1992). Association of biologic false-positive reactions for syphilis with human immunodeficiency virus infection. *J Infect Dis* 165(6):1124–6.

42 Joyanes P, Borobio MV, Arquez JM, Perea EJ (1998). The association of false-positive rapid plasma reagin results and HIV infection. *Sex Transmitt Dis* 25(10):569–71.

43 Radolf JD, Kaplan RP (1988). Unusual manifestations of secondary syphilis and abnormal humoral immune response to *Treponema pallidum* antigens in a homosexual man with asymptomatic human immunodeficiency virus infection. *J Am Acad Dermatol* 18(2 Pt 2):423–8.

44 Hutchinson CM, Rompalo AM, Reichart CA, Hook EW 3rd (1991). Characteristics of patients with syphilis attending Baltimore STD clinics. Multiple high-risk subgroups and interactions with human immunodeficiency virus infection. *Arch Internal Med* 151(3):511–16.

45 Johnson PD, Graves SR, Stewart L, *et al.* (1991). Specific syphilis serological tests may become negative in HIV infection. *AIDS* 5(4):419–23.

46 Tikjob G, Russel M, Petersen CS, *et al.* (1991). Seronegative secondary syphilis in a patient with AIDS: identification of *Treponema pallidum* in biopsy specimen. *J Am Acad Dermatol* 24(3):506–8.

47 Marra CM, Longstreth WT Jr, Maxwell CL, Lukehart SA (1996). Resolution of serum and cerebrospinal fluid abnormalities after treatment of neurosyphilis. Influence of concomitant human immunodeficiency virus infection. *Sex Transmitt Dis* 23(3):184–9.

48 Yinnon AM, Coury-Doniger P, Polito R, Reichman RC (1996). Serologic response to treatment of

syphilis in patients with HIV infection. *Arch Internal Med* 156(3):321–5.

49 Goeman J, Kivuvu M, Nzila N, *et al.* (1995). Similar serological response to conventional therapy for syphilis among HIV-positive and HIV-negative women. *Genitourinary Med* 71(5):275–9.

50 US Department of Health and Human Services, PHS (2000). Tracking the hidden epidemics: trends in STDs in the United States 2000. Atlanta. Centers for Disease Control:1–36.

51 Jajosky RA, Hall PA, Adams DA, *et al.* (2006). Summary of notifiable diseases – United States, 2004. *MMWR* 53(53):1–79.

52 Schulte JM, Martich FA, Schmid GP (1992). Chancroid in the United States, 1981–1990: evidence for underreporting of cases. *MMWR CDC Surveill Summ* 41(3):57–61.

53 Bogaerts J, Ricart CA, Van Dyck E, Piot P (1989). The etiology of genital ulceration in Rwanda. *Sex Transmitt Dis* 16(3):123–6.

54 Goens JL, Schwartz RA, De Wolf K (1994). Mucocutaneous manifestations of chancroid, lymphogranuloma venereum and granuloma inguinale. *Am Fam Phys* 49(2):415–18, 23–5.

55 Ortiz-Zepeda C, Hernandez-Perez E, Marroquin-Burgos R (1994). Gross and microscopic features in chancroid: a study in 200 new culture-proven cases in San Salvador. *Sex Transmitt Dis* 21(2):112–7.

56 Buntin DM, Rosen T, Lesher JL Jr, *et al.* (1991). Sexually transmitted diseases: bacterial infections. Committee on Sexually Transmitted Diseases of the American Academy of Dermatology. *J Am Acad Dermatol* 25(2 Pt 1): 287–99.

57 Chapel TA, Brown WJ, Jeffres C, Stewart JA (1977). How reliable is the morphological diagnosis of penile ulcerations? *Sex Transmitt Dis* 4(4):150–2.

58 Werman BS, Herskowitz LJ, Olansky S, *et al.* (1983). A clinical variant of chancroid resembling granuloma inguinale. *Arch Dermatol* 119(11):890–4.

59 Sturm AW, Stolting GJ, Cormane RH, Zanen HC (1987). Clinical and microbiological evaluation of 46 episodes of genital ulceration. *Genitourinary Med* 63(2):98–101.

60 Joseph AK, Rosen T (1994). Laboratory techniques used in the diagnosis of chancroid, granuloma

inguinale, and lymphogranuloma venereum. *Dermatol Clin* **12**(1):1–8.

61 Manget Velasco CS, Borbujo Martinez J, Manzano de Arostegui JA, *et al.* (1993). Soft chancroid: 4 clinical cases. *Aten Primaria* **12**(10):667–70.

62 Tyndall MW, Plourde PJ, Agoki E, *et al.* (1993). Fleroxacin in the treatment of chancroid: an open study in men seropositive or seronegative for the human immunodeficiency virus type 1. *Am J Med* **94**(3A):85S–8S.

63 Kimani J, Bwayo JJ, Anzala AO, *et al.* (1995). Low-dose erythromycin regimen for the treatment of chancroid. *East Afr Med J* **72**(10):645–8.

64 King R, Choudhri SH, Nasio J, *et al.* (1998). Clinical and in situ cellular responses to Haemophilus ducreyi in the presence or absence of HIV infection. *Int J STD AIDS* **9**(9):531–6.

65 Magro CM, Crowson AN, Alfa M, *et al.* (1996). A morphological study of penile chancroid lesions in human immunodeficiency virus (HIV)-positive and -negative African men with a hypothesis concerning the role of chancroid in HIV transmission. *Hum Pathol* **27**(10):1066–70.

66 Quale J, Teplitz E, Augenbraun M (1990). Atypical presentation of chancroid in a patient infected with the human immunodeficiency virus. *Am J Med* **88**(5N):43N–4N.

67 MacDonald KS, Cameron DW, D'Costa L, *et al.* (1989). Evaluation of fleroxacin (RO 23-6240) as single-oral-dose therapy of culture-proven chancroid in Nairobi, Kenya. *Antimicrob Agents Chemother* **33**(5):612–14.

68 Plourde PJ, D'Costa LJ, Agoki E, *et al.* (1992). A randomized, double-blind study of the efficacy of fleroxacin versus trimethoprim–sulfamethoxazole in men with culture-proven chancroid. *J Infect Dis* **165**(5):949–52.

69 Tyndall MW, Agoki E, Plummer FA, *et al.* (1994). Single dose azithromycin for the treatment of chancroid: a randomized comparison with erythromycin. *Sex Transmitt Dis* **21**(4):231–4.

70 Lal S, Nicholas C (1970). Epidemiological and clinical features in 165 cases of granuloma inguinale. *Br J Vener Dis* **46**(6):461–3.

71 Mitchell KM, Roberts AN, Williams VM, Schneider J (1986). Donovanosis in Western Australia. *Genitourinary Med* **62**(3):191–5.

72 O'Farrell N (2002). Donovanosis. *Sex Transmitt Infect* **78**(6):452–7.

73 Rosen T, Tschen JA, Ramsdell W, *et al.* (1984). Granuloma inguinale. *J Am Acad Dermatol* **11**(3):433–7.

74 Hudson BJ, van der Meijden WI, Lupiwa T, *et al.* (1994). A survey of sexually transmitted diseases in five STD clinics in Papua New Guinea. *P N G Med J* **37**(3):152–60.

75 World Health Organization National AIDS Council, National Department of Health, Papua New Guinea (2000). Consensus report on STI, HIV and AIDS epidemiology Papua New Guinea 2000. Papua New Guinea. (http://www.wpro.who.int/NR/rdonlyres/EEC64817-5D9F-4E72-9F7C-6014887E3483/0/Consensus_Report_PNG_2000.pdf).

76 Begg K, Roche P, Owen R, *et al.* (2006). Australia's Notifiable Diseases Status (2006). Annual Report of the National Notifiable Diseases Surveillance System (http://www.health.gov.au/internet/main/publishing.nsf/content/cda-cdi3202-pdf-cnt.htm/$FILE/cdi3202a.pdf).

77 Brown TJ, Yen-Moore A, Tyring SK (1999). An overview of sexually transmitted diseases. Part I. *J Am Acad Dermatol* **41**(4):511–32.

78 Govender D, Naidoo K, Chetty R (1997). Granuloma inguinale (donovanosis): an unusual cause of otitis media and mastoiditis in children. *Am J Clin Pathol* **108**(5):510–14.

79 Packer H, Goldberg J (1950). Studies of the antigenic relationship of *D. grandulomatis* to members of the tribe Eschericheae. *Am J Syph Gonorrhea Vener Dis* **34**(4):342–50.

80 Ramachander M, Jayalaxmi S, Pankaja P (1967). A study of donovanosis in Guntur. *Ind J Dermatol, Venereol, Leprol* **33**:236–44.

81 Sehgal VN, Sharma NL, Bhargava NC, *et al.* (1979). Primary extragenital disseminated cutaneous donovanosis. *Br J Dermatol* **101**(3):353–6.

82 Hart G (1997). Donovanosis. *Clin Infect Dis* **25**(1):24–30; quiz 31–2.

83 Maddocks I, Anders EM, Dennis E (1976). Donovanosis in Papua New Guinea. *Br J Vener Dis* **52**(3):190–6.

84 Brigden M, Guard R (1980). Extragenital granuloma inguinale in North Queensland. *Med J Aust* **2**(10):565–7.

85 Hoosen AA, Draper G, Moodley J, Cooper K (1990). Granuloma inguinale of the cervix: a carcinoma look-alike. *Genitourinary Med* **66**(5):380–2.

86 Hacker P, Fisher BK, Dekoven J, Shier RM (1992). Granuloma inguinale: three cases diagnosed in Toronto, Canada. *Int J Dermatol* **31**(10):696–9.

87 Kharsany AB, Hoosen AA, Kiepiela P, *et al.* (1996). Culture of *Calymmatobacterium granulomatis*. *Clin Infect Dis* **22**(2):391.

88 Carter J, Hutton S, Sriprakash KS, *et al.* (1997). Culture of the causative organism of donovanosis (*Calymmatobacterium granulomatis*) in HEp-2 cells. *J Clin Microbiol* **35**(11):2915–7.

89 Manders SM, Baxter JD (1997). Granuloma inguinale and HIV: a unique presentation and novel treatment regimen. *J Am Acad Dermatol* **37**(3 Pt 1):494–6.

90 Jamkhedkar PP, Hira SK, Shroff HJ, Lanjewar DN (1998). Clinico-epidemiologic features of granuloma inguinale in the era of acquired immune deficiency syndrome. *Sex Transmitt Dis* **25**(4):196–200.

91 Hoosen AA, Mphatsoe M, Kharsany AB, *et al.* (1996). Granuloma inguinale in association with pregnancy and HIV infection. *Int J Gynaecol Obstet* **53**(2):133–8.

92 Sanders CJ (1998). Extragenital donovanosis in a patient with AIDS. *Sex Transmitt Infect* **74**(2):142–3.

93 Schachter J (1978). Chlamydial infections (first of three parts). *N Engl J Med* **298**(8):428–35.

94 Schachter J, Osoba AO (1983). Lymphogranuloma venereum. *Br Med Bull* **39**(2):151–4.

95 Moodley P, Sturm PD, Vanmali T, *et al.* (2003). Association between HIV-1 infection, the etiology of genital ulcer disease, and response to syndromic management. *Sex Transmitt Dis* **30**(3):241–5.

96 Bauwens JE, Orlander H, Gomez MP, *et al.* (2002). Epidemic lymphogranuloma venereum during epidemics of crack cocaine use and HIV infection in the Bahamas. *Sex Transmitt Dis* **29**(5):253–9.

97 (No authors listed) (2004). Lymphogranuloma venereum among men who have sex with men – Netherlands, 2003–2004. *MMWR* **53**(42):985–8.

98 van de Laar MJ, Fenton KA, Ison C

(2005). Update on the European lymphogranuloma venereum epidemic among men who have sex with men. *Euro Surveill* **10**(6):E050602 1.

99 Ahdoot A, Kotler DP, Suh JS, *et al.* (2006). Lymphogranuloma venereum in human immunodeficiency virus-infected individuals in New York City. *J Clin Gastroenterol* **40**(5):385–90.

100 Halioua B, Bohbot JM, Monfort L, *et al.* (2006). Ano-rectal lymphogranuloma venereum: 22 cases reported in a sexually transmited infections center in Paris. *Eur J Dermatol* **16**(2):177–80.

101 Perenboom RM (2006). Lymphogranuloma venereum proctitis: an emerging sexually transmitted disease in HIV-positive men in the Netherlands. *Drugs Today (Barc.)* **42**(Suppl A):43–5.

102 Williams D, Churchill D (2006). Ulcerative proctitis in men who have sex with men: an emerging outbreak. *BMJ* **332**(7533):99–100.

103 Spaargaren J, Fennema HS, Morre SA, *et al.* (2005). New lymphogranuloma venereum *Chlamydia trachomatis* variant, Amsterdam. *Emerg Infect Dis* **11**(7):1090–2.

104 Spaargaren J, Schachter J, Moncada J, *et al.* (2005). Slow epidemic of lymphogranuloma venereum L2b strain. *Emerg Infect Dis* **11**(11):1787–8.

105 de Vries HJ, Fennema JS, Morre SA (2006). Lymphogranuloma venereum among men having sex with men; what have we learned so far? *Sex Transmitt Infect* **82**(4):344.

106 Morre SA, Spaargaren J, Fennema JS, *et al.* (2005). Real-time polymerase chain reaction to diagnose lymphogranuloma venereum. *Emerg Infect Dis* **11**(8):1311–12.

107 Scieux C, Barnes R, Bianchi A, *et al.* (1989). Lymphogranuloma venereum: 27 cases in Paris. *J Infect Dis* **160**(4):662–8.

108 Speers D (1999). Lymphogranuloma venereum presenting with a psoas abscess. *Aust NZ J Med* **29**(4):563–4.

109 Kellock DJ, Barlow R, Suvarna SK, *et al.* (1997). Lymphogranuloma venereum: biopsy, serology, and molecular biology. *Genitourinary Med* **73**(5):399–401.

110 Mostad S, Welch M, Chohan B, Reilly M, *et al.* (1994). Cofactors for heterosexual transmission of HIV to prostitutes in Mombasa, Kenya. *Ninth International Conference on AIDS and STD in Africa. Kampala, Uganda* Dec 10–14.

111 Mroczkowski TF, Martin DH (1994). Genital ulcer disease. *Dermatol Clin* **12**(4):753–64.

112 Burgoyne RA (1990). Lymphogranuloma venereum. *Prim Care* **17**(1):153–7.

113 Greaves AB (1963). The frequency of lymphogranuloma venereum in persons with perirectal abscesses, fistulae in ano, or both, with particular reference to the relationship between perirectal abscesses of lymphogranuloma origin in the male and Inversion. *Bull World Health Organ* **29**:797–801.

114 Quinn TC, Goodell SE, Mkrtichian E, *et al.* (1981). *Chlamydia trachomatis* proctitis. *N Engl J Med* **305**(4):195–200.

115 Lynch CM, Felder TL, Schwandt RA, Shashy RG (1999). Lymphogranuloma venereum presenting as a rectovaginal fistula. *Infect Dis Obstet Gynecol* **7**(4):199–201.

116 Faro S (1989). Lymphogranuloma venereum, chancroid, and granuloma inguinale. *Obstet Gynecol Clin North Am* **16**(3):517–30.

117 Kraus SJ (1990). Diagnosis and management of acute genital ulcers in sexually active patients. *Semin Dermatol* **9**(2):160–6.

118 Mittal A, Sachdeva KG (1993). Monoclonal antibody for the diagnosis of lymphogranuloma venereum: a preliminary report. *Br J Biomed Sci* **50**(1):3–7.

119 Van Dyck E, Piot P (1992). Laboratory techniques in the investigation of chancroid, lymphogranuloma venereum and donovanosis. *Genitourinary Med* **68**(2):130–3.

120 Thompson SE, Washington AE (1983). Epidemiology of sexually transmitted *Chlamydia trachomatis* infections. *Epidemiol Rev* **5**:96–123.

121 Treharne JD, Forsey T, Thomas BJ (1983). Chlamydial serology. *Br Med Bull* **39**(2):194–200.

122 Stephens RS, Kuo CC, Tam MR (1982). Sensitivity of immunofluorescence with monoclonal antibodies for detection of *Chlamydia trachomatis* inclusions in cell culture. *J Clin Microbiol* **16**(1):4–7.

123 Aldridge KE, Cammarata C, Martin DH (1993). Comparison of the *in vitro* activities of various parenteral and oral antimicrobial agents against endemic *Haemophilus ducreyi*. *Antimicrob Agents Chemother* **37**(9):1986–8.

124 Parkash S, Radhakrishna K (1986). Problematic ulcerative lesions in sexually transmitted diseases: surgical management. *Sex Transmitt Dis* **13**(3):127–33.

125 Nieuwenhuis RF, Ossewaarde JM, van der Meijden WI, Neumann HA (2003). Unusual presentation of early lymphogranuloma venereum in an HIV-1 infected patient: effective treatment with 1 g azithromycin. *Sex Transmitt Infect* **79**(6):453–5.

126 Spornraft-Ragaller P, Luck C, Straube E, Meurer M (2006). Lymphogranuloma venereum. Two cases from Dresden. *Hautarzt* **57**(12):1095–100.

127 Van der Bij AK, Spaargaren J, Morre SA, *et al.* (2006). Diagnostic and clinical implications of anorectal lymphogranuloma venereum in men who have sex with men: a retrospective case–control study. *Clin Infect Dis* **42**(2):186–94.

128 Hammer GP, Kellogg TA, McFarland WC, *et al.* (2003). Low incidence and prevalence of hepatitis C virus infection among sexually active nonintravenous drug-using adults, San Francisco, 1997–2000. *Sex Transmitt Dis* **30**(12):919–24.

129 Roy KM, Goldberg DJ, Hutchinson S, *et al.* (2004). Hepatitis C virus among self-declared noninjecting sexual partners of injecting drug users. *J Med Virol* **74**(1):62–6.

130 Bodsworth NJ, Cunningham P, Kaldor J, *et al.* (1996). Hepatitis C virus infection in a large cohort of homosexually active men: independent associations with HIV-1 infection and injecting drug use but not sexual behaviour. *Genitourinary Med* **72**(2):118–22.

131 Alary M, Joly JR, Vincelette J, *et al.* (2005). Lack of evidence of sexual transmission of hepatitis C virus in a prospective cohort study of men who have sex with men. *Am J Public Health* **95**(3):502–5.

132 Gotz HM, van Doornum G, Niesters HG, *et al.* (2005). A cluster of acute hepatitis C virus infection among men who have sex with men – results from contact tracing and public health implications. *AIDS* **19**(9):969–74.

133 zur Hausen, H (2000).

Papillomaviruses causing cancer: evasion from host-cell control in early events in carcinogenesis. *J Natl Cancer Inst* **92**(9):690–8.

134 de Villiers EM, Gunst K, Stein H, Scherubl H (2004). Esophageal squamous cell cancer in patients with head and neck cancer: prevalence of human papillomavirus DNA sequences. *Int J Cancer* **109**(2):253–8.

135 Meyer T, Arndt R, Christophers E, *et al.* (1998). Association of rare human papillomavirus types with genital premalignant and malignant lesions. *J Infect Dis* **178**(1):252–5.

136 Trottier H, Franco EL (2006). The epidemiology of genital human papillomavirus infection. *Vaccine* **24**(Suppl 1):S1–15.

137 Heaton CL (1995). Clinical manifestations and modern management of condylomata acuminata: a dermatologic perspective. *Am J Obstet Gynecol* **172**(4 Pt 2):1344–50.

138 Chuang TY, Perry HO, Kurland LT, Ilstrup DM (1984). Condyloma acuminatum in Rochester, Minn., 1950–1978. I. Epidemiology and clinical features. *Arch Dermatol* **120**(4):469–75.

139 Koutsky LA, Wolner-Hanssen P (1989). Genital papillomavirus infections: current knowledge and future prospects. *Obstet Gynecol Clin North Am* **16**(3):541–64.

140 von Krogh G (1991). Genitoanal papillomavirus infection: diagnostic and therapeutic objectives in the light of current epidemiological observations. *Int J STD AIDS* **2**(6):391–404.

141 Koutsky LA, Galloway DA, Holmes KK (1988). Epidemiology of genital human papillomavirus infection. *Epidemiol Rev* **10**:122–63.

142 Beutner KR, Tyring SK, Trofatter KF Jr, *et al.* (1998). Imiquimod, a patient-applied immune-response modifier for treatment of external genital warts. *Antimicrob Agents Chemother* **42**(4):789–94.

143 Edwards L, Ferenczy A, Eron L, *et al.* (1998). Self-administered topical 5% imiquimod cream for external anogenital warts. HPV Study Group. Human PapillomaVirus. *Arch Dermatol* **134**(1):25–30.

144 Syrjanen K, Vayrynen M, Castren O, *et al.* (1984). Sexual behaviour of women with human papillomavirus (HPV) lesions of the uterine cervix. *Br J Vener Dis* **60**(4):243–8.

145 Daling JR, Sherman KJ, Weiss NS (1986). Risk factors for condyloma acuminatum in women. *Sex Transmitt Dis* **13**(1):16–18.

146 Kataja,V, Syrjanen S, Yliskoski M, *et al.* (1993). Risk factors associated with cervical human papillomavirus infections: a case–control study. *Am J Epidemiol* **138**(9):735–45.

147 Hippelainen M, Syrjanen S, Hippelainen M, *et al.* (1993). Prevalence and risk factors of genital human papillomavirus (HPV) infections in healthy males: a study on Finnish conscripts. *Sex Transmitt Dis* **20**(6):321–8.

148 Habel LA, Van Den Eeden SK, Sherman J, *et al.* (1998). Risk factors for incident and recurrent condylomata acuminata among women. A population-based study. *Sex Transmitt Dis* **25**(6):285–92.

149 Stone KM (1995). Human papillomavirus infection and genital warts: update on epidemiology and treatment. *Clin Infect Dis* **20**(Suppl 1): S91–7.

150 Luchtefeld MA (1994). Perianal condylomata acuminata. *Surg Clin North Am* **74**(6):1327–38.

151 Handsfield HH (1997). Clinical presentation and natural course of anogenital warts. *Am J Med* **102**(5A):16–20.

152 Ferenczy A (1995). Epidemiology and clinical pathophysiology of condylomata acuminata. *Am J Obstet Gynecol* **172**(4 Pt 2):1331–9.

153 Kaufman RS, Balogh K (1969). Verrucas and juvenile laryngeal papillomas. *Arch Otolaryngol* **89**(5):748–9.

154 Sundararaj AS, Williams J, Deivam S, *et al.* (1991). Anal and laryngeal papillomata in an 8-month-old child. *Int J STD AIDS* **2**(3):213–14.

155 Williams LR, Webster G (1991). Warts and molluscum contagiosum. *Clin Dermatol* **9**(1):87–93.

156 Tang CK, Shermeta DW, Wood C (1978). Congenital condylomata acuminata. *Am J Obstet Gynecol* **131**(8):912–13.

157 Laraque D (1989). Severe anogenital warts in a child with HIV infection. *N Engl J Med* **320**(18):1220–1.

158 Woolley P (1995). Identifying and treating genital warts. *Practitioner* **239**(1554):542–6.

159 Douglas JM Jr, Werness BA (1989). Genital human papillomavirus infections. *Clin Lab Med* **9**(3):421–44.

160 Tseng CJ, Pao CC, Lin JD, *et al.*

(1999). Detection of human papillomavirus types 16 and 18 mRNA in peripheral blood of advanced cervical cancer patients and its association with prognosis. *J Clin Oncol* **17**(5):1391–6.

161 Arany I, Tyring SK, Stanley MA, *et al.* (1999). Enhancement of the innate and cellular immune response in patients with genital warts treated with topical imiquimod cream 5%. *Antiviral Res* **43**(1):55–63.

162 Nicholls PK, Moore PF, Anderson DM, *et al.* (2001). Regression of canine oral papillomas is associated with infiltration of CD4+ and CD8+ lymphocytes. *Virology* **283**(1):31–9.

163 Penn I (1986). Cancers of the anogenital region in renal transplant recipients. Analysis of 65 cases. *Cancer* **58**(3):611–16.

164 Fennema JS, van Ameijden EJ, Coutinho RA, van den Hoek AA (1995). HIV, sexually transmitted diseases and gynaecologic disorders in women: increased risk for genital herpes and warts among HIV-infected prostitutes in Amsterdam. *AIDS* **9**(9):1071–8.

165 Petry KU, Kochel H, Bode U, *et al.* (1996). Human papillomavirus is associated with the frequent detection of warty and basaloid high-grade neoplasia of the vulva and cervical neoplasia among immunocompromised women. *Gynecol Oncol* **60**(1):30–4.

166 Palefsky JM (1997). Cutaneous and genital HPV-associated lesions in HIV-infected patients. *Clin Dermatol* **15**(3):439–47.

167 Steenbergen RD, de Wilde J, Wilting SM, *et al.* (2005). HPV-mediated transformation of the anogenital tract. *J Clin Virol* **32**(Suppl 1):S25–33.

168 Stern PL (2005). Immune control of human papillomavirus (HPV) associated anogenital disease and potential for vaccination. *J Clin Virol* **32**(Suppl 1):S72–81.

169 Beckmann AM, Sherman KJ, Myerson D, *et al.* (1991). Comparative virologic studies of condylomata acuminata reveal a lack of dual infections with human papillomaviruses. *J Infect Dis* **163**(2):393–6.

170 von Krogh G, Gross G (1997). Anogenital warts. *Clin Dermatol* **15**(3):355–68.

171 Cobb MW (1990). Human papillomavirus infection. *J Am Acad Dermatol* **22**(4):547–66.

172 de Villiers EM (1994). Human

pathogenic papillomavirus types: an update. *Curr Top Microbiol Immunol* **186**:1–12.

173 Steinberg JL, Cibley LJ, Rice PA (1993). Genital warts: diagnosis, treatment, and counseling for the patient. *Curr Clin Top Infect Dis* **13**:99–122.

174 Martin DH, Mroczkowski TF (1994). Dermatologic manifestations of sexually transmitted diseases other than HIV. *Infect Dis Clin North Am* **8**(3):533–82.

175 Rogozinski TT, Janniger CK (1988). Bowenoid papulosis. *Am Fam Phys* **38**(1):161–4.

176 Park KC, Kim KH, Youn SW, et al. (1998). Heterogeneity of human papillomavirus DNA in a patient with bowenoid papulosis that progressed to squamous cell carcinoma. *Br J Dermatol* **139**(6):1087–91.

177 Porter WM, Francis N, Hawkins D, et al. (2002). Penile intraepithelial neoplasia: clinical spectrum and treatment of 35 cases. *Br J Dermatol* **147**(6):1159–65.

178 Williams GR, Lu QL, Love SB, et al. (1996). Properties of HPV-positive and HPV-negative anal carcinomas. *J Pathol* **180**(4):378–82.

179 Frisch M, Fenger C, van den Brule AJ, et al. (1999). Variants of squamous cell carcinoma of the anal canal and perianal skin and their relation to human papillomaviruses. *Cancer Res* **59**(3):753–7.

180 Daling JR, Madeleine MM, Johnson LG, et al. (2004). Human papillomavirus, smoking, and sexual practices in the etiology of anal cancer. *Cancer* **101**(2):270–80.

181 Daling JR, Madeleine MM, Schwartz SM, et al. (2002). A population-based study of squamous cell vaginal cancer: HPV and cofactors. *Gynecol Oncol* **84**(2):263–70.

182 Rubin MA, Kleter B, Zhou M, et al. (2001). Detection and typing of human papillomavirus DNA in penile carcinoma: evidence for multiple independent pathways of penile carcinogenesis. *Am J Pathol* **159**(4):1211–18.

183 Ferreux E, Lont AP, Horenblas S, et al. (2003). Evidence for at least three alternative mechanisms targeting the p16INK4A/cyclin D/Rb pathway in penile carcinoma, one of which is mediated by high-risk human papillomavirus. *J Pathol* **201**(1):109–18.

184 Pecorelli S, Favalli G, Zigliani L,

Odicino F (2003). Cancer in women. *Int J Gynaecol Obstet* **82**(3):369–79.

185 Dunne EF, Markowitz LE (2006). Genital human papillomavirus infection. *Clin Infect Dis* **43**(5):624–9.

186 van Muyden RC, ter Harmsel BW, Smedts FM, et al. (1999). Detection and typing of human papillomavirus in cervical carcinomas in Russian women: a prognostic study. *Cancer* **85**(9):2011–16.

187 Walboomers JM, Jacobs MV, Manos MM, et al. (1999). Human papillomavirus is a necessary cause of invasive cervical cancer worldwide. *J Pathol* **189**(1):12–19.

188 Munoz N, Bosch FX, de Sanjose S, et al. (2003). Epidemiologic classification of human papillomavirus types associated with cervical cancer. *New Engl J Med* **348**(6):518–27.

189 Zielinski GD, Snijders PJ, Rozendaal L, et al. (2003). The presence of high-risk HPV combined with specific p53 and p16INK4a expression patterns points to high-risk HPV as the main causative agent for adenocarcinoma *in situ* and adenocarcinoma of the cervix. *J Pathol* **201**(4):535–43.

190 McDonald LL, Stites PC, Buntin DM (1997). Sexually transmitted diseases update. *Dermatol Clin* **15**(2):221–32.

191 Moscicki AB, Shiboski S, Hills NK, et al. (2004). Regression of low-grade squamous intraepithelial lesions in young women. *Lancet* **364**(9446):1678–83.

192 Buntin DM (1994). The 1993 sexually transmitted disease treatment guidelines. *Semin Dermatol* **13**(4):269–74.

193 Gross G, Von Krogh G (1997). Therapy of anogenital HPV-induced lesions. *Clin Dermatol* **15**(3):457–70.

194 Petersen CS, Weismann K (1995). Quercetin and kaempherol: an argument against the use of podophyllin? *Genitourinary Med* **71**(2):92–3.

195 Wilson L, Bamburg JR, Mizel SB, et al. (1974). Interaction of drugs with microtubule proteins. *Fed Proc* **33**(2):158–66.

196 Beutner KR (1990). Bridging the gap. Notes of a wart watcher. *Arch Dermatol* **126**(11):1432–5.

197 Snoeck R, Bossens M, Parent D, et al. (2001). Phase II double-blind, placebo-controlled study of the

safety and efficacy of cidofovir topical gel for the treatment of patients with human papillomavirus infection. *Clin Infect Dis* **33**(5):597–602.

198 Garland SM, Sellors JW, Wikstrom A, et al. (2001). Imiquimod 5% cream is a safe and effective self-applied treatment for anogenital warts – results of an open-label, multicentre Phase IIIB trial. *Int J STD AIDS* **12**(11):722–9.

199 Carrasco D, vander Straten M, Tyring SK (2002). Treatment of anogenital warts with imiquimod 5% cream followed by surgical excision of residual lesions. *J Am Acad Dermatol* **47**(4 Suppl):S212–6.

200 Lacey CJ (2005). Therapy for genital human papillomavirus-related disease. *J Clin Virol* **32**(Suppl 1): S82–90.

201 Kreuter A, Hochdorfer B, Stucker M, et al. (2004). Treatment of anal intraepithelial neoplasia in patients with acquired HIV with imiquimod 5% cream. *J Am Acad Dermatol* **50**(6):980–1.

202 Kreuter A, Brockmeyer NH, Weissenborn SJ, et al. (2006). 5% imiquimod suppositories decrease the DNA load of intra-anal HPV types 6 and 11 in HIV-infected men after surgical ablation of condylomata acuminata. *Arch Dermatol* **142**(2):243–4.

203 Myers ER (2006). HPV vaccines: now that they're here, how do we maximize their benefit? *Contraception* **74**(4):277–9.

204 European Cervical Cancer Association Report, April 2009. http://www.ecca.info/fileadmin/user_upload/HPV_Vaccination/ECCA_HPV_Vaccination_April_2009.pdf

205 (No authors listed) (2005). WHO consultation on human papillomavirus vaccines. *Wkly Epidemiol Rec* **80**(35):299–302.

206 Kiviat N, Rompalo A, Bowden R, et al. (1990). Anal human papillomavirus infection among human immunodeficiency virus-seropositive and -seronegative men. *J Infect Dis* **162**(2):358–61.

207 Critchlow CW, Holmes KK, Wood R, et al. (1992). Association of human immunodeficiency virus and anal human papillomavirus infection among homosexual men. *Arch Internal Med* **152**(8):1673-6.

208 Palefsky JM, Shiboski S, Moss A (1994). Risk factors for anal human papillomavirus infection and anal cytologic abnormalities in HIV-

positive and HIV-negative homosexual men. *J Acquir Immune Defic Syndr* **7**(6):599–606.

209 Williams AB, Darragh TM, Vranizan K, *et al.* (1994). Anal and cervical human papillomavirus infection and risk of anal and cervical epithelial abnormalities in human immunodeficiency virus-infected women. *Obstet Gynecol* **83**(2):205–11.

210 Breese PL, Judson FN, Penley KA, Douglas JM Jr. (1995). Anal human papillomavirus infection among homosexual and bisexual men: prevalence of type-specific infection and association with human immunodeficiency virus. *Sex Transmitt Dis* **22**(1):7–14.

211 Aynaud O, Piron D, Barrasso R, Poveda JD (1998). Comparison of clinical, histological, and virological symptoms of HPV in HIV-1 infected men and immunocompetent subjects. *Sex Transmitt Infect* **74**(1):32–4.

212 Vernon SD, Reeves WC, Clancy KA, *et al.* (1994). A longitudinal study of human papillomavirus DNA detection in human immunodeficiency virus type 1-seropositive and -seronegative women. *J Infect Dis* **169**(5):1108–12.

213 Sun XW, Ellerbrock TV, Lungu O, *et al.* (1995). Human papillomavirus infection in human immunodeficiency virus-seropositive women. *Obstet Gynecol* **85**(5 Pt 1):680–6.

214 Chopra KF, Tyring SK (1997). The impact of the human immunodeficiency virus on the human papillomavirus epidemic. *Arch Dermatol* **133**(5):629–33.

215 Arany I, Evans T, Tyring SK (1998). Tissue specific HPV expression and downregulation of local immune responses in condylomas from HIV seropositive individuals. *Sex Transmitt Infect* **74**(5):349–53.

216 Arany I, Tyring SK (1998). Systemic immunosuppression by HIV infection influences HPV transcription and thus local immune responses in condyloma acuminatum. *Int J STD AIDS* **9**(5):268–71.

217 Rabkin CS, Yellin F (1994). Cancer incidence in a population with a high prevalence of infection with human immunodeficiency virus type 1. *J Natl Cancer Inst* **86**(22):1711–16.

218 Castro KG, John W. Ward JW, Slutsker L, *et al.* (1992). 1993 revised classification system for HIV infection and expanded surveillance case definition for AIDS among adolescents and adults. www.cdc.gov **41**(RR-17):1–19. (http://www.cdc.gov/mmwr/preview/mmwrhtml/00018871.htm).

219 Bower M, Palmieri C, Dhillon T (2006). AIDS-related malignancies: changing epidemiology and the impact of highly active antiretroviral therapy. *Curr Opin Infect Dis* **19**(1):14–9.

220 De Panfilis G, Melzani G, Mori G, *et al.* (2002). Relapses after treatment of external genital warts are more frequent in HIV-positive patients than in HIV-negative controls. *Sex Transmitt Dis* **29**(3):121–5.

221 Silverberg MJ, Ahdieh L, Munoz A, *et al.* (2002). The impact of HIV infection and immunodeficiency on human papillomavirus type 6 or 11 infection and on genital warts. *Sex Transmitt Dis* **29**(8):427–35.

222 Xiang Y, Moss B (2001). Correspondence of the functional epitopes of poxvirus and human interleukin-18-binding proteins. *J Virol* **75**(20):9947–54.

223 Agromayor M, Ortiz P, Lopez-Estebaranz JL, *et al.* (2002). Molecular epidemiology of molluscum contagiosum virus and analysis of the host-serum antibody response in Spanish HIV-negative patients. *J Med Virol* **66**(2):151–8.

224 Garvey TL, Bertin J, Siegel RM, *et al.* (2002). Binding of FADD and caspase-8 to molluscum contagiosum virus MC159 v-FLIP is not sufficient for its antiapoptotic function. *J Virol* **76**(2):697–706.

225 Becker TM, Blount JH, Douglas J, Judson FN (1986). Trends in molluscum contagiosum in the United States, 1966–1983. *Sex Transmitt Dis* **13**(2):88–92.

226 Janniger CK, Schwartz RA (1993). Molluscum contagiosum in children. *Cutis* **52**(4):194–6.

227 Vander Straten M, Tyring SK (2002). Mucocutaneous manifestations of viral diseases in children. *Clin Dermatol* **20**(1):67–73.

228 Porter CD, Blake NW, Archard LC, *et al.* (1989). Molluscum contagiosum virus types in genital and non-genital lesions. *Br J Dermatol* **120**(1):37–41.

229 Epstein WL (1992). Molluscum contagiosum. *Semin Dermatol* **11**(3):184–9.

230 Porter CD, Archard LC (1992). Characterisation by restriction mapping of three subtypes of molluscum contagiosum virus. *J Med Virol* **38**(1):1–6.

231 Thompson CH (1998). Immunoreactive proteins of molluscum contagiosum virus types 1, 1v, and 2. *J Infect Dis* **178**(4):1230–1.

232 Yamashita H, Uemura T, Kawashima M (1996). Molecular epidemiologic analysis of Japanese patients with molluscum contagiosum. *Int J Dermatol* **35**(2):99–105.

233 Niizeki K, Kano O, Kondo Y (1984). An epidemic study of molluscum contagiosum. Relationship to swimming. *Dermatologica* **169**(4):197–8.

234 Ghura HS, Camp RD (2001). Scarring molluscum contagiosum in patients with severe atopic dermatitis: report of two cases. *Br J Dermatol* **144**(5):1094–5.

235 Billstein SA, Mattaliano VJ Jr (1990). The 'nuisance' sexually transmitted diseases: molluscum contagiosum, scabies, and crab lice. *Med Clin North Am* **74**(6):1487–505.

236 Brown ST, Nalley JF, Kraus SJ (1981). Molluscum contagiosum. *Sex Transmitt Dis* **8**(3):227–34.

237 Bugert JJ, Darai G (1997). Recent advances in molluscum contagiosum virus research. *Arch Virol Suppl* **13**:35–47.

238 Hawley TG (1970). The natural history of molluscum contagiosum in Fijian children. *J Hyg (Lond)* **68**(4):631–2.

239 Whitaker SB, Wiegand SE, Budnick SD (1991). Intraoral molluscum contagiosum. *Oral Surg Oral Med Oral Pathol* **72**(3):334–6.

240 Ingraham HJ, Schoenleber DB (1998). Epibulbar molluscum contagiosum. *Am J Ophthalmol* **125**(3):394–6.

241 Silverberg NB, Sidbury R, Mancini AJ (2000). Childhood molluscum contagiosum: experience with cantharidin therapy in 300 patients. *J Am Acad Dermatol* **43**(3):503–7.

242 Kipping HF (1971). Molluscum dermatitis. *Arch Dermatol* **103**(1):106–7.

243 Takematsu H, Tagami H (1994). Proinflammatory properties of molluscum bodies. *Arch Dermatol Res* **287**(1):102–6.

244 Ive FA (1985). Follicular molluscum contagiosum. *Br J Dermatol* 113(4):493–5.

245 Brandrup F, Asschenfeldt P (1989). Molluscum contagiosum-induced comedo and secondary abscess formation. *Pediatr Dermatol* 6(2):118–21.

246 Curtin BJ, Theodore FH (1955). Ocular molluscum contagiosum. *Am J Ophthalmol* 39(3):302–7.

247 Ha SJ, Park YM, Cho SH, *et al.* (1998). Solitary giant molluscum contagiosum of the sole. *Pediatr Dermatol* 15(3):222–4.

248 Pandhi D, Singhal A (2005). Giant molluscum contagiosum. *Indian Pediatr* 42(5):488–9.

249 Penneys NS, Matsuo S, Mogollon R (1986). The identification of molluscum infection by immunohistochemical means. *J Cutan Pathol* 13(2):97–101.

250 Thompson CH, Biggs IM, de Zwart-Steffe RT (1990). Detection of molluscum contagiosum virus DNA by *in situ* hybridization. *Pathology* 22(4):181–6.

251 (No authors listed) (1999). National guideline for the management of molluscum contagiosum. Clinical Effectiveness Group (Association of Genitourinary Medicine and the Medical Society for the Study of Venereal Diseases). *Sex Transmitt Infect* 75(Suppl 1):S80–1.

252 Allen AL, Siegfried EC (2001). Management of warts and molluscum in adolescents. *Adolesc Med* 12(2):vi, 229–42.

253 Michel JL (2004). Treatment of molluscum contagiosum with 585 nm collagen remodeling pulsed dye laser. *Eur J Dermatol* 14(2):103–6.

254 Dabis R, Rosbotham J, Jones L, Knowles S, Harland CC (2006). Potassium titanyl phosphate (KTP) laser treatment for molluscum contagiosum. *J Dermatolog Treat* 17(1):45–7.

255 Garrett SJ, Robinson JK, Roenigk HH Jr (1992). Trichloroacetic acid peel of molluscum contagiosum in immunocompromised patients. *J Dermatol Surg Oncol* 18(10):855–8.

256 Longstaff E, von Krogh G (2001). Condyloma eradication: self-therapy with 0.15–0.5% podophyllotoxin versus 20–25% podophyllin preparations – an integrated safety assessment. *Regul Toxicol Pharmacol* 33(2):117–37.

257 von Krogh G, Longstaff E (2001). Podophyllin office therapy against condyloma should be abandoned. *Sex Transmitt Infect* 77(6):409–12.

258 Papa, CM, Berger RS (1976). Venereal herpes-like molluscum contagiosum: treatment with tretinoin. *Cutis* 18(4):537–40.

259 Kono T, Kondo S, Pastore S, *et al.* (1994). Effects of a novel topical immunomodulator, imiquimod, on keratinocyte cytokine gene expression. *Lymphokine Cytokine Res* 13(2):71–6.

260 Testerman TL, Gerster JF, Imbertson LM, *et al.* (1995). Cytokine induction by the immunomodulators imiquimod and S-27609. *J Leukocyt Biol* 58(3):365–72.

261 Buckley R, Smith K (1999). Topical imiquimod therapy for chronic giant molluscum contagiosum in a patient with advanced human immunodeficiency virus 1 disease. *Arch Dermatol* 135(10):1167–9.

262 Brown CW Jr, O'Donoghue M, Moore J, Tharp M (2000). Recalcitrant molluscum contagiosum in an HIV-afflicted male treated successfully with topical imiquimod. *Cutis* 65(6):363–6.

263 Liota E, Smith KJ, Buckley R, *et al.* (2000). Imiquimod therapy for molluscum contagiosum. *J Cut Med Surg* 4(2):76–82.

264 Barba AR, Kapoor S, Berman B (2001). An open label safety study of topical imiquimod 5% cream in the treatment of molluscum contagiosum in children. *Dermatol Online J* 7(1):20.

265 Reichert CM, O'Leary TJ, Levens DL, *et al.* (1983). Autopsy pathology in the acquired immune deficiency syndrome. *Am J Pathol* 112(3):357–82.

266 Matis WL, Triana A, Shapiro R, *et al.* (1987). Dermatologic findings associated with human immunodeficiency virus infection. *J Am Acad Dermatol* 17(5 Pt 1):746–51.

267 Hira SK, Wadhawan D, Kamanga J, *et al.* (1988). Cutaneous manifestations of human immunodeficiency virus in Lusaka, Zambia. *J Am Acad Dermatol* 19(3):451–7.

268 Coldiron BM, Bergstresser PR (1989). Prevalence and clinical spectrum of skin disease in patients infected with human immunodeficiency virus. *Arch Dermatol* 125(3):357–61.

269 Koopman RJ, van Merrienboer FC, Vreden SG, Dolmans WM (1992). Molluscum contagiosum; a marker for advanced HIV infection. *Br J Dermatol* 126(5):528–9.

270 Reynaud-Mendel B, Janier M, Gerbaka J, *et al.* (1996). Dermatologic findings in HIV-1-infected patients: a prospective study with emphasis on CD4+ cell count. *Dermatology* 192(4):325–8.

271 Schaub N, Gilli L, Rufli T, *et al.* (1996). Epidemiology of skin diseases in HIV-infected patients: a prospective cohort study. *Schweiz Rundsch Med Prax* 85(38):1162–6.

272 Husak R, Garbe C, Orfanos CE (1997). Mollusca contagiosa in HIV infection. Clinical manifestation, relation to immune status and prognostic value in 39 patients. *Der Hautarzt*; *Zeitschrift Derm Venerol Gebiete* 48(2):103–9.

273 Mahe A, Bobin P, Coulibaly S, Tounkara A (1997). Skin diseases disclosing human immunodeficiency virus infection in Mali. *Ann Dermatol Venereol* 124(2):144–50.

274 Munoz-Perez MA, Rodriguez-Pichardo A, Camacho F, Colmenero MA (1998). Dermatological findings correlated with CD4 lymphocyte counts in a prospective 3 year study of 1161 patients with human immunodeficiency virus disease predominantly acquired through intravenous drug abuse. *Br J Dermatol* 139(1):33–9.

275 Jung AC, Paauw DS (1998). Diagnosing HIV-related disease: using the CD4 count as a guide. *J Gen Intern Med* 13(2):131–6.

276 Konya J, Thompson CH (1999). Molluscum contagiosum virus: antibody responses in persons with clinical lesions and seroepidemiology in a representative Australian population. *J Infect Dis* 179(3):701–4.

277 Ficarra G, Cortes S, Rubino I, Romagnoli P (1994). Facial and perioral molluscum contagiosum in patients with HIV infection. A report of eight cases. *Oral Surg Oral Med Oral Pathol* 78(5):621–6.

278 Thompson CH, de Zwart-Steffe RT, Donovan B (1992). Clinical and molecular aspects of molluscum contagiosum infection in HIV-1 positive patients. *Int J STD AIDS* 3(2):101–6.

279 Schwartz JJ, Myskowski PL (1992b). Molluscum contagiosum in patients with human immunodeficiency virus infection. A review of twenty-seven patients. *J*

Am Acad Dermatol **27**(4):583–8.

280 Redfield RR, James WD, Wright DC, *et al.* (1985). Severe molluscum contagiosum infection in a patient with human T cell lymphotrophic (HTLV-III) disease. *J Am Acad Dermatol* **13**(5 Pt 1):821–4.

281 Betlloch I, Pinazo I, Mestre F, *et al.* (1989). Molluscum contagiosum in human immunodeficiency virus infection: response to zidovudine. *Int J Dermatol* **28**(5):351–2.

282 Biswas J, Therese L, Kumarasamy N, *et al.* (1997). Lid abscess with extensive molluscum contagiosum in a patient with acquired immunodeficiency syndrome. *Indian J Ophthalmol* **45**(4):234–6.

283 Leahey AB, Shane JJ, Listhaus A, Trachtman M (1997). Molluscum contagiosum eyelid lesions as the initial manifestation of acquired immunodeficiency syndrome. *Am J Ophthalmol* **124**(2):240–1.

284 Gottlieb SL, Myskowski PL (1994). Molluscum contagiosum. *Int J Dermatol* **33**(7):453–61.

285 Felman YM (1984). Molluscum contagiosum. *Cutis* **33**(1):113–14, 117.

286 Fivenson DP, Weltman RE, Gibson SH (1988). Giant molluscum contagiosum presenting as basal cell carcinoma in an acquired immunodeficiency syndrome patient. *J Am Acad Dermatol* **19**(5 Pt 1):912–14.

287 Cockerell CJ (1990). Cutaneous manifestations of HIV infection other than Kaposi's sarcoma: clinical and histologic aspects. *J Am Acad Dermatol* **22**(6 Pt 2):1260–9.

288 Schwartz JJ, Myskowski PL (1992). HIV-related molluscum contagiosum presenting as a cutaneous horn. *Int J Dermatol* **31**(2):142–4.

289 Itin PH, Gilli L (1994). Molluscum contagiosum mimicking sebaceous nevus of Jadassohn, ecthyma and giant condylomata acuminata in HIV-infected patients. *Dermatology* **189**(4):396–8.

290 Feuilhade de Chauvin M, Revuz J, Deniau M (1983). Histoplasma duboisii histoplasmosis. Skin lesions simulating molluscum contagiosum. *Ann Dermatol Venereol* **110**(9):715–16.

291 Rico MJ, Penneys NS (1985). Cutaneous cryptococcosis resembling molluscum contagiosum in a patient with AIDS. *Arch Dermatol* **121**(7):901–2.

292 Concus AP, Helfand RF, Imber MJ, *et al.* (1988). Cutaneous cryptococcosis mimicking molluscum contagiosum in a patient with AIDS. *J Infect Dis* **158**(4):897–8.

293 Cavicchini S, Brezzi A, Alessi E (1993). Ultrastructural findings in mucocutaneous infections of patients seropositive to HIV. *Am J Dermatopathol* **15**(4):320–5.

294 Smith KJ, Skelton HG 3rd, Yeager J, *et al.* (1992). Molluscum contagiosum. Ultrastructural evidence for its presence in skin adjacent to clinical lesions in patients infected with human immunodeficiency virus type 1. Military Medical Consortium for Applied Retroviral Research. *Arch Dermatol* **128**(2):223–7.

295 Birthistle K, Carrington D (1997). Molluscum contagiosum virus. *J Infect* **34**(1):21–8.

296 Cronin TA Jr, Resnik BI, Elgart G, Kerdel FA (1996). Recalcitrant giant molluscum contagiosum in a patient with AIDS. *J Am Acad Dermatol* **35**(2 Pt 1):266–7.

297 de Waard-van der Spek FB, Oranje AP, Lillieborg S, *et al.* (1990). Treatment of molluscum contagiosum using a lidocaine/prilocaine cream (EMLA) for analgesia. *J Am Acad Dermatol* **23**(4 Pt 1):685–8.

298 Mayumi M, Yamaoka K, Tsutsui T, *et al.* (1986). Selective immunoglobulin M deficiency associated with disseminated molluscum contagiosum. *Eur J Pediatr* **145**(1-2):99–103.

299 Nelson MR, Chard S, Barton SE (1995). Intralesional interferon for the treatment of recalcitrant molluscum contagiosum in HIV antibody positive individuals—a preliminary report. *Int J STD AIDS* **6**(5):351–2.

300 Strauss RM, Doyle EL, Mohsen AH, Green ST (2001). Successful treatment of molluscum contagiosum with topical imiquimod in a severely immunocompromised HIV-positive patient. *Int J STD AIDS* **12**(4):264–6.

301 Nehal KS, Sarnoff DS, Gotkin RH, Friedman-Kien A (1998). Pulsed dye laser treatment of molluscum contagiosum in a patient with acquired immunodeficiency syndrome. *Dermatol Surg* **24**(5): 533–5.

302 Yoshinaga IG, Conrado LA, Schainberg SC, Grinblat M (2000). Recalcitrant molluscum contagiosum in a patient with AIDS: combined treatment with CO(2) laser, trichloroacetic acid, and pulsed dye laser. *Lasers Surg Med* **27**(4):291–4.

303 Calista D (2000). Topical cidofovir for severe cutaneous human papillomavirus and molluscum contagiosum infections in patients with HIV/AIDS. A pilot study. *JEADV* **14**(6):484–8.

304 Baxter KF, Highet AS (2004). Topical cidofovir and cryotherapy—combination treatment for recalcitrant molluscum contagiosum in a patient with HIV infection. *J Eur Acad Dermatol Venereol* **18**(2):230–1.

305 Matteelli A, Beltrame A, Graifemberghi S, *et al.* (2001). Efficacy and tolerability of topical 1% cidofovir cream for the treatment of external anogenital warts in HIV-infected persons. *Sex Transmitt Dis* **28**(6):343–6.

306 Hicks CB, Myers SA, Giner J (1997). Resolution of intractable molluscum contagiosum in a human immunodeficiency virus-infected patient after institution of antiretroviral therapy with ritonavir. *Clin Infect Dis* **24**(5):1023–5.

307 Horn CK, Scott GR, Benton EC (1998). Resolution of severe molluscum contagiosum on effective antiretroviral therapy. *Br J Dermatol* **138**(4):715–17.

308 Zancanaro PC, McGirt LY, Mamelak AJ, *et al.* (2006). Cutaneous manifestations of HIV in the era of highly active antiretroviral therapy: an institutional urban clinic experience. *J Am Acad Dermatol* **54**(4):581–8.

309 Chang Y, Cesarman E, Pessin MS, *et al.* (1994). Identification of herpesvirus-like DNA sequences in AIDS-associated Kaposi's sarcoma. *Science* **266**(5192):1865–9.

310 Ansari MQ, Dawson DB, Nador R, *et al.* (1996). Primary body cavity-based AIDS-related lymphomas. *Am J Clin Pathol* **105**(2):221–9.

311 Soulier J, Grollet L, Oksenhendler E, *et al.* (1995). Kaposi's sarcoma-associated herpesvirus-like DNA sequences in multicentric Castleman's disease. *Blood* **86**(4):1276–80.

312 Corbellino M, Poirel L, Aubin JT, *et al.* (1996). The role of human herpesvirus 8 and Epstein–Barr virus in the pathogenesis of giant lymph node hyperplasia (Castleman's disease). *Clin Infect*

Dis **22**(6):1120–1.

313 Walker GJ, Johnstone PW (2000). Interventions for treating scabies. *Cochrane Database Syst Rev*(3):CD000320.

314 Landwehr D, Keita SM, Ponnighaus JM, Tounkara C (1998). Epidemiologic aspects of scabies in Mali, Malawi, and Cambodia. *Int J Dermatol* **37**(8):588–90.

315 Christophersen J (1978). The epidemiology of scabies in Denmark, 1900 to 1975. *Arch Dermatol* **114**(5):747–50.

316 Church RE, Knowelden J (1978). Scabies in Sheffield: a family infestation. *Br Med J* **1**(6115):761–3.

317 Bukh J, Miller RH, Purcell RH (1995). Genetic heterogeneity of hepatitis C virus: quasispecies and genotypes. *Semin Liver Dis* **15**(1):41–63.

318 Choo L, Kuo G, Weiner AJ, *et al.* (1989). Isolation of a cDNA clone derived from a blood-borne non-A, non-B viral hepatitis genome. *Science* **244**(4902):359–62.

319 Shepard CW, Finelli L, Alter MJ (2005). Global epidemiology of hepatitis C virus infection. *Lancet Infect Dis* **5**(9):558–67.

320 Armstrong GL, Wasley A, Simard EP, *et al.* (2006). The prevalence of hepatitis C virus infection in the United States, 1999 through 2002. *Ann Internal Med* **144**(10):705–14.

321 Terrault NA (2002). Sexual activity as a risk factor for hepatitis C. *Hepatology* **36**(5 Suppl 1):S99–105.

322 Vandelli C, Renzo F, Romano L, *et al.* (2004). Lack of evidence of sexual transmission of hepatitis C among monogamous couples: results of a 10-year prospective follow-up study. *Am J Gastroenterol* **99**(5):855–9.

323 Kane A, Lloyd J, Zaffran M, *et al.* (1999). Transmission of hepatitis B, hepatitis C and human immunodeficiency viruses through unsafe injections in the developing world: model-based regional estimates. *Bull World Health Organ* **77**(10):801–7.

324 Hauri AM, Armstrong GL, Hutin YJ (2004). The global burden of disease attributable to contaminated injections given in health care settings. *Int J STD AIDS* **15**(1):7–16.

325 Kiyosawa K, Sodeyama T, Tanaka E, *et al.* (1991). Hepatitis C in hospital employees with needlestick injuries. *Ann Internal Med* **115**(5):367–9.

326 Mitsui T, Iwano K, Masuko K, *et al.* (1992). Hepatitis C virus infection in medical personnel after needlestick accident. *Hepatology* **16**(5):1109–14.

327 Alter HJ, Purcell RH, Shih JW, *et al.* (1989). Detection of antibody to hepatitis C virus in prospectively followed transfusion recipients with acute and chronic non-A, non-B hepatitis. *N Engl J Med* **321**(22):1494–500.

328 Aach RD, Stevens CE, Hollinger FB, *et al.* (1991). Hepatitis C virus infection in post-transfusion hepatitis. An analysis with first- and second-generation assays. *N Engl J Med* **325**(19):1325–9.

329 Koretz RL, Abbey H, Coleman E, Gitnick G (1993). Non-A, non-B post-transfusion hepatitis. Looking back in the second decade. *Ann Internal Med* **119**(2):110–15.

330 (No authors listed) (1998). Recommendations for prevention and control of hepatitis C virus (HCV) infection and HCV-related chronic disease. *Centers for Disease Control and Prevention* **47**(RR-19):1–39.

331 Esteban JI, Lopez-Talavera JC, Genesca J, *et al.* (1991). High rate of infectivity and liver disease in blood donors with antibodies to hepatitis C virus. *Ann Internal Med* **115**(6):443–9.

332 Seeff LB, Buskell-Bales Z, Wright EC, *et al.* (1992). Long-term mortality after transfusion-associated non-A, non-B hepatitis. The National Heart, Lung, and Blood Institute Study Group. *N Engl J Med* **327**(27):1906–11.

333 Shakil AO, Conry-Cantilena C, Alter HJ, *et al.* (1995). Volunteer blood donors with antibody to hepatitis C virus: clinical, biochemical, virologic, and histologic features. The Hepatitis C Study Group. *Ann Internal Med* **123**(5):330–7.

334 Liang TJ, Jeffers L, Reddy RK, *et al.* (1993). Fulminant or subfulminant non-A, non-B viral hepatitis: the role of hepatitis C and E viruses. *Gastroenterology* **104**(2):556–62.

335 Wright TL (1993). Etiology of fulminant hepatic failure: is another virus involved? *Gastroenterology* **104**(2):640–3.

336 Alter MJ, Margolis HS, Krawczynski K, *et al.* (1992). The natural history of community-acquired hepatitis C in the United States. The Sentinel Counties Chronic non-A, non-B Hepatitis Study Team. *N Engl J Med* **327**(27):1899–905.

337 Benvegnu, L, Fattovich G, Noventa F, *et al.* (1994). Concurrent hepatitis B and C virus infection and risk of hepatocellular carcinoma in cirrhosis. A prospective study. *Cancer* **74**(9):2442–8.

338 Thomas DL, Shih JW, Alter HJ, *et al.* (1996). Effect of human immunodeficiency virus on hepatitis C virus infection among injecting drug users. *J Infect Dis* **174**(4):690–5.

339 Schiff ER (1997). Hepatitis C and alcohol. *Hepatology* **26**(3 Suppl 1):39S–42S.

340 Collier J, Heathcote J (1998). Hepatitis C viral infection in the immunosuppressed patient. *Hepatology* **27**(1):2–6.

341 Corrao G, Arico S (1998). Independent and combined action of hepatitis C virus infection and alcohol consumption on the risk of symptomatic liver cirrhosis. *Hepatology* **27**(4):914–19.

342 Seeff LB (2002). Natural history of chronic hepatitis C. *Hepatology* **36**(5 Suppl 1):S35–46.

343 Kenny-Walsh E (1999). Clinical outcomes after hepatitis C infection from contaminated anti-D immune globulin. Irish Hepatology Research Group. *N Engl J Med* **340**(16):1228–33.

344 Blackard JT, Kemmer N, Sherman KE (2006). Extrahepatic replication of HCV: insights into clinical manifestations and biological consequences. *Hepatology* **44**(1):15–22.

345 Cacoub P, Poynard T, Ghillani P, *et al.* (1999). Extrahepatic manifestations of chronic hepatitis C. MULTIVIRC Group. Multidepartment Virus C. *Arthritis Rheum* **42**(10):2204–12.

346 Korkij W, Chuang TY, Soltani K (1984). Liver abnormalities in patients with lichen planus. A retrospective case-control study. *J Am Acad Dermatol* **11**(4 Pt 1):609–15.

347 Mobacken, H, Nilsson LA, Olsson R, Sloberg K (1984). Incidence of liver disease in chronic lichen planus of the mouth. *Acta Derm Venereol* **64**(1):70–3.

348 Rebora A, Rongioletti F (1984). Lichen planus and chronic active hepatitis. *J Am Acad Dermatol* **10**(5 Pt 1):840–1.

349 Katz M, Pisanti S (1985). Oral erosive lichen planus and chronic active hepatitis. *J Am Acad Dermatol* **12**(4):719.

350 Monk B (1985). Lichen planus and the liver. *J Am Acad Dermatol* **12**(1 Pt 1):122–4.

351 Rebora A (1992). Lichen planus and the liver. *Int J Dermatol* **31**(6):392–5.

352 Cribier B, C Garnier, D Laustriat, E Heid (1994). Lichen planus and hepatitis C virus infection: an epidemiologic study. *J Am Acad Dermatol* **31**(6):1070–2.

353 Dupin N, Chosidow O, Lunel F, Fretz C, Szpirglas H, Frances C (1997). Oral lichen planus and hepatitis C virus infection: a fortuitous association? *Arch Dermatol* **133**(8):1052–3.

354 Nagao Y, Sata M, Tanikawa K, *et al.* (1995). Lichen planus and hepatitis C virus in the northern Kyushu region of Japan. *Eur J Clin Invest* **25**(12):910–14.

355 Bellman B, Reddy RK, Falanga V (1995). Lichen planus associated with hepatitis C. *Lancet* **346**(8984):1234.

356 Imhof M, Popal H, Lee JH, *et al.* (1997). Prevalence of hepatitis C virus antibodies and evaluation of hepatitis C virus genotypes in patients with lichen planus. *Dermatology* **195**(1):1–5.

357 Cribier B, Samain F, Vetter D, *et al.* (1998). Systematic cutaneous examination in hepatitis C virus infected patients. *Acta Derm Venereol* **78**(5):355–7.

358 Fargion S, Piperno A, Cappellini MD, *et al.* (1992). Hepatitis C virus and porphyria cutanea tarda: evidence of a strong association. *Hepatology* **16**(6):1322–6.

359 DeCastro M, Sanchez J, Herrera JF, *et al.* (1993). Hepatitis C virus antibodies and liver disease in patients with porphyria cutanea tarda. *Hepatology* **17**(4):551–7.

360 Ferri C, Baicchi U, la Civita L, *et al.* (1993). Hepatitis C virus-related autoimmunity in patients with porphyria cutanea tarda. *Eur J Clin Invest* **23**(12):851–5.

361 Herrero C, Vicente A, Bruguera M, *et al.* (1993). Is hepatitis C virus infection a trigger of porphyria cutanea tarda? *Lancet* **341**(8848):788–9.

362 Lacour JP, Bodokh I, Castanet J, *et al.* (1993). Porphyria cutanea tarda and antibodies to hepatitis C virus. *Br J Dermatol* **128**(2):121–3.

363 Koester G, Feldman J, Bigler C (1994). Hepatitis C in patients with porphyria cutanea tarda. *J Am Acad Dermatol* **31**(6):1054.

364 Pawlotsky JM, Dhumeaux D, Bagot M (1995). Hepatitis C virus in dermatology. A review. *Arch Dermatol* **131**(10):1185–93.

365 Hadziyannis SJ (1996). Nonhepatic manifestations and combined diseases in HCV infection. *Dig Dis Sci* **41**(12 Suppl):63S–74S.

366 Agnello V, Chung RT, Kaplan LM (1992). A role for hepatitis C virus infection in type II cryoglobulinemia. *N Engl J Med* **327**(21):1490–5.

367 Cacoub P, Fabiani FL, Musset L, *et al.* (1994). Mixed cryoglobulinemia and hepatitis C virus. *Am J Med* **96**(2):124–32.

368 Levey JM, Bjornsson B, Banner B, *et al.* (1994). Mixed cryoglobulinemia in chronic hepatitis C infection. A clinicopathologic analysis of 10 cases and review of recent literature. *Medicine (Baltimore)* **73**(1):53–67.

369 Ferri C, Sebastiani M, Giuggioli D, *et al.* (2004). Mixed cryoglobulinemia: demographic, clinical, and serologic features and survival in 231 patients. *Semin Arthritis Rheum* **33**(6):355–74.

370 Cacoub P, Saadoun D, Limal N, Sene D, Lidove O, Piette JC (2005). PEGylated interferon alfa-2b and ribavirin treatment in patients with hepatitis C virus-related systemic vasculitis. *Arthritis Rheum* **52**(3):911–15.

371 Alter MJ, Evatt BL, Margolis HS, *et al.* (1991). Public Health Service interagency guidelines for screening donors of blood, plasma, organs, tissues, and semen for evidence of hepatitis B and hepatitis C. *www.cdc.gov* **40**(RR-4):1–17. (http://www.cdc.gov/mmwr/preview/mmwrhtml/00043883.htm)

372 Kleinman S, Alter H, Busch M, *et al.* (1992). Increased detection of hepatitis C virus (HCV)-infected blood donors by a multiple-antigen HCV enzyme immunoassay. *Transfusion* **32**(9):805–13.

373 Alter MJ, Kuhnert WL, Finelli L (2003). Guidelines for laboratory testing and result reporting of antibody to hepatitis C virus. *Centers for Disease Control and Prevention* **52**(RR-3):1–13, 15; quiz CE1–4.

374 (No authors listed) (1997). National Institutes of Health Consensus Development Conference Panel statement: management of hepatitis C. *Hepatology* **26**(3 Suppl 1):2S–10S.

375 Schvarcz R, Yun ZB, Sonnerborg A, Weiland O (1995). Combined treatment with interferon alpha-2b and ribavirin for chronic hepatitis C in patients with a previous nonresponse or nonsustained response to interferon alone. *J Med Virol* **46**(1):43–7.

376 Schalm SW, Brouwer JT, Chemello L, *et al.* (1996). Interferon-ribavirin combination therapy for chronic hepatitis C. *Dig Dis Sci* **41**(12 Suppl):131S–34S.

377 Puoti M, Spinetti A, Ghezzi A, *et al.* (2000). Mortality for liver disease in patients with HIV infection: a cohort study. *J Acquir Immune Defic Syndr* **24**(3):211–17.

378 Tedder RS, Gilson RJ, Briggs M, *et al.* (1991). Hepatitis C virus: evidence for sexual transmission. *BMJ* **302**(6788):1299–302.

379 Pasquier C, Bujan L, Daudin M, *et al.* (2003). Intermittent detection of hepatitis C virus (HCV) in semen from men with human immunodeficiency virus type 1 (HIV-1) and HCV. *J Med Virol* **69**(3):344–9.

380 Greub G, Ledergerber B, Battegay M, *et al.* (2000). Clinical progression, survival, and immune recovery during antiretroviral therapy in patients with HIV-1 and hepatitis C virus coinfection: the Swiss HIV Cohort Study. *Lancet* **356**(9244):1800–5.

381 Chung RT, Evans SR, Yang Y, *et al.* (2002). Immune recovery is associated with persistent rise in hepatitis C virus RNA, infrequent liver test flares, and is not impaired by hepatitis C virus in co-infected subjects. *AIDS* **16**(14):1915–23.

382 De Luca A, Bugarini R, Lepri AC, *et al.* (2002). Coinfection with hepatitis viruses and outcome of initial antiretroviral regimens in previously naive HIV-infected subjects. *Arch Internal Med* **162**(18):2125–32.

383 Sulkowski MS, Moore RD, Mehta SH, *et al.* (2002). Hepatitis C and progression of HIV disease. *JAMA* **288**(2):199–206.

384 Soto B, Sanchez-Quijano A, Rodrigo L, *et al.* (1997). Human immunodeficiency virus infection

modifies the natural history of chronic parenterally-acquired hepatitis C with an unusually rapid progression to cirrhosis. *J Hepatol* **26**(1):1–5.

385 Benhamou Y, Bochet M, Di Martino V, *et al.* (1999). Liver fibrosis progression in human immunodeficiency virus and hepatitis C virus coinfected patients. The Multivirc Group. *Hepatology* **30**(4):1054–8.

386 Lesens O, Deschenes M, Steben M, *et al.* (1999). Hepatitis C virus is related to progressive liver disease in human immunodeficiency virus-positive hemophiliacs and should be treated as an opportunistic infection. *J Infect Dis* **179**(5):1254–8.

387 Martin-Carbonero L, Benhamou Y, Puoti M, *et al.* (2004). Incidence and predictors of severe liver fibrosis in human immunodeficiency virus-infected patients with chronic hepatitis C: a European collaborative study. *Clin Infect Dis* **38**(1):128–33.

388 Soriano V, Garcia-Samaniego J, Bravo R, *et al.* (1996). Interferon alpha for the treatment of chronic hepatitis C in patients infected with human immunodeficiency virus. Hepatitis-HIV Spanish Study Group. *Clin Infect Dis* **23**(3):585–91.

389 Mauss S, Klinker H, Ulmer A, *et al.* (1998). Response to treatment of chronic hepatitis C with interferon alpha in patients infected with HIV-1 is associated with higher CD4+ cell count. *Infection* **26**(1):16–19.

390 Dane DS, Cameron CH, Briggs M (1970). Virus-like particles in serum of patients with Australia-antigen-associated hepatitis. *Lancet* **1**(7649):695–8.

391 Ganem D (1991). Assembly of hepadnaviral virions and subviral particles. *Curr Top Microbiol Immunol* **168**:61–83.

392 Allain JP (2006). Epidemiology of Hepatitis B virus and genotype. *J Clin Virol* **36**(Suppl 1): S12–7.

393 (No authors listed) (1991). Hepatitis B virus: a comprehensive strategy for eliminating transmission in the United States through universal childhood vaccination. Recommendations of the Immunization Practices Advisory Committee (ACIP). www.cdc.gov/19 **40**(RR-13):1–25. (http://www.cdc.gov/mmwr/preview/ mmwrhtml/00033405.htm)

394 West DJ, Margolis HS (1992). Prevention of hepatitis B virus

infection in the United States: a pediatric perspective. *Pediatr Infect Dis J* **11**(10):866–74.

395 (No authors listed) (2004). National, state, and urban area vaccination coverage among children aged 19–35 months – United States, 2003. *MMWR* **53**(29):658–61.

396 (No authors listed) (2004). Incidence of acute hepatitis B – United States, 1990–2002. *MMWR* **52**(51-52):1252–4.

397 Alter MJ, Ahtone J, Weisfuse I, *et al.* (1986). Hepatitis B virus transmission between heterosexuals. *JAMA* **256**(10):1307–10.

398 Alter MJ, Coleman PJ, Alexander WJ, *et al.* (1989). Importance of heterosexual activity in the transmission of hepatitis B and non-A, non-B hepatitis. *JAMA* **262**(9):1201–5.

399 Kingsley LA, Rinaldo CR Jr, Lyter DW, *et al.* (1990). Sexual transmission efficiency of hepatitis B virus and human immunodeficiency virus among homosexual men. *JAMA* **264**(2):230–4.

400 Rosenblum L, Darrow W, Witte J, *et al.* (1992). Sexual practices in the transmission of hepatitis B virus and prevalence of hepatitis delta virus infection in female prostitutes in the United States. *JAMA* **267**(18):2477–81.

401 de Franchis R, Meucci G, Vecchi M, *et al.* (1993). The natural history of asymptomatic hepatitis B surface antigen carriers. *Ann Internal Med* **118**(3):191–4.

402 Stevens CE, Beasley RP, Tsui J, Lee WC (1975). Vertical transmission of hepatitis B antigen in Taiwan. *N Engl J Med* **292**(15):771–4.

403 Chisari FV, Ferrari C (1995). Hepatitis B virus immunopathogenesis. *Annu Rev Immunol* **13**:29–60.

404 Sarkany I (1988). The skin–liver connection. *Clin Exp Dermatol* **13**(3):151–9.

405 Ganem D, Prince AM (2004). Hepatitis B virus infection – natural history and clinical consequences. *N Engl J Med* **350**(11):1118–29.

406 Baron JL, Gardiner L, Nishimura S, *et al.* (2002). Activation of a nonclassical NKT cell subset in a transgenic mouse model of hepatitis B virus infection. *Immunity* **16**(4):583–94.

407 Weiss TD, Tsai CC, Baldassare AR, Zuckner J (1978). Skin lesions in viral hepatitis: histologic and immunofluorescent findings. *Am J*

Med **64**(2):269–73.

408 Dienstag JL, Rhodes AR, Bhan AK, *et al.* (1978). Urticaria associated with acute viral hepatitis type B: studies of pathogenesis. *Ann Internal Med* **89**(1):34–40.

409 Popp JW Jr, Harrist TJ, Dienstag JL, *et al.* (1981). Cutaneous vasculitis associated with acute and chronic hepatitis. *Arch Internal Med* **141**(5):623–9.

410 Parsons ME, Russo GG, Millikan LE (1996). Dermatologic disorders associated with viral hepatitis infections. *Int J Dermatol* **35**(2):77–81.

411 Gocke DJ, Hsu K, Morgan C, *et al.* (1970). Association between polyarteritis and Australia antigen. *Lancet* **2**(7684):1149–53.

412 Trepo CG, Zucherman AJ, Bird RC, Prince AM (1974). The role of circulating hepatitis B antigen/antibody immune complexes in the pathogenesis of vascular and hepatic manifestations in polyarteritis nodosa. *J Clin Pathol* **27**(11):863–8.

413 Chan G, Kowdley KV (1995). Extrahepatic manifestations of chronic viral hepatitis. *Compr Therap* **21**(4):200–5.

414 Losowsky MS (1980). The clinical course of viral hepatitis. *Clin Gastroenterol* **9**(1):3–21.

415 Levo Y, Gorevic PD, Kassab HJ, *et al.* (1977). Association between hepatitis B virus and essential mixed cryoglobulinemia. *N Engl J Med* **296**(26):1501–4.

416 Heim LR (1979). Cryoglobulins: characterization and classification. *Cutis* **23**(3):259–66.

417 McElgunn PS (1983). Dermatologic manifestations of hepatitis B virus infection. *J Am Acad Dermatol* **8**(4):539–48.

418 Maggiore G, Grifeo S, Marzani MD (1983). Erythema nodosum and hepatitis B virus (HBV) infection. *J Am Acad Dermatol* **9**(4):602–3.

419 Rebora A, Rongioletti F (1984). Lichen planus and chronic active hepatitis. A retrospective survey. *Acta Derm Venereol* **64**(1):52–6.

420 Divano MC, Parodi A, Rebora A (1992). Lichen planus, liver kidney microsomal (LKM1) antibodies and hepatitis C virus antibodies. *Dermatology* **185**(2):132–3.

421 Gower RG, Sausker WF, Kohler PF, *et al.* (1978). Small vessel vasculitis caused by hepatitis B virus immune complexes. Small vessel vasculitis and HBsAG. *J Allergy Clin*

Immunol 62(4):222–8.

422 Green LK, Hebert AA, Jorizzo JL, *et al.* (1985). Pyoderma gangrenosum and chronic persistent hepatitis. *J Am Acad Dermatol* 13(5 Pt 2):892–7.

423 Pittsley RA, Shearn MA, Kaufman L (1978). Acute hepatitis B simulating dermatomyositis. *JAMA* 239(10):959.

424 Colombo M, Rumi MG, Sagnelli E, *et al.* (1986). Acute hepatitis B in children with papular acrodermatitis. *Pediatr Pathol* 6(2-3):249–57.

425 Hoofnagle JH (1981). Serologic markers of hepatitis B virus infection. *Annu Rev Med* 32:1–11.

426 Wright TL, Lau JY (1993). Clinical aspects of hepatitis B virus infection. *Lancet* 342(8883):1340–4.

427 Kajino K, Jilbert AR, Saputelli J, *et al.* (1994). Woodchuck hepatitis virus infections: very rapid recovery after a prolonged viremia and infection of virtually every hepatocyte. *J Virol* 68(9):5792–803.

428 Koff RS, Slavin MM, Connelly JD, Rosen DR (1977). Contagiousness of acute hepatitis B. Secondary attack rates in household contacts. *Gastroenterology* 72(2):297–300.

429 Weinberger KM, Wiedenmann E, Bohm S, Jilg W (2000). Sensitive and accurate quantitation of hepatitis B virus DNA using a kinetic fluorescence detection system (TaqMan PCR). *J Virol Methods* 85(1–2):75–82.

430 Tedder RS, Ijaz S, Gilbert N, *et al.* (2002). Evidence for a dynamic host-parasite relationship in e-negative hepatitis B carriers. *J Med Virol* 68(4):505–12.

431 Beasley RP (1988). Hepatitis B virus. The major etiology of hepatocellular carcinoma. *Cancer* 61(10):1942–56.

432 Yang HI, Lu SN, Liaw YF, *et al.* (2002). Hepatitis B e antigen and the risk of hepatocellular carcinoma. *N Engl J Med* 347(3):168–74.

433 Matsubara K, Tokino T (1990). Integration of hepatitis B virus DNA and its implications for hepatocarcinogenesis. *Mol Biol Med* 7(3):243–60.

434 Kim CM, Koike K, Saito I, *et al.* (1991). HBx gene of hepatitis B virus induces liver cancer in transgenic mice. *Nature* 351(6324):317–20.

435 Lauer U, Weiss L, Hofschneider PH, *et al.* (1992). The hepatitis B virus pre-S/S(t) transactivator is generated by 3' truncations within a defined region of the S gene. *J Virol* 66(9):5284–9.

436 Wong DK, Cheung AM, O'Rourke K, *et al.* (1993). Effect of alpha-interferon treatment in patients with hepatitis B e antigen-positive chronic hepatitis B. A meta-analysis. *Ann Internal Med* 119(4):312–23.

437 Dienstag JL, Schiff ER, Wright TL, *et al.* (1999). Lamivudine as initial treatment for chronic hepatitis B in the United States. *N Engl J Med* 341(17):1256–63.

438 Puoti M, Airoldi M, Bruno R, *et al.* (2002). Hepatitis B virus co-infection in human immunodeficiency virus-infected subjects. *AIDS Rev* 4(1):27–35.

439 Villeneuve JP, Condreay LD, Willems B, *et al.* (2000). Lamivudine treatment for decompensated cirrhosis resulting from chronic hepatitis B. *Hepatology* 31(1):207–10.

440 Perrillo R, Schiff E, Yoshida E, *et al.* (2000). Adefovir dipivoxil for the treatment of lamivudine-resistant hepatitis B mutants. *Hepatology* 32(1):129–34.

441 Ying C, De Clercq E, Nicholson W, *et al.* (2000). Inhibition of the replication of the DNA polymerase M550V mutation variant of human hepatitis B virus by adefovir, tenofovir, L-FMAU, DAPD, penciclovir and lobucavir. *J Viral Hepat* 7(2):161–5.

442 Ristig MB, Crippin J, Aberg JA, *et al.* (2002). Tenofovir disoproxil fumarate therapy for chronic hepatitis B in human immunodeficiency virus/hepatitis B virus-coinfected individuals for whom interferon-alpha and lamivudine therapy have failed. *J Infect Dis* 186(12):1844–7.

443 Nelson M, Portsmouth S, Stebbing J, *et al.* (2003). An open-label study of tenofovir in HIV-1 and Hepatitis B virus co-infected individuals. *AIDS* 17(1):F7–10.

444 Alter MJ (2006). Epidemiology of viral hepatitis and HIV coinfection. *J Hepatol* 44(1 Suppl):S6–9.

445 Denis F, Adjide CC, Rogez S, *et al.* (1997). Seroprevalence of HBV, HCV and HDV hepatitis markers in 500 patients infected with the human immunodeficiency virus. *Pathol Biol (Paris)* 45(9):701–8.

446 Thio CL, Seaberg EC, Skolasky R Jr, *et al.* (2002). HIV-1, hepatitis B virus, and risk of liver-related mortality in the Multicenter Cohort Study (MACS). *Lancet* 360(9349):1921–6.

447 Kellerman SE, Hanson DL, McNaghten AD, Fleming PL (2003). Prevalence of chronic hepatitis B and incidence of acute hepatitis B infection in human immunodeficiency virus-infected subjects. *J Infect Dis* 188(4):571–7.

448 Hess G, Rossol S, Voth R, *et al.* (1989). Modification of the immune response against hepatitis B virus by the human immunodeficiency virus. *Rheumatol Int* 9(3-5):175–9.

449 Bodsworth NJ, Cooper DA, Donovan B (1991). The influence of human immunodeficiency virus type 1 infection on the development of the hepatitis B virus carrier state. *J Infect Dis* 163(5):1138–40.

450 Hadler SC, Judson FN, O'Malley PM, *et al.* (1991). Outcome of hepatitis B virus infection in homosexual men and its relation to prior human immunodeficiency virus infection. *J Infect Dis* 163(3):454–9.

451 Scharschmidt BF, Held MJ, Hollander HH, *et al.* (1992). Hepatitis B in patients with HIV infection: relationship to AIDS and patient survival. *Ann Internal Med* 117(10):837–8.

452 Horvath J, Raffanti SP (1994). Clinical aspects of the interactions between human immunodeficiency virus and the hepatotropic viruses. *Clin Infect Dis* 18(3):339–47.

453 Herrero Martinez E (2001). Hepatitis B and hepatitis C co-infection in patients with HIV. *Rev Med Virol* 11(4):253–70.

454 Gilson RJ, Tedder RS, Weller IV (1989). Hepatitis B: reactivation or reinfection associated with HIV-1 infection. *Lancet* 2(8675):1330.

455 Vento S, di Perri G, Luzzati R, *et al.* (1989). Clinical reactivation of hepatitis B in anti-HBs-positive patients with AIDS. *Lancet* 1(8633):332–3.

456 Sulkowski MS, Thomas DL, Mehta SH, *et al.* (2002). Hepatotoxicity associated with nevirapine or efavirenz-containing antiretroviral therapy: role of hepatitis C and B infections. *Hepatology* 35(1):182–9.

457 Manegold C, Hannoun C, Wywiol A, *et al.* (2001). Reactivation of hepatitis B virus replication accompanied by acute hepatitis in patients receiving highly active antiretroviral therapy. *Clin Infect Dis* 32(1):144–8.

458 Hofer M, Joller-Jemelka HI, Grob PJ, *et al.* (1998). Frequent chronic hepatitis B virus infection in HIV-infected patients positive for antibody to hepatitis B core antigen only. Swiss HIV Cohort Study. *Eur J Clin Microbiol Infect Dis* **17**(1):6–13.

459 Grob P, Jilg W, Bornhak H, *et al.* (2000). Serological pattern 'anti-HBc alone': report on a workshop. *J Med Virol* **62**(4):450–5.

460 Piroth L, Binquet C, Vergne M, *et al.* (2002). The evolution of hepatitis B virus serological patterns and the clinical relevance of isolated antibodies to hepatitis B core antigen in HIV-infected patients. *J Hepatol* **36**(5):681–6.

CHAPTER 14

1 Coogan MM, Greenspan J, Challacombe SJ (2005) Oral lesions in infection with human immunodeficiency virus. *Bull World Health Org* **83**:700–6.

2 Greenspan JS, Greenspan D (2002) The epidemiology of the oral lesions of HIV infection in the developed world. *Oral Dis* **8**:34–9.

3 Lifson AR, Hilton JF, Westenhouse JL, *et al.* (1994). Time from HIV seroconversion to oral candidiasis or hairy leukoplakia among homosexual and bisexual men enrolled in three prospective cohorts. *AIDS* **8**:73–9.

4 Hodgson TA, Greenspan D, Greenspan JS (2006). Oral lesions of HIV disease and HAART in industrialized countries. *Adv Dent Res* **19**(1):57–62.

5 Patton LL, McKaig R, Strauss R, *et al.* (2000). Changing prevalence of oral manifestations of human immuno-deficiency virus in the era of protease inhibitor therapy. *Oral Surg Oral Med Oral Pathol Oral Radiol Endod* **89**:299–304.

6 Schmidt-Westhausen AM, Priepke F, Bergmann FJ, *et al.* (2000). Decline in the rate of oral opportunistic infections following introduction of highly active antiretroviral therapy. *J Oral Pathol Med* **29**:336–41.

7 Tappuni AR, Fleming GJ (2001). The effect of antiretroviral therapy on the prevalence of oral manifestations in HIV-infected patients: a UK study. *Oral Surg Oral Med Oral Pathol Oral Radiol Endod* **92**:623–8.

8 Flanagan MA, Barasch A, Koenigsberg SR, *et al.* (2000). Prevalence of oral soft tissue lesions in HIV-infected minority children treated with highly active antiretroviral therapies. *Pediatr Dent* **22**:287–91.

9 Khongkunthian P, Grote M, Isaratanan W, *et al.* (2001). Oral manifestations in 45 HIV-positive children from Northern Thailand. *J Oral Pathol Med* **30**:549–52.

10 Greenspan D, Canchola AJ, MacPhail LA, *et al.* (2001). Effect of highly active antiretroviral therapy on frequency of oral warts. *Lancet* **357**:1411–12.

11 Ramírez-Amador V, Esquivel-Pedraza L, Sierra-Madero J, *et al.* (2003). The changing clinical spectrum of human immunodeficiency virus (HIV)-related oral lesions in 1,000 consecutive patients. A twelve-year study in a referral center in Mexico. *Medicine* **82**:39–50.

12 Dull JS, Sen P, Raffanti S, Middleton JR (1991). Oral candidiasis as a marker of acute retroviral illness. *Southern Med J* **84**:733–9.

13 Klein RS, Harris CA, Small CR, *et al.* (1984). Oral candidiasis in high-risk patients as the initial manifestation of the aquired immunodeficiency syndrome. *N Engl J Med* **311**:354–8.

14 Torssander J, Morfeldt-Manson L, Biberfield G, *et al.* (1987). Oral *Candida albicans* in HIV infection. *Scand J Infect Dis* **19**:291–295.

15 Korting HC, Ollert M, Georgii A, Froschl M (1989). *In vitro* susceptibilities and biotypes of *Candida albicans* isolated from the oral cavities of patients infected with human immunodeficiency virus. *J Clin Microbiol* **26**:2626–31.

16 Franker CT, Lucartorto FM, Johnson BS, Jacobson JJ (1990). Characterization of the mycoflora from oral mucosal surfaces of some HIV-infected patients. *Oral Surg Oral Med Oral Pathol* **69**:683–7.

17 Samaranayake LP, Holmstrup P (1989). Oral candidiasis and human immunodeficiency virus infection. *J Oral Pathol Med* **18**:554–64.

18 Moss AR, Bacchetti P, Osmond D, *et al.* (1988). Seropositivity fro HIV and the development of AIDS or AIDS related condition: three year follow up of the San Francisco General Hospital Cohort. *Br Med J* **296**:745–50.

19 Feigal DW, Katz MH, Greenspan D, *et al.* (1991). The prevalence of oral lesions in HIV-infected homosexual and bisexual men: three San Francisco epidemiology cohorts. *AIDS* **5**:519–25.

20 Samaranayake LP, Holmstrup P (1989). Oral candidiasis and human immunodeficiency virus infection. *J Oral Pathol Med* **18**(10):554–64.

21 Greenspan D, Greenspan JS (1996). Oral manifestations of HIV infection. In: *Color Atlas of AIDS*, 2nd edn. Friedman-Kien AE, Cockerell CJ (eds). WB Saunders, Philadelphia, pp.160–1.

22 Greenspan JS, Greenspan D (1992). Oral lesions associated with HIV Infection. In: *AIDS and Other Manifestations of HIV Infection*, 2nd edn. GP Wormser (ed). Raven Press, New York, pp. 489–98.

23 Greenspan JS (1997). Sentinels and signposts: the epidemiology and significance of the oral manifestations of HIV disease. *Oral Dis* **3**: S13–17.

24 Dodd CL, Greenspan D, Katz MH, *et al.* (1991). Oral candidiasis in HIV infection: Pseudomembranous and erythematous candidiasis show similar rates of progression to AIDS. *AIDS* **5**:1339–43.

25 Phelan JA (1997). Oral manifestations of human immunodeficiency virus infection. *Med Clin North Am* **81**:511–31.

26 Greenspan D (1994). Treatment of oral candidiasis in HIV infection. *Oral Surg Oral Med Oral Pathol* **78**:211–15.

27 Just-Nubling G, Gentschew G, Meisner K, *et al.* (1991). Fluconazole prophylaxis of recurrent oral candidiasis in HIV-positive patients. *Eur J Clin Infect Dis* **10**:917–21.

28 McCreary C, Bergin C, Pilkington R (1995). Clinical parameters associated with recalcitrant oral candidosis in HIV infection: A preliminary study. *Int J STD AIDS* **6**:204–7.

29 Chinn H, Chernoff DN, Migliorati CA, *et al.* (1995). Oral histoplasmosis in HIV-infected patients: A report of two cases. *Oral Surg Oral Med Oral Pathol Oral Radiol Endod* **79**:710–14.

30 Cole MC, Grossman ME (1995). Disseminated histoplasmosis presenting as tongue nodules in a patient infected with human immunodeficiency virus. *Cutis* **55**:104–6.

31 Heinic GS, Greenspan D, MacPhail LA, *et al.* (1992). Oral *Histoplasma capsulatum* infection in association

with HIV infection: a case report. *J Oral Pathol Med* 21:85–9.

32 Oda D, McDougal L, Fritsche T (1990). Oral histoplasmosis as a presenting disease in acquired immunodeficiency syndrome. *Oral Surg Oral Med Oral Pathol* 70:631–6.

33 Lynch DP, Naftolin LZ (1987). Oral *Cryptococcus neoformans* infection in AIDS. *Oral Surg Oral Med Oral Pathol* 64:449–53.

34 Schmidt-Westhausen A, Grunewald T, Reichart PA, Pohle HD (1995). Oral cryptococcosis in a patient with AIDS: a case report. *Oral Dis* 1:77–9.

35 Rubin MM, Jui V, Sadoff RS (1990). Oral aspergillosis in a patient with acquired immunodeficiency syndrome. *J Oral Maxillofac Surg* 48:997–9.

36 Eisenberg E, Krutchkoff D, Yamase H (1992). Incidental oral hairy leukoplakia in immunocompetent persons. *Oral Surg Oral Med Oral Pathol* 4:332–3.

37 King GN, Healy CM, Glover MT, et al. (1994). Prevalence and risk factors associated with leukoplakia, hairy leukoplakia, erythematous candidiasis and gingival hyperplasia in renal transplant recipients. *Oral Surg Oral Med Oral Pathol* 78:718–26.

38 Zakrzewska JM, Aly Z, Speight PM (1995). Oral hairy leukoplakia in a HIV-negative asthmatic patient on systemic steroids. *J Oral Pathol Med* 24:282–4.

39 Greenspan D, Conant M, Silverman S, et al. (1984). Oral 'hairy' leukoplakia in male homosexuals: evidence of association with both papillomavirus and a herpes-group virus. *Lancet* 2:831–4.

40 Katz MH, Greenspan D, Westenhouse J, et al. (1992). Progression to AIDS in HIV-infected homosexual and bisexual men with hairy leukoplakia and oral candidiasis. *AIDS* 6:95–100.

41 Greenspan D, Greenspan JS, Hearst NG, et al. (1987). Relation of oral hairy leukoplakia to infection with the human immunodeficiency virus and the risk of developing AIDS. *J Infect Dis* 155:475–81.

42 Greenspan JS, Barr CE, Sciubba JJ, Winkler JR (1992). Oral manifestations of HIV infection: definitions, diagnostic criteria, and principles of therapy. *Oral Surg Oral Med Oral Pathol* 73:142–4.

43 Mendoza N, Diamantis M, Arora A, et al. (2008). Mucocutaneous manifestations of Epstein–Barr virus infection. *Am J Clin Dermatol* 9(5):295–305.

44 Resnick L, Herbst JS, Ablashi DV, et al. (1988). Regression of oral hairy leukoplakia after orally administered acyclovir therapy. *JAMA* 259:384–88.

45 Gowdey G, Lee RK, Carpenter WM (1995). Treatment of HIV-related hairy leukoplakia with podophyllum resin 25% solution. *Oral Surg Oral Med Oral Pathol Oral Radiol Endod* 79:64–7.

46 Greenspan D, De Souza YG, Conant MA, et al. (1990). Efficacy of desciclovir in the treatment of Epstein–Barr virus infection in oral hairy leukoplakia. *J Acquir Immune Defic Syndr* 3:571–8.

47 Kessler HA, Benson CA, Urbanski P (1988). Regression of oral hairy leukoplakia during zidovudine therapy. *Arch Internal Med* 148:2496–7.

48 Katz MH, Greenspan D, Heinic GS, et al. (1991). Resolution of hairy leukoplakia: an observational trial of zidovudine versus no treatment. *J Infect Dis* 164:1240–1.

49 Schofer H, Ochsendorf FR, Helm EB, Milbracht R (1987). Treatment of oral 'hairy' leukoplakia in AIDS patients with vitamin A acid (topically) or acyclovir (systemically). *Dermatologica* 174:150–1.

50 Silverman S, Migliorati CA, Lozada-Nur F, et al. (1986). Oral findings in people with or at risk for AIDS: a study of 375 homosexual males. *J Am Dental Assoc* 112:187–92.

51 Reichart PA, Gelderblom HR, Becker J, Kuntz A (1987). AIDS and the oral cavity: the HIV infection – virology, etiology, origin, immunology, precautions and clinical observations in 110 patients. *Int J Oral Maxillofac Surg* 16:129–53.

52 Silverman S Jr, Migliorati CA, Lozada-Nur F, et al. (1986). Oral findings in people with or at high risk for AIDS: a study of 375 homosexual males. *J Am Dent Assoc* 112:187–92.

53 Phelan JA, Saltzman BR, Friedland GH, Klein RS (1987). Oral findings in patients with acquired immunodeficiency syndrome. *Oral Surg Oral Med Oral Pathol* 64:50–6.

54 Quinnan GV, Masur H, Rook AH, et al. (1984). Herpes virus infection in the acquired immunodeficiency syndrome. *J Am Med Assoc* 252:72–7.

55 Stoopler ET, Greenberg MS (2003). Update on herpesvirus infections. *Dent Clin North Am* 47:517–32.

56 (No authors listed) (1992). Centers for Disease Control and Prevention: 1993 revised classification system for HIV infection and expanded surveillance case definition for AIDS among adolescents and adults. *MMWR* 41:1–19.

57 Johnson NW (2010). The mouth in HIV/AIDS: markers of disease status and management challenges for the dental profession. *Aust Dent J* 55(Suppl 1):85–102.

58 Lavelle CL (1993). Acyclovir: is it an effective virostatic agent for orofacial infections? *J Oral Pathol Med* 22:391–401.

59 MacPhail LA, Greenspan D, Schiodt M, et al. (1989). Acyclovir-resistant, foscarnet-sensitive oral herpes simplex type 2 lesion in a patient with AIDS. *Oral Surg Oral Med Oral Pathol* 67:427–32.

60 Malvy D, Treilhaud M, Bouee S, et al. (2005). A retrospective, case-control study of acyclovir resistance in herpes simplex virus. *Clin Infect Dis* 41:320–6.

61 Chilukuri S, Rosen T (2003). Management of acyclovir-resistant herpes simplex virus. *Dermatol Clin* 21:311–20.

62 Volter C, He Y, Delius H, et al. (1996). Novel HPV types present in oral papillomatous lesions from patients with HIV infection. *Int J Cancer* 66:453–6.

63 Greenspan D, de Villiers EM, Greenspan JS, et al. (1988). Unusual HPV types in the oral warts in association with HIV infection. *J Oral Pathol* 17:482–7.

64 de Villiers EM (1989). Prevalence of HPV 7 papillomas in the oral mucosa and facial skin of patients with human immunodeficiency virus. *Arch Dermatol* 125:1590.

65 Melbye M, Grossman RJ, Goedert RJ, et al. (1987). Risk of AIDS after herpes zoster. *Lancet* 1:728–31.

66 Colebunders R, Mann J, Francis H, et al. (1988). Herpes zoster in African patients: a clinical predictor of human immunodeficiency virus infection. *J Infect Dis* 157:314–18.

67 Dodd CL, Winkler JR, Heinic GS, et al. (1993). Cytomegalovirus infection presenting as acute periodontal infection in a patient infected with the human

immunodeficiency virus. *J Clin Periodontol* 20:282–5.

68 Jones AC, Freedman PD, Phelan JA, *et al.* (1993). Cytomegalovirus infections of the oral cavity: a report of six cases with review of the literature. *Oral Surg Oral Med Oral Pathol* 75:76–85.

69 Langford A, Kunze R, Timm H, *et al.* (1990). Cytomegalovirus-associated oral ulcerations in HIV-infected patients. *J Oral Pathol Med* 18:71–6.

70 Kanas RJ, Jensen JL, Abrams AM, *et al.* (1987). Oral mucosal cytomegalovirus as a manifestation of the acquired immune deficiency syndrome. *Oral Surg Oral Med Oral Pathol* 64:1839.

71 Holmstrup P, Westergaard J (1994). Periodontal diseases in HIV-infected patients. *J Clin Periodontol* 21:270–80.

72 Zambon JJ, Reynolds HS, Genco RJ (1990). Studies of the subgingival microflora in patients with acquired immunodeficiency syndrome. *J Periodontol* 61:699–704.

73 Paster BJ, Russell MK, Alpagot T, *et al.* (2002). Bacterial diversity in necrotizing ulcerative periodontitis in HIV-positive subjects. *Ann Periodontol* 7:8–16.

74 Lopez de Blanc S, Sambuelli R, Femopase F, *et al.* (2000). Bacillary angiomatosis affecting the oral cavity. Report of two cases and review. *J Oral Pathol Med* 29:91–6.

75 Salama C, Finch D, Bottone EJ (2004). Fusospirochetosis causing necrotic oral ulcers in patients with HIV infection. *Oral Surg Oral Med Oral Pathol Oral Radiol Endod* 98:321–3.

76 Jones AC, Gulley ML, Freedman PD (2000). Necrotizing ulcerative stomatitis in human immuno-deficiency virus-seropositive individuals: a review of the histopathologic, immunohistochemical, and virologic characteristics of 18 cases. *Oral Surg Oral Med Oral Pathol Oral Radiol Endod* 89:323–32.

77 Ficarra G, Berson Am, Silverman S, *et al.* (1988). Kaposi's sarcoma of the oral cavity: a study of 134 patients with a review of the pathogenesis, epidemiology, clinical aspects, and treatment. *Oral Surg Oral Med Oral Pathol* 66:543–50.

78 Ramirez-Amador V, Esquivel-Pedraza L, Lozada-Nur F, *et al.* (2002). Intralesional vinblastine *vs.* 3% sodium tetradecyl sulfate for the treatment of oral Kaposi's sarcoma. A double blind, randomized clinical trial. *Oral Oncol* 38:460–7.

79 Lester R, Li C, Phillips P, *et al.* (2004). Improved outcome of human immunodeficiency virus-associated plasmablastic lymphoma of the oral cavity in the era of highly active antiretroviral therapy: a report of two cases. *Leuk Lymphoma* 45:1881–5.

80 Zieglar JL, Beckstead JA, Volderbing PA, *et al.* (1984). Non-Hodgkins lymphoma in 90 homosexual men: Relation to generalized lymphadenopathy and the acquired immunodeficiency syndrome. *N Engl J Med* 311:565–70.

81 Dodd CA, Greenspan D, Schiødt M, *et al.* (1992). Unusual oral presentation of non-Hodgkin's lymphoma in association with HIV infection. *Oral Surg Oral Med Oral Pathol* 73:603–8.

82 Kerr AR, Ship JA (2003). Management strategies for HIV-associated aphthous stomatitis. *Am J Clin Dermatol* 4:669–80.

83 Scully C, Gorsky M, Lozada-Nur F (2003). The diagnosis and management of recurrent aphthous stomatitis: a consensus approach. *J Am Dent Assoc* 134:200–7.

84 Lugo RI, Fornatora ML, Reich RF, Freedman PD (1999). Linear gingival erythema in an HIV-seropositive man. *AIDS Read* 9:97–9.

85 Greenberg RG, Berger TG (1990). Nail and mucocutaneous hyperpigmentation with azidothymidine therapy. *J Am Acad Dermatol* 22:327–30.

86 Ramos-Gomez FJ, Flaitz C, Catapano P, *et al.* (1999). Classification, diagnostic criteria, and treatment recommendations for orofacial manifestations in HIV-infected pediatric patients. Collaborative Workgroup on Oral Manifestations of Pediatric HIV Infection. *J Clin Pediatr Dent* 23:85–96.

87 Greenspan JS, Mastrucci MT, Leggott PJ, *et al.* (1988). Hairy leukoplakia in a child. *AIDS* 2:143.

88 Exposito-Delgado AJ, Vallejo-Bolanos E, Martos-Cobo EG (2004). Oral manifestations of HIV infection in infants: a review article. *Med Oral Pathol Oral Cir Buccal* 9:410–20.

89 Ramos-Gomez FJ, Petru A, Hilton JF, *et al.* (2000). Oral manifestations and dental status in paediatric HIV infection. *Int J Paediatr Dent* 10:3–11.

90 Hodgson TA, Naidoo S, Chidzonga M, *et al.* (2006). Identification of oral health care needs in children and adults, management of oral diseases. *Adv Dent Res* 19(1):106–17.

91 Jabs DA, Quinn TC (1996). Acquired immunodeficiency syndrome. In: *Ocular Infection & Immunity*. JS Pepose, GN Holland, KR Wilhelmus (eds). Mosby, St. Louis, pp. 289–310.

92 Sanjay S, Huang P, Lavanya R (2011). Herpes zoster ophthalmicus. *Curr Treat Options Neurol* 13(1):79–91.

93 Ormerod LD, Larkin JA, Margo CA, *et al.* (1998). Rapidly progressive herpetic retinal necrosis: a blinding disease characteristic of advanced AIDS. *Clin Infect Dis* 26:34–45.

94 Tyring S, Engst R, Corriveau C, *et al.* (2001). Famciclovir for ophthalmic zoster: a randomised aciclovir controlled study. *Br J Ophthalmol* 85:576–81.

95 Colin J, Prisant O, Cochener B, *et al.* (2000). Comparison of the efficacy and safety of valaciclovir and acyclovir for the treatment of herpes zoster ophthalmicus. *Ophthalmology* 107:1507–11.

96 Rivaud E, Massiani MA, Vincent F, *et al.* (2000). Valacyclovir hydrochloride therapy and thrombotic thrombocytopenic purpura in an HIV-infected patient. *Arch Internal Med* 160:1705–6.

97 Schwartz JJ, Myskowski PL (1992). Molluscum contagiosum in patients with human immunodeficiency virus infection: a review of twenty-seven patients. *J Am Acad Dermatol* 27:583–8.

98 Bardenstein DS, Elmets C (1995). Hyperfocal cryotherapy of multiple molluscum contagiosum lesions in patients with the acquired immune deficiency syndrome. *Ophthalmology* 102:1031–4.

99 Moiin A (2003). Photodynamic therapy for molluscum contagiosum infection in HIV-coinfected patients: review of 6 patients. *J Drugs Dermatol* 2:637–9.

100 Brun SC, Jakobiec FA (1997). Kaposi's sarcoma of the ocular adnexa. *Int Ophthalmol Clin* 37:25–38.

101 Ateenyi-Agaba C (1995). Conjunctival squamous-cell

carcinoma associated with HIV infection in Kampala, Uganda. *Lancet* 345:695–6.

102 Nakamura Y, Mashima Y, Kameyama K, *et al.* (1997). Detection of human papillomavirus infection in squamous tumours of the conjunctiva and lacrimal sac by immunohistochemistry, *in situ* hybridization, and polymerase chain reaction. *Br J Ophthalmol* 81:308–13.

103 Eng HL, Lin TM, Chen SY, *et al.* (2002). Failure to detect human papillomavirus DNA in malignant epithelial neoplasms of conjunctiva by polymerase chain reaction. *Am J Clin Pathol* 117:429–36.

104 Antle CM, White VA, Horsman DE, Rootman J (1990). Large cell orbital lymphoma in a patient with acquired immune deficiency syndrome. Case report and review. *Ophthalmology* 97:1494–8.

105 Akduman L, Pepose JS (1995). Anterior segment manifestations of acquired immunodeficiency syndrome. *Semin Ophthalmol* 10:111–18.

106 Cunningham ET, Margolis TP (1998). Current concepts: ocular manifestations of HIV infection. *N Engl J Med* 339:236–44.

107 Silverstein BE, Chandler D, Neger R, Margolis TP (1997). Disciform keratitis: a case of herpes zoster sine herpete. *Am J Ophthalmol* 123:254–5.

108 Karbassi M, Raizman MB, Schuman JS (1992). Herpes zoster ophthalmicus. *Surv Ophthalmol* 36:395–410.

109 Almagro M, del Pozo J, Garcia-Silva J, *et al.* (2003). Eyelash length in HIV-infected patients. *AIDS* 17:1695–6.

110 Howe L, Jones NS (2004). Guidelines for the management of periorbital cellulitis/abscess. *Clin Otolaryngol Allied Sci* 29:725–8.

111 Ikoona E, Kalyesubula I, Kawuma M (2003). Ocular manifestations in paediatric HIV/AIDS patients in Mulago Hospital, Uganda. *Afr Health Sci* 3:83–6.

112 Wiznia AA, Lambert G, Pavlakis S (1996). Pediatric HIV infection. *Med Clin North Am* 80:1309–36.

113 Marion RW, Wiznia AA, Hutcheon RG, Rubinstein A (1987). Fetal AIDS syndrome score: correlation between severity of dysmorphism and age at diagnosis of immunodeficiency. *Am J Dis Child* 141:429–31.

CHAPTER 15

1 Wiwanitkit V (2004). Prevalence of dermatological disorders in Thai HIV-infected patients correlated with different CD4 lymphocyte count statuses: a note on 120 cases. *Int J Dermatol* 43(4):265–8.

2 Smith KJ, Skelton HG, DeRusso D, *et al.* (1996). Clinical and histopathologic features of hair loss in patients with HIV-1 infection. *J Am Acad Dermatol* 34(1):63–8.

3 Calista D, Boschini A (2000). Cutaneous side-effects induced by indinavir. *Eur J Dermatol* 10(4):292–6.

4 Schonwetter RS, Nelson EB (1986). Alopecia areata and the acquired-immunodeficiency-syndrome-related complex. *Ann Internal Med* 104(2):287.

5 Munoz-Perez MA, Rodriguez-Pichardo A, Camacho F, *et al.* (1998). Dermatologic findings correlated with CD4 lymphocyte counts in a prospective 3 year study of 1161 patients with human immunodeficiency virus disease predominantly acquired through intravenous drug abuse. *Br J Dermatol*139:33–9.

6 Kumarasamy N, Solomon S, Madhivanan P, *et al.* (2000). Dermatologic manifestations among human immunodeficiency virus patients in south India. *Int J Dermatol* 39(3):192–5.

7 Sadick NS (1993). Clinical and laboratory evaluation of AIDS trichopathy. *Int J Dermatol* 32(1):33–8.

8 Almagro M, del Pozo J, Garcia-Silva J, *et al.* (2002). Telogen effluvium as a clinical presentation of human immunodeficiency virus infection. *Am J Med* 112(6):508–9.

9 Barcaui CB, Goncalves da Silva AM, Sotto MN, Genser B (2006). Stem cell apoptosis in HIV-1 alopecia. *J Cut Pathol* 33(10):667–71.

10 d'Arminio Monforte A, Testa L, Gianotto M, *et al.* (1998). Indinavir-related alopecia. *AIDS* 12(3):328.

11 Bouscarat F, Prevot MH, Matheron S (1999). Alopecia associated with indinavir therapy. *N Engl J Med* 12(3):328.

12 Harry TC, Matthews M, Salvary I (2000). Indinavir use: associated reversible hair loss and mood disturbance. *Int J STD AIDS* 11(7):474–6.

13 Ginarte M, Losada E, Prieto A, *et al.* (2002). Generalized hair loss induced by indinavir plus ritonavir therapy. *AIDS* 16(12):1695–6.

14 Bongiovanni M, Chiesa E, Monforte A, Bini T (2003). Hair loss in a HIV-infected woman receiving lopinavir plus ritonavir therapy as first line HAART. *Dermatol Online J* 9(5):28.

15 Hardcastle NJ, Tunbridge AJ, Shum KW, *et al.* (2005). Alopecia in association with severe seborrheic dermatitis following combination antiretroviral therapy for acute retroviral syndrome. *J Eur Acad Dermatol Venereol* 19(5):631–3.

16 Carr A, Samaras K, Chisholm, *et al.* (1998). Pathogenesis of HIV-1 protease inhibitor-associated peripheral lipodystrophy, hyperlipidemia, and insulin resistance. *Lancet* 351:181–3.

17 Cockerell CJ, Friedman-Kien AE (1999). Cutaneous manifestations of HIV infection. In: *Textbook of AIDS Medicine*, 2nd edn. TC Merigan, JG Bartlett, D Bolognesi (eds). William & Wilkins, Baltimore, p. 499.

18 Bergfeld WA (1992). Hair disorders. In: *Moschella Dermatology*, 3rd edn. SL Moschella, HJ Hurley (eds). WB Saunders, Philadelphia, p.1543.

19 Sperling LC (2009). Telogen effluvium. In: *An Atlas of Hair Pathology*. Informa Healthcare USA, Inc. New York, pp 43–6.

20 Olsen E A (2003). Hair. In: *Fitzpatrick's Dermatology in General Medicine, Volume I*, 6th edn. IM Freedber, AZ Eisen, KF Austen, *et al.* (eds). McGraw Hill, New York, p. 640.

21 Stewart MI, Smoller BR (1993). Alopecia universalis in an HIV-positive patient: possible insight into pathogenesis. *J Cut Pathol* 20:180–3.

22 Lafeuillade A, Quilichi R, Chaffanjon P, *et al.* (1990). Alopecia universalis in a homosexual man seropositive for the human immunodeficiency virus [Letter]. *J Acquir Immune Defic Syndr* 3:1019.

23 Prose NS, Abson KG, Scher RK (1992). Disorders of the nails and hair associated with human immunodeficiency virus infection. *Int J Dermatol* 31:453–7.

24 Cho M, Cohen PR, Duvic M (1995). Vitiligo and alopecia areata in patients with human immunodeficiency virus infection. *Southern Med J* 88(4):489–91.

25 Grossman MC, Cohen PR, Grossman ME (1996). Acquired eyelash trichomegaly and alopecia

areata in a human immunodeficiency virus infected patient. *Dermatology* 193:52–3.

26 Randall VA (2001). Is alopecia areata an autoimmune disease? *Lancet* 358:1922–5.

27 Gilhar A, Kalish RS (2006). Alopecia areata: a tissue specific autoimmune disease of the hair follicle. *Autoimm Rev* 5:64–9.

28 Nagai H, Oniki S, Oka M, *et al.* (2006). Induction of cellular immunity against hair follicle melanocyte causes alopecia. *Arch Dermatol Res* 298(3):131–4.

29 Ostlere LS, Langtry JA, Staughton RC, *et al.* (1992). Alopecia universalis in a patient seropositive for the human immunodeficiency virus. *J Am Acad Dermatol* 27:630–1.

30 Whiting DA (2001) The histopathology of alopecia areata in vertical and horizontal sections. *Dermatol Therapy* 14:297–305.

31 Geletko SM, Segarra M, Mikolich DJ (1996). Alopecia associated with zidovudine therapy. *Pharmacotherapy* 16(1):79–81.

32 Sereti I, Sarlis NJ, Arioglu E, *et al.* (2001). Alopecia universalis and Graves' disease in the setting of immune restoration after highly active antiretroviral therapy. *AIDS* 15(1):138–40.

33 Alkhalifah A, Alsantali A, Wang E, *et al.* (2010). Alopecia areata update: part I. Clinical picture, histopathology, and pathogenesis. *J Am Acad Dermatol* 62(2):177–88, quiz 189–90.

34 Wasserman D, Guzaman-Sanchez DA, Scott K (2007). Alopecia areata. *Int J Dermatol* 46:121–31.

35 Madani S, Shapiro J (2000). Alopecia areata update. *J Am Acad Dermatol* 42:549–70.

36 Tan E, Tay YK, Goh CL, Chin Giam Y (2002). The pattern and profile of alopecia areata in Singapore – a study of 219 Asians. *Int J Dermatol* 41(11):748–53.

37 Marques AR, Struas SE (2003). Herpes simplex. In: *Fitzpatrick's Dermatology in General Medicine*, 6th edn. IM Freedberg, AZ Elsen, K Wolff *et al.* (eds). McGraw Hill, New York, p. 2063.

38 Eudy G, Solomon AR (2006). The histopathology of noncicatricial alopecia. *Semin Cut Med Surg* 25:35–40.

39 Ross EK, Shapiro J (2005). Management of hair loss. *Dermatol Clin* 23:227–43.

40 Mohamed Z, Bhouri A, Jallouli A, *et al.* (2005). Alopecia areata treatment with phototoxic dose of UVA and topical 8-methoxypsoralen. *J Eur Acad Dermatol Venereol* 19(5):552–5.

41 Baranda L, Layseca-Espinosa E, Abud-Mendoza C, *et al.* (2004). Severe and unresponsive HIV-associated alopecia areata successfully treated with thalidomide [Letter]. *Acta Derm Venereol* 85:277–8.

42 Skurkovich S, Korotky NG, Sharova, NM, Skurkovich B (2005). Treatment of alopecia areata with anti-interferon antibodies. *J Investig Dermatol Symp Proc* 10(3):283–4.

43 Heffernan MP, Hurley MY, Martin KS, *et al.* (2005). Alefacept for alopecia areata. *Arch Dermatol* 141(12):1513–16.

44 Joly P (2006). The use of methotrexate alone or in combination with low doses of oral corticosteroids in the treatment of alopecia totalis or universalis. *J Am Acad Dermatol* 55(4)632–6.

45 Kaelin U, Hassan AS, Braathen LR, Yawalkar N (2006). Treatment of alopecia areata partim universalis with efalizumab. *J Am Acad Dermatol* 55(3):529–32.

46 Hordinsky MK (2006). Medical treatment of noncicatricial alopecia. *Semin Cut Med Surg* 25:51–5.

47 Casanova JM, Puig T, Rubio M (1987). Hypertrichosis of the eyelashes in acquired immunodeficiency syndrome. *Arch Dermatol* 123(12):1599–601.

48 Janier M, Schwartz C, Dontenville MN, *et al.* (1987). Hypertrichose des cils au cours du SIDA. *Ann Dermatol Venereol* 114:1490.

49 Straka BF, Whitaker DL, Morrison SH, *et al.* (1988). Cutaneous manifestations of the acquired immunodeficiency syndrome in children. *J Am Acad Dermatol* 18:1089–102.

50 Patrizi A, Neri I, Trestini D, *et al.* (1998). Acquired trichomegaly of the eyelashes in a child with human immunodeficiency virus infection. *J Eur Acad Venereol* 11(1):89–91.

51 Kaplan MH, Sadick NS, Talmor M (1991). Acquired trichomegaly of the eyelashes: a cutaneous marker of acquired immunodeficiency syndrome. *J Am Acad Dermatol* 25:801–4.

52 Klutman NE, Hinthorn DR (1991). Excessive growth of eyelashes in a patient with AIDS being treated with zidovudine. *N Engl J Med* 324(26):1896.

53 Graham DA, Sires BS (1997). Acquired trichomegaly associated with acquired immunodeficiency syndrome. *Arch Ophthalmol* 115(4):557–8.

54 Mirmirani P, Hessol NA, Maurer TA, *et al.* (2003). Hair changes in women from the women's interagency HIV study. *Arch Dermatol* 139:105–6.

55 Almagro M, del Pozo J, Garcia-Silva J, *et al.* (2003). Eyelash length in HIV-infected patients. *AIDS* 17:1695–707.

56 Baccard M, Morel P (1994). Excessive growth of eyelashes in patients with acquired immunodeficiency syndrome. *Cutis* 53(2):83–4.

57 Leonidas J (1987). Hair alteration in black patients with the acquired immunodeficiency syndrome. *Cutis* 39:537–8.

58 Kinchelow T, Schmidt U, Ingato S (1988). Changes in the hair of black patients with AIDS. *J Infect Dis* 157(2):394.

59 Sing NT, Schneiderman H (1992). AIDS and straightening of kinked hair. *J Gen Internal Med* 7(1):124.

60 Fischer BK, Warner LC (1987). Cutaneous manifestations of the acquired immunodeficiency syndrome. *Int J Dermatol* 26:615–30.

61 Farthing CF, Brown SE, Staughton RCD (1986). *A Colour Atlas of AIDS*. Wolfe Medical Publications, London, pp. 24–37.

62 Duvic M, Rapini R, Hoots WK, *et al.* (1987). Human immunodeficiency virus-associated vitiligo: expression of autoimmunity with immunodeficiency? *J Am Acad Dermatol* 17:656–62.

63 Tosti A, Gaddoni G, Peluso AM, *et al.* (1993). Acquired hairy pinnae in a patient infected with the human immunodeficiency virus. *J Am Acad Dermatol* 28(3):513.

64 Harindra V, Sivapalan S, Roy RB (1993). Increased nail and hair growth in a patient with AIDS. *Br J Clin Prac* 27(4):215–16.

65 Valenzano L, Giacalone B, Grillo LR, *et al.* (1988). Compromisione ungueale in corso de AIDS. *G Ital Dermatol Venereol* 123:527–8.

66 Cribier B, Mena ML, Rey D, *et al.* (1998). Nail changes in patients infected with human immunodeficiency virus. A prospective controlled study. *Arch*

Dermatol **134**:1216–20.

67 Cockerell CJ, Odom R (1995). The differential diagnosis of nail disease. *AIDS Patient Care* **9**:S5–S8.

68 Nelson MM, Martin AG, Heffernan MP (2003). Superficial fungal infections: dermatophytosis, onychomycosis, tinea nigra, piedra. In: *Fitzpatrick's Dermatology in General Medicine*, 6th edn. IM Freeberg, AZ Elsen, K Wolff, *et al.* (eds). McGraw-Hill, New York, p. 2001.

69 Gupta AK, Taborda P, Taborda V, *et al.* (2000). Epidemiology and prevalence of onychomycosis in HIV-positive individuals. *Int J Dermatol* **39**(10):746–53.

70 Korting HC, Blecher P, Stallmann D, *et al.* (1993). Dermatophytes on the feet of HIV-infected patients: frequency, species distribution, localization and antimicrobial susceptibility. *Mycoses* **36**:271–4.

71 Uthayakumar S, Nandwani R, Drinkwater T, *et al.* (1997). The prevalence of skin disease in HIV infection and its relationship to the degree of immunosupression. *Br J Dermatol* **137**:595–8.

72 Gregory N (1996). Special patient populations: onychomycosis in the HIV-positive patient. *J Am Acad Dermatol* **35**:S13–S16.

73 Tosti A, Baran R, Dawber RPR (2001). The nail in systemic diseases. In: *Baran and Dawber's Diseases of the Nails and their Management*, 3rd edn. Baran R, Dawber RPR, de Berker DAR, Haneke E, Tosti A (eds). Blackwell Science, Oxford, pp. 223–31.

74 Hay RJ, Baran R, Haneke E, *et al.* (2001). Fungal and other infections In: *Diseases of the Nails and their Management*, 3rd edn. R Baran, RPR Dawber, de Berker, *et al.* (eds). Blackwell Science, Oxford, p. 160.

75 Tosti A, Piraccini BA (2003). Nail disorders. In: *Dermatology*. JL Bolognia, JL Jorizzio, RP Rapini (eds). Mosby, Edinburgh, ch 71, pp..

76 Martins CR, Al-Hariri J (2001). Human immunodeficiency virus In: *Cutaneous Medicine, Cutaneous Manifestations of Systemic Disease.* TT Provost, JA Flynn (eds). BC Decker Inc, Hamilton, p. 634.

77 Robayna MG, Herranz P, Rubio RA, *et al.* (1997). Destructive herpetic whitlow in AIDS: report of three cases. *Br J Dermatol* **137**:812–15.

78 Cockerell CJ (1990). Cutaneous manifestations of HIV infection other than Kaposi's sarcoma: clinical and histologic aspects. *J Am Acad Dermatol* **22**:1260–9.

79 El Hachem M, Bernardi S, Giraldi L, *et al.* (2005). Herpetic whitlow as a harbinger of pediatric HIV-1 infection. *Pediatr Dermatol* **22**(2):119–21.

80 Baden LA, Bigby M, Kwan T (1991). Persistent necrotic digits in a patient with the acquired immunodeficiency syndrome. *Arch Dermatol* **121**:113–16.

81 Zuretti AR, Schwartz IS (1990). Gangrenous herpetic whitlow in a human immunodeficiency virus-positive patient. *Am J Clin Pathol* **93**:828–30.

82 Norris SA, Kessler HA, Fife KH (1988). Severe, progressive herpetic whitlow caused by an acyclovir-resistant virus in a patient with AIDS. *J Infect Dis* **157**:209–10.

83 Nogueira ML, Oliveira AF, Araujo JG *et al.* (1998). PCR-based diagnosis of herpetic whitlow in an AIDS patient. *Rev Inst Med Trop de São Paulo* **40**(5):317–19.

84 Bowling JC, Saha M, Bunker CB (2005). Herpetic whitlow: a forgotten diagnosis. *Clin Exp Dermatol* **30**(5):609–10.

85 Chernosky ME, Finley VK (1985). Yellow nail syndrome in patients with acquired immunodeficiency disease. *J Am Acad Dermatol* **13**:731–6.

86 Goodman DS, Teplitz ED, Wishner A, *et al.* (1987). Prevalence of cutaneous disease in patients with acquired immunodeficiency syndrome (AIDS) or AIDS-related complex. *J Am Acad Dermatol* **17**:210–20.

87 Morfeldt-Manson L, Julander I, Nilsson B (1989). Dermatitis of the face, yellow toe nail changes, hairy leukoplakia and oral candidiasis are clinical indicators of progression to AIDS/opportunistic infection in patients with HIV infection. *Scand J Infec Dis* **21**(5):497–505.

88 Daniel CR (1986). Yellow nail syndrome and acquired immunodeficiency disease. *J Am Acad Dermatol* **14**:844–6.

89 Haas A, Dover JS (1986). Yellow nail syndrome and acquired immunodeficiency (letter). *J Am Acad Dermatol* **14**(5):845.

90 Scher RK (1988). Acquired immunodeficiency syndrome and yellow nails. *J Am Acad Dermatol* **18**:758–9.

91 Norton LA (1986). Yellow nail syndrome controlled by vitamin E therapy. *J Am Acad Dermatol* **15**:714–16.

92 Samman PD, White WF (1964). The 'yellow nail' syndrome. *Br J Dermatol* **76**:153–7.

93 Ayres S (1986). Yellow nail syndrome controlled by vitamin E therapy. *J Am Acad Dermatol* **15**(4):714–15.

94 Azon-Masoliver A, Mallolas J, Gatell J, *et al.* (1988). Zidovudine induced nail pigmentation. *Arch Dermatol* **124**:1570–1.

95 Anders KH, Abele DC (1989). Development of nail pigmentation during zidovudine therapy. *J Am Acad Dermatol* **21**:792–3.

96 Fischer CA, McPoland PR (1989). Azidothymidine-induced nail pigmentation. *Cutis* **43**:552–4.

97 Groark SP, Hood AF, Nelson K (1989). Nail pigmentation associated with zidovudine. *J Am Acad Dermatol* **21**:1032–3.

98 Don PC, Fusco F, Fried P, *et al.* (1990). Nail dyschromia associated with zidovudine. *Ann Internal Med* **112**:145–6.

99 Greenberg RG, Berger TG (1990). Nail and mucocutaneous hyperpigmentation with azidothymidine therapy. *J Am Acad Dermatol* **22**:327–30.

100 Grau-Massanes M, Millan F, Ferber MI, *et al.* (1990). Pigmented nail bands and mucocutaneous pigmentation of HIV positive patients trated with zidovudine. *J Am Acad Dermatol* **44**:687–90.

101 Sahai J, Conway B, Cameron D, *et al.* (1991). Zidovudine-associated hypertrichosis and nail pigmentation in an HIV-infected patient. *AIDS* **5**(11):1395–6.

102 Rahav G, Mayaan S (1992). Nail pigmentation associated with zidovudine. *Scand J Infect Dis* **24**:557–61.

103 Furth PA, Kazakis AM (1987). Nail pigmentation changes associated with azidothymidine (zidovudine). *Ann Internal Med* **107**:350.

104 Pappert AS, Scher RK, Cohen JL (1991). Longitudinal pigmented nail bands. *Dermatol Clin* **9**(4):703–16.

105 Jeanmougin M, Civatte J (1983). Nail dyschromia. *Int J Dermatol* **22**(5):279–90.

106 Glaser DA, Reminger K (1996). Blue nails and acquired immunodeficiency syndrome: not always associated with azidothymidine use. *Cutis* **57**:243–4.

107 Panwalker AP (1987). Nail pigmentation in the acquired immunodeficiency syndrome (AIDS). *Ann Internal Med* 107:943–4.

108 Smith KJ, Skelton HG, Yeager J, *et al.* (1994). Cutaneous finding in HIV-1 positive patients: a 42-month prospective study. *J Am Acad Dermatol* 31:746–54.

109 Garcia-Silva J, Almagro M, Pena-Penabad C, *et al.* (2002). Indinavir-induced retinoid like effects: incidence, clinical features and management. *Drug Safety* 25:993–1003.

110 Bouscarat F, Bouchard C, Bouhour D (1998). Paronychia and pyogenic granuloma of the great toes in patients with indinavir. *N Engl J Med* 338(24):1776–7.

111 Tosti A, Piraccini BM, D'Antuono A, *et al.* (1999). Paronychia associated with antiretroviral therapy. *Br J Dermatol* 140(6):1165–8.

112 Sass JO, Solder J, Heitger A, *et al.* (2000). Paronychia with pyogenic granuloma in a child treated with indinavir: the retinoid-mediated side-effect theory revisited. *Dermatology* 200:40–2.

113 Colson AE, Sax PE, Keller MJ, *et al.* (2001). Paronychia in association with indinavir treatment. *Clin Infect Dis* 32(1):140–3.

114 Zerboni R, Angius AG, Cusini M, *et al.* (1998). Lamivudine-induced paronychia. *Lancet* 351(9111):1256.

115 Russo F, Collantes C, Guerrero J (1999). Severe paronychia due to zidovudine-induced neutropenia in a neonato. *J Am Acad Dermatol* 40(2 Pt 2):322–4.

116 Dauden E, Pascual-Lopez M, Martinez-Garcia C, *et al.* (2000). Paronychia and excess granulation tissue of the toes and finger in a patient treated with indinavir. *Br J Dermatol* 142(5):1063–4.

117 James CW, McNelis KC, Cohen DM, *et al.* (2001). Recurrent ingrown toenails secondary to indinavir/ritonavir combination therapy. *Ann Pharmacotherap* 35(7–8):881–4.

118 Kang-Birken SL, Prichard JG (1999). Paronychia of the great toes associated with protease inhibitors. *Am J Healthy-System Pharm* 56:1674–5.

119 Hawkins T (2006). Appearance-related side-effects of HIV-1 treatment. *AIDS Patient Care STDs* 20(1):6–18.

120 High WA, Tyring SK, Taylor RS (2003). Rapidly enlarging growth of the proximal nail fold. *Dermatol Surg* 29(9):984–6.

121 Tosti A, La Placa M, Fanti PA, *et al.* (1994). Human papillomavirus type 16-associated periungual squamous cell carcinoma in a patient with acquired immunodeficiency syndrome. *Acta Derm Venereol* 74(6):478–9.

122 Kreuter A, Brockmeyer NH, Pfister H, *et al.* (2005). Human papillomavirus type 26-associated periungual squamous cell carcinoma *in situ* in a HIV-infected patient with concomitant penile and anal intraepithelial neoplasia. *J Am Acad Dermatol* 53(4):737–9.

123 Graham SM, Daley HM, Ngwira B (1997). Finger clubbing and HIV infection in Malawian children. *Lancet* 349(9044):31.

124 Zar HJ, Hussey G (2001). Finger clubbing in children with human immunodeficiency virus infection. *Ann Trop Paediatr* 21:15–19.

125 Belzunegui J, Gonzalez C, Figueroa M (1997). Clubbing in patients with human immunodeficiency virus infection. *Br J Rheumatol* 36(1):142–3.

126 Boonen A, Schrey G, Van der Linden S (1996). Clubbing in human immunodeficiency virus infection. *Br J Rheumatol* 35(3):292–4.

127 Granel F, Truchetet F, Grandidier M (1997). Pigmentation diffuse (ungueale, buccale, cutanee) associée a une infection par le virus de l'immunodéficience humaine (VIH). *Ann Dermatol Venereol* 124:460–2.

128 Rizos E, Drosos AA, Loannidis JPA (2003). Nail pigmentation and fatigue in a 39-year-old woman. *Clin Infect Dis* 36:378–9.

129 Gallais V, Lacour JP, Perrin C, *et al.* (1992). Acral hyperpigmented macules and longitudinal melanonychia in AIDS patients. *Br J Dermatol* 126:387–91.

130 Chandrasekar P (1989). Nail discoloration and human immunodeficiency virus infection. *Am J Med* 86:506–7.

131 Leppard B (1999). Blue nails are a sign of HIV infection. *Int J STD AIDS* 10:479–82.

132 de Carvalho VO, da Cruz CR, Marinoni LP, *et al.* (2006). Transverse leukonychia and AIDS. *Arch Dis Child* 91:326.

133 Perchere M, Krischer J, Rosay A (1996). Red fingers syndrome in patients with HIV and hepatitis C infection. *Lancet* 348:196–7.

134 Battegay M, Itin PH (1996). Red fingers syndrome in HIV patients. *Lancet* 348(9029):763.

135 Ruiz-Avila P, Tercedor J, Rodenas JM (1997). Periungual erythema in HIV-infected patients. *J Am Acad Dermatol* 37(6):1018–19.

INDEX